Textbook of
Dermatology
and Sexually Transmitted Diseases

with **HIV Infections**

Textbook of
Dermatology
and Sexually Transmitted Diseases

with **HIV Infections**

Editor

Kabir Sardana MD, DNB, MNAMS
Professor of Skin and VD
Central Health Services, MOH & FW
Post Graduate Institute of Medical Education & Research and Dr RML Hospital
New Delhi
Professor of Dermatology, Indraprastha University, Delhi
Associate Professor of Dermatology, Delhi University

Assistant Editor

Pallavi Ailawadi MD, DNB
Ex-Senior Resident
Maulana Azad Medical College and Lok Nayak Hospital
New Delhi

CBS

CBS Publishers & Distributors Pvt Ltd

New Delhi • Bengaluru • Chennai • Kochi • Kolkata • Mumbai
Bhopal • Bhubaneswar • Hyderabad • Jharkhand • Nagpur • Patna • Pune • Uttarakhand • Dhaka (Bangladesh)

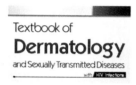

Textbook of
Dermatology
and Sexually Transmitted Diseases
with HIV Infections

ISBN: 978-93-88327-55-8

First Edition: 2019

Published by Satish Kumar Jain and produced by Varun Jain for

CBS Publishers & Distributors Pvt Ltd
4819/XI Prahlad Street, 24 Ansari Road, Daryaganj, New Delhi 110 002, India.
Ph: 23289259, 23266861, 23266867   Fax: 011-23243014   Website: www.cbspd.com
e-mail: delhi@cbspd.com; cbspubs@airtelmail.in.
Corporate Office: 204 FIE, Industrial Area, Patparganj, Delhi 110 092
Ph: 4934 4934   Fax: 4934 4935   e-mail: publishing@cbspd.com; publicity@cbspd.com

Branches

- **Bengaluru:** Seema House 2975, 17th Cross, K.R. Road,
Banasankari 2nd Stage, Bengaluru 560 070, Karnataka
Ph: +91-80-26771678/79   Fax: +91-80-26771680   e-mail: bangalore@cbspd.com
- **Chennai:** 7, Subbaraya Street, Shenoy Nagar, Chennai 600 030, Tamil Nadu
Ph: +91-44-26680620, 26681266   Fax: +91-44-42032115   e-mail: chennai@cbspd.com
- **Kochi:** 42/1325, 1326, Power House Road, Opposite KSEB Power House,
Ernakulam 682 018, Kochi, Kerala
Ph: +91-484-4059061-65   Fax: +91-484-4059065   e-mail: kochi@cbspd.com
- **Kolkata:** 6/B, Ground Floor, Rameswar Shaw Road, Kolkata-700 014, West Bengal
Ph: +91-33-22891126, 22891127, 22891128   e-mail: kolkata@cbspd.com
- **Mumbai:** 83-C, Dr E Moses Road, Worli, Mumbai-400018, Maharashtra
Ph: +91-22-24902340/41   Fax: +91-22-24902342   e-mail: mumbai@cbspd.com

Representatives

- **Bhopal**   0-8319310552   • **Bhubaneswar** 0-9911037372   • **Hyderabad** 0-9885175004   • **Jharkhand** 0-9811541605
- **Nagpur**   0-9021734563   • **Patna**   0-9334159340   • **Pune**   0-9623451994   • **Uttarakhand** 0-9716462459
- **Dhaka (Bangladesh)** 01912-003485

Printed at Nutech Print Services, Faridabad, India

"Weather is a great metaphor for life—sometimes it's good, sometimes it's bad, and there's nothing much you can do about it but carry an umbrella or choose to dance in the rain"

—Terri Guillemets

to
_____

the people and places who stood by me in the **times of strife**—which mirrors the famous saying,
"In life it's not where you go, it is who goes with you".

My wife Dr Supriya Mahajan in whom "I found a woman, stronger than anyone I know, she shares my dreams, I hope that someday I'll share her dreams too". My daughter Zoya—who personifies the best of us and is trying to follow our footsteps into this profession, my parents—the strongest and the most honest people I have seen—Maj Gen KN Sardana and Amba Sardana who are away from the pollution infested capital, at the valley station, Dehradun.

Certain people and spirits (Shri Raman Maharishi) that showed up in my life when I needed them most, these were my gifts from God, a proof that He exists

Shri Najeeb Jung, Mr Ashok Chaturvedi, CMD, Flex Industries, Shri Anshu Prakash, Dr Vinay Kamal, Mr AP Singh, Flex Industries Mr Rajiv Aggarwal, Shri SK Srivastava, Shri AK Jha, Mr Gaya Prasad, Mr SM Routray, Mr Lalit Kumar

Dr DM Rao, Dr RP Gupta, Dr VK Upadhyaya, Dr RK Gautam, Dr KD Barman

My students all over the place…

Shri Brijesh Sharma, Shri RK Tyagi and the innumerable officers at various levels in Delhi Government, Central Health Services and MAMC establishment.

Surajpur Bird Sanctuary, the most peaceful place in NCR, And, of course, CBS Publishers and Distributors who stood by me and piled me up with book projects!

And the people who were with me in the **good times**

God, almost everyone else and my colleagues in the Department of Dermatology at MAMC and RML Hospital

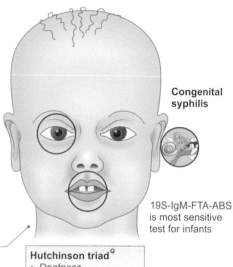

Congenital syphilis

19S-IgM-FTA-ABS is most sensitive test for infants

Diagrammatic Depiction

Hutchinson triad^Q
• Deafness
• Keratitis
• Dental abnormalities

A

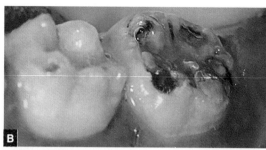

B

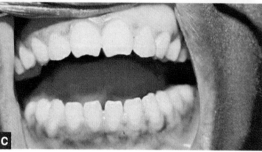

C

Fig. 31.3A to C: (A) Depiction of the Hutchinson triad; (B) Mulberry molars; (C) Upper and lower middle incisors shaped in the form of the head of a screwdriver, known as Hutchinson's teeth

from **page** 449

Pemphigus Group

Pemphigus refers to a group of disorders with loss of intraepidermal adhesion because of autoantibodies directed against proteins of the desmosomal complex that hold keratinocytes together. The desmosome is a complex structure, with many of its components targets for autoantibodies. In pemphigus, desmogleins 1 and 3 are important and they have a variable distribution in the epidermis.

Important Questions ^{Q}

The **1** (Dsg 1) is more at the **top** (stratum granulosum), while the **3** (Dsg 3) is more at the **bottom** (S. basale).^{Q}

Desmoglein 3 is crucial for cell adhesion and is found in the oral mucosa and the lower layers of the epidermis, while desmoglein 1 is almost only present in the skin and most expressed in the upper layers. Thus pemphigus foliaceus never involves the mucosa and has superficial erosions, while pemphigus vulgaris often presents with oral disease and may have full-thickness acantholysis (*see* Fig. 17.9).

*3OL: **D**esmoglein 3, **O**ral mucosa, **L**ower epidermis.*

Mnemonic

from **page** 228

Syphilis

 Key Points in Syphilis

Key Points

• Dory-flop sign^Q—chancre on the prepuce, being cartilaginous in consistency flips back suddenly on retraction of prepuce
• Rash, generalized lymphadenopathy, condylomata lata (most classical, most infectious), snail track ulcers, moth-eaten alopecia are all features of secondary syphilis.
• Buschke-Ollendorf sign^Q—pressure with a blunt instrument on the lesions over palms and soles elicits tenderness.
• Pseudochancre redux—gumma occurring over site of chancre
• Chancre redux^Q—inadequate treatment leading to formation of chancre at the site of healed chancre.

from **page** 449

Acne

The basic **principles of treatment** are:
• The primary aim of acne treatment is to prevent or minimize scarring, once scarred, the skin will never return to normal.

Clinical Applications

The patient should apply these medications to the entire affected area (e.g. the entire face) rather than just to the individual lesions.^{Q}

from **page** 333

Herpes Simplex Virus Infections

Clinical Features

There are many uncommon sites of involvement like on the fingers (herpetic whitlow),^{Q} in wrestlers (herpes gladiatorum),^{Q} HSV encephalitis (most common cause of viral encephalitis in adults, 95% HSV-1) and eye (herpes keratitis---Fig. 4.5).

An overview of the salient features is given in Box 4.1.^{Q}

Disease Summary

Box 4.1	Overview of common HSV infections

Primary infection:
• HSV-1 usually occurs in children, subclinical in 90% of cases.
• 10% of infected children have acute gingivostomatitis.
Lips (herpes labialis): Caused by HSV-1
Genitals and buttocks: HSV-2.
Recurrence (genital): Less with HSV-1 (14%) than with HSV-2 (60%)

from **page** 58

Contributors

Abhishek Bhardwaj MD
Associate Professor (DVL)
AIIMS, Jodhpur
(*Chapter 31*)

Ajeet Singh MBBS
PG IIIrd year
PGIMER and Dr RML Hospital
(*Questions*)

Ananta Khurana MD, DNB, MNAMS
Associate Professor
Department of Dermatology and STDs
PGIMER, Dr Ram Manohar Lohia Hospital
New Delhi
(*Chapters 13 and 24 Co-author*)

Anuva Bansal MD
Senior Resident
Maulana Azad Medical College and Lok Nayak Hospital, New Delhi
(*Chapter 32 Co-Author*)

Chander Grover MD, DNB, MNAMS
Professor, Department of Dermatology and STD
University College of Medical Sciences and GTB Hospital
Delhi
(*Chapter 25*)

Devendra Mishra MD
Professor, Department of Pediatrics
Maulana Azad Medical College and Lok Nayak Hospital
New Delhi
(*Chapter 4*)

Devika Choudhry MBBS
PG IIIrd year
PGIMER and Dr RML Hospital
(*Questions*)

Isha Narang MD
Specialist Registrar
Department of Dermatology
University Hospitals of Derby and Burton
Derby, DE22 3NE
United Kingdom
(*Chapter 32 Author*)

Jyoti Yadav MBBS
PG IInd year
Maulana Azad Medical College, New Delhi
(*Questions*)

Kabir Sardana MD, DNB, MNAMS
Professor of Skin and VD
Central Health Services, MOH & FW
Post Graduate Institute of Medical Education & Research and
Dr RML Hospital
New Delhi

Krishna Deb Barman MD
Professor
Department of Dermatology and Venereology
Maulana Azad Medical College and Associated Hospital
New Delhi 110002
(*Chapter 18*)

Lalit Gupta MD, FAAD
Sr Professor, Department of Dermatology
RNT Medical College
Udaipur 313001
(*Chapter 16*)

Mahima Agrawal MBBS (MAMC, Delhi), MD (LHMC, Delhi), DNB
Senior Resident, Department of Dermatology and STD
Lady Hardinge Medical College and Associated Hospitals
New Delhi
(*Questions*)

Masarat Jabeen MD, DNB
Fellow in Aesthetic Medicine (University of Griefswald, Germany)
Lecturer
Department of Dermatology and Venereology
Government Medical College, Jammu
(*Chapter 24*)

Neirita Hazarika MD
Associate Professor
Department of Dermatology
AIIMS, Rishikesh
(*Chapter 22*)

Nilay Kanti Das MD
Professor
Department of Dermatology
Bankura Sammilani Medical College
Bankura, West Bengal
(*Arsenicosis*)

Pallavi Ailawadi MD, DNB
Ex-Senior Resident
Maulana Azad Medical College and Lok Nayak Hospital
New Delhi

Pooja Arora Mrig MD, DNB, MNAMS
Associate Professor
Department of Dermatology
PGIMER, Dr Ram Manohar Lohia Hospital, New Delhi
(*Chapter 18 Co-Author*)

Premanshu Bhushan MD
Senior Consultant
Skin Institute and School of Dermatology
N Block, Greater Kailash, New Delhi
(*Chapter 7 Co-Author*)

Sandeep Garg MD
Professor of Medicine
Maulana Azad Medical College and Lok Nayak Hospital, New Delhi
(*Chapter 26*)

Shikha Chugh MD
Ex-Senior Resident
Maulana Azad Medical College
New Delhi
(*Chapter 30 Co-Author*)

Snigdha Saxena MBBS
PG IIIrd year
PGIMER and Dr RML Hospital, New Delhi
(*Questions*)

Vikrant Choubey MD
Senior Resident
Maulana Azad Medical College
New Delhi
(*Chapter 27*)

Foreword

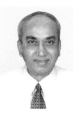

The dermatology outpatient department is the busiest and most crowded place in any hospital. So too has the interest in dermatology soared in the past few years, making dermatology one of the most preferred choices for postgraduation by young medical graduates. Keeping pace with this current surge of interest is the growing Indian dermatology literature in the form of books and listed journals. This book is an attempt to simplify and demystify a subject that often baffles a young undergraduate student, and attempts to create an interest in the subject by presenting it in an easy to read way. The book has 32 chapters contributed by 23 experienced dermatologists, each sharing the wealth of their experience on the subject. There is no attempt to discuss all the skin conditions that we know exist, but to give the reader a sense of the essential features of some of the more common conditions, an ideal aid for a student of dermatology in the undergraduate and early postgraduate days. Dermatology is a visual science, and to facilitate its understanding, there are 100-artist drawn images and a large number of clinical photographs for a better appreciation of the conditions. The book is also a very useful companion for those aspiring to appear for the postgraduate entrance test as there is an emphasis on those topics of importance together with mnemonics for certain of the must know facts. I hope this book will help students and doctors treat their patients with skin diseases better.

Rui J Fernandez MD, DVD, DDV
National President, Indian Association of Dermatologists, Venereologists and Leprologists
Honorary Professor and Head, Seth Gordhandas Sunderdas Medical College, Mumbai
Honorary Consultant Dermatologist, King Edward Memorial Hospital, Mumbai
Honorary Consultant Dermatologist, Dr RN Cooper Hospital, Mumbai
Honorary Professor of Dermatology, Dr DY Patil Medical College, Mumbai
Honorary Consultant Dermatologist, Holy Family Hospital, Mumbai

Foreword

I feel privileged to write this Foreword for the book entitled *Textbook of Dermatology and Sexually Transmitted Diseases* by Prof Kabir Sardana. He is known to me since last 20 years. He is well recognized as a fine clinician, researcher and sincere academician.

I found his present book, concised but full of knowledge. All the chapters are well written by experienced authors. It has been planned in such a way that those who intend to appear in UG/PG competitive examinations, will be benefitted more and shall be able to revise dermatology quickly. Additional advantage is that contents and clinical diseases are well explained with tables, diagrams and clinical photographs, making it suitable for postgraduates, clinicians of other specialities as well as for practising physicians.

I am hopeful that this book will fulfil aspirations of all those who wish to learn clinical dermatology, including differential diagnosis, investigation and management.

I congratulate Prof Kabir Sardana for this well-written book and wish him good luck and success in this venture.

RP Sharma MD, DVD, MNAMS
Professor and Head
Department of Dermatology and STD
LLRM Government Medical College, Meerut, UP
Former Faculty at SN Medical College, Agra, UP

Foreword

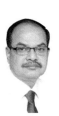

I was very happy to receive the mail and invitation from Prof Kabir Sardana to write the Foreword for his book *Textbook of Dermatology and Sexually Transmitted Diseases*. The reason was more than my friendship with Prof Kabir Sardana, I consider him as one of the few academician dermatologists of the present generation in our speciality.

Dermatology is a developing medical science. *Textbook of Dermatology and Sexually Transmitted Diseases* brings you the most practical and comprehensive information on the clinical features, pathogenesis and treatment. The book has 32 chapters covering all sections of dermatological disorders from 23 of experienced contributors. The book targets undergraduates, first year postgraduates and primary physicians. There are more than 100-artist drawn images with a plethora of clinical photographs. Dermatology being visual speciality, it is easier to understand a picture than to read and process words on a page (Da Vinci's reason for favoring images over words).

This book shall cater to needs of 'NEET' appearing MBBS graduates as authors have made it easy for students to locate important part of text by placing '*Q*' mark.

Mnemonics and boxed clinical pearls embedded in the chapters help the students understand the subject in an easier way. Addition of 'further reading' would have made the book more complete.

In this new age of rapid development of science, evolving better management strategies for various skin disorders and competition to excel in entrance examinations like NEET, it is necessary to provide an all-inclusive book to professionals, UG and PG students, with state-of-the-art knowledge on the frontiers in 'dermoscience'. This book is a good step in that direction.

Hope to see the book to reach all the intended target audience and 'Happy reading to all'.

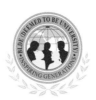

Arun C Inamadar MD, FRCP (Edinburgh)
Professor and Head
Department of Dermatology
Shri BM Patil Medical College,
Hospital and Research Centre, Vijayapura
BLDE (Deemed to be University)

Foreword

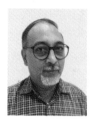

It is such a delight to write the Foreword for Prof Kabir Sardana's *Textbook of Dermatology and Sexually Transmitted Diseases*. Prof Kabir Sardana has come out with this book which should now tick all the right boxes, of both the discerning undergraduate students and graduate doctors seeking specialization. It is studded with plentiful of illustrations, diagrams and pictures, all created under the watchful supervision of experienced teachers who are themselves skilled communicators and have contributed the chapters. Interesting and key facts are highlighted in boxes enabling easy revision and serve as memory aids. Points that are important for NEET can now hardly escape the student's notice.

Dermatology continues to be a neglected area in the evolving MBBS curriculum. The MBBS student is given more time and opportunity in the curriculum to learn about things that he/she is not expected to deal with as a primary care doctor, whereas in dermatology, simple diseases of which he/she is expected to diagnose and manage, he/she is only allowed six weeks and thirty lectures of exposure to the subject in the entire MBBS course. This continues to leave both the primary care physicians as well as non-dermatologist specialists largely unprepared to deal with primary care dermatological conditions.

Prof Kabir Sardana has put together a galaxy of co-authors who well understand the dynamics of teaching dermatology and the expectations of today's students and this resulting book has a great future ahead.

The discriminating MBBS student, and later, the non-dermatologist and who needs a stand alone book, that gives a well-rounded understanding of dermatology from molecular genetics and pathogenesis to advanced therapeutics, that he/she can continue to consult and utilize even while practising other specializations after MBBS, now need not look any further.

SN Bhattacharya
Director, Professor and Head
Department of Dermatology and STD
UCMS and GTB Hospital
New Delhi

Preface

Dermatology today is a much sought after branch which most students are unable to get. This is possibly as they spend more time in coaching institutes than the college which defeats the very aim of MBBS training. This book aims at solving that by inculcating in one book both teaching of basic skills with impressive illustrations and important questions so that they can read the book through their MBBS training and their PG entrance preparation days!

Skin problems are hugely variable (>2500 diagnoses), but this book with its rich diagrams and photographs will help you to make sense of what you find in the wards and will provide you with a framework for analysing clinical signs and disorders.

We have added Q marks to enable the reader know what is important. We have purposely *not added MCQ* as that restricts learning. There are *mnemonics* and *clinical applications* throughout the book (*see* How to use the book).

Dermatology trainees should find the book particularly useful, as may hospital doctors in other medical specialties including medicine and pediatrics. It is a great summary read for first year PGs in dermatology.

Our contributors range from faculty of dermatology, medicine and pediatrics, postgraduate students, former students. Dr Pallavi Ailawadi who has used her skills in teaching at various coaching institutes in adding the common questions asked in the entrance examinations.

A big thanks to the fabulous team at CBS Publishers & Distributors, Mr YN Arjuna Senior Vice-President—Publishing, Editorial and Publicity, and their team, Mrs Ritu Chawla General Manager—Production, the patient and dedicated reformatting by Mr Vikrant Sharma, the artistic depiction and image balancing of Mr Ram Murti, copy editing of Mr Surendra Jha and Mr Prasenjit Paul. CBS is one of the few publishers who have invested in an advanced preproduction software that matches the quality of print before it is out. This has been possible due to the ingenuity of Mr SK Jain CMD, Mr Varun Jain, Director, Mr SK Verma and Mr Sunil Dutt. And the whole office staff of the office where I spend more than 3 months on and off for this onerous task, of course, after duty hours!

And for those who finally do not get dermatology in their PGs, remember the famous quote of Albert Einstein.

"Everybody is a genius. But if you judge a fish by its ability to climb a tree, it will live its whole life believing that it's stupid". And you are already in the toughest course in the world—that's an achievement in itself and the rest as Shri Raman Maharishi said, is destiny!

We hope that you will find this book useful. Please send back your comments or criticisms, so that we can improve the book in future editions. You can send your comments to us at the mail id kabirijdvl@gmail.com and apallavi99@gmail.com.

Kabir Sardana
Pallavi Ailawadi

Contents

Introduction to Skin Disorders

Structure and Function of Skin

The skin is the interface between humans and their environment. It weighs an average of 4 kg and covers an area of 2 m². It acts as a barrier, protecting the body from harsh external conditions and preventing the loss of important body constituents, especially water.

> The study of skin disorders and the practice of dermatology have become a much sought after branch and interestingly most students may not even get the branch for their MD.

EMBRYOLOGY

The skin consists of the epidermis with layers of variously differentiated keratinocytes and an underlying dermis with adnexal structures, vessels, and nerves, as well as subcutaneous fat. The skin develops from the ectoderm and mesoderm (Fig. 1.1). Initially, there is a single layer of ectodermal cells, but by around 8 weeks, a flattened outer layer (periderm) appears. By birth, the complex epidermis is present. Melanocytes[Q] migrate into the skin from the neural crest, as do nerves. The dermis, with its connective tissue, derives from the mesenchyme.

The adnexal structures develop from interaction between epidermal invaginations and supporting mesenchymal structures.

STRUCTURE AND FUNCTION

The skin has three layers. The outer one is the *epidermis*, which is firmly attached to, and supported by connective tissue in the underlying *dermis*. It adheres to the dermis at the basement membrane where downward projections **(epidermal rete ridges or pegs)** interlock with upward projections of the dermis **(dermal papillae)**. This is akin to the interlocking of the hands and it gives stability to the epidermis. This interdigitation is responsible for the ridges seen most readily on the fingertips (as fingerprints). Beneath the dermis is loose connective tissue, the *subcutis* or *hypodermis*, which usually contains abundant fat (Fig. 1.2).

EPIDERMIS

Keratinocytes

The epidermis is the outer layer of the skin. It is formed by **keratinocytes** which are arranged into multiple layers: The word keratinocyte literally means cells coated by keratin.[Q]

> The thickness can vary from less than **0.1** mm on the eyelids to nearly **1 mm** on the palms and soles.[Q] That's why an injury even minor around eye leads to a ugly black eye!

- *Stratum basale (stratum germinativum) (single layer)*: Anchors the epidermis to the dermis and contains cuboidal cells which continuously divide, allowing for replacement of the epidermis. The basal surfaces are attached to the basement membrane zone via fine processes and hemidesmosomes,[Q] anchoring them to the lamina densa of the basement membrane. They contain housekeeping granules.[Q]
- *Stratum spinosum (8–10 cells)*: Thickest layer of epidermis[Q] so named because connecting desmosomes[Q] appear as 'spines' under the microscope. These cells contain lamellar granules.
- *Stratum granulosum (2–5 cells)*: This is so-called due to presence of keratohyalin granules and Odland

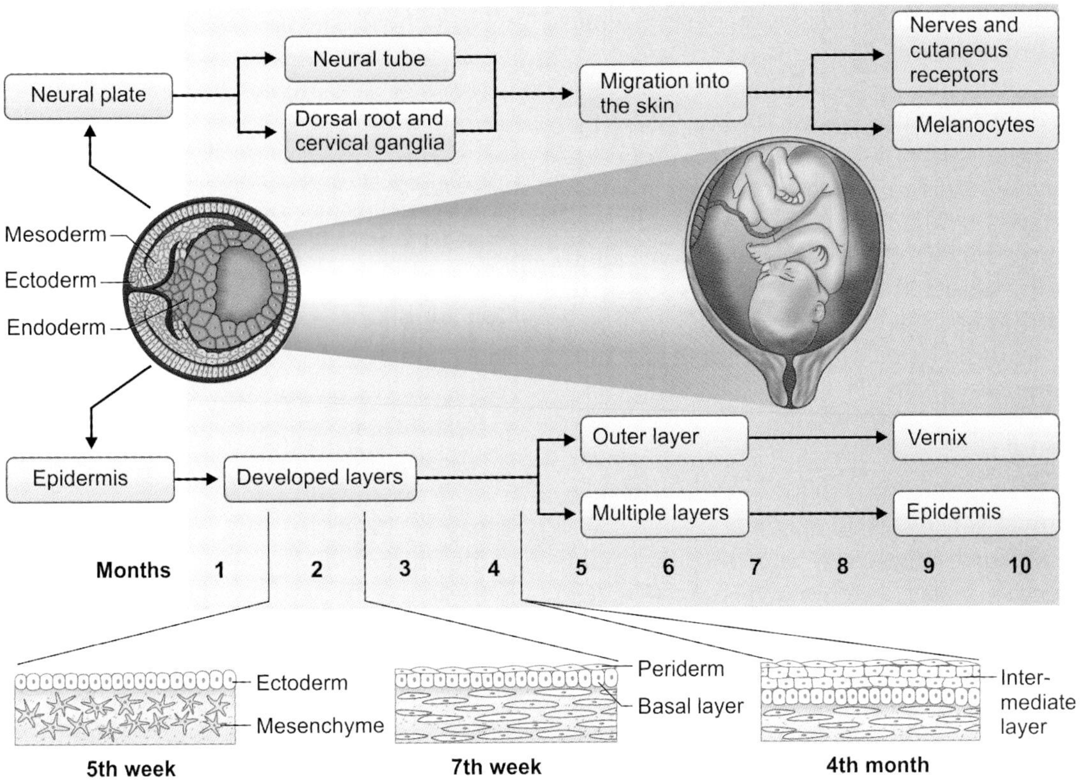

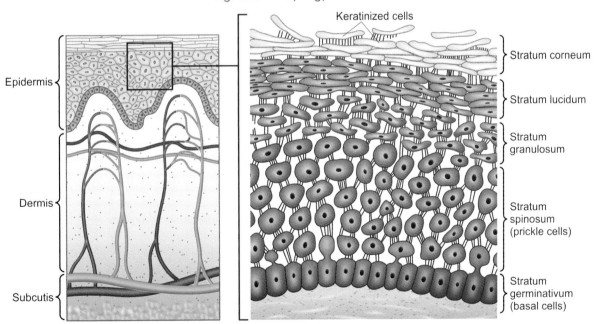

Fig. 1.1: Embryology of the skin

Fig. 1.2: Components of the skin

bodies, which contain profilaggrin and lipids, respectively.[Q] These help in completing the process of keratinization. The last is important as its defect leads to atopic dermatitis.[Q]
- *Stratum lucidum:* An amorphous band between the stratum granulosum and stratum corneum, only seen in the palms and soles.[Q]
- *Stratum corneum (20–25 cells):* Remnants of keratinocytes, consisting of keratin and cell walls without nuclei.

The typical 'basket weave' appearance of the horny layer in routine histological sections is artefactual. In fact, cells deep in the horny layer stick tightly together and only those at the surface flake off, thus process is called desquamation.[Q] This is in part caused by the activity of cholesterol sulfatase and this is deficient in X-linked recessive ichthyosis.[Q]

The stratum basale and stratum spinosum together are called stratum malpighii, which along with stratum granulosum are the living layers of skin, while stratum corneum is the dead layer.[Q]

The journey of terminal differentiation towards the dead stratum corneum takes about **30 days**[Q] and the stratum basale eventually becomes the stratum corneum, much like our own human body, but of course much faster! This process is called **keratinization**, and in this, the keratin fibrils in the cells of the horny layer align and aggregate, under the influence of filaggrin. Cysteine, found in keratins of the horny layer, allows cross-linking of fibrils to give the epidermis strength to withstand injury.

Other Epidermal Cells

Three other cells are found in the normal epidermis; also called immigrant cells (Fig. 1.3):[Q]

- *Melanocytes*, which synthesize melanin, the main photoprotective factor. (Melanocytes are derived from the neural crest).
- *Langerhans cells*, which are the antigen-presenting cells of the skin, part of innate immunity (800 Langerhans cells per mm²). It also lacks desmosomes and tonofibrils, but has a lobulated nucleus. The specific granules within the cell look like a tennis racket (Birbeck granules).[Q] Topical or systemic glucocorticoids reduce the density of epidermal Langerhans cells as does ultraviolet radiation.

- *Merkel cells*, which are neuroendocrine cells, that function as mechanoreceptors and mediate touch.[Q] (Merkel cells are derived from the neural crest).

> Of these cells, the pigmented races, like in India, are hell bent on removing the melanocyte in a bid to get fairer, but this cell still luckily bounces back! This is good for us, they serve as an effective natural sunscreen in tropical countries!

Cell Junctions

There are several types of cell junctions in the epidermis. Each plays an important pathophysiologic role:

- Desmosomes complex structures with many proteins holding cells together (Fig. 1.4). They are composed of transmembranous desmoglein–desmocollin pairs.[Q] There are four types of desmoglein found in the epidermis. Desmoglein (Dsg) 1 is expressed in the upper epidermis while Dsg 3 is mostly expressed in the basal epidermis (*'1' number top of epidermis, '3' number down in the epidermis*).[Q] Dsg 1 is not present in mucosal epithelium. The pemphigus group features dissolution of the epidermis due to damage by autoantibodies against the desmogleins (Dsg 1/3).[Q] Staphylococcal scalded skin syndrome is caused by bacterial toxins that damage desmogleins (Dsg 1).[Q]
- The other cell junctions are adherent, gap and tight junctions.

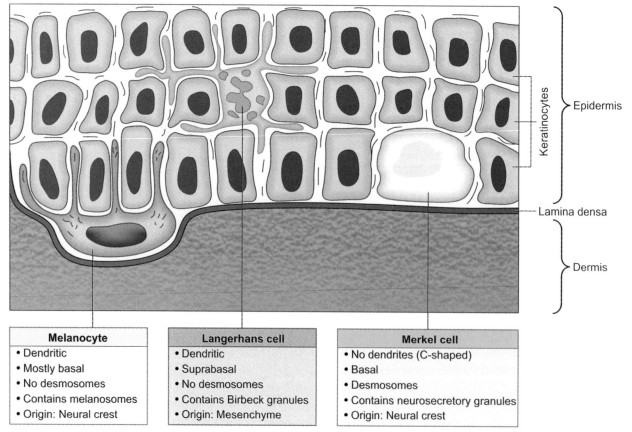

Melanocyte	Langerhans cell	Merkel cell
• Dendritic	• Dendritic	• No dendrites (C-shaped)
• Mostly basal	• Suprabasal	• Basal
• No desmosomes	• No desmosomes	• Desmosomes
• Contains melanosomes	• Contains Birbeck granules	• Contains neurosecretory granules
• Origin: Neural crest	• Origin: Mesenchyme	• Origin: Neural crest

Fig. 1.3: A depiction of the three immigrant cells in the epidermis[Q]

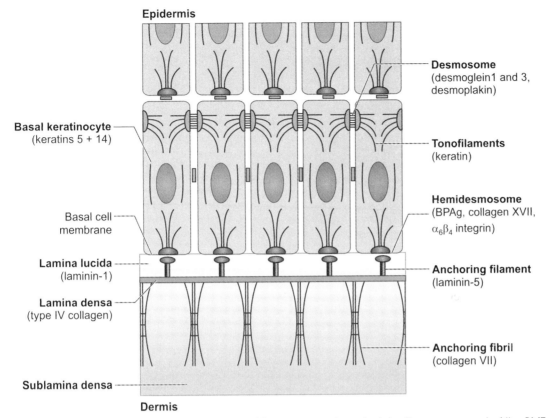

Fig. 1.4: An overview of the basement membrane zone and its component, each defective component of the BMZ is linked to a skin disorder

THE BASEMENT MEMBRANE ZONE

Different proteins interact to anchor the epidermis to the dermis. Key components of the basement membrane zone (BMZ) are hemidesmosomes, structures in the lower pole of basal cells sharing many features with desmosomes, and the basal membrane, made up of the lamina lucida and lamina densa (Fig. 1.4). The hemidesmosomes are made up of bullous pemphigoid antigens 1 (a 230 kDa plakin) and 2 (180 kDa collagen XVII) (*1 is more important than 2; 230 >180 kDa*), plectin and $\alpha_6\beta_4$ integrin.[Q] The BMZ contributes the barrier function, allowing molecules to diffuse to and from the dermis.

- [Q]Damage via mutations in proteins of the BMZ leads to epidermolysis bullosa, a family of diseases featuring easy blistering.
- Another condition affected by this zone an autoimmune bullous disease, bullous pemphigoid (BPAg 1 and 2).

DERMIS

The dermis is the major structural component of the skin. The predominant cells are fibroblasts, which are responsible for the synthesis of collagen and elastin, the main dermal fibers (Fig. 1.5).

The dermis has two main compartments:
- Superficial or papillary dermis (1/10th of dermis)
- Deeper or reticular dermis (9/10th of dermis).

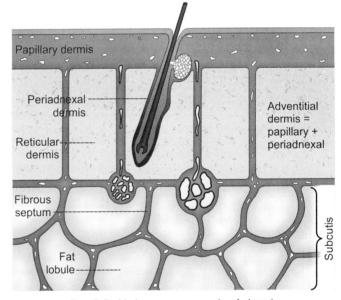

Fig. 1.5: Various components of dermis

Collagen: Collagen is an ubiquitous structural protein which accounts for 70% of the dry weight of the dermis (collagen 1–70% and collagen 3–15%).[Q] There are some major collagens and their defects can cause certain disorders as described in Table 1.1.

Elastic fibers: Elastic fibers account for only 2–3% of the dry weight of skin and they impart a resilience and stretchability to the skin.

Table 1.1 Types of collagen in the skin and their defects

I	Main structural protein	
III	Blood vessels, skin	Ehlers-Danlos syndrome (joint hypermotility and skin extensibility, also blood vessel instability)
IV	Essential component of the BMZ	
VII	Anchoring fibrils in the upper dermis	Dystrophic epidermolysis bullosa,[Q] EB acquisita
XVII	Hemidesmosomes[Q]	Junctional epidermolysis bullosa, bullous pemphigoid, pemphigoid gestations

Abnormalities in elastin can lead to saggy skin cutis laxa. Disorders in copper metabolism, e.g. Menkes syndromes, can affect the elastic fiber. Ultraviolet (UV) light induces changes in elastic fibers, which play a major role in cutaneous aging.

- The use of 'fillers' in the beauty industry and various moisturizers are aimed at plumping up the dermis, but the results are temporary!
- For a fair skin type, like those who live in the hills, the intense sunlight and the damage to the dermis is the reason for early ageing.

Extrafibrillary matrix: The main constituents are proteoglycans, composed of core proteins and glycosaminoglycans (GAGs), which are also known as mucopolysaccharides because of their slimy, tenacious nature.

ADNEXA

The adnexal structures include hair, nails, and glands.

Adnexal Glands

Eccrine Glands (Sweat Glands)

These are active since birth. These are widely distributed, but are most concentrated on the palms and soles. They are not found on the lips, external ear canal, clitoris, glans penis and labia minora.[Q] Each individual has several millions. They consist of a coiled secretory portion and a long duct coursing through the dermis to open onto the epidermis (Fig. 1.6) and work through merocrine secretion.[Q]

Eccrine sweat is usually **clear** and **odorless**, so the eccrine glands are to some extent 'the skin's kidneys.'[Q]

Apocrine Glands

These glands are associated with hair follicles; their secretory duct empties into the upper part of the hair follicle.[Q] They are richest in the axillae, nipple areola complex and groin.[Q] They function via 'decapitation secretion',[Q] where the free luminal end of the cell is shed with the secretory products. Apocrine sweat is odoriferous; their function may be to produce

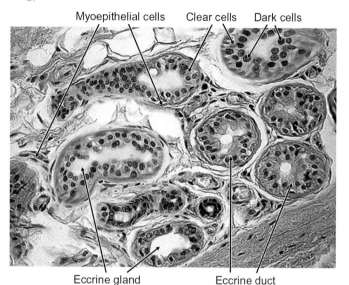

Fig. 1.6: Histology of the eccrine gland

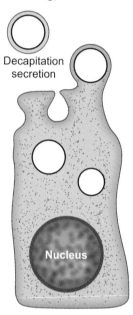

Fig. 1.7: Apocrine gland with decapitation secretion

pheromones for sexual attraction and other messaging (Fig. 1.7). Although present since birth, they develop around puberty, as they are androgen sensitive.[Q]

Apoecrine Glands

These glands are found in the axillae of adults and have overlapping features of eccrine and apocrine glands, with both types of secretory cells found in the coiled gland. They open directly on the skin surface, not via hair follicles.

Sebaceous Glands

These glands are also intimately associated with hair follicles, as their oily secretion lubricates the follicle to allow the hair shaft to grow outwards against less resistance. Sebaceous glands are very androgen sensitive. When they function to excess, the skin becomes oily and of course they cause **acne**.

Temperature Control

Eccrine glands are intimately involved in temperature control. In a resting state, evaporative loss of water through the skin is approximately **900 mL** daily.^{Q} This insensitive water loss provides about 20% of the cooling effect of the skin. Apocrine glands have no role in thermoregulation.^{Q}

Core temperature: The body maintains a central temperature at 37°C. By varying skin blood flow, the heat lost by convection and radiation (dry heat loss) can be manipulated over a wide range. For example, digital blood flow can change 500-fold between warm and mid temperatures. Shunts in the digital circulation controlled by contractile glomus cells **(Sucquet-Hoyer anastomosis)**^{Q} make this variation possible. The main control of core temperature is in the preoptic nucleus of hypothalamus.^{Q}

Sweating: When the ambient temperature rises, less dry heat loss can occur, so sweating assumes a major role. Sweating is an active process controlled by cholinergic sympathetic fibers.^{Q} With increased temperature and physical activity, sweat volumes of 1–4 L/hour are possible. Because the eccrine sweat is rich in electrolytes, attention must be paid to replacing not only fluids but also sodium chloride and other ingredients.

When one lives in a warm climate baseline sweating increases, electrolyte concentration in sweat decreases, and thirst increases. No such adjustments are possible in cold climates. Furred and feathered animals can increase their insulation by fluffing their outer coats. 'Goose bumps' in humans are residual ineffective attempts to fluff the hairs!

THE INNERVATION

Cutaneous Innervation

The skin is the largest sensory organ; it is served by a variety of nerves, including somatic sensory nerves and autonomic sympathetic fibers (Fig. 1.8). The autonomic nerves help control vessel and sweat gland function. The sensory nerves transmit information about the periphery (skin) to the central nervous system (CNS).

Dermatomes: Sensory nerves follow a dermatomal pattern, best seen in herpes zoster.

Nerve fibers: *C fibers* are slow polymodal unmyelinated fibers that can sense and transmit pain, itch, touch, heat, cold, and movement. *A fibers* are myelinated and have a higher conduction velocity. They interact with a variety of receptors:

- **Free nerve endings** are widespread, found extending into the epidermis and around hair follicles. Known as nociceptors,^{Q} they sense pain, motion, touch, heat, and cold.
- **Meissner's corpuscles**—superficial mechanoreceptors, most common on the digits, sensitive to Touch.^{Q}
- **Pacinian corpuscles**—deep mechanoreceptors with a 'cut onion' pattern, sensitive to Pressure.^{Q}
- **Hair disks**—complexes of Merkel cells and free nerve endings, most common on the face; they are not seen on ordinary histology but stain with cytokeratin.
- **Golgi-Mazzoni corpuscle:** SC tissue of fingers laminated structure.
- **Krause end bulb:** Encapsulated swelling of myelinated fibers, superficial dermis.

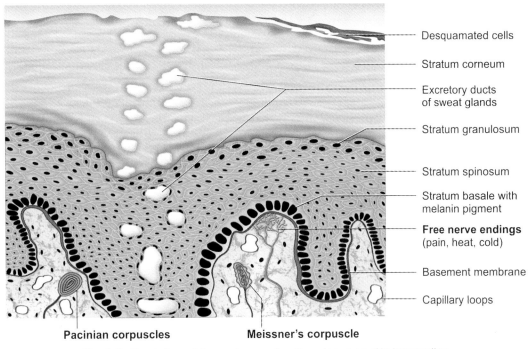

Desquamated cells

Stratum corneum

Excretory ducts of sweat glands

Stratum granulosum

Stratum spinosum

Stratum basale with melanin pigment

Free nerve endings (pain, heat, cold)

Basement membrane

Capillary loops

Pacinian corpuscles   **Meissner's corpuscle**

Fig. 1.8: Depiction of the various cells with a focus on skin innervation

ADIPOSE TISSUE

The subcutis contains numerous connective-tissue septa which carry lymphatics, blood vessels, and nerves. The network of septa keeps the lobules of fat in place and provides support. The smallest functional unit is the microlobule which is nourished by an arteriole.

The vast majority of fat is known as white fat. It serves as a site for energy storage, as well as providing thermal insulation and padding. Newborns have about **5% brown fat**, which is more rapidly metabolized producing heat directly. Brown fat is usually located on the back and along large vessels. Adults have only rudimentary deposits. Brown fat has smaller lipid droplets and is rich in mitochondria. The rapid production of heat is necessary for infants, who cannot shiver as adults do routinely when exposed to cold.

HAIR AND NAILS

Hair

Human hair plays a major role in forming one's image and also has biological functions. Scalp hairs provide *sun protection* as skin cancers are more common on bald scalps. The density varies from $615/cm^2$ at age 25 to $425/cm^2$ after 70 years of age. The eyelashes, eyebrows, and hairs in the anterior nares help to protect these orifices from airborne particles.

The first hair follicles appear in the 10th week of embryonic life,[Q] resulting from an interaction between the epithelial hair germ and the underlying hair papillae, a condensation of mesenchymal cells. Further follicular epithelial regions differentiate into the sebaceous glands, apocrine glands, and the bulge or regenerating region of the hair follicle. The hair papilla determines the size of the hair bulb and thus the hair thickness. The activity of the melanocytes within the matrix determines the hair color.

Parts of Hair

The *infundibulum* starts where the sebaceous duct enters the follicle. Just below this, the outer root sheath thickens at the site of attachment of the arrector pili muscle into the *bulge region*, which contains epithelial stem cells. It also blends with the epidermis at the distal end of the follicle (isthmus) (Fig. 1.9). If the bulge region is damaged, scarring alopecia results (**scarring** also known as cicatricial).[Q]

The hair shaft consists of a medulla, cortex, and cuticle. The cortex is the main component of hair; it contains cornified hair matrix cells analogous to the stratum corneum but formed into a cylindrical mass. The outer layer of the hair shaft is the cuticle, whose overlapping shingle-like cells *interlock* with the cuticle of the inner root sheath, anchoring the hair in the follicle (Fig. 1.10).

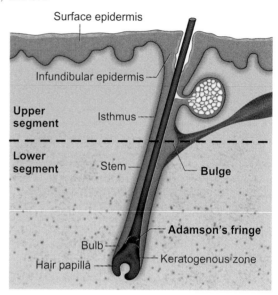

Fig. 1.9: A depiction of the components of hair

Types of Hair

Lanugo hairs are fetal hairs and only seen in premature infants. They are long, thin, non-medullated, soft, and usually without pigment.

Vellus hairs are the normal body hairs, usually <2 cm thin, non-medullated and colorless.

Terminal hairs are long, thick, pigmented hairs with a medulla. They are present at birth on the scalp, as well as forming eyelashes and eyebrows.

Sexual hairs are specialized terminal hairs which appear during puberty as androgens influence vellus hairs in certain body areas, such as the axilla, genitalia, and beard area of men.

Hair Cycle

Hair growth occurs in repetitive cycles. The **3–6 years** period with stable hair growth and maximal follicular size, with high mitotic activity in the matrix, is known as the **anagen** phase.[Q] Next, the hair follicle enters a short 2-week transitory period known as the **catagen phase**, with apoptosis of the hair bulb region and regression to about one-third of its previous length as the hair papilla condenses and moves upward and forms the club hair. After 2–4 months of the telogen or resting phase, the club hair is pushed aside by the next anagen hair developing from the interaction between the bulge region and the papilla, and then shed. Normally, more than 80% of hairs are anagen and less than 20% telogen,[Q] with only a fraction of a percent catagen (Fig. 1.11).

Nails

The nail unit develops between the 9th and 20th embryonal week as pocket-like invagination of the epidermis at the distal end of the digits.

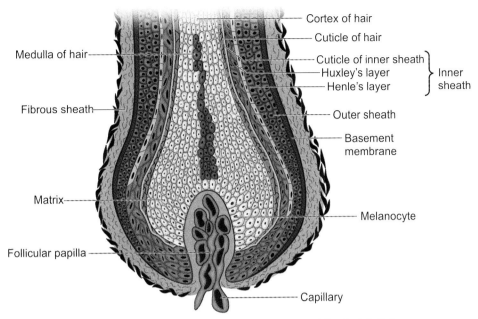

Fig. 1.10: A depiction of the various layers of the hair follicle

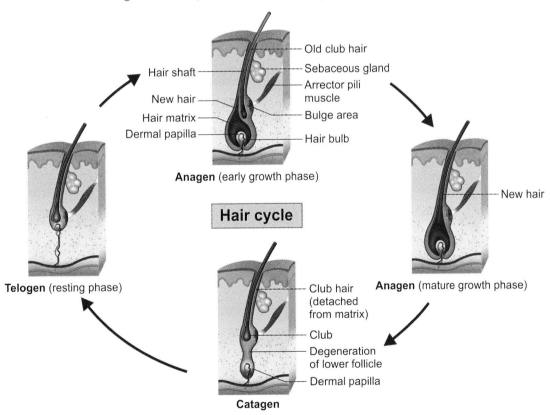

Fig. 1.11: Various phases of the hair cycle

Parts of Nail

It consists of the nail matrix, nail plate, nail bed and periungual skin or paronychium.

The nail stabilizes and projects the fingers and toes, serves as an important tool, and has significant cosmetic effects. In many animals and some humans, it is an effective weapon!

The **nail matrix** is the **growth zone** of the nail; it extends for 3–6 mm beneath the proximal nail fold. The proximal part of the nail fold forms the superficial third of the nail plate, while the more distal part forms the rest of the plate. The nail plate is sealed proximally by the **cuticle (eponychium)** and laterally by the nail folds.

Nail bed: Dermal tissue beneath nail plate, 2–5-cell layer thick.

At its distal end, the 0.5–1.0 mm yellow-brown **onychodermal band** marks the site where the nail plate loses its adherence to the nail bed. Distal to this attachment, the free nail appears white because of the underlying air, and covers the **hyponychium**, a thin stripe of skin without dermatoglyphics or adnexal structures. The **lunula**[Q] is a half-moon-shaped white zone covering the distal matrix at the base of the thumb nails and sometimes other nails (Fig. 1.12).

> Nails grow slowly; a finger nail requires **4–6 months** to replace itself, while a toe nail needs **12–18 months**. That is why for onychomycosis, griseofulvin, a fungistatic drug, has to be given for 12 months!

Nails grow **faster** at night than during the day, in summer than in winter, in young individuals than in the elderly, and in men than in women.

Disorders and Nail

Skin diseases may be associated with more rapid nail growth (psoriasis) or slowed nail growth (atopic dermatitis). The capillaries are visible through the transparent nail plate and cuticle. Using capillary microscopy, vessel changes can be visualized in the nail fold, helping diagnose collagen-vascular diseases such as systemic sclerosis and dermatomyositis.[Q]

Anemia (pale), methemoglobulinemia (blue-gray) and pigmented disorders (melanin deposits, melanocytic nevus, or melanoma) can be seen through the nail, as can subungual tumors such as glomus tumors.

About 10–20% of visible light, 5–10% of UVA and 1–3% of UVB pass through a normal nail plate and reach the nail bed.

IMPORTANT FUNCTIONAL CHANGES

Keratinization

The transition from the cuboidal cells of the basal layer to the scales of the stratum corneum is a complex one. The change from a **basal layer** keratinocyte to a corneocyte takes **14 days** and then the loss of this cell remnant, as scales occur after another **14 days**.[Q] Total 4 weeks (28–30 days).

The main component of the epidermis is keratins and they are arranged in a pair, one acidic and the other basic. This rule of nature that opposites attract is seen down to the molecular level! These two cytokeratins, one basic and one acidic, combine to form a keratin filament[Q] (tonofilament), a hallmark of epithelial cells.

The main events during keratinization:[Q]
1. Cell size increases, cell flattens
2. Nucleus size decreases
3. Metabolism becomes focused

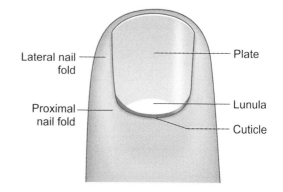

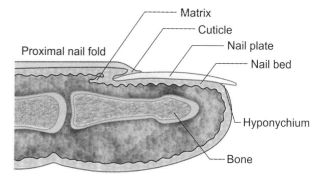

Fig. 1.12: Parts of the nail

4. Dehydration of the cell
5. Finally, apoptosis

Different pairs of keratin are transcribed and expressed at different levels of the epidermis (Fig. 1.13).

They are important as any dysfunction of these pairs can lead to skin disorders (Table 1.2).

There are three important aspect of the process of keratinization, one involves keratin, second filaggrin and third Odland bodies (Fig. 1.14).

- Odland bodies (keratinosomes), which discharge epidermal lipids into the intercellular spaces of the stratum corneum.[Q]
- Profilaggrin, which is synthesized by keratinocytes in the stratum spinosum; it is the precursor of filaggrin, which binds together with keratin to form keratohyalin granules.[Q]

> **Clinical correlate:** Mutations in filaggrin are important in both **atopic dermatitis and ichthyosis vulgaris**.[Q]

- **Involucrin**, which is the main component of the cornified envelope, is linked by transglutaminase.

Table 1.2	Keratin pairs in skin
Keratins 5 and 14	Basal layer[Q]
Keratins 1 and 10	Spinous layer[Q]
Keratins 6 and 16	Psoriasis
Keratins 4 and 13	Mucosa
Keratins 6a, 6b, 16, and 17	Hair and nails
Keratins 31–40 and 81–86	Hair

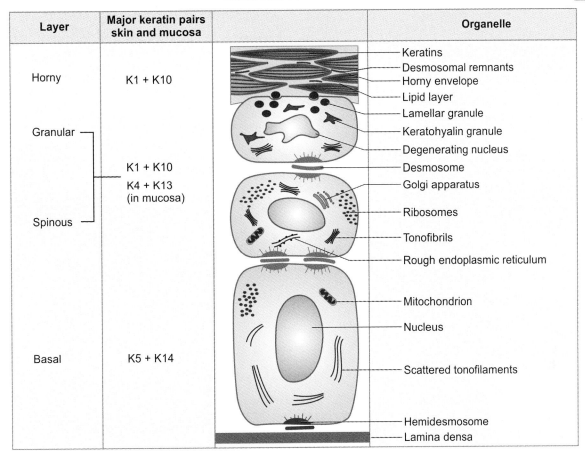

Layer	Major keratin pairs skin and mucosa	Organelle
Horny	K1 + K10	Keratins Desmosomal remnants Horny envelope Lipid layer Lamellar granule Keratohyalin granule Degenerating nucleus Desmosome
Granular Spinous	K1 + K10 K4 + K13 (in mucosa)	Golgi apparatus Ribosomes Tonofibrils Rough endoplasmic reticulum Mitochondrion Nucleus
Basal	K5 + K14	Scattered tonofilaments Hemidesmosome Lamina densa

Fig. 1.13: An overview of the keratin pairs with their location in the epidermis

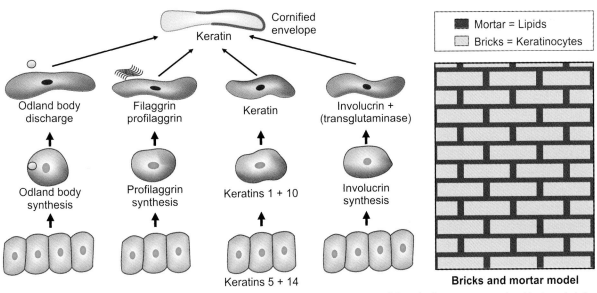

Fig. 1.14: An overview of the process of keratinization. Though the composition of the stratum corneum is akin to a brick wall, the keratinocytes (bricks) and the intercellular space (mortar) undergo metamorphosis and are dynamic

Melanization

Melanocytes

Melanocytes are derived from the neural crest and migrate into the epidermis.[Q] On light microscopy, they are dendritic cells located in the basal layer. About every 10th basal layer, cell is a melanocyte **(ratio of melanocyte to basal cells—1:10)**.[Q]

Melanogenesis

Melanocytes manufacture melanin, the key pigment of the skin. The synthesis of melanin is complex starting with tyrosine; the most important enzyme is tyrosinase.[Q] An important intermediate is DOPA (a precursor of dopamine). Two major forms of melanin are:

- **Eumelanin (brown-black)** (*EBB—eumelanin, brown, black*).
- **Pheomelanin:** It contains sulfur (red-yellow; copper) (*PC—pheomelanin; copper*).

The melanin is packaged into melanosomes in the Golgi apparatus and then transferred to keratinocytes. Melanocytes have long cell extension (dendrites) and transfer pigment to approximately 36 keratinocytes (Fig. 1.15).[Q]

(*Epidermal melanin unit → 1:36*).

Defects in Melanogenesis (Fig. 1.16)

- **Albinism**—lack or reduced function of tyrosinase or other enzymes leading to defective production of melanin; often associated with visual problems.
- **Transfer defect**—'ash-leaf' macules of tuberous sclerosis result from abnormal transfer of melanosomes.
- **Piebaldism**—congenital absence of melanocytes because of aberrant cell migration secondary to loss of function mutations in the tyrosine kinase (Kit)[Q] receptor; causes white streaks of hair (poliosis) or hypopigmented patches of skin; it may be coupled with deafness **(Waardenburg syndrome)**.

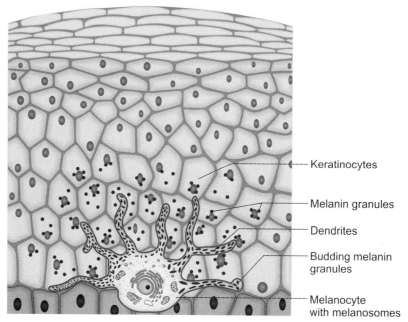

Fig. 1.15: Localization of the melanocyte and its interaction with the keratinocytes

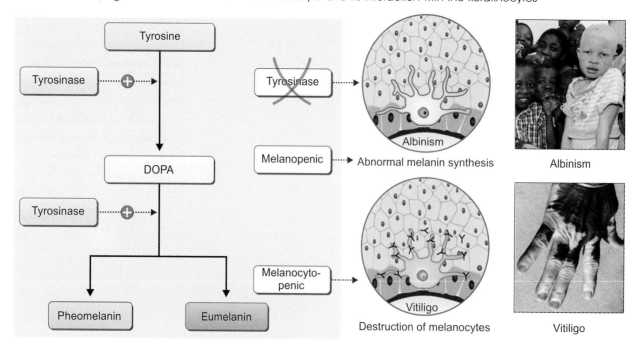

Fig. 1.16: Common defects in melanogenesis and their clinical effect

- **Vitiligo**—an autoimmune disease with localized destruction of melanocytes.

Skin Color and Type

Very minor differences in melanogenesis lead to major variations in skin color. **Skin color** is determined by the *type of melanin* and by the nature of the *melanosomes*, NOT *by the number* of melanocytes.[Q] In black skin, the melanosomes are larger, more highly pigmented and more slowly degraded; they primarily contain eumelanin (Fig. 1.17).

Brown and black hairs have eumelanin, while blond and red hairs contain more pheomelanin. Red hair also contains trichrome melanin.

Melanin is crucial as it provides protection against ultraviolet (UV) irradiation. It functions as a free-radical scavenger and can be called the **'umbrella' of the skin.**[Q] Fitzpatrick identified six different skin types, based on tendency to burn or tan. Type I individuals burn always, never tan, and are at increased risk for both melanoma and other skin cancers. Indians are Type IV, but we try to use products to make our skin fairer, a mistake, as it is our protection against UV damage.

Diagnosis of skin color disorders can be made of two questions:
Q. Hyperpigmented lesions—increased melanin or increased melanocytes? Pigment in the epidermis or dermis?
Q. Hypopigmented lesions—absent melanocytes or defects in melanin production and transfer?

IMMUNOLOGY OF SKIN

The purpose of the immune system is to protect the body against potentially damaging influences like microbes or toxins. The first step is the mechanical barrier and biologic barriers, which prevent entry of the noxious agents into the body. When these agents penetrate the skin defense, the immune system is activated (Fig. 1.18).

There are two types of immune responses, the *inborn* or also called the *innate immunity* and when this cannot contain the outside agent the *acquired immunity* is activated.

Innate Immunity

Some immune cells can phagocytose and destroy damaged cells or microorganisms. Cell damage appears to release alarm signals, which trigger the immune response and later also enhance the effector functions

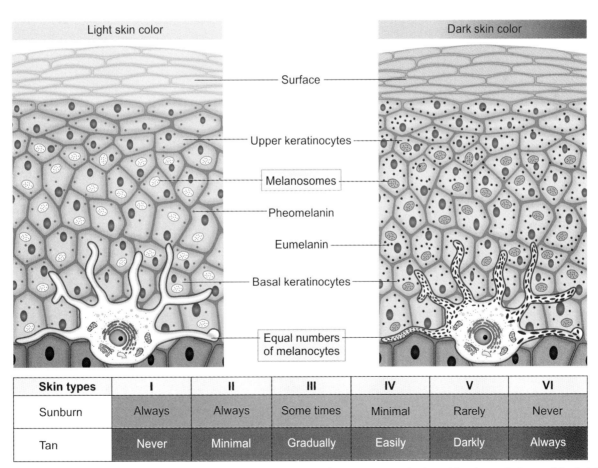

Skin types	I	II	III	IV	V	VI
Sunburn	Always	Always	Some times	Minimal	Rarely	Never
Tan	Never	Minimal	Gradually	Easily	Darkly	Always

Fig. 1.17: Comparison of a light skin and dark skin patient. It is the *melanosomes* content and the type of pigment that determine skin color. Indians are lucky to have this natural sunscreen and are of Type IV skin. The sad part is that we keep trying to reduce our natural skin color to become fairer, fighting natures protective mechanism

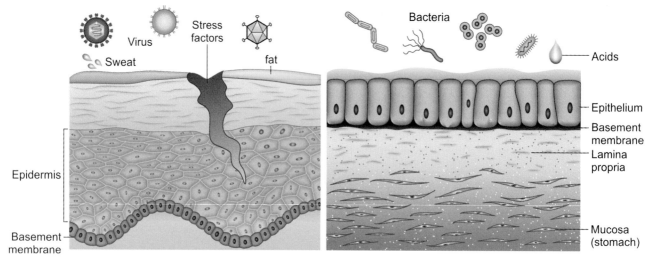

Fig. 1.18: The physical barriers that determine skin and mucosal defense

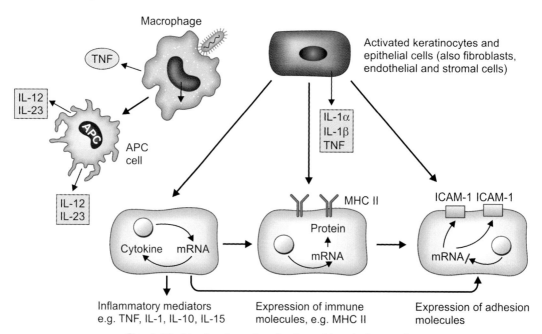

Fig. 1.19: Mechanism of activation of innate immunity

of the defense. All the cells that can be attacked by exogenous agents contribute to the innate response. In the skin, they include the keratinocyte; in the mucosa, epithelial cells, and in the liver, hepatocytes; in addition, fibroblasts and glial cells can also raise an alarm (Fig. 1.18).

a. The cells react to the stress signals by releasing a group of *alarm cytokines*, mainly interleukin-1 **(IL-1)**.

b. In the *skin*, inflammation starts with the activation of the *inflammasome*.

c. This activation leads to the transcription, processing and cleavage of **IL-1α** and **IL-1β**.

d. These activate the other interleukins (IL-6, IL-18), tumor necrosis factor-α (TNF-α) and chemokines, which attract and activate antigen-presenting cells (APCs).

Thus, the innate immune response is set into motion (Fig. 1.19).

Specific (Acquired) Immunity

a. Activated APCs carrying foreign antigen migrate to the regional lymph nodes, where they use chemokines to attract naive CD4+ helper T cells and CD8 cytotoxic T cells (Fig. 1.20).

b. The APCs present their antigens or haptens to these cells. The naive T cells that recognize the antigens on the basis of their receptor structure are then activated to 'blast' forms.

c. With the help of the cytokine **IL-2**, these activated T cells can increase by a factor of 10,000 within a few days. In the lymph nodes, activated T cells interact with B cells and signal them to start producing immunoglobulin.

d. The T cells then leave the lymph nodes and return via the bloodstream to the site of initial injury, guided

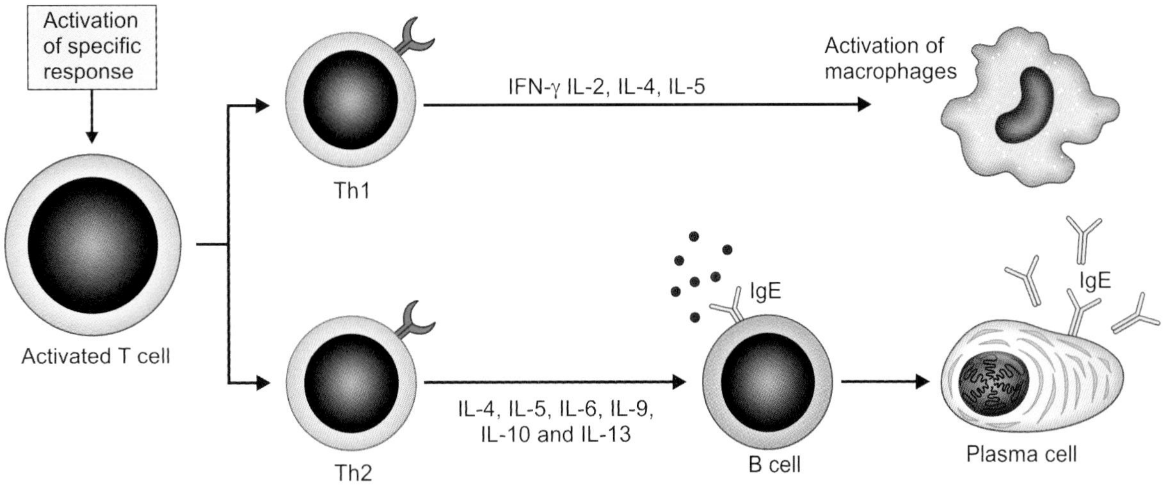

Fig. 1.20: Specific immune response and the role of Th1 and Th2 cells

by a variety of cell messengers. As part of the innate response, an inflammatory reaction is initiated, which leads to the production of adhesion molecules. These enable the activated T cells to attach to vessel walls, migrate through the walls, and move into the inflamed tissue. There they are further stimulated by antigen-carrying macrophages and monocytes, to produce a group of proinflammatory mediators.

e. Interferon-γ **(IFN-γ)** plays a central role, as it induces macrophages to produce important inflammatory mediators, cranking up the entire response process by stimulating the tissue cells to produce vast amounts of free oxygen radicals, TNF, and all the other factors with which they initially signaled alarm. In contrast to the initiation phase, both the number and quantity of cytokines are now much greater.

The initially nonspecific defense mechanisms are so effectively enhanced by the appearance of immune cells specifically directed against the triggering antigen or hapten, that the process of cleaning up can begin, with the killing and phagocytosis of the invading substances. This is dominated either by lymphocytes and macrophages or neutrophils (Fig. 1.20).

T Cell Response and Activation

T cells are the binding link between the innate and specific immune responses. They are characterized by the membrane-bound T cell receptor (TCR). T cells can only be activated by APCs that present, with their MHC molecule, a peptide that fits the highly specific TCR.

There are broadly two types of cells (Fig. 1.21):

1. **CD4+ or helper T cells (Th)** can induce or suppress the inflammatory immune responses via cytokines (Th1,Th2, Th17 response) or via the T reg.
2. **CD8+ or cytotoxic T cells (Tc)** can destroy virally infected target cells.

The CD4 and CD8 molecules are membrane coreceptors that determine which MHC molecules the T cells interact with. The MHC class I molecules are expressed by almost all cells, while MHC class II molecules are only expressed by APCs.

- **CD4+ cells** [Th] interact with **MHC class II** (HLA-DR and HLA-DQ) molecules, which primarily present *exogenous* antigens (such as allergens or haptens) to T cells.
- Cytotoxic **CD8+ cells** (Tc) interact with **MHC class I** (HLA-A and HLA-B) molecules; primarily *endogenous* antigens such as viral and tumor peptides.

The selection of those T cells that are allowed to circulate in the body, as well as the association of a TCR with a CD4 or CD8 molecule, occurs in the thymus. The average adult has around 10^{12} T cells available, with around 10^9 different TCRs, which circulate as naive T cells until they meet their specific antigen in association with an APC and are then activated. Thus the T cell repertoire is capable of recognizing 10^9 different peptides.

APC: The initiation of a specific immune response requires the stimulation of naive T cells by activated APCs in the lymph nodes. The Th cells then have the task of initiating the production of immunoglobulin by B cells in the lymph nodes, and of further activating the nonspecific effector cells, such as macrophages and monocytes, in the tissue. For this apart from TCR and MHC molecules, adhesion molecules are essential for cell affinity—they include intracellular adhesion molecule (ICAM)-1 and lymphocyte function antigen (LFA)-1. Costimulatory molecules are then required for T cell activation.

Important representatives are CD28 and CTLA-4 on T cells, and their partners CD80 and CD86 on APCs (Fig. 1.22).

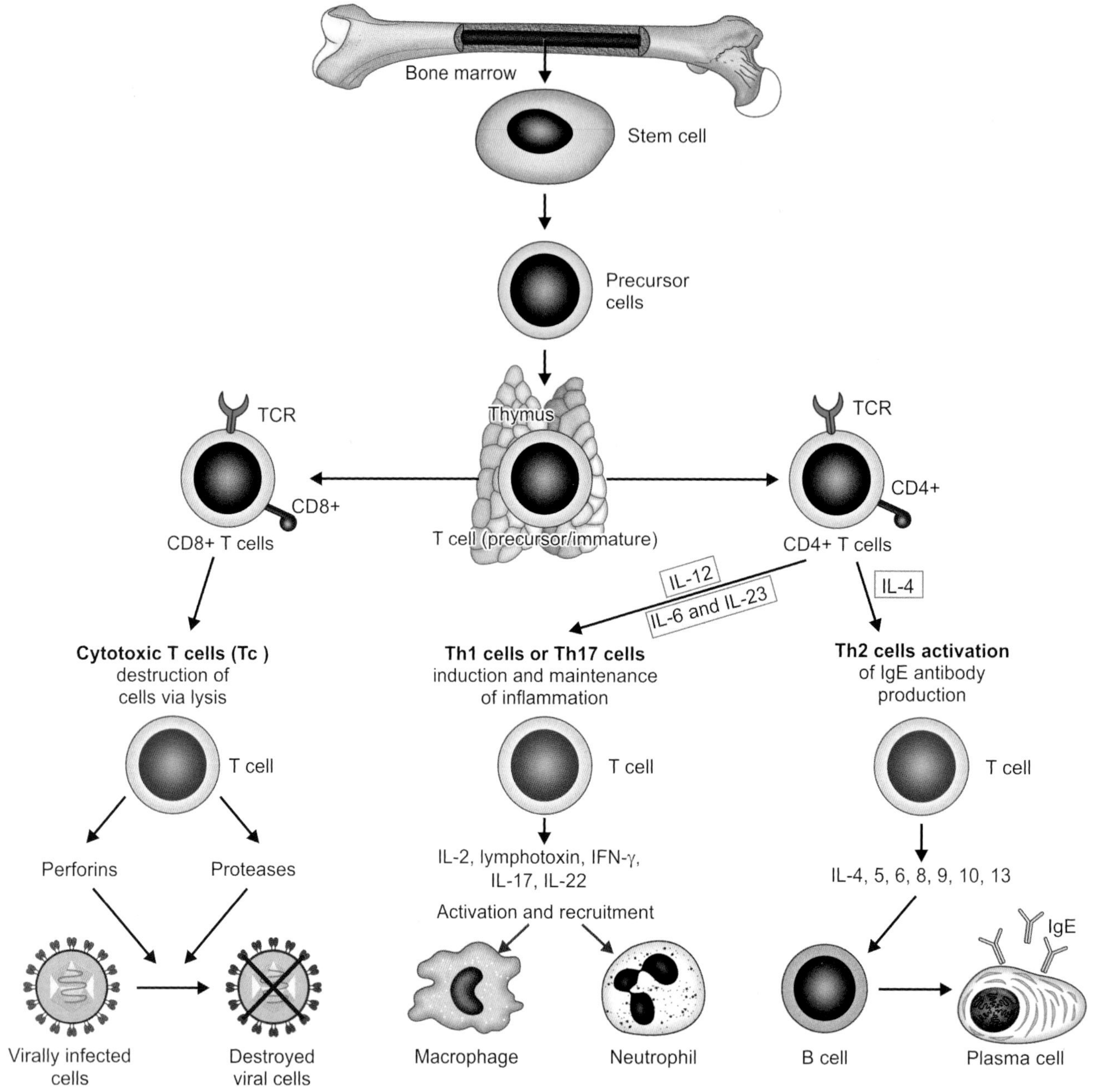

Fig. 1.21: A depiction of the T cell origin and differentiation

Cytokines: For adequate activation and clonal expansion of T cells, both IL-2 and IL-15 are required. In addition, cytokines direct the differentiation of T cells (Fig. 1.23A).

a. **IL-12** promotes the development of naïve Tc cells into cytotoxic Tc 1 cells, and naive Th cells into proinflammatory Th1 cells.

b. **IL-1**, **IL-6**, and **IL-23** induce IL-17-secreting Th17 cells.

c. **IL-4** induces Th cells to the Th2 cells which counterbalances the Tc, Th1 and Th17 cells.

d. Th2 cells induce IgE production by B cells, and activate and attract eosinophils, playing an essential role in all forms of immediate allergy.

Th17 cells: The importance of Th17 cells was recognized with the observation that both IL-17 and IL-23 play a central role in the development of autoimmune inflammatory diseases. These cells produce interleukin IL-17A and recruit neutrophils.

This cell is important both in the causation and treatment of psoriasis[Q] and multiple sclerosis. Recent data suggest that Th17 cells in coordination with the Th1 cells play a role in delayed-type hypersensitivity reactions, such as allergic contact dermatitis and many other inflammatory diseases.

During inflammation, the Th17 cells is produced with the Th1 cells but are activated by different cytokines. IL-12 is important for the differentiation of naive CD4+

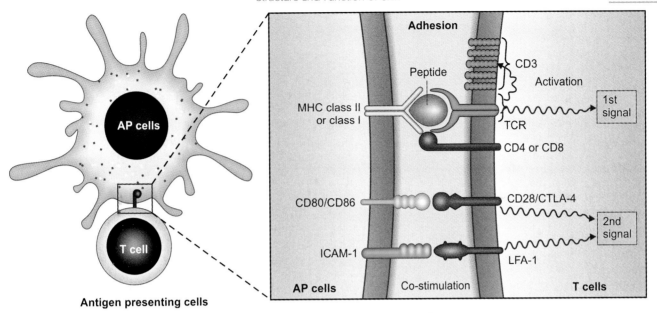

Fig. 1.22: Interaction of T cells and APC

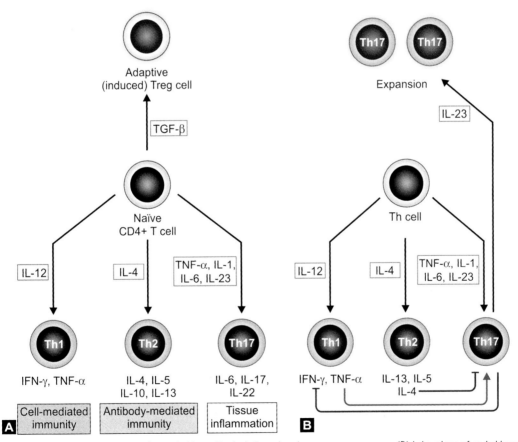

Fig. 1.23A and B: (A) A depiction of the major cytokines that determine immune response; (B) Interplay of cytokines and Th1, Th2, and Th17 cells

T cells into a Th1 phenotype. In contrast, IL-1, IL-6, and IL-23 are required for the induction of Th17 cells, while IL-23 (a subtype of IL-12) is needed for their expansion. IFN-γ and IL-4 suppress the differentiation of Th17 cells (Fig. 1.23B). IFN-γ suppresses angiogenesis, while IL-17 stimulates it.[Q]

T regulatory cells: The most important counterbalance to the Th1, Th2 and Th17 cells are the T reg cells. These are activated CD4+ T cells which express the IL-2 receptor CD 25 on their surface apart from the transcription factor FOXp3 (forkhead box p3). They keep the other cells in balance primarily by cell-cell contact. The inhibition is via soluble mediators like IL-10 and TGF-β.

Their use stems from the fact that they mediate the aggravated allergic response in conditions like asthma, a classic type I allergy, allergic alveolitis, and severe forms of allergic rhinoconjunctivitis, and can arrest the progression to asthma, the 'atopic march'.[Q] There is good evidence that hyposensitization therapy or allergen-specific immunotherapy against type I allergies involves the induction of specific T reg cells.

B Cells and Antibody Production

B cells are responsible for Ab production. To differentiate into Ig-secreting plasma cells, B cells must be stimulated by Th cells, usually in the lymph node follicles. With their ability to present peptide antigens with MHC class II molecules, and to produce cytokines for the innate immune response, B cells also function as weak APCs in the regulation of the T cell response. They appear to suppress cell-mediated immune reactions and facilitate the differentiation of T cells into Th2 cells or regulatory (T reg) cells.

Antibodies (immunoglobulins): Antibodies are immunoglobulins that react with antigens.

- Immunoglobulin G (IgG) is responsible for long-lasting humoral immunity. It can cross the placenta, and binds complement to activate the classic complement pathway. IgG can coat neutrophils and macrophages and acts as an opsonin by cross-bridging antigen.
- IgM is the largest immunoglobulin molecule. It is the first antibody to appear after immunization or infection. Like IgG, it can fix complement but unlike IgG it cannot cross the placenta.
- IgA is the most common immunoglobulin in secretions. It acts as a protective paint in the gastrointestinal and respiratory tracts. It does not bind complement but can activate it via the alternative pathway.
- IgE binds to Fc receptors on mast cells and basophils, where it sensitizes them to release inflammatory mediators in type I immediate hypersensitivity reactions.

Mediators of Immune System

Immune cells interact via both direct cell-cell contacts and soluble molecules known as mediators. They include a broad spectrum of different molecular classes and are a crucial component of the signaling system that leads to an effective immune response.

The ultimate effect of these mediators on the cells can be variable. IFN-α and IFN-β bind to the same receptor, but transmit in part different signals, so IFN-α is used for *immunostimulation* and IFN-β for *immunosuppression*.

Important mediators include:
- Cytokines
- Chemokines
- Soluble surface molecules.

Cytokines

The cytokines are a large family of soluble mediators which include interleukins (ILs), growth factors (GFs) and IFNs (Figs 1.21, 1.23 and 1.24).

- **Basic mediators:** Tumor necrosis factor (TNF), IL-1, and IL-6 are rapidly released by macrophages in all forms of inflammation. Blocking IL-1 or TNF inhibits many aspects of inflammation.
- **T cell:** T cell cytokines, which confusingly can also be secreted by other cells, regulate the course of the immune response via T cells. IL-2 is the most important T cell growth factor. The function of T cells is determined by the cytokine pattern.

IL-2 and IFN-γ are **Th1** cytokines that have the following effects:
a. Formation of TNF and free radicals in macrophages.
b. Convert CD8+ T cells into cytotoxic cells.
c. Drive B cells to isotype switch to produce complement-binding immunoglobulins.

Th1, cytokines and **IL-17**, the main cytokines of the **Th17** cells, initiate the cell-mediated or delayed-type immune response.

The **Th2 cytokines** are IL-4, IL-9, and IL-13, and have the following actions:
a. Suppress the proinflammatory properties of macrophages.
b. Drive B cells to isotype switch producing IgG4 and IgE.
c. Support immediate-type allergies or type I reactions, including airway hypersecretion and increased smooth muscle tone.

Additional important cytokines are IL-10, IL-12, and IL-23, which are secreted by APCs. **IL-10** can block immune responses, while **IL-12** and **IL-23** can induce strong delayed-type hypersensitivity reactions, **IL-31** seems to induce itch.

Chemokines

Chemokines help in migration and homing of different immune cells, in cooperation with IL-1 and TNF, which induce the expression of adhesion molecules by endothelial cells. This facilitates the attachment of immune cells to the vessel wall and then migration through the wall. The chemokines guide the successful migrants to the site of inflammation. The chemokine pattern determines the type of infiltrate. For example, eotaxin binds to chemokine receptor 3 (CCR3), thus attracting eosinophils and Th2 cells (Fig. 1.25).

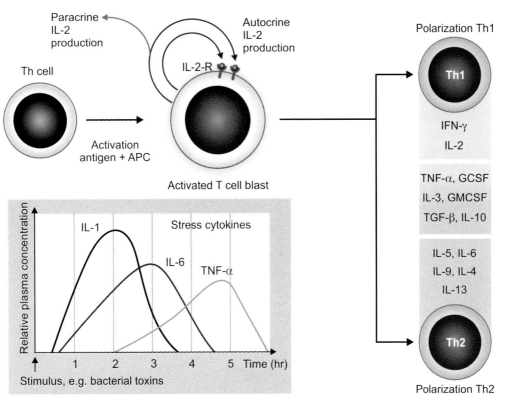

Fig. 1.24: A depiction of various cytokines and their role in Th1 and Th2 polarization and response to stress

Surface Molecules

In addition to the classic soluble mediators, cell surface molecules and receptors can have a similar function when they are separated.

For example, in severe inflammation, the soluble TNF receptor is released into serum and has an anti-inflammatory effect by binding to TNF.

Types of Immune Reaction

Specific immune responses enable a targeted and amplified inflammatory response. As shown above, a close and intricate interaction between the antigen and the APC is needed. This leads to certain specific kinds of response which were divided into 4 types using the original classification of Coombs and Gell.

Their basic classification is still useful:
- Type I—immediate
- Type II—cytotoxic
- Type III—immune-complex mediated
- Type IV—cell-mediated or delayed-type hypersensitivity reaction

Immediate Reaction (Type I)

This immune reaction is mediated by IgE antibodies. They are directed against soluble protein antigens (allergens); typical examples are pollen, animal dander, house dust mites, foods, and arthropod toxins. Allergen contact leads to linking of IgE molecules on the surface of mast cells or basophils, and triggers a cascade of events:
- Release of immediate mediators such as histamine or TNF.
- Synthesis and release of leukotrienes and prostaglandins.
- Synthesis of proallergic cytokines like IL-4 or IL-5.

These can trigger disorders like allergic rhinitis, asthma, or urticaria.

Cytotoxic Reaction (Type II)

Here, IgG antibodies react with antigens that sit on the cell surface. The antigens are medications (such as penicillin) bound to erythrocyte membranes, cell components like the Rhesus D antigen (RhD), or basement membrane components. The IgG mediates cytotoxic effects through complement and phagocytosis.

Examples of type II reactions include medication- or RhO-mediated hemolysis, heparin-induced thrombocytopenia (HIT), glomerulonephritis, and urticaria caused by anti-Fcϵ-receptor antibodies.

Immune-complex Reaction (Type III)

The responsible IgG antibodies are directed against soluble antigens. Examples include:
- Injected serum
- Fragments of pathogenic microbes, e.g. in bacterial endocarditis or viral hepatitis
- Molds or components of hay or that are inhaled.

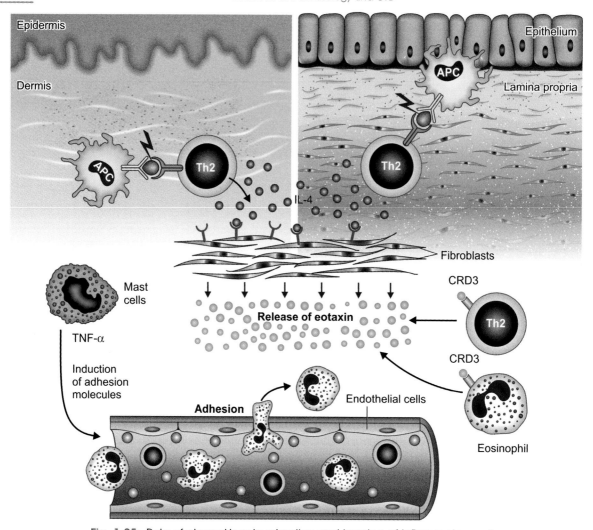

Fig. 1.25: Role of chemokines in migration and homing of inflammatory cells

The resultant antigen–antibody complexes (immune complex) can cause local or systemic reactions. Effector mechanisms include complement binding and activation, as well as activation of granulocytes and macrophages with vessel wall and tissue damage.

Clinical examples are serum sickness or localized Arthus reaction to injected products, vasculitis affecting the skin, joints, and kidneys, persistent viral hepatitis, and allergic alveolitis (farmer's lung).Q

Delayed Reaction (Type IV)

Antigen-specific T cells mediate the delayed-type hypersensitivity or cell-mediated reaction. Triggers include metal ions (such as nickel or chromium) or low molecular weight substances such as fragrances or preservatives, which can bind to body proteins to form complete antigens. Protein antigens from mycobacteria, bacteria, yeasts, and dermatophytes can also induce delayed reactions. The allergen contact is mediated by antigen-presenting dendritic cells and monocytes macrophages, leading to stimulation of T cells. Released cytokines trigger the inflammation, with T cells returning to the site of antigen exposure.

Clinical examples include allergic contact dermatitis and dermal erythematous papules, as in a tuberculin reaction when the allergen bypasses the epidermis.

Diagnosis of Skin Disorders

Though most seasoned clinicians perform what is called the **blink diagnosis** in most skin disorders, the general method of diagnosis is like that in medicine with a proper history and examination. The steps that are to be followed are as follows:

Steps in dermatologic diagnosis

1. History
2. Physical examination: Identify the morphology of basic lesion
3. Configuration or distribution of lesions (when applicable)
4. Investigations and laboratory tests
5. Diagnostic tools
6. Consider clinicopathologic correlations

This said it must be understood that dermatology is a visual specialty, and diagnosis rests heavily on skin inspection. Thus examination is crucial and a full examination is a must. Like physicians rely on a stethoscope, here one must rely on our 'eyes'. We need to train our eyes to see the skin lesions before us and ultimately be able to recognize them. That in turn needs a knowledge of the skin disorder, hence the off-stated statement "the eyes will not see, what the mind does not know".

HISTORY

In medicine, the traditional approach is to take the history before performing the physical examination. Some dermatologists prefer to reverse this order. A useful method is to ask history in conjunction with examination. In a case of urticaria in a child, a history of ingestants, food and infection can be asked while examining the patient as the diagnosis is obvious. But in an STD case, history may be needed to elicit the course of the infection (Fig. 2.1A and B).

Chief Complaint

An open-ended question, such as, "What is your skin problem?", is a useful initial point.

History of Present Illness

The history should include the following:
- How lesions **appeared** at the start
- How **long** they have been present
- How they have **changed**
- Whether **pruritic** or not

> - Nighttime pruritus is typical for **scabies**,[Q] while pruritus after a warm bath is a sign of **polycythemia vera**.[Q]
> - Many dermatoses are typically pruritic like atopic dermatitis, lichen planus, prurigo simplex and lichen simplex chroncius.

- **Systemic** complaints
- Exposures, occupation, travel
- Any relation to light or physical stress
- What **treatments** have been tried.

The last is crucial as in Indian patients usually use OTC steroids even though they are a Schedule H drug. Many cases of recalcitrant tinea and acne have been complicated by steroids use. More worrying is the use of oral steroids.

Another issue is that some medicines have already been used by the patient. This is relevant in, say acne, where a patient may have used tetracyclines, here isotretinoin would be a good option.

Family History

This should include:
- Anyone with similar lesions
- Others with other skin diseases

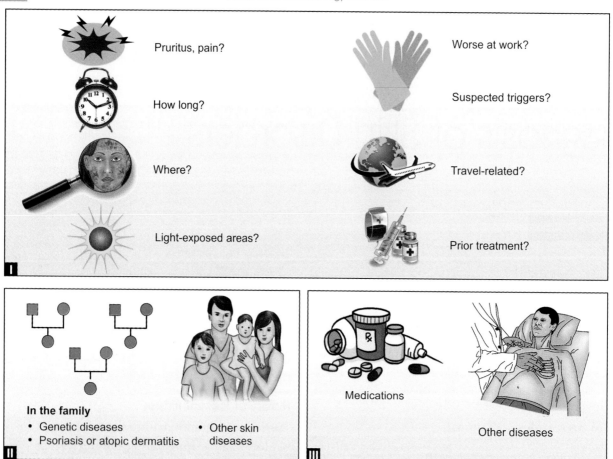

Fig. 2.1A: An overview of the salient features in the history: (I) History of present illness; (II) Family history; (III) Past medical history

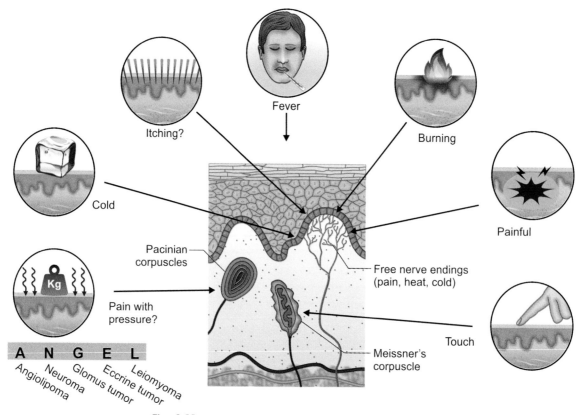

Fig. 2.1B: Important clinical symptoms in the history

- Predisposition to psoriasis, atopic dermatitis.
  Examples:
  - In a child with a chronic itching eruption in the **antecubital and popliteal fossae**, atopic dermatitis is suspected.[Q] A positive family history for atopic diseases (atopic dermatitis, asthma, hay fever) supports the diagnosis.
  - In a youngster with multiple café-au-lait spots, a diagnosis of neurofibromatosis[Q] is considered. A positive family history for this disorder, substantiated by examination of family members, helps to support the diagnosis of this dominantly inherited disorder.
  - Scabies patients invariably have a family history.

Social and Skin Exposure History

This would indicate the social environment of the patient. A chronic skin ulcer from persistent herpes simplex infection is a sign of immunosuppression, and is also an AIDS defining condition. Therefore, a patient with such an ulceration should be asked about high-risk factors for acquiring AIDS, including sexual behavior, intravenous drug abuse, and exposure to blood products.

Contact dermatitis, the big mimicker, is also an occasion for probing into a patient's social history. Patients encounter potentially sensitizing materials both at work and at play. Like a jeweller is sensitized to nickel.[Q] Housewives are exposed to detergents, soaps and vegetables and this leads to chronic hand dermatitis.[Q]

Past Medical History

Ask about
- Medications
- Underlying diseases.

In a patient with a generalized erythematous rash or hives, systemic drugs should be high on the list of possible causes. Also certain foods trigger attacks of episodic liver.

Systemic Illness

In a patient with a malar rash, a diagnosis of systemic lupus erythematosus should be considered, and history regarding other systems may be advisable. This includes history of Raynaud's phenomenon, photosensitivity, hair loss, mouth ulcers, and arthritis. In a patient with a generalized maculopapular eruption, the two most common causes are drugs and viruses, so symptoms of the latter, such as fever, malaise, and upper respiratory or gastrointestinal symptoms should be elicited.

PHYSICAL EXAMINATION

A patient with scaly plaques on the knees, if seen as an adjunct to similarly demarcated lesions on the palms,

Box 2.1	Salient features in examination of skin

1. Complete skin examination is recommended at the first visit.
2. Good lighting is critical.
3. Describe the morphology and distribution of the eruption.

is strongly suggestive of psoriasis. In most cases, a hand lens, Wood's lamp and a dermatoscope are sufficient for diagnosis of most skin disorders (Box 2.1).

Distribution of Lesions and Examination Sequence

It is advisable always. Start at the top and work your way down (Fig. 2.2A).

This can be diagnostic in some disorders. For example, an area of seborrheic dermatitis may look very like an area of atopic dermatitis; but the key to diagnosis lies in the location. Seborrheic dermatitis affects the scalp, forehead, eyebrows, nasolabial folds and central chest;[Q] atopic dermatitis typically affects the antecubital and popliteal fossae. Figures 2.2B and 2.2C show the typical distribution of some common skin conditions.

Some eruptions have peculiar predilections:
- Photo-exposed sites (e.g. lupus erythematosus (Fig. 2.2D), polymorphic light eruption).[Q]
- Sites of trauma, the Koebner phenomenon[Q] (e.g. psoriasis, lichen planus; Fig. 2.2E).
- Possible contact allergy (e.g. nickel earrings, kumkum—Fig. 2.2F, leather or rubber shoes).

Look for **symmetry** which implies a systemic origin, whereas **unilaterality** or **asymmetry** implies an external cause (Fig. 2.2C). Look in the mouth and remember to check the hair and the nails.

Scalp

- Think about the scalp and the hair separately
- Feel the scalp as the hair may be too thick to see much
- Part the hair to see the scalp
- Any baldness? If yes, any alopecia areata 'exclamation mark' hairs?
- Any **scarring** (flat shiny bald areas free of follicle openings)?
- Any unusual hair thickness or twistiness?

Ears

External pinnae
- Signs of solar damage especially at the edge.
- Scaliness suggesting seborrheic dermatitis.
- Discrete tender area on prominent ridge suggesting chondrodermatitis.

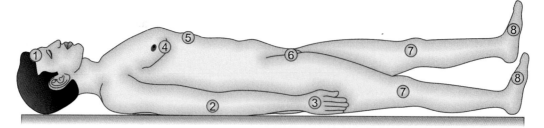

Fig. 2.2A: A step-by-step approach of examination to diagnose skin disorders, starting from the head (1) to the foot (8)

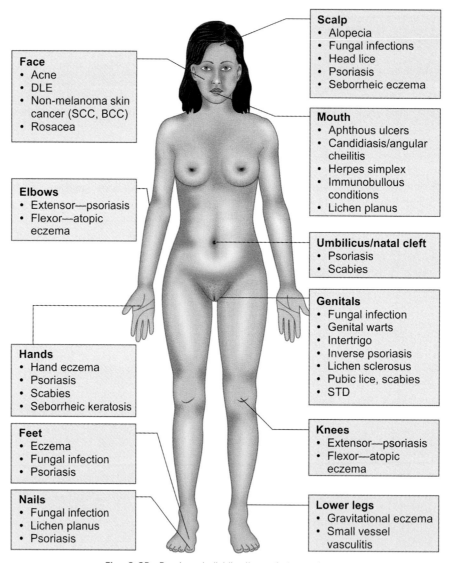

Face
• Acne
• DLE
• Non-melanoma skin cancer (SCC, BCC)
• Rosacea

Elbows
• Extensor—psoriasis
• Flexor—atopic eczema

Hands
• Hand eczema
• Psoriasis
• Scabies
• Seborrheic keratosis

Feet
• Eczema
• Fungal infection
• Psoriasis

Nails
• Fungal infection
• Lichen planus
• Psoriasis

Scalp
• Alopecia
• Fungal infections
• Head lice
• Psoriasis
• Seborrheic eczema

Mouth
• Aphthous ulcers
• Candidiasis/angular cheilitis
• Herpes simplex
• Immunobullous conditions
• Lichen planus

Umbilicus/natal cleft
• Psoriasis
• Scabies

Genitals
• Fungal infection
• Genital warts
• Intertrigo
• Inverse psoriasis
• Lichen sclerosus
• Pubic lice, scabies
• STD

Knees
• Extensor—psoriasis
• Flexor—atopic eczema

Lower legs
• Gravitational eczema
• Small vessel vasculitis

Fig. 2.2B: Regional distribution of dermatoses

External auditory meatus

• Psoriasis
• Eczema

Face

• Examine areas of maximum sun damage: Forehead, upper cheeks and nose. Any sign of skin cancer?
• Hair growth normal (also eyelashes, eyebrows)?
• Eyes: Mucosal surfaces.

• Lips, mouth: Check tongue, gums and buccal mucosal surface inside cheeks (e.g. white net-like pattern of lichen planus).

Neck, Axillae and Arms

Flexures

• Axillae: Erythrasma, hidradenitis suppurativa, fungal infection, flexural psoriasis, seborrheic dermatitis?
• Antecubital fossae: Atopic eczema?

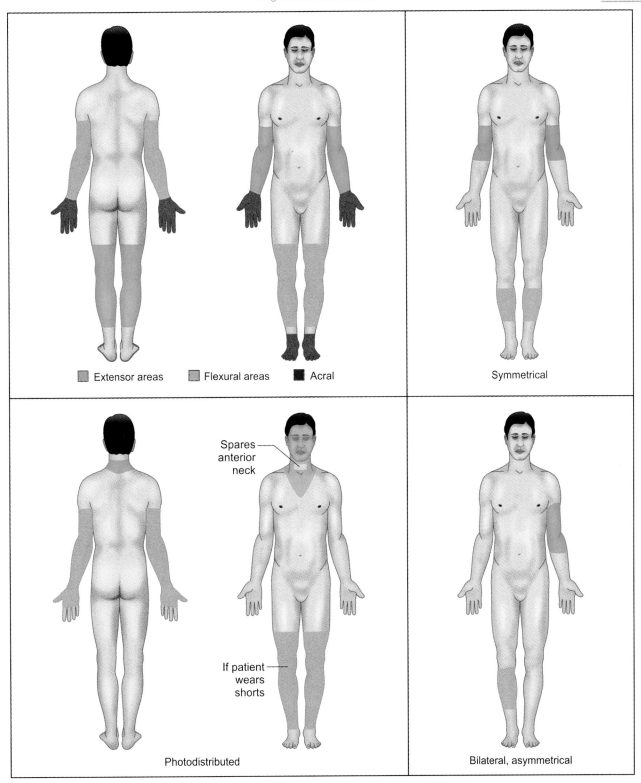

Extensor areas Flexural areas ■ Acral

Symmetrical

Spares anterior neck

If patient wears shorts

Photodistributed

Bilateral, asymmetrical

Fig. 2.2C: Common patterns of skin disorders

Extensors
- Elbows: Psoriasis?

Hands
- Wrists: Scabies?
- Finger webs: Irritant contact dermatitis, scabies?
- Nails: Fungal infection, psoriasis?

Trunk: Back, Chest, Abdomen and Buttocks
- Upper trunk: Acne?
- Flexures: Intertrigo?
- Nipples: Atopic eczema, contact dermatitis, Paget's disease?
- Umbilicus: Psoriasis?

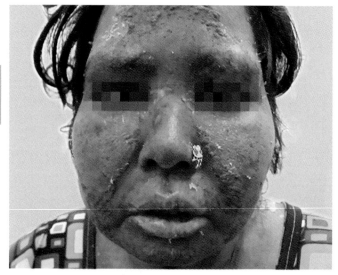

Fig. 2.2D: Acute rash of SLE. Note the marked involvement of the face and neck. Unlike in fairer skin type, in Indian skin, the erythema is less marked

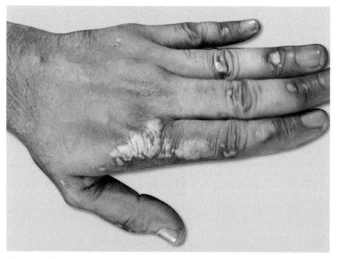

Fig. 2.2E: Violaceous papules of lichen planus with lesions linearly distributed localized to the area of scratching

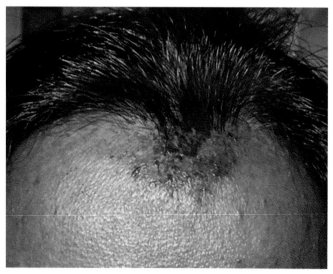

Fig. 2.2F: Contact dermatitis due to kumkum

Genitalia, Perineum, Groins and Perianal Skin
- Contact dermatitis
- Fungal infection
- Intertrigo
- Genital warts or discharge

Legs
- Flexures: Atopic eczema?
- Knees: Psoriasis?
- Lower legs: Varicose veins?
- Ankles: Venous eczema?

Feet
- Soles: Pustular psoriasis?
- Toe webs: Fungal infection?
- Toe nails: Fungal infection, onychogryphosis?

Terminology of Skin Lesions

The definition of skin lesions has 2 parts, first is the type of lesion, second is the features that define it. A combination of the two can help define the lesion. A few important signs can then be used to qualify the lesion.

Types of Lesions

1. **Primary lesions:** The size in many of the definitions given below is arbitrary and it is often helpful to record the actual measurement.

   A **macule** is a small flat area, less than 0.5 cm in diameter, of altered color or texture (Fig. 2.3A to G).
   - Petechiae are pinhead-sized macules of blood in the skin (Fig. 2.3F).
   - The term purpura describes a larger macule or papule of blood in the skin. Such blood-filled lesions do not blanch, if a glass lens is pushed against them.
   - An ecchymosis (bruise) is a larger extravasation of blood into the skin and deeper structures (Fig. 2.3G).

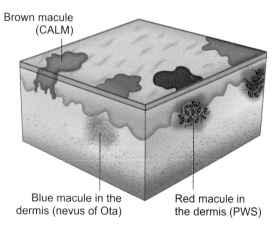

Fig. 2.3A: Various types of macule

Fig. 2.3B to G: (B) Port-wine stain on the face; (C) Nevus of Ota on the face; (D) Vitiligo; (E) Lentigines; (F) Petechiae in a child with ITP; (G) A case of ecchymosis with purpura in a patient with meningococcemia

A **papule** is a small solid elevation of skin, less than 0.5 cm in diameter (Fig. 2.4A and B).
* A burrow^Q is a linear or curvilinear papule, with some scaling, caused by a scabies mite. It lies in the straum corneum^Q (Fig. 2.5).

A **plaque** is an elevated area of skin greater than 0.5 cm in diameter but without substantial depth (Fig. 2.6).

A **nodule** is a solid mass in the skin, usually greater than 0.5 cm in diameter, in both width and depth, which can be seen to be elevated (exophytic) or can be palpated (endophytic) (Fig. 2.7).

A **vesicle** is a circumscribed elevation of skin, less than 0.5 cm in diameter, and containing fluid (Fig. 2.8).

A **bulla** is a circumscribed elevation of skin greater than 0.5 cm in diameter and containing fluid (Fig. 2.8).

A **pustule** is a visible accumulation of pus in the skin (Fig. 2.9A and B).^Q

A **wheal** is an elevated white compressible evanescent^Q area produced by dermal edema. It is often surrounded by a red axon-mediated flare. Although usually less than 2 cm in diameter, some wheals are huge (Fig. 2.9C and D).

2. **Secondary lesions:** These evolve from primary lesions.

A **scale** is a visible flake arising from the horny layer. Scales may be seen on the surface of many

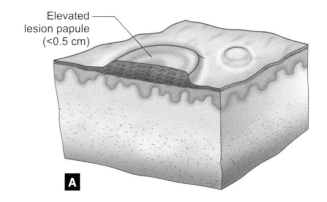

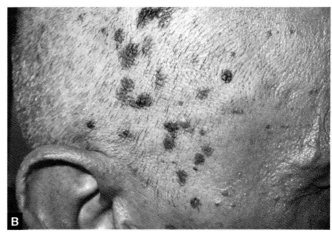

Fig. 2.4A and B: (A) Papule; (B) Multiple plane warts on the face (papules)

primary lesions. It is usually representative of hyperkeratosis (Fig. 2.10).

A **keratosis** is a horn-like thickening of the stratum corneum.

A **crust** may look like a scale, but is composed of dried blood or tissue fluid (Fig. 2.11).

An **ulcer** is an area of skin from which the whole of the epidermis and at least the upper part of the dermis have been lost (Fig. 2.12).

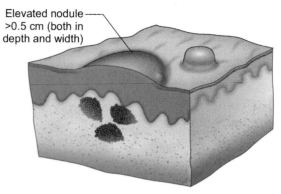

Fig. 2.7A: Nodules

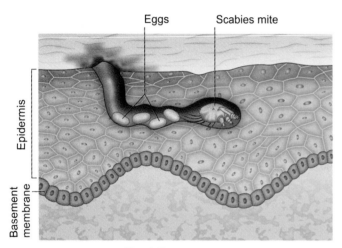

Fig. 2.5: A burrow

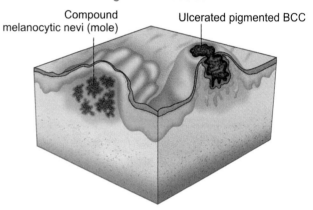

Fig. 2.7B: Two examples of nodules

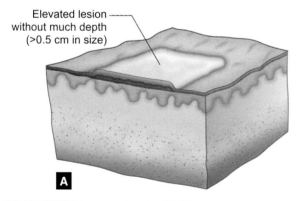

A

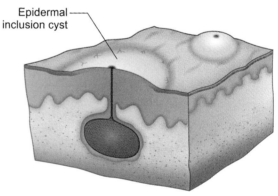

Fig. 2.7C: Epidermal inclusion cyst with a punctum, an example of nodule

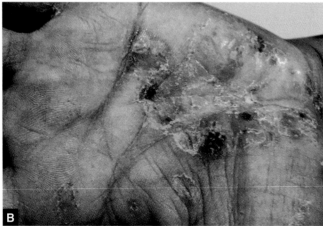

B

Fig. 2.6A and B: (A) Plaque; (B) Multiple scaly and crusted plaques in a case of hand eczema

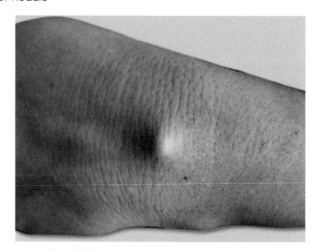

Fig. 2.7D: A ganglion better felt than seen

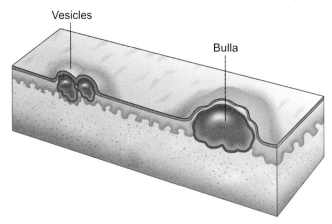

Fig. 2.8A: Vesicle and bulla

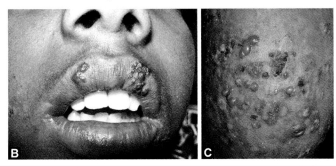

Fig. 2.8B and C: (B) Vesicles of herpes simplex; (C) Bulla in bullous pemphigoid

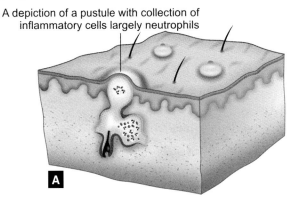

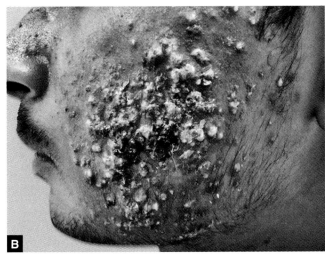

Fig. 2.9A and B: (A) Pustule in acne; (B) Multiple pustules in a case of acne

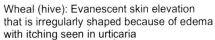

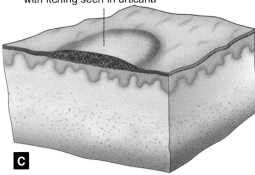

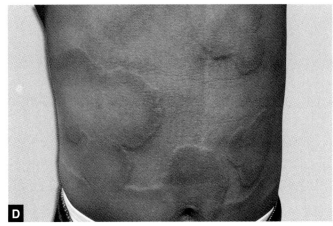

Fig. 2.9C and D: (C) Wheal in urticaria; (D) Erythema, edema and itchy and transient lesion (wheal)Q

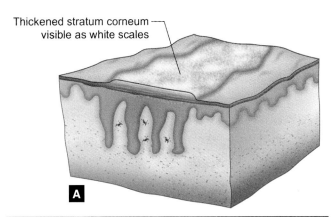

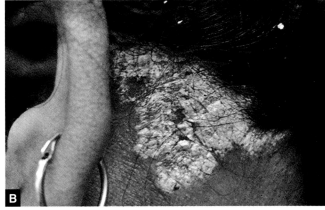

Fig. 2.10A and B: (A) Scale; (B) Scaly plaque in psoriasis

Crust: Secondary lesion due to dried blood or exudate — Oozing of serum

Ulcer is a defect that extends to the dermis

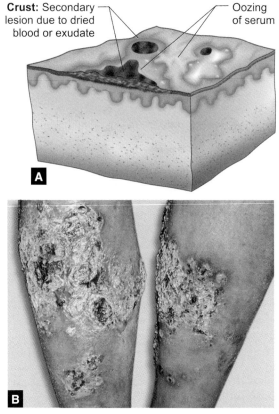

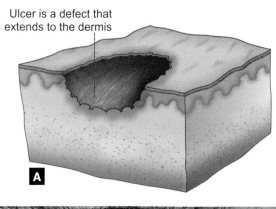

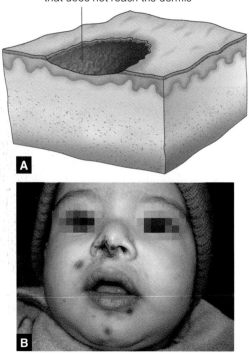

Fig. 2.11A and B: (A) Oozing serum leads to crust; (B) Crusted plaques on the lower limb in ecthyma pyogenicum

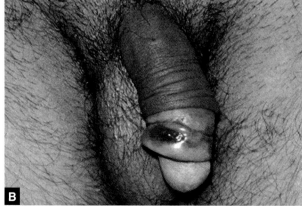

Fig. 2.12A and B: (A) Ulcer; (B) Primary chancre, painless ulcer in syphilis

An **erosion** is an area of skin denuded by a complete or partial loss of only the epidermis. Erosions heal without scarring (Fig. 2.13).

Erosion is a defect in the epidermis that does not reach the dermis

An **excoriation** is an ulcer or erosion produced by scratching (Fig. 2.14).

A **fissure** is a slit in the skin which is usually localized to the epidermis (Fig. 2.15).

A **scar** is a result of healing, where normal structures are permanently replaced by fibrous tissue (Fig. 2.16).

Fig. 2.13A and B: (A) Erosion; (B) Erosions in a case of impetigo

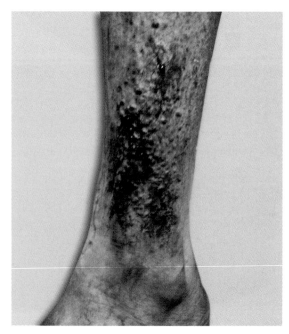

Fig. 2.14: A case of prurigo nodularis with excoriations

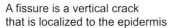

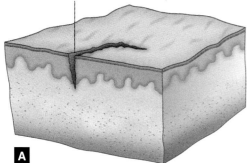

Fig. 2.15A and B: (A) Fissure; (B) Hand eczema with scaly fissured plaques

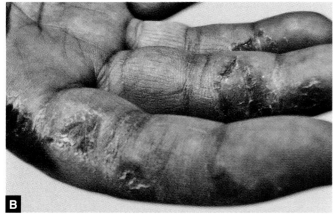

Fig. 2.16: Elevated scar due to road traffic accident

Atrophy is a thinning of skin caused by diminution of the epidermis, dermis or subcutaneous fat. When the epidermis is atrophic it may crinkle like cigarette paper, appear thin and translucent, and lose normal surface markings. Blood vessels may be easy to see in both epidermal and dermal atrophies (Fig. 2.17).

Lichenification is an area of thickened skin with increased markings (Fig. 2.18).

Pustule: It can be both primary and secondary skin lesions.[Q]

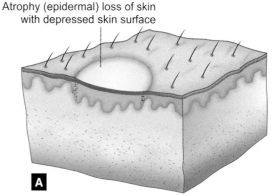

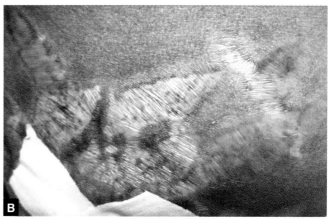

Fig. 2.17A and B: (A) Atrophy; (B) Atrophic depressed skin with 'cigarette paper' wrinkling[Q] in a case of *lichen sclerosus* et atrophicus

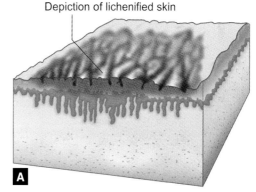

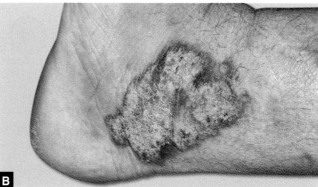

Fig. 2.18A and B: (A) Lichenification; (B) Thick hyperkeratotic skin with increased surface marking in a case of lichen simplex chronicus

Morphology of Lesions

1. **Description:** Color, size, margin (well-defined or ill-defined; regular/irregular—Fig. 2.19), and consistency.
2. **Number of lesions:** Solitary or multiple; if multiple, confluent or distinct?
3. **Arrangement:** A diagrammatic depiction is given in Fig. 2.20A and clinical photographs of these patterns are given in Fig. 2.20B to L.

   Linear:
   - Dermatomal: Following cutaneous sensory nerves, as in herpes zoster[Q] (Fig. 2.20B).
   - Lines of Blaschko[Q]: Following lines of embryonic skin development, as in epidermal nevi (Fig. 2.20D).
   - Other examples: Contact dermatitis, psoriasis, lichen planus (Fig. 2.20E), flat warts.

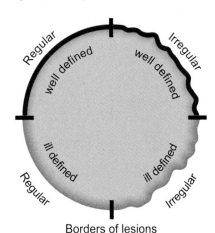

Borders of lesions

Fig. 2.19: A depiction of the margins of skin lesions

Annular: Papules grouped in circular pattern, as in granuloma annulare (Fig. 2.20F). Other examples—tinea corporis/cruris (Fig. 2.20G and H), secondary syphilis and subacute cutaneous lupus erythematosus.

Herpetiform: Grouped vesicles, as in herpes simplex. Other examples are herpes (simplex and zoster), insect bites, leiomyomas.

Other adjectives include:
- *Nummular* means round or coin-like.
- *Circinate* means circular.
- *Arcuate* means curved.
- *Discoid* means disk-like (Fig. 2.20I).
- *Gyrate* means wave-like.
- *Retiform* and *reticulate* mean net-like (Fig. 2.20J).
- *Targetoid* means target-like or 'bull's eye' (Fig. 2.20K).
- *Polycyclic* means formed from coalescing circles, or incomplete rings.

4. Surface contour (e.g. dome-shaped, umbilicated, spire-like; Fig. 2.21A to G).
5. The lesion should always be assessed for the following properties (Fig. 2.22):
   - Tenderness
   - Temperature
   - Consistency (firm, soft)
   - Mobile or fixed
   - Estimation of the depth or level of involvement (epidermis, dermis, subcutis).

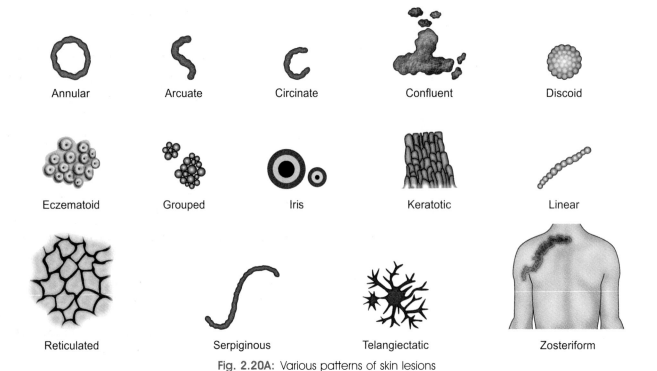

| Annular | Arcuate | Circinate | Confluent | Discoid |

| Eczematoid | Grouped | Iris | Keratotic | Linear |

| Reticulated | Serpiginous | Telangiectatic | Zosteriform |

Fig. 2.20A: Various patterns of skin lesions

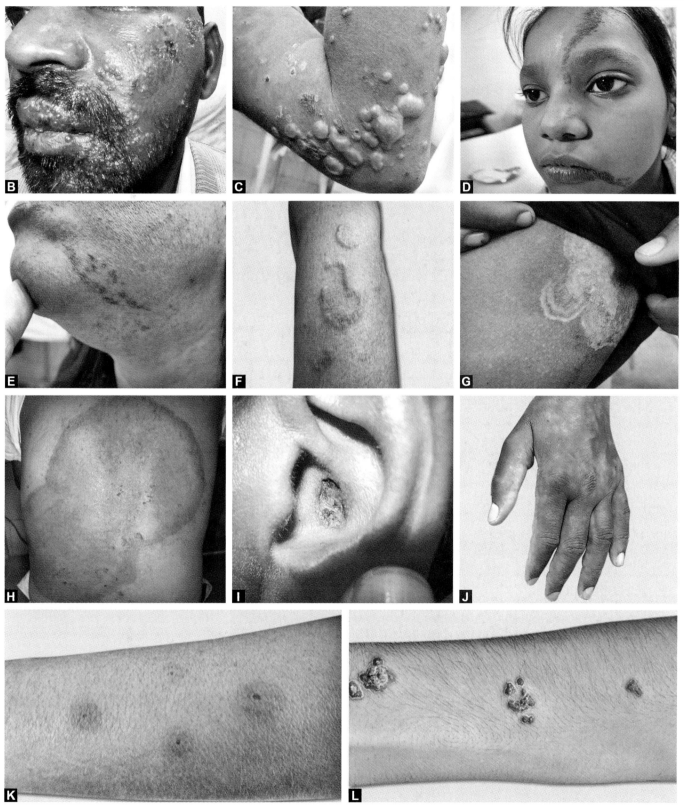

Fig. 2.20B to L: (B) Grouped vesicles with crusting along a dermatome: Herpes zoster; (C) Grouped bullae in a child with linear IgA disease; (D) Epidermal nevi along lines of Blaschko; (E) Linear lichen planus; (F) Annular and arcuate plaques with the border studded with papules in a case of granuloma annulare; (G) Annular plaques with central clearing—*tinea cruris*; (H) Large circinate and annular plaque of *tinea corporis*; (I) A discoid plaque with follicular plugging and atrophy in a case of *discoid lupus erythematosus*; (J) Reticulate pigmentation in a case of *erythema ab igne*; (K) Erythematous plaque with central *dusky pigmentation*, 'iris lesion'ᵠ of erythema multiformeᵠ; (L) Grouped crusted papules and plaques in a case of Reiter's syndrome (reactive arthritis)

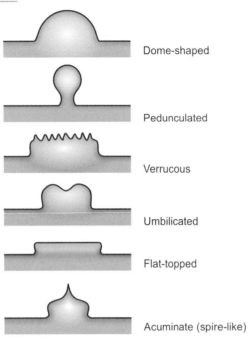

Dome-shaped

Pedunculated

Verrucous

Umbilicated

Flat-topped

Acuminate (spire-like)

Fig. 2.21A: Surface contours of lesion

Clinical Signs

Look for specific clinical signs:

a. **Dermographism:** The development of urticarial lesions when the skin is stroked or written on 'red dermographism'[Q] seen in physical urticaria.

   'White dermographism' is the reverse and a white line is seen on stroking, seen in atopic dermatitis.[Q]

'*Black dermographism*'[Q] designates the fact that under certain conditions, a well-defined black line appears where the skin is stroked with certain metals (nickel).[Q]

b. **Sweat test:** The diagnosis of cholinergic urticaria is confirmed with a sweat test.[Q] A hot bath (40–41°C, 10 minutes) or physical activity in a sweat suit is used to induce tiny wheals.

c. **Pathergy:** Skin trauma (needle stick, insect bite, biopsy) can trigger lesion in pyoderma gangrenosum Sweet's syndrome and Behçet's syndrome.[Q]

   It is performed as follows: Inject 0.1 mL of physiologic NaCl with fine needle on forearm; read after 24–48 hours. Pustule or papule suggests diagnosis; histology shows neutrophilic infiltrate or vasculitis.[Q]

d. **Nikolsky sign:**[Q]
   • True Nikolsky sign: Gentle rubbing allows one to separate upper layer of epidermis from lower, producing blister or erosion—fairly specific for pemphigus.

e. **Bulla spread sign (Asboe-Hansen sign):** Enlargement of intact blister by application of mechanical pressure on its roof. The advancing border in BP is rounded.

f. **Darier sign:** Darier sign is positive when lesions easily urticate, releasing mast cell mediators and is seen in mastocytosis (Fig. 2.23).[Q]

g. **Koebner phenomenon:** Trauma-induced skin dermatoses.

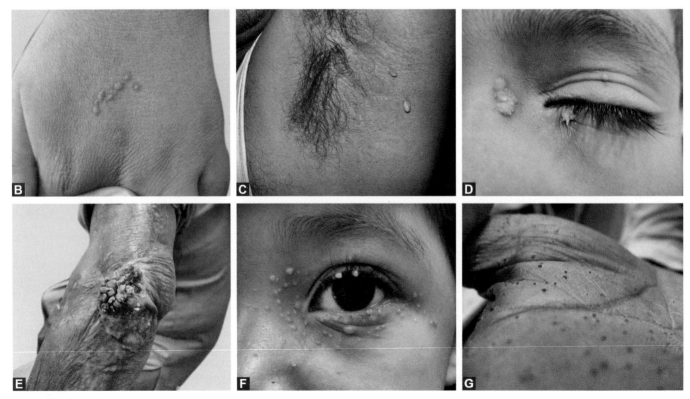

Fig. 2.21B to G: (B) Flat-topped papules in lichen planus; (C) Pedunculated skin tags; (D) Verrucous surface—verruca vulgaris; (E) Squamous cell carcinoma; (F) Umbilicated lesions in molluscum contagiosum; (G) Acuminate papules in spiny keratoderma

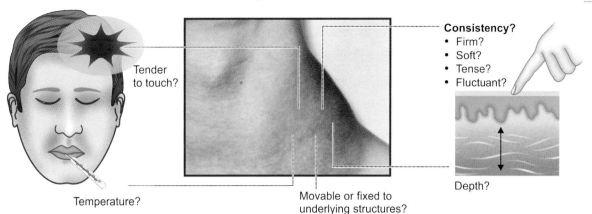

Fig. 2.22: Clinical evaluation in skin lumps

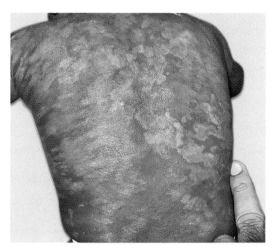

Fig. 2.23: A case of mastocytosis. Note the urticated raised wheals with plaques in the background. The raised wheals are consequent to rubbing—'Darier's sign'

Boyd and Neldner have classified all reported cases of Koebner phenomenon into four different groups:

1. **True isomorphic phenomenon:** There appear to be three disease processes that display the true isomorphic response of Koebner: Psoriasis, lichen planus (Fig. 2.2E) and vitiligo.ᵠ
2. **Pseudoisomorphic phenomenon:** This Koebner phenomenon is seen in infectious diseases, due to autoinoculation of the virus, e.g. warts (Fig. 2.24), molluscum contagiosum and herpes.ᵠ
3. **Occasionally occurring isomorphic phenomenon:** In this category, diseases occasionally localize to sites of trauma, e.g. cancer (gastric, testicular or mammary), Darier's disease, erythema multiforme,ᵠ Kaposi's sarcoma, Kyrle's disease, lichen sclerosus et atrophicus, pellagra, perforating folliculitis, reactive perforating collagenosis, and Hailey-Hailey disease.
4. **Questionable isomorphic phenomenon:** There are many conditions that have been associated with the Koebner phenomenon, many of which are single case reports like vasculitis.

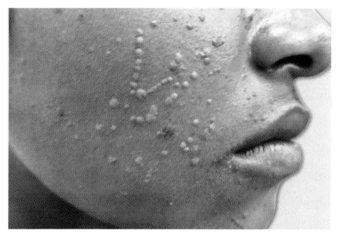

Fig. 2.24: Koebner phenomenon in a case of verruca plana

DIAGNOSTIC METHODS

a. A magnifying lens is a helpful aid to diagnosis because subtle changes in the skin become more apparent when enlarged.
b. **Wood's lamp:** UV radiation from a mercury-vapor source is passed through a filter (Ba silicate and 9% NiO_2),ᵠ producing light at a wavelength of about 365 nm.ᵠ

Usesᵠ

1. *Dermatophyte infection:* Microsporum species that infect hairs impart a green fluorescence.ᵠ Wood's light can be used for screening or for control of therapy.
   Caution: Both sebum and salicylic acid preparations may have blue-green fluorescence; also the scales do not fluoresce, just infected hairs. In addition, Trichophyton infections do not fluoresce.
2. *Favus: Trichophyton schoenleinii* imparts a green fluorescence.ᵠ
3. *Erythrasma:* Coral red fluorescence.ᵠ
4. *Trichomycosis axillaris:* Blue-white fluorescence.
5. *Tinea versicolor:* Blue-white fluorescence.
6. *Pseudomonas:* Green fluorescence.

7. *Porphyrin:* Red fluorescence of skin and teeth in some porphyrias;[Q] fluorescence of urine in others.

8. *Pigment abnormalities:* Hypopigmentation can be distinguished from depigmentation. Thus vitiligo[Q] can be more readily seen, ash leaf macules in tuberous sclerosis and café-au-lait macules in neurofibromatosis are also accentuated.

9. *Tetracycline:* Can be identified in teeth, keratin plugs.

10. *Contact allergens:* Some allergens fluoresce and can be found on the skin or in cosmetics; examples include halogenated salicylanilides and furocoumarins.

11. *Mineral oil:* Remains in hair follicles and can be seen after washing (as in oil acne).

12. *Miscellaneous:* Topical medications or protective creams can be labeled with fluorescent marker, allowing control of usage patterns.

c. **Diascopy** is the name given to the technique in which a (or two) glass slide or clear plastic spoon is pressed on vascular lesions to blanch them and verify that their redness is caused by vasodilatation and to unmask their underlying color.

- Diascopy is also used to confirm the presence of extravasated blood in the dermis (i.e. petechia and purpura, the appearance of which does not change on pressure).[Q]

- This technique may also be helpful in the diagnosis of granulomatous conditions (e.g. sarcoidosis with grain-like nodules)[Q]. Also in lupus vulgaris, the apple jelly nodules can be seen.[Q]

d. **Dermatoscopy** (also known as dermoscopy, epiluminescence microscopy, skin surface microscopy) is a non-invasive technique, now common in the clinic or office setting. It has many potential uses: Not least as an aide in the diagnosis of pigmented lesions (benign and malignant); the visualization of scabies mites in their burrows; and in deciding, if alopecia is scarring or non-scarring.

e. **Patch testing:** Patch testing is used to identify allergens that could potentially be responsible for the **allergic contact dermatitis** (not for irritant contact dermatitis),[Q] variant of delayed hypersensitivity, a type IV reaction.

Procedure: Test substances are placed in small aluminum (Finn) chambers, taped to the back with hypoallergenic tape. Some allergens are available in impregnated test strips. The patches are left on the back for **48 hours**,[Q] during which time the area must be kept dry. The sites are read 20 minutes after the patches have been removed (to allow reaction to the tape to resolve) and again after another 24–72 hours to capture late reactions.[Q]

If multiple ≥5 positive reactions occur to unrelated substances, **'angry back'** syndrome should be suspected, with a state of excessive reactivity because of subclinical inflammation. In such a case, each individual allergen should be tested separately.

If patch tests are negative but clinical suspicion is high, then either repeated testing or a controlled-usage test is required. The latter involves applying the suspected substances twice daily to the inner forearm and then observing for a reaction after 5–7 days. This is useful for household and daily use items.

f. **Mycological diagnosis**
- Diagnosis of dermatophyte infections.
- The step by step approach is shown in Figure 2.25. Histologic examination of a skin biopsy, or more commonly nail clippings, using PAS stain is another way to demonstrate dermatophytes.
- Diagnosis of yeast infections. *Candida* spp. can be cultured at 37°C over 3 days. Speciation of the yeast colonies is made using a germ-tube test[Q] (immediate identification of *C. albicans*).
- *Malassezia* spp. are easily identified on KOH examination by the typical short hyphae and spherical yeast (spaghetti and meatballs).[Q] Culture on media containing olive oil is possible.

g. **Bacteriologic diagnosis:** Bacteria can be directly identified in smears or biopsies. Smears are applied to a microscope slide, stained, and examined.

- Gram stain employs a basic aniline dye such as gentian violet or crystal violet, which helps both identify and classify the bacteria.
- Ziehl-Neelsen and Fite stains are used to identify mycobacteria.
- Warthin-Starry and Dieterle stains are used for spirochetes.
- Dark-field examination is used for diagnosing early syphilis.

h. **Sonography:** Sonography (also known as ultrasonography or ultrasound) is a noninvasive method of imaging structures by recording the reflections of ultrasonic waves directed into tissues. The higher the frequency of the waves, the better the resolution and the worse the penetration.

1. *High-frequency sonography:* The superficial structures of the skin can be imaged (skin sonography) using frequencies of 20–100 MHz[Q]. The maximum penetration with 20 MHz is 8 mm. This modality is primarily used to measure the tumor thickness of melanomas prior to surgery, and is also used for monitoring the therapeutic response of scleroderma.[Q]

2. *7.5 MHz sonography:* This form is used primarily to evaluate subcutaneous lymph nodes and vessels. With frequencies of 7.5–3.5 MHz, depths up to 7 cm can be imaged.

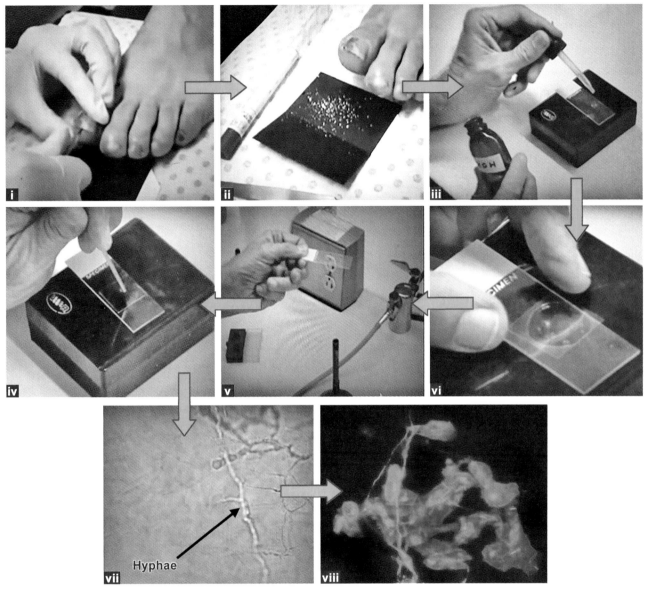

Fig. 2.25: Steps in detection of fungal element in sample; i. Scraping of nail sample; ii. Collection of sample on a sterile black paper; iii. A portion of scraping is put on clean glass slide and a drop of 10% KOH is added; iv. A coverslip is put on KOH preparation; v. The slide is gently warmed (not boiled); vi. Coverslip gently pressed to make a single layer of cells; vii. Detection of fungal element (hyphae) in sample when observed under 40X in bright field microscopy; and viii. Use of calcofluor—highlights the apple green fluorescence of hyphal elements (*Courtesy*: Dr Shukla Das, UCMS, GTB Hospital, Delhi)

BIOPSY AND HISTOLOGY

The following steps will maximize information obtained from the biopsy (Figs 2.26 and 2.27):

- Choose a fresh lesion that is not scratched or ulcerated.
- The type of biopsy depends on the lesion. Punch, shave, or excisional biopsy may be appropriate. Shave biopsies are ideal for benign exophytic lesions; they should be avoided, if melanoma is suspected.
- Do not grasp the specimen with forceps; crush artifact destroys much cellular detail (Fig. 2.27).
- A punch biopsy can usually be popped out and lifted up with scissors. Excisions should only be handled at the edge (Fig. 2.27).

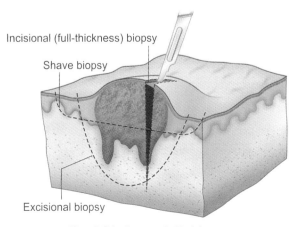

Fig. 2.26: Types of skin biopsy

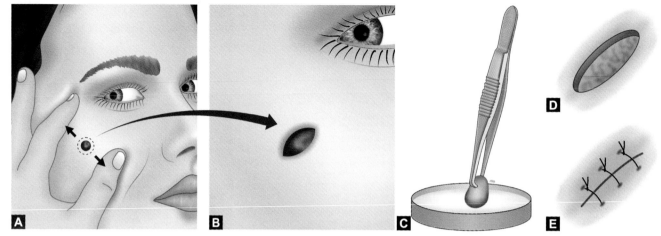

Fig. 2.27: Steps of skin biopsy. Punch biopsy: (A) Stretch the skin at right angles to the intended direction of the scar; (B) Remove the lesion by cutting; (C) Do not crush the specimen; (D and E) The defect is then sutured

Histological Features

Specific terms are applied to a variety of pathologic changes. These are detailed below. Apart from this, the type of the infiltrate and the localization are also important.

Epidermal Changes

- **Epidermal atrophy:** Thinning of the entire epidermis, to just 2–4 cell layers thick.
- **Acanthosis:** Thickened stratum spinosum of the epidermis with enlarged cells (Fig. 2.28).^{Q}

 An increase in thickness of the epidermis consequent to an increase in thickness of the malpighian zone secondary usually to an increase in number of cells, but occasionally, to an increase in size of cells or both of them concurrently.

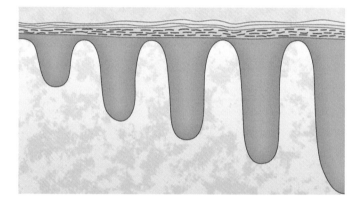

Fig. 2.28: Acanthosis: Thickening of malphigian layer

> - Increase in number of spinous cells is **psoriasis**.^{Q}
> - Increase in size of spinous cells is seen in **lichen planus**.^{Q}
> - Increase in number and in size of spinous cells are seen together in some examples of **lichen simplex chronicus**.

- **Hyperkeratosis:** Thickened stratum corneum (Fig. 2.29)^Q is of two types:
  1. Orthokeratosis, in which no nuclei are visible in cornified cells.
  2. Parakeratosis,^{Q} in which nuclei are retained overtly by cornified cells.

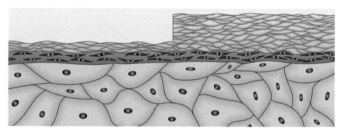

Fig. 2.29: Normal epidermis (left) and hyperkeratosis (right)

It results either from acceleration in epidermopoiesis (e.g. in **psoriasis**)^Q or from faulty maturation of keratocytes (e.g. in **Bowen's disease**).^{Q}

- **Abscess:** Clinically, a circumscribed collection of pus and histopathologically a localized collection of neutrophils.

 Examples:
  - Abscesses of non-infectious nature are seen histopathologically in eruptive lesions of psoriasis, **'pustular' psoriasis** being an exaggerated histo-

logical response of such a neutrophilic^Q collection which is named depending on the site, Munro's microabscess (stratum corneum) and spongiform pustule of Kogoj (stratum spinulosum).^{Q}

  - Abscesses in eccrine units, designated neutrophilic eccrine hidradenitis, are seen in various conditions including insect 'bite' reaction and in response to treatment for cancer by chemotherapeutic agents, such as cytarabine.
  - Eosinophilic abscess—pemphigus vegetans^Q
  - Lymphocytic abscess—Pautrier's abscess^Q seen in mycosis fungoides.

- **Hypergranulosis:** The stratum granulosum is thickened (lichen planus)^Q (Fig. 2.30).

Hypergranulosis is a finding stereotypical for **lichen planus**, in which the granular zone tends to assume a wedge shape[Q] as a result of accentuation of keratohyaline-containing keratocytes in infundibula and acrosyringia.

Hypergranulosis can also be seen in other disorders like **lichen simplex chronicus** and bullous congenital ichthyosiform erythroderma.

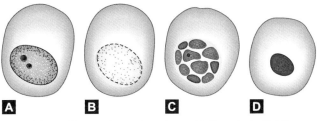

Fig. 2.32A to D: (A) Normal nucleus; (B) Karyolysis; (C) Karyorrhexis; (D) Pyknosis

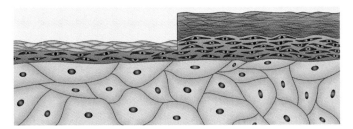

Fig. 2.30: Hypogranulosis (left) and hypergranulosis (right)

- **Hypogranulosis** (Fig. 2.30): A thinned granular zone as a consequence of a decreased number of cells containing keratohyaline granules. It may occur across the entire front of a lesion, such as in ichthyosis vulgaris or in foci of diseases as different as psoriasis,[Q] inflammatory linear verrucous epidermal nevus, and solar keratosis.
- **Dyskeratosis:** Cornification abnormally of individual keratocytes within the epidermis and epithelial structures of adnexa. Dyskeratotic cells have pyknotic nuclei and eosinophilic cytoplasm (Fig. 2.31), the latter is consequent to the filaments of keratin in perinuclear aggregation.

  Examples:
  – Grover's disease[Q]
  – Verrucous stage of incontinentia pigmenti
  – Neoplastic diseases, such as Bowen's disease[Q] and subungual keratoacanthoma
  – Genodermatoses such as Darier's disease[Q]
  – Cystic conditions such as warty dyskeratoma.
- **Karyolysis** (ghosts of nuclei), **karyorrhexis** (fragmentation of nuclei), and **pyknosis** (shrinkage and darkening of nuclei) are the three cardinal signs of necrosis (Fig. 2.32). Karyolysis may be observed in herpes virus infection and pilomatricoma.

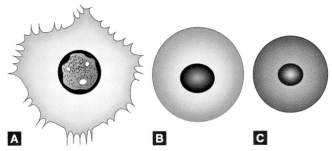

Fig. 2.31A to C: (A) Normal cell; (B) Acantholytic cell; and (C) Dyskeratotic cell

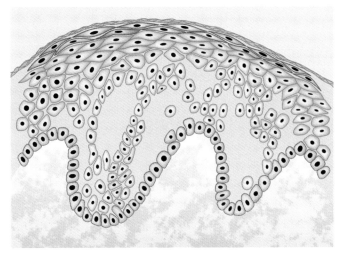

Fig. 2.33: Separation of cells with acantholysis

- **Apoptosis:** Individual cell death, leaving eosinophilic cells (lichen planus, GVHD).
- **Acantholysis:** Loss of connections between keratinocytes (Fig. 2.33). This can be either primary or secondary.[Q]
  Primary:[Q] Damage occurs to the intercellular adhesion (pemphigus, Hailey-Hailey disease).
  Secondary:[Q] Damage occurs to the cell directly (SCC, herpes infections, warty dyskeratoma, the solitary keratosis).

  When acantholysis occurs rapidly in an inflammatory disease, such as in pemphigus vulgaris, the cells affected die rapidly, becoming necrotic. When, however, acantholysis develops more slowly in an inflammatory disorder, such as in **Hailey-Hailey[Q] disease**, the cells then separated from their neighbors die more slowly, permitting time for cornification to occur in the form of acantholytic dyskeratotic cells, those tending to be polygonal rather than round.
- **Hydropic or vacuolar change:** Damage to the basal layer (lupus erythematosus).
- **Ballooning degeneration** (Fig. 2.34)[Q]: 'Intracellular edema' of epidermis and epithelial structures of adnexa, recognizable morphologically as swollen pale cytoplasm of affected spinous cells. Rupture of the ballooned keratocytes leads to formation of a pattern of epidermis that resembles a net and, therefore, is termed reticular alteration.

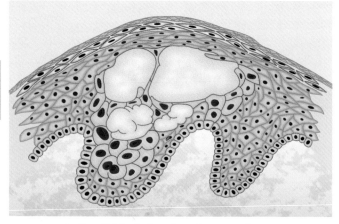

Fig. 2.34: Ballooning degeneration

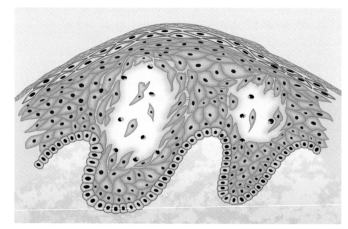

Fig. 2.35: Spongiosis with separation of cells seen in eczema

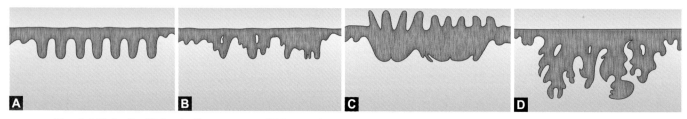

Fig. 2.36A to D: (A) Psoriasiform—even; (B) Psoriasiform—uneven; (C) Papillomatous; (D) Pseudocarcinomatous

Examples: This is seen in herpes,^{Q} pox, and coxsackie viruses infection as also in erythema multiforme, fixed drug eruption, and Mucha-Habermann disease.

- **Spongiosis:** Epidermal edema with exocytosis of inflammatory cells (Fig. 2.35).
- **Proliferation:** An increase in number, usually of cells. A proliferation of epithelial cells in skin may be divided into those that are epidermal and those that are adnexal.
  i. A proliferation of epidermal keratocytes may be **psoriasiform^Q evenly** (Fig. 2.36A), i.e. elongated rete ridges of about equal length, those alternating with dermal papillae of about equal length, as in psoriasis.
  ii. **Psoriasiform unevenly** (Fig. 2.36B), i.e. elongated rete ridges that are not of uniform length, jagged, i.e. serrations at the base of a thickened epidermis, as in lichen planus.
  iii. Papillated (Fig. 2.36C) or digitated, i.e. the surface of the epidermis resembling breasts, nipples, or fingers, respectively, as in some examples of nevus sebaceous, acanthosis nigricans, and verruca vulgaris, respectively. 'Verrucous' is a synonym for 'digitate'. It is also called "church-spire pattern of epidermis".^{Q}
  iv. Proliferation of cells of epithelial structures of adnexa, i.e. the upper part of eccrine ducts (and of infundibular epidermis) may be slight or marked, the latter sometimes simulating squamous carcinoma (pseudocarcinomatous) (Fig. 2.36D), as seen in some examples of

halogenodermas, infections by deep fungi and atypical mycobacteria, and the verrucous stage of incontinentia pigmenti.

Dermal Changes

- **Grenz zone:** Uninvolved and largely cell-free area of dermis beneath the epidermis or adjacent to a hair follicle (border zone) seen classically in leprosy and granuloma faciale.^{Q}
- **Lichenoid:** Clinically, flat-topped papules and, histopathologically, a band-like infiltrate, usually of lymphocytes mostly, in a papillary dermis thickened by it.

  Nearly always, lichenoid infiltrates of an inflammatory process consist of lymphocytes, as in lichen planus, lichenoid discoid lupus erythematosus, and lichenoid purpura of Gougerot and Blum.

  As a rule, lichenoid infiltrates of inflammatory diseases obscure the dermoepidermal interface where they are accompanied by vacuolar alteration and necrotic keratocytes.
- **Incontinence of pigment (basement pigment degeneration):** Melanin falls into the dermis following inflammation of the dermal-epidermal junction (DEJ). *Example:* Lichen planus.^{Q}
- **Solar elastosis:** Basophilic change in collagen after chronic sun exposure.
- **Fibrosis:** Thickening of the dermis through increased numbers of collagen fibers. *Example:* Morphea, scleroderma (Fig. 2.37A) Collagen bundles thicker than normal and oriented perpendicular to the epidermis (Fig. 2.37B) is seen

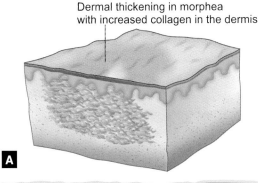

Dermal thickening in morphea with increased collagen in the dermis

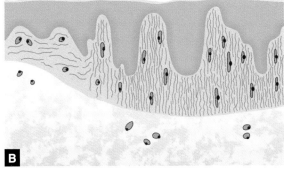

Fig. 2.37A and B: (A) Depiction of dermal thickening causing bound down skin; (B) Vertical bands of collagen in pruritic disorders

in conditions where there is constant rubbing or itching and is seen in persistent forceful rubbing of skin, as occurs in lichen simplex chronicus and its variant, prurigo nodularis.

- **Atrophy:** Thinning of the dermis.
- **Granuloma:** A collection of histiocytes, usually epithelioid ones (Fig. 2.38).

Cells:

a. Epithelioid histiocytes (so termed because of their resemblance to epithelial cells, namely oval nuclei, readily discernable eosinophilic cytoplasm, and some tendency to seeming cohesiveness) are seen in granulomas of tuberculoid leprosy.

b. Foamy histiocytes are seen in lepromatous leprosy, in xanthomas and xanthogranulomas.[Q]

c. Both epithelioid histiocytes and foamy histiocytes are present together in granulomas of dimorphous leprosy.

d. Multinucleate histiocytes,[Q] as well as mononuclear ones, may be found in a granuloma, and they have been given different names depending on nuances on cytopathology with regard to how the nuclei are dispersed, e.g. Langhans, Touton, and foreign body, none of which has either specificity or is pathognomonic for any disease.

Types of granuloma:[Q]

a. Sarcoidal granuloma: A granuloma devoid of inflammatory cells other than epithelioid histiocytes is termed sarcoidal granuloma ('naked' tubercle)[Q], and that surrounded by a dense mantle of lymphocytes, and sometimes plasma cells, is designated tuberculoid granuloma. Sarcoidal granulomas are found in (Fig. 2.38A):
   - Sarcoidosis
   - Foreign body responses to materials such as silica and beryllium.

b. Tuberculoid granulomas are encountered in infectious diseases like (Fig. 2.38B):
   - Tuberculosis
   - Tuberculoid leprosy
   - Recidivans manifestation of leishmaniasis
   - Rosacea
   - Perioral/periocular dermatitis.

c. Palisading granuloma: When epithelial histiocytes are aligned in the manner of stakes in a stockade, the arrangement is referred to as palisading, seen in Fig. 2.38C:
   - Granuloma annulare
   - Necrobiosis lipoidica
   - Necrobiotic xanthogranuloma
   - Rheumatoid nodule.

When histiocytes are dispersed between and among bundles of collagen, the pattern is designated interstitial, the exemplar of it being the interstitial manifestation of granuloma annulare.

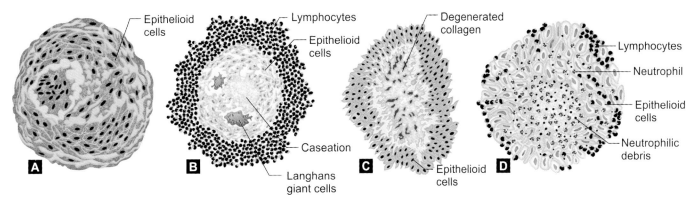

Fig. 2.38A to D: Types of granuloma: (A) Sarcoidal; (B) Tuberculoid; (C) Palisading; (D) Suppurative

Table 2.1 Common cells and their special stains

Cells	Special stains[Q]
Mast cell	Giemsa
Fungal elements BMZ	PAS
Melanin	Masson-Fontan
Connective tissue stains	Masson's trichrome stain
Elastic stain	Orcein
Collagen, smooth muscles	van Giemsa
Amyloid[1]	Congo red
Calcium	von Kossa
Lipids	Oil red O
	Sudan black
	Osmium tetroxide
Melanocytes, nerves, Langerhans cells	S-100
Langerhans cells	CD 1a
Spirochetes	Warthin-Starry
Fungi	PAS, Grocott's methenamine silver (GMS)

[1]Congo red, Thioflavin T, Crystal violet.

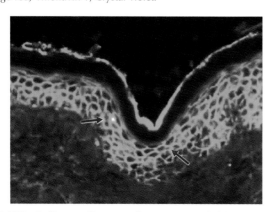

Fig. 2.39A: Patterns of immunofluorescence A: Intercellular 'fish net' pattern in pemphigus vulgaris

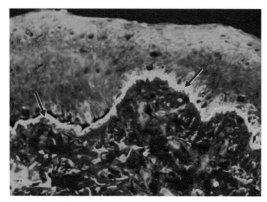

Fig. 2.39B: Linear pattern on the basement membrane zone—bullous pemphigoid

d. Suppurative granuloma: When an abscess is present in a collection of epithelioid histiocytes, as is common in infectious processes such as

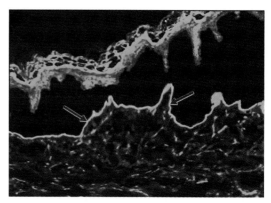

Fig. 2.39C: Salt split IF

those initiated by atypical mycobacteria and deep fungi, the granuloma is known as suppurative (Fig. 2.38D).

Stains

A list of the common stains used in dermatology is given in Table 2.1.

Immunofluorescence (IF)

This is a method of identification of antibodies in the skin. There are two types of IF:

a. **Direct IF (DIF):** Tissue specimen from the patient is stained with labeled antibody that specifically recognizes an antigen that characterizes either a cell or an intra- or extracellular glycoprotein.

Two common patterns are:

1. Intercellular Ab in a **fish net pattern**—pemphigus vulagaris (Fig. 2.39A)[Q]
2. Linear Ab seen in the BMZ—bullous pemphigoid (Fig. 2.39B)[Q]

Dermatitis herpetiformis shows granular deposits of IgA in the dermal papillae.[Q]

b. **Indirect IF (IIF):** The patient serum is applied to control tissue (monkey esophagus, salt-split human skin), which is then counterstained with secondary antibody.

c. **Salt split method**[Q] is used for diagnosing EB acquisita from bullous pemphigoid (Fig. 2.39C). Salt-split skin employs normal human skin incubated in 1 M (molar) NaCl; the split occurs at the level of the lamina lucida; bullous pemphigoid antibodies are found above the split, while epidermolysis bullosa acquisita and others are below it.

ELISA

Both ELISA and immunoblotting can replace IIF to identify serum antibodies. Commercially available ELISA tests for desmoglein 1 and 3, as well as the bullous pemphigoid antigens BP180 and BP230 have made diagnosis of pemphigus vulgaris and bullous pemphigoid more precise.

Infections and Infestations

CHAPTER 3

Bacterial Infections

Chapter Outline

- Staphylococci Infections
- Streptococci Infections
- Toxin-mediated Syndromes

- Corynebacteria Infection
- Miscellaneous Infection

Bacterial infections of the skin are one of the most common problems in tropical countries. For convenience, they are divided into **primary** and **secondary** infections. Another more useful method is based on the **organism** implicated, though some of the pyodermas can have multiple causes (Box 3.1).

STAPHYLOCOCCI INFECTIONS

Staphylococci are a common Gram-positive group of bacteria. The main pathogen is coagulase-positive *Staphylcoccus aureus*;[Q] in contrast, *S. epidermidis* is part of normal flora.

There is increasing trend of MRSA (methicillin-resistant *S. aureus*). Though these infections were initially hospital acquired, now community-acquired MRSA (CAMRSA) are commonly seen. The therapy of most of them is similar with minor variations except in special scenarios (like MRSA) (Fig. 3.1).

The treatment of methicillin-sensitive *S. aureus* (MSSA) is given below.

- First-generation cephalosporin, e.g. cephalexin 250–500 mg PO three or four times a day.
- Dicloxacillin 250–500 mg PO four times a day.

Folliculitis

It is infection of hair follicle and can have many causes but the most commonly caused by bacteria.

Superficial folliculitis: Bockhart's impetigo.[Q]

Clinical Features

Tiny pustules with erythematous border localized in superficial aspect (infundibulum) of follicle.
- *Superficial*: 1- to 4-mm pustules on an erythematous base (Fig. 3.2).

Box 3.1	Common Gram-positive bacterial infections[Q]
Staphylococcus aureus	Skin: Folliculitis, furuncle, furunculosis, carbuncle, impetigo, cellulitis, paronychia Other sites: Chalazion[Q] (granulomatous inflammation of the Meibomian gland) Hordeolum[Q] (*S. aureus* folliculitis of the eyelid) Toxin-mediated diseases[Q] (staphylococcal scalded skin syndrome)
Streptococcus pyogenes (group A, β-hemolytic) *Streptococcus viridans*	Erysipelas, impetigo (less often), scarlet fever, ecthyma, lymphangitis, necrotizing fasciitis, purpura fulminans
Corynebacteria	Erythrasma—*Corynebacterium minutissimum* *Corynebacterium tenuis*—trichomycosis axillaris[Q]

Note: Impetigo can be caused by both *Staphylococcus* and *Streptococcus*.

- *Deep*: Also referred to as sycosis—tender, erythematous papulonodules, often with a central pustule (Fig. 3.3A). Sycosis barbae is a deep folliculitis involving the beard region, usually in males (Fig. 3.3B).

Site

In children, usually scalp; in adults, trunk, buttocks, thighs, beard area.

Therapy

Topical antiseptics or antibiotics (fusidic acid or mupirocin acid). If lack of response, systemic antibiotics (penicillinase-resistant penicillins or first-generation cephalosporin for 7–10 days).

Outpatient management of skin and soft tissue infections in the era of community-associated MRSA

Patient present with signs/ symptoms of skin infection:
- Redness
- Swelling
- Warmth
- Pain/tenderness

 YES

Are any of the following signs present
- Fluctuance–palpable fluid-filled cavity, movable, compressible
- Yellow or white center
- Central point or "head"
- Draining pus
- Possible to aspirate pus with needle and syringe

 NO

Possible cellulitis without abscess:
- Provide antimicrobial therapy with coverage for *Streptococcus* spp. and/or other suspected pathogens
- Maintain close follow-up
- Consider adding coverage for MRSA (if not provided initially), if patient does not respond

 YES

1. Drain the lesion
2. Send wound drainage for culture and susceptibility testing
3. Advise patient on wound care and hygiene
4. Discuss follow-up plan with patient

Abbreviations:
I & D—incision and drainage
MRSA—methicillin-resistant *S. aureus*
SSTI—skin and soft tissue infection

If systemic symptoms, severe local symptoms, immunosuppression, or failure to respond to I & D, consider antimicrobial therapy with coverage for MRSA in addition to I & D.

Options for empiric outpatient antimicrobial treatment of SSTIs when MRSA is a consideration

Drug name	Considerations	Precautions
Clindamycin	• FDA-approved to treat serious infections due to *S. aureus* • D-zone test should be performed to identify inducible clindamycin resistance in erythromycin-resistant isolates	• *Clostridium difficile*-associated disease, while uncommon, may occur more frequently in association with clindamycin compared to other agents
Tetracycline • Doxycycline • Minocycline	• Doxycycline is FDA-approved to treat *S. aureus* skin infections	• ***Not*** recommended during pregnancy • ***Not*** recommended for children under the age of 8 • Activity against group A Streptococcus, a common cause of cellulitis, unknown
Trimethoprim sulfamethoxazole	• Not FDA-approved to treat any staphylococcal infection	• May not provide for group A Streptococcus, a cause of cellulitis • ***Not*** recommended for women in the *third trimester of pregnancy* • ***Not*** recommended for infants less than 2 months
Rifampin	• Use only in combination with other agents	• Drug-drug interactions are common
Linezolid	• FDA-approved to treat complicated skin infections, including those caused by MRSA	• Has been associated with myelosuppression[a], neuropathy and lactic acidosis during prolonged therapy

- MRSA is resistant to all currently available beta-lactam agents (penicillins and cephalosporins)
- Fluoroquinolones (e.g. ciprofloxacin, levofloxacin) and macrolides (erythromycin, clarithromycin, azithromycin) are not optimal for treatment of MRSA SSTIs because resistance is common or may develop rapidly

Role of decolonization
Regimens intended to eliminate MRSA colonization should not be used in patients with active infections. Decolonization regimens may have a role in preventing recurrent infections, but more data are needed to establish their efficacy and to identify optimal regimens for us in community settings.

Fig. 3.1: An overview of management of SSTI and MRSA

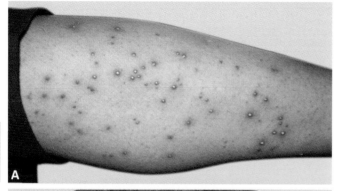

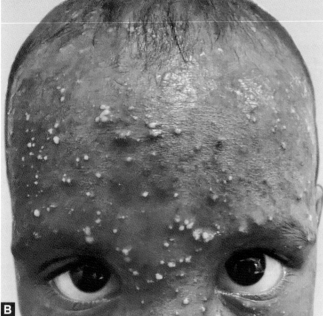

Fig. 3.2A and B: Folliculitis: (A) This patient had an eruption of follicular pustules post-waxing; (B) Patient with superficial folliculitis on the face

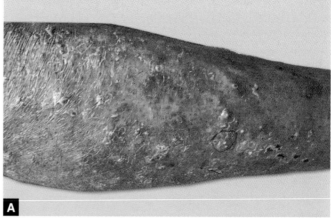

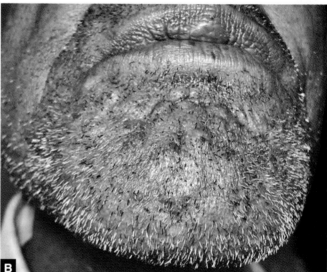

Fig. 3.3A and B: (A) Deep folliculitis; (B) Sycosis barbae

Furuncle

Clinical Features

Deep infection of hair follicle with involvement of surrounding tissue that starts as firm red nodule which rapidly becomes painful and then, after a few days, fluctuant (Fig. 3.4A and B). It is also known as a boil.[Q]

Therapy

Same as for folliculitis.

In case of recurrent folliculitis, think of MRSA (Fig. 3.1) and also search for predisposing factors:

- Diabetes mellitus
- Immunosuppression
- Perineal or nasal carriage of *Staphylococcus aureus* (20% of patients are carriers and 60% are transient carriers)[Q]

The management of skin carriage is given in Box 3.2.

Carbuncle

Confluence of multiple furuncles (Fig. 3.5); the patient is often sick and may require bed rest as well as incision and drainage.

Folliculitis, furuncle and carbuncle can be understood as a process of progressive horizontal spread with follicular, then perifollicular followed by coalescing of multiple furuncles (Fig. 3.6).

The commonest site is the neck[Q] as this area has a horizontal fascia that causes the infection to spread laterally causing confluence of furuncles.

Therapy: Same as for MSSA.

Bullous Impetigo

Cause

Staphylococci of phage group II produce a toxin, exfoliatin[Q] (coded by the phage virus) which is capable of splitting the epidermis in the stratum granulosum (acting on desmoglein 1)[Q]. This action produces large superficial blisters may contain pus (Fig. 3.7) or more diffuse superficial skin loss.

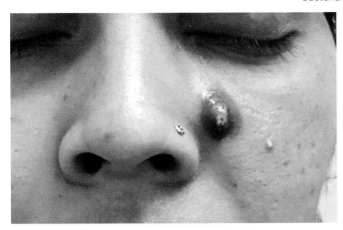

Fig. 3.4A: Furuncle presenting as painful erythematous nodule over the face of a young female

Common conditions with subcorneal split[Q] **FCI**—**P**emphigus **F**oliaceous, Sub**c**orneal pustular dermatoses, **I**mpetigo.

Box 3.2	Management of carrier state of *S. aureus*

- Meticulous attention to handwashing and other personal hygiene.
- Disinfectant soaps and shampoos, used daily.
- Wash body with chlorhexidine, bathe in diluted hydrogen peroxide once or twice a week.
- Mupirocin ointment applied b.i.d. for 5 days, and then twice weekly, is the most effective prophylactic measure.[Q]
- Mupirocin 2% cream to major body folds, e.g. axillae, groin, inframammary, as well as umbilicus.
- Treat as for MRSA.

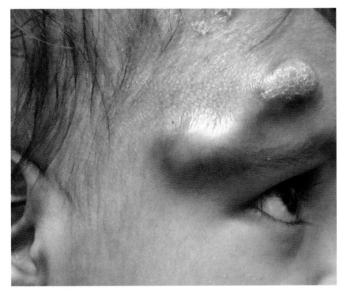

Fig. 3.4B: Large boils in a child

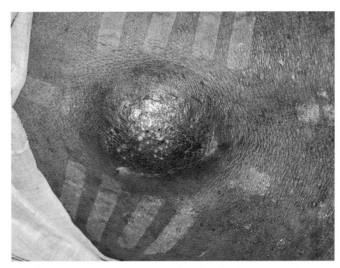

Fig. 3.5: Multiple furuncles coalescing to form a carbuncle. Note the multiple orifices on the lesion with discharge of pus

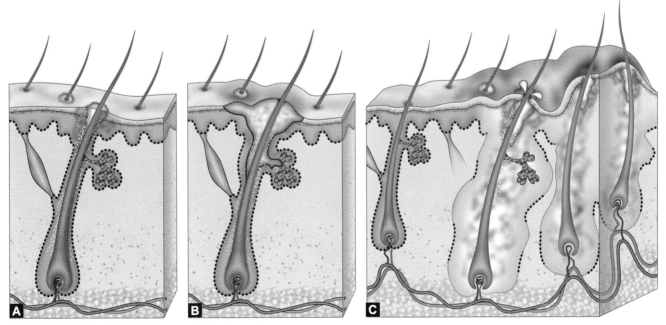

Fig. 3.6A to C: A depiction of the horizontal spread of infection from folliculitis to carbuncle (A) Folliculitis; (B) Furuncle; (C) Carbuncle

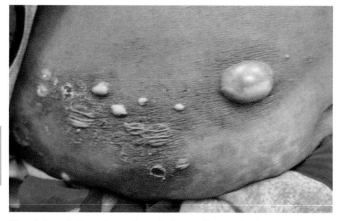

Fig. 3.7A: Bullous impetigo: Bullae with purulent content seen over the abdomen

Clinical Features

Seen in children with sudden appearance of small blisters that rapidly enlarge; little associated erythema. Soon form yellow crusts.

Therapy: Same as for MSSA

Staphylococcal Scalded Skin Syndrome (SSSS)

This is a serious infection with widespread superficial skin loss caused by exfoliation (Fig. 3.7B), due to hematogenous dissemination of the toxin.

Clinical Features

It is seen in newborns or small infants.

• Rapid onset (sometimes with prodrome) of diffuse erythema and fever.

• After 12 hours, Nikolsky phenomenon positive[Q]—stratum corneum can be pushed over underlying layers (Fig. 3.8A and B).

• A distant source of infection, i.e. otitis externa or folliculitis may be present.

The organism usually **cannot be cultured**[Q] from the *skin*, but often from pharynx or other sites. Biopsy with frozen section is diagnostic.

> In SSSS, the skin biopsy shows a very **superficial epidermal (granular layer) split**, whereas in toxic epidermal necrolysis, there is **full-thickness epidermal necrosis**.[Q]
>
> SSSS → Mucosa not involved, SJS/TEN → Mucosa involved.

Therapy

Needs hospital admission:

• Attention to fluid replacement, electrolytes, temperature control.

• Vancomycin: Drug of choice.[Q]

• Systemic antibiotics (penicillinase-resistant penicillins or first-generation cephalosporins; as soon as possible, culture and sensitivity-directed choice of agents).

• Search for staphylococcal carrier among parents or especially nursing personnel in case of nursery epidemics.

Paronychia

Painful infection of the nailfold with *S. aureus*, often because of damaged protective cuticle (Fig. 3.9). It causes nail dystrophy. Deeper paronychia is known as

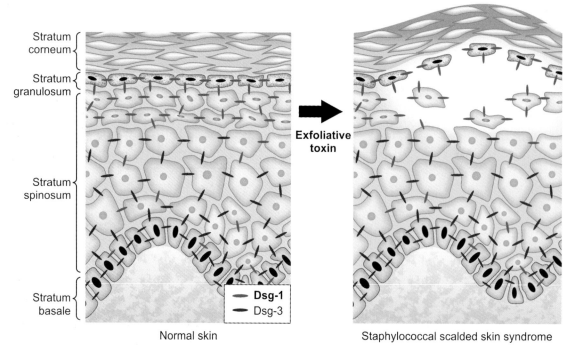

Stratum corneum
Stratum granulosum
Stratum spinosum
Stratum basale

Exfoliative toxin

— Dsg-1
— Dsg-3

Normal skin   Staphylococcal scalded skin syndrome

Fig. 3.7B: A depiction of SSSS with the toxin targeting Desmogelin 1[Q] causing a superficial split

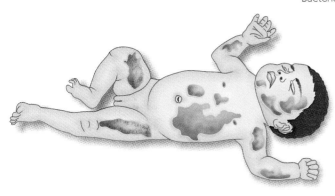

Fig. 3.8A: There is erythema with denudation of skin in SSSS

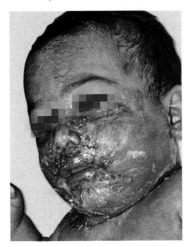

Fig. 3.8B: A child with impetigo on the face and peeling of normal skin on the face and neck, a case of suspected SSSS

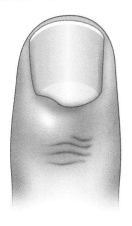
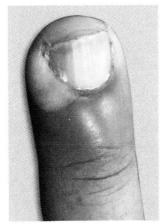

Fig. 3.9: Acute pyogenic paronychia with a painful swelling of the nail fold

felon^Q and carries the risk of infecting the tendon sheath, so immediate surgical management and systemic antibiotics are required.

STREPTOCOCCI INFECTIONS

Though in most cases these infections overlap with staphylococcal infections, some of them have a unique morphology. An overview of the therapy is given in Box 3.3.

| **Box 3.3** | **Therapy of streptococcal infections** |

a. Mild infections (impetigo, scarlet fever, mild erysipelas):
  • Penicillin V 250 mg p.o. 4–6 × daily.
  • If mixed staphylococcal infection is suspected, dicloxacillin 500–1000 mg p.o. q 8 h.
  • Erythromycin 500 mg p.o. q.i.d. or clindamycin 150–300 mg p.o. t.d.s
b. Severe infections (widespread erysipelas, necrotizing fasciitis):
  • Hospital admission, culture and sensitivity, infectious disease consultation.
  • If mixed staphylococcal infection is suspected, give penicillin or cephalosporins. In severe cases, vancomycin 1.0–1.5 g IV daily.

p.o.—per oral

Impetigo (Non-Bullous)

It is commonly caused by group A streptococci (*Streptococcus pyogenes*), as well as by mixed infections with *Staphylococcus aureus*.

Clinical Features

Yellowish crusts (honey colored)^Q develop from tiny blisters and superficial pustules on the face or hands (Fig. 3.10). Some of the streptococci causing impetigo also cause glomerulonephritis, so patients' renal status should be checked initially then 2–4 weeks later.^{Q}

Relevant test: Diagnostic approach: Antistreptolysin (ASL) and antistreptodornase-B (ADB) titers elevated.

Ecthyma

Clinical Features

Punched-out ulcers, usually on legs, presumably at sites of minor trauma (Fig. 3.11). Healing is slow and with scarring.

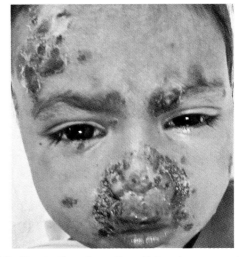

Fig. 3.10: Non-bullous impetigo: Yellow-brown crusts on an erythematous base seen on the face (especially around the nose and mouth) in a 2-year-old child. The ideal therapy would involve administering cefadroxil

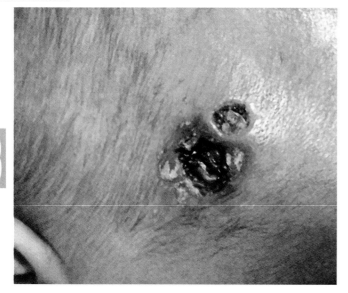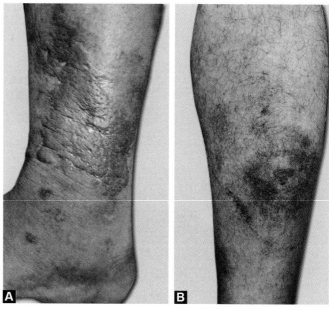

Fig. 3.11: A child with deep punched out lesions of ecthyma

Fig. 3.12A and B: (A) Diffuse erythema with pain and swelling with raised border (erysipelas); (B) Diffuse erythema and pain with linear radiating lymphangitis (cellulitis)

Erysipelas

Acute superficial infection involving dermal lymphatics;[Q] caused by group A streptococci.

Cause

There is usually a portal for entry. On the face, it is often herpes simplex; on the legs, interdigital tinea with maceration.

Complications

On the face, there is a risk of **cavernous sinus thrombosis**. In recurrent erysipelas, chronic damage to the lymphatics leads to persistent **lymphedema**.

Clinical Features

Bright red, sharply demarcated, rapidly spreading erythematous patch (Fig. 3.12A). The border of the involved area is more sharply demarcated in classic erysipelas than in cellulitis, and the surface looks more like an orange peel.[Q] There is associated fever, chills, malaise.

Cellulitis

Deep infection involving dermis and subcutaneous fat.

Etiology

- Staphylococci and streptococci are the most common causes
- *Clostridium* (gas gangrene)
- *Haemophilus influenzae* (facial cellulitis)[Q]

Clinical Features

Localized deep erythematous process usually associated with systemic signs and symptoms. The border is indistinct[Q] (Fig. 3.12B).

Necrotizing Fasciitis

In this, the infection involves the subcutaneous fat and muscle.

Etiology

Usually caused by group A streptococci; less often by MRSA or Gram-negative bacteria.

Clinical Features

Usually involves legs. Starts with erythema, edema, and warmth. After 2–3 days, red-blue color blisters, and widespread dermal necrosis with vessel thrombosis which can spread to involve the deep fascia and muscles, producing compartment syndrome (Fig. 3.13).

Therapy

- Debridement
- Antibiotic cover

Scarlet Fever

Scarlet fever is a streptococcal infection with production of erythrogenic toxin. It is usually associated with pharyngitis.

Clinical Features

- IP: 3–5 days.
- Fever, headache, sore throat
- Exanthem: Starts in the flexures and then spreads to the trunk (Fig. 3.14)
  1. Lesions are fine follicular lesions which resemble **rough sandpaper**[Q] and there is facial erythema with sparing of the perioral region.

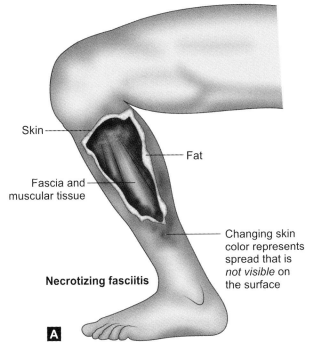

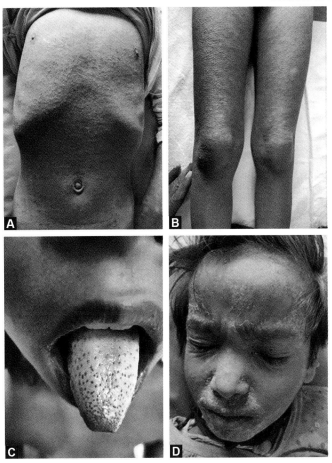

Fig. 3.14A to D: (A and B) Diffuse sandpaper-like rash on the trunk and limbs; (C) Prominent lingual papilla; (D) Desquamative phase of scarlet fever

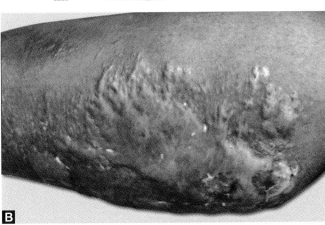

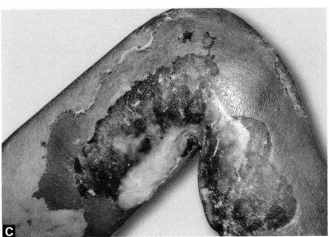

Fig. 3.13A to C: (A) A depiction of necrotizing fasciitis; (B) Swelling pain with overlying bulla in a case of incipient necrotizing fasciitis; (C) A full blown case of necrotizing fasciitis with pus, necrosis and visible fascia

2. Petechiae and later desquamation of the tips of the fingers and toes.

Oral Findings

Denuded tongue with prominent papillae **(strawberry tongue).**^Q

TOXIN-MEDIATED SYNDROMES

Toxic erythema is a cutaneous response to a circulating toxin. For example, in case of scarlet fever, erythrogenic toxin is secreted by group A streptococci, usually infecting the pharynx. In staphylococcal scarlatiniform eruption, staphylococcal scalded skin syndrome, and toxic shock syndrome, the responsible toxins are secreted by *Staphylococcus aureus* infection or colonization (Fig. 3.15A and B). Rarely toxic shock-like syndrome can be seen with group A streptococci. In Kawasaki syndrome, also called mucocutaneous lymph node syndrome (Fig. 3.15C), the toxin has not been identified.

An overview of the main toxin syndromes is given in Table 3.1, but the hallmark features of all toxin syndromes are:
• Distant infection (such as streptococcal pharyngitis) causes cutaneous findings (scarlet fever). Thus the bacteria are usually not found in the skin.

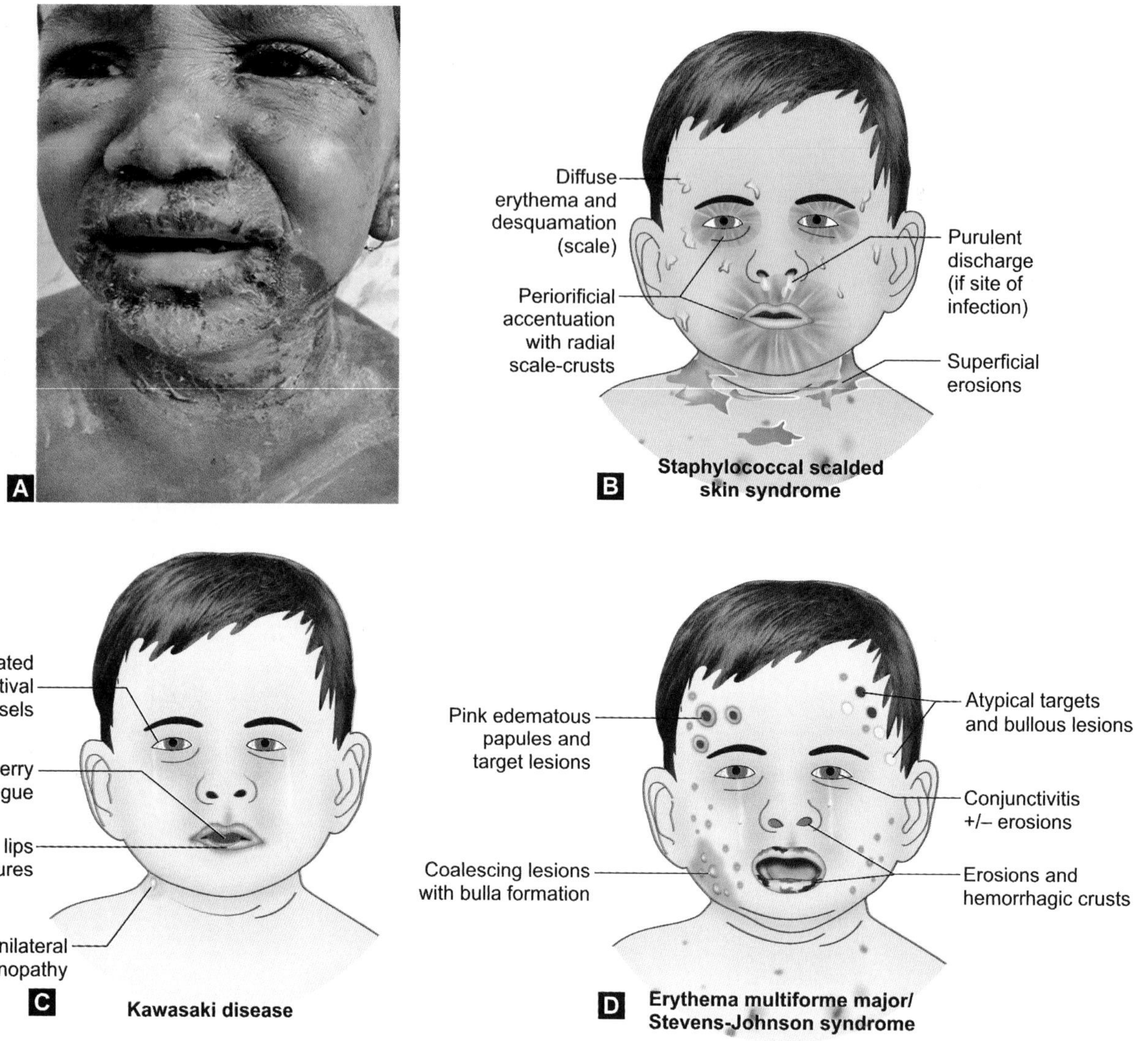

Fig. 3.15A to D: (A) A case of staphylococcal scalded skin syndrome with the classical 'sad man facies' (Dr Gaurish Load, Goa); (B to D) Staphylococcal scalded skin syndrome, facial findings in Kawasaki disease and erythema multiforme major/Stevens-Johnson syndrome

Etiology	Toxin	Type
Streptococcus pyogenes	Pyrogenic toxins	• Scarlet fever • Streptococcal toxic shock syndrome
Staphylococcus aureus	TSST-1	Toxic shock syndrome
	Exfoliatins	• Bullous impetigo • Staphylococcal scalded skin syndrome • Staphylococcal scarlet fever • Recalcitrant erythematous desquamating disorder (REDD syndrome)
Multiple infections, autoimmune?	Vasculitis	Kawasaki disease

Table 3.1 Overview of the toxin syndromes

- The actual infection is mild or limited, but secondary effects of toxins are severe.
- The toxins act as super antigens.

Epidemiology

Toxic erythemas are still uncommon, and in children all can be seen, except for toxic shock syndrome, which usually occurs in adults. After the advent of antibiotics, scarlet fever is less commonly seen.

Neonates are at highest risk for SSSS because of decreased toxin clearance by kidneys and lack of antibody to the toxin.

Clinical Features

The toxin syndromes have similar findings:
1. A rash that is 'Sandpapery'
2. Accentuated in flexural folds
3. Followed by desquamation

For all of these disorders, post-inflammatory desquamation usually occurs in 1 to 2 weeks. It is most striking on the hands and feet, where stratum corneum often sheds in large sheets.

The features are given below, but there is a lot of overlap in various disorders (Fig. 3.15D).

- **SSSS:** Mucous membrane involvement is usually striking, occurring in all toxic eruptions except SSSS. In SSSS, patients may have a history of a local staphylococcal infection causing conjunctivitis, cutaneous abscess, or external otitis. This disorder is now more frequently found in postoperative patients. The focus of infection for staphylococcal toxic shock syndrome is usually the skin,[Q] most commonly an area of painful cellulitis on an extremity.
- **Scarlet fever:** The patients with scarlet fever have a history of a sore throat preceding the rash by 1 to 2 days have acute streptococcal pharyngitis and a 'strawberry tongue', which starts with a white exudate studded with prominent red papillae (white strawberry). After several days, the tongue becomes 'beefy red' (red strawberry).[Q]
- In **toxic shock syndrome**, mucous membrane hyperemia frequently affects the conjunctivae, oral pharynx, or vagina. This is characterized by hypotension, vomiting, diarrhea, severe myalgia, and encephalopathy with mental confusion.
- In **Kawasaki syndrome**,[Q] patients usually have marked erythema of the lips (cherry-red lips), tongue (strawberry tongue), and conjunctivae. In this disease, a symmetric lymphadenopathy[Q] occurs in approximately 75% of patients—hence the name *mucocutaneous lymph node syndrome*. They also frequently experience abdominal pain, diarrhea, arthralgia, and other systemic symptoms.

The diagnostic criteria of TSS and Kawasaki syndrome are given in Table 3.2.

Laboratory Findings
- Bacterial cultures from potential foci of infection are mandatory. In suspected cases of scarlet fever, a throat culture should be taken. The same is true for staphylococcal toxic erythemas. In women with suspected toxic shock syndrome, vaginal cultures should be obtained.
- In seriously ill patients, blood cultures should be taken.
- The focus of infection in patients with streptococcal toxic shock syndrome most often is a severe, necrotizing cellulitis.

Leukocytosis with neutrophilia, ESR/CRP, hepatic transaminase levels, thrombocytosis (2nd or 3rd week),

Table 3.2 Criteria of toxic shock and Kawasaki syndromes

Toxic shock syndrome	Kawasaki syndrome
Fever of ≥38.9°C	Fever for ≥5 days
Scarlatiniform rash	Red palms and soles with edema, then desquamation
Desquamation of skin 1–2 weeks after onset	Exanthem on trunk
Hypotension	Conjunctivitis
Clinical or laboratory abnormalities of at least three organ systems	Mucosal erythema (lips, tongue, or pharynx)
Absence of other causes of the illness	Cervical lymphadenopathy
(All six are required for diagnosis)	**(Fever plus four of the remaining five criteria are required for diagnosis)**

hypoalbuminemia and occasionally thrombocytopenia are seen.

> In toxic shock syndrome, thrombocytopenia occurs early; in Kawasaki disease, thrombocytosis occurs late.

Differential Diagnosis
- Viral exanthem
- Drug eruption
- TEN

Therapy
- Hospitalization for supportive and ancillary care
- Antibiotics for infections
- Aspirin and γ-globulin for Kawasaki syndrome.

Scarlet fever follows a relatively benign course, with complete recovery usually within 5 to 10 days. Rarely post-streptococcal glomerulonephritis may occur.

Death has occurred in patients with toxic shock syndrome as a result of severe hypotension, sepsis, or multisystem organ failure. The death rate for streptococcal toxic shock syndrome is higher[Q] than that for staphylococcal toxic shock syndrome (70% versus 30%, respectively).

Death can result from Kawasaki syndrome, usually the result of coronary artery aneurysm and thrombosis.[Q] This complication occurs in up to 20%[Q] of patients and can be delayed by 1 year or more after the acute episode.

CORYNEBACTERIA INFECTION

Erythrasma

Etiology

Corynebacterium minutissimum.[Q]

Clinical Features

Asymptomatic: Red-brown superficial patches with fine scale, seen in intertriginous areas (groin, axillae (Fig. 3.16A and B)).

Diagnosis is by clinical suspicion and coral-red fluorescence[Q] on Wood's light examination. Microscopy is difficult; culture is impossible. Commonly seen in diabetic and immunosuppressed patients.[Q]

Differential Diagnosis

- **Tinea cruris:** Patches more infiltrated with active border and usually more itchy.
- **Candidiasis:** Patches more macerated with satellite pustules.

Therapy

Topical erythromycin solution or cream; topical imidazoles; meticulous hygiene. If resistant, then erythromycin 250 mg p.o. qid for 5–7 days.

Trichomycosis Axillaris

Axillary hair infection with *Corynebacterium tenuis*.[Q]

Clinical Features

The axillary hairs are coated by tiny bacterial colonies (Fig. 3.17A) which are orange-brown color (secreted by the corynebacteria), there is associated malodor.

Therapy

Shaving of axillary hairs, apart from the measures listed above.

Pitted Keratolysis

This is consequent to a combination of sweaty feet and occlusive shoes that encourages the growth of diphtheroid organisms that can digest keratin.[Q]

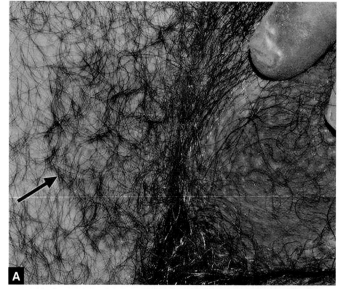

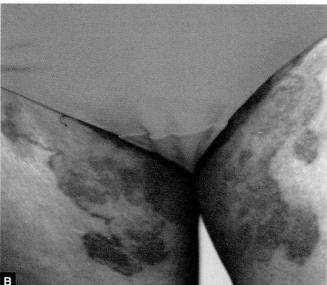

Fig. 3.16A and B: (A) Erythematous 'relatively' non-itchy lesion of erythrasma; (B) A case of tinea cruris

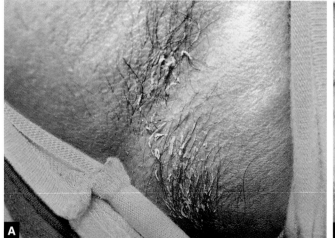

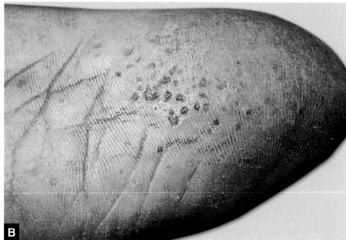

Fig. 3.17A and B: (A) Yellowish concretions on the axillary hair in a case of trichomycosis axillaris; (B) Multiple pits, associated with foul odor and hyperhidrosis (pitted keratolysis)

Clinical Features

There is a cribriform pattern of fine punched-out depressions on the plantar surface (Fig. 3.17B), with a foul smell (of methane thiol).[Q]

MISCELLANEOUS INFECTION

There are numerous other bacterial infections and an overview is given in Table 3.3 as a ready reckoner. Out of these, toe-web infection and Gram-negative folliculitis (seen in acne vulgaris) are commonly encountered (Figs 3.18 and 3.19).

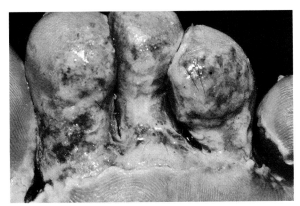

Fig. 3.18: A case of tinea pedis with superadded infection of the toe-web, with erythema and erosions. This is often co-treated with antibiotics but rarely is the Gram-negative flora covered

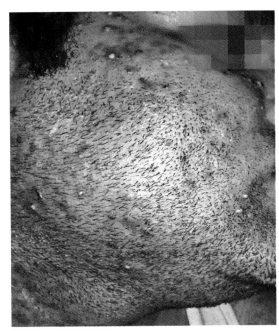

Fig. 3.19: A case of acne on long-term antibiotics with nodules and pustules that grew pure colonies of E. coli (Gram-negative folliculitis)

Table 3.3	Overview of other bacterial infections affecting the skin	
Erysipeloid *Erysipelothrix rhusiopathiae*	Contact with animal products like bones and skin	Painful boggy red plaque Usually on the finger
Actinomycosis *Actinomyces israelii*	Part of normal oral flora and usually found in mixed infection with *Actinobacillus actinomycetemcomitans* only the combination[Q] is pathogenic.	• Cervicofacial form with woody induration of the soft tissues of the neck or cheeks. Fistulas drain yellow granules (called sulfur granules,[Q] which are masses of organisms). • Abdominal and thoracic actinomycosis (postoperative) • Genitourinary (IUDs)
Nocardia spp.	Trauma	• Swelling, draining sinuses and sulfur granules • Sporotrichoid lesions with lymphangitic spread. • Mycetoma
Gram-negative folliculitis	Superficial lesions are usually caused by *Klebsiella* and *Proteus*	Recurrent paranasal and perioral pustules occur as a complication of long-term antibiotic use, mainly in acne[Q] (Fig. 3.18)
Gram-negative toe-web infection (*P. aeruginosa* and a mixture of other Gram-negative organisms, such as *E. coli* and *Proteus* are usually present)	Underlying cause is hyperhidrosis	There is interdigital erythema, erosions, and maceration (Fig. 3.19)
Bite injuries (most dangerous are human bites[Q])	Dog bites (*Pasteurella multocida*) Cat bites Human bites (*Streptococci, staphylococci, Eikenella corrodens,* and *Haemophilus spp.*)	• Dog bites are more dramatic but generally superficial tears • Cat bites involve deep puncture wounds, often endangering the tendons of the hand • Human bite: More common is clenched fist-tooth conflict where the fist usually loses out. Hand infections are the common result.
Pseudomonas aeruginosa	• Immunosuppression • Trauma	• Hot tub folliculitis[Q] • Ecthyma gangrenosum[Q] • Paronychia

CHAPTER 4

Viral Infections

Chapter Outline

- Poxvirus Infections
- Herpesvirus Infections
- Human Papillomaviruses

- Picornavirus Infections
- Viral Exanthem

The viral infections constitute an important disorder in clinical practice and an elaborate list is given in Table 4.1, but we will restrict to the common conditions in this section.

Table 4.1 An overview of common viral infections[Q]

Poxvirus	
Molluscum contagiosum virus	Molluscum contagiosum
Cowpox	Cowpox
Paravaccinia	Milker's nodule
Parapoxvirus	Orf (ecthyma contagiosum)
Herpesvirus	
Herpes simplex virus (HSV-1, HSV-2)	Herpes simplex
Varicella-zoster virus (VZV)	Chickenpox, herpes zoster
Human cytomegalovirus	Gianotti-Crosti syndrome
Epstein-Barr virus	Infectious mononucleosis
Human herpesvirus 6	Exanthem subitum[Q]
Human herpesvirus 8	Kaposi sarcoma[Q]
Papillomavirus	
Human papillomaviruses (HPV)	Warts, condylomata, cervical carcinoma
Picornavirus	
Coxsackieviruses	Hand-foot-and-mouth disease[Q]; herpangina; various exanthems
Paramyxovirus	
Measles virus	Measles
Mumps virus	Mumps
Togavirus	
Rubella	Rubella
Hepadnavirus	
HBV	Gianotti-Crosti syndrome[Q]
Parvoviruses	
Parvovirus B19	Erythema infectiosum

POXVIRUS INFECTIONS

- Molluscum contagiosum virus—molluscum contagiosum
- Paravaccinia virus—milker's nodule
- Parapoxvirus ovis (PPOV)—orf
- Variola virus—smallpox
- Cowpox/catpox virus—cowpox

Molluscum Contagiosum

This is a common infections seen in children cause by MCV-1 and 2.[Q]

Predisposing factors: Atopic dermatitis, immune defects, immunosuppression, HIV/AIDS.

Clinical Features

Incubation period—days to several months. Pearly white, dome shaped, 1–5 mm **umbilicated papules**,[Q] often arranged in groups or linear fashion (pseudo Koebner's phenomenon after autoinoculation[Q]) (Fig. 4.1). On extirpation, a 'cheesy' core can be expressed.

This unstained material readily reveals numerous oval molluscum bodies (Henderson-Peterson bodies[Q]—largest inclusion body) (Fig. 4.2) when examined with a microscope. In fact, the molluscum virus is the largest known virus[Q] and hence can be seen under a light microscope!

Spontaneous remission often occurs within 6 to 9 months. Complications include, eczema, secondary infection, meibomianitis.[Q] Individual lesions can become secondarily inflamed and may resemble furuncles.

Sites: Various in children; genital region in adults; disseminated and larger in size in atopic dermatitis or HIV/AIDS (Fig. 4.3).

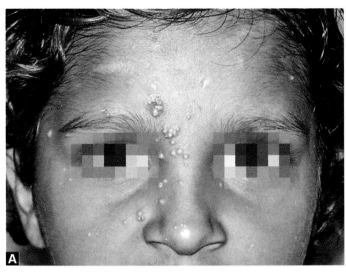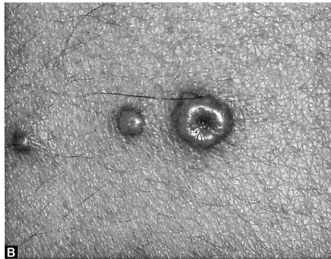

Fig. 4.1A and B: (A) Multiple pearly white dome-shaped umbilicated papules seen on the face; (B) A close up of the central umbilication in molluscum contagiosum

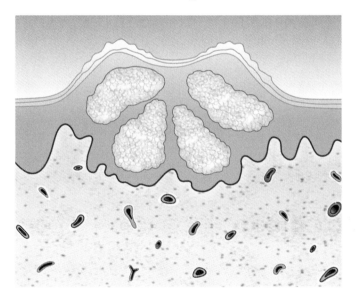

Fig. 4.2: Histology with thickened epidermis with "molluscum bodies"

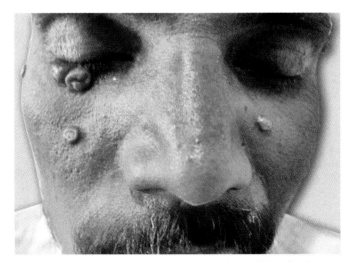

Fig. 4.3: Multiple facial molluscum seen in an HIV patient. Note the larger size of the lesions in this case

Therapy

This is one condition where possibly treatment may be deferred awaiting spontaneous resolution but children often manipulate the lesion and this itself helps to spread the lesion. The various options include:

- Extirpation of the molluscum body and destruction of the lesion by TCA
- Treatment by cryotherapy
- Topical salicylic acid preparations or tretinoin
- Curettage
- Imiquimod cream 5% applied daily has also been successful.

Milker's Nodule

Source: Infected cows (less often sheep or goats) (Fig. 4.4).[Q]

Clinical Features

Firm, dome-shaped nodules, several centimeters in diameter with an erythematous periphery, usually on the hands.

Orf (Ecthyma Contagiosum)

Source: Sheep or goats to contact persons.[Q]

The infected animals have a stomatitis, so infection requires contact other than milking. With sheep, those nursing the young lambs are at risk, as are the shepherds caring for sick animals.

Clinical features: Identical to milker's nodule.

HERPESVIRUS INFECTIONS (Table 4.2)

Herpes Simplex Virus Infections

These are infections caused by herpes simplex virus type 1 (HSV-1) or type 2 (HSV-2).

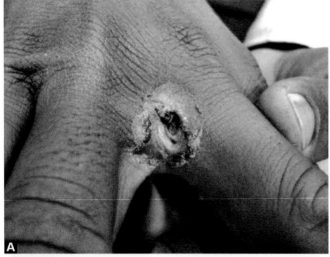

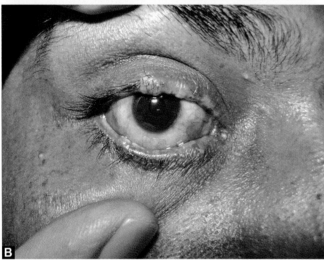

Fig. 4.4A and B: A milk man with an ulcer in the web space with autoinoculation of the eye (milker's nodule)

Table 4.2	Overview of viral infections[Q]
Herpes virus	
Herpes simplex virus (HSV-1, HSV-2):	Herpes simplex
Varicella-zoster virus (VZV)	Varicella (chickenpox), zoster
Human cytomegalovirus (CMV)	Infections in immunosuppressed patients, neonates; Gianotti-Crosti syndrome
Epstein-Barr virus	Infectious mononucleosis (often with ampicillin/amoxicillin rash);[Q] Gianotti-Crosti syndrome[Q]
Human herpesvirus 6	Exanthema subitem[Q]
Human herpesvirus 8	Kaposi sarcoma[Q]

Almost everyone suffers from HSV-1 infection; the first infection is silent in 90%, non-specific in 9%, and clinically manifest in only 1%. Infection occurs in childhood. HSV-2 appears after start of sexual activity and affects 25–50% of population.

Pathogenesis

Initial infection: HSV enters via small defects in skin or mucosa and starts to replicate locally; then spreads via axons to sensory ganglia where further replication occurs. Through centrifugal spread via other nerves, affects wider areas. After resolution of the primary infection, the virus remains latent in the sensory ganglia.

Recurrent infection: Reactivation of virus by various stimuli **(UV light, fever)** as well as local or systemic immunosuppression leads to seeding of the virus into area served by the sensory ganglia and thus to local recurrences.

- In the genital area, the recurrence rate for HSV-2 infections is 10× greater than for HSV-1.[Q]
- In the orofacial infections, HSV-1 has a significantly higher recurrence rate.[Q]

Clinical Features

There are many uncommon sites of involvement like on the fingers (herpetic whitlow),[Q] in wrestlers (herpes gladiatorum),[Q] HSV encephalitis (most common cause of viral encephalitis in adults, 95% HSV-1) and eye (herpes keratitis—Fig. 4.5). Post-herpetic erythema[Q] multiforme can be seen in over 95% of patients with recurrent erythema multiforme have recurrent HSV as trigger.

An overview of the salient features is given in Box 4.1.[Q]

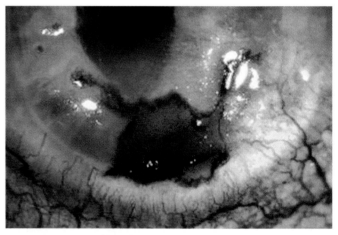

Fig. 4.5: Herpetic keratitis

Box 4.1	Overview of common HSV infections

Primary infection:
- HSV-1 usually occurs in children, subclinical in 90% of cases.
- 10% of infected children have acute gingivostomatitis.

Lips (herpes labialis): Caused by HSV-1

Genitals and buttocks: HSV-2.

Recurrence (genital): Less with HSV-1 (14%) than with HSV-2 (60%)

a. Orofacial HSV infections:

- *Primary infection:* Herpetic gingivostomatitis. Usually in infants; extensive erosions with hemorrhagic crusts on lips and oral mucosa; difficulty feeding, foul smelling breath, systemic signs and symptoms.

  Recurrences: These are commoner than the primary infection.

  Small grouped blisters on erythematous base, rapidly become pustules and then eroded; often painful with dysesthesias and neuralgias. *Common sites*: Lips (herpes labialis), chin, cheeks, periorbital region (Figs 4.6 to 4.8).

- *Eczema herpeticum:* Patients with atopic dermatitis[Q] can develop extensive orofacial HSV infections which disseminate, especially favoring areas of active dermatitis (Kaposi varicelliform eruption).[Q]

b. Herpes genitalis:

Primary infection:

- Disseminated, rapidly eroded vesicles leading to small painful superficial ulcers as well as bilateral lymphadenopathy.

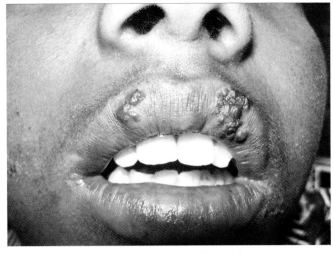

Fig. 4.8: Grouped vesicles on an erythematous base (herpes labialis)

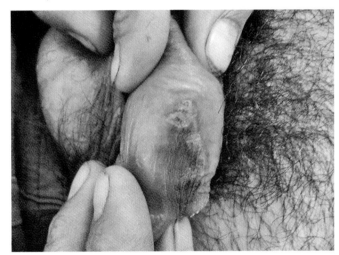

Fig. 4.9: Multiple erosions on the shaft of penis in recurrent herpes genitalis

- Burning or pain on urination common.
- Cervix involved in 80% of women.
- Systemic signs and symptoms; malaise, fever, headache.
- Healing after 2–3 weeks.

Recurrences: Grouped blisters or pustules on erythematous base (Fig. 4.9). This is commoner than the primary infection.[Q] Women often have minimal symptoms. In 80% of patients, caused by HSV-2.

c. Neonatal HSV infections:

- HSV-2 (and increasingly HSV-1) in birth canal with direct transfer to newborn and potential for HSV sepsis. Two-thirds of affected infants have mucocutaneous manifestations of HSV infection.
- Genital HSV recurrences in women are **asymptomatic in 70%**[Q] of cases, making diagnosis most difficult.
- Course of HSV in newborns tends to be severe because of incomplete immune response. The

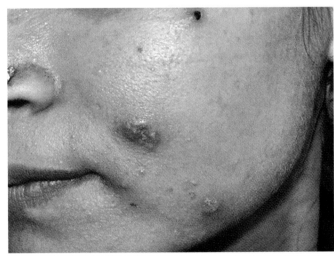

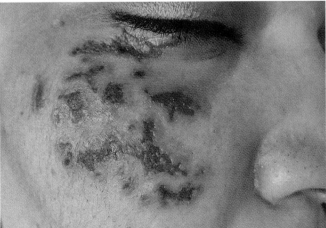

Figs 4.6 and 4.7: Recurrent herpes on the face. Note the vesicles and the erosions

fatality rate without treatment is **50%** and **50%** have neurological complications.

Significant reduction of mortality and morbidity occurs with acyclovir treatment. For women who have evidence of active HSV infection at delivery, cesarean section is recommended.[Q]

Investigation

Tzanck smear: It can be confirmed with a Tzanck smear, which reveals multinucleated giant cells (Tzanck cell) (Fig. 4.10).[Q]

• Deroof fresh blister and scrape base with blade
• Smear blade material onto glass slide
• Examine microscopically in lab after Giemsa staining for multinucleated giant cells

The positivity of the Tzanck preparation varies with the lesion sampled[Q]: Vesicle, 67%; pustule, 55%; and crusted ulcer, 16.7%.

Culture ideally is better[Q]: Vesicle, 100%; pustule, 73%; and crust-ulcer, 33%.

Treatment

The mode of action of acyclovir is via inhibition of thymidine kinase.[Q]

This enzyme converts acyclovir to acyclovir triphosphate which in turn inhibits viral DNA polymerase and replication of viral DNA. It is effective against replicating virus but does not eliminate latent virus.[Q]

Valaciclovir is a prodrug that is better absorbed than its metabolite aciclovir.[Q] Famciclovir, also a prodrug, is metabolized to penciclovir, a synthetic acyclic guanosine derivative.

In active infections, these antiviral drugs decrease the duration of viral shedding, accelerate healing of the lesions, and may reduce local and systemic symptoms.

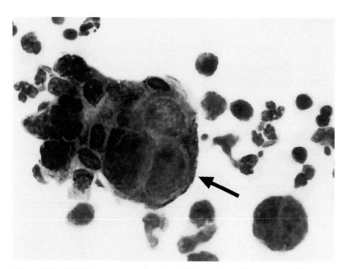

Fig. 4.10: Multinucleate giant cell (Tzanck cell; seen on Giemsa stain)

Table 4.3	Therapy for herpes simplex

Initial

First episode—primary
• Aciclovir: 400 mg tid for 7 days, 5–10 mg/kg IV every 8 h for 5–7 days
• Valaciclovir: 1000 mg bid for 7 days
• Famciclovir: 250 mg tid for 7 days

Recurrent
• Aciclovir: 800 mg tid for 2 days, 5% ointment every 2 h for 7 days
• Valaciclovir: 2000 mg bid for 1 day
• Famciclovir: 1 g bid for 1 day
• Aciclovir 5% ointment: Six times daily for 7 days
• Penciclovir 1% cream: Every 2 h while awake for 4 days
• Docosanol 10% cream: Five times daily until healed

Chronic suppressive
• Aciclovir: 400 mg bid
• Valaciclovir: 1000 mg daily
• Famciclovir: 250 mg bid

Alternative
• Foscarnet 40 mg/kg every 8–12 h for 1–2 weeks

For genital herpes infection, condom use can prevent transmission of HSV-2 by 50% and should be encouraged for individuals with active and asymptomatic shedding of the virus.

For resistant case, foscarnet is an alternative drug, if aciclovir fails.

An overview of treatment is given in Table 4.3.

Varicella (Chickenpox)

This is a highly infectious childhood disease, though in 30% it may be clinically nonapparent.

Chickenpox occurs throughout the year, but the incidence peaks sharply in March, April, and May.

Clinical Features

After a 10–14-day incubation period, a 2- to 3-day prodrome precedes the rash. The patient is infectious for approximately **1 week**[Q] (**1–2 days** before the rash and a further **4–5 days** after the vesicles have become crusted).

Starts with a centripetal rash—red maculae on trunk, oral mucosa and scalp, which converts to a vesicular lesion and then pustular lesion. The rash is polymorphic.[Q] The vesicles are described as 'dewdrop on a rose petal' appearance (Fig. 4.11).[Q]

Treatment

Treatment of chickenpox is largely symptomatic and antihistamines and topical agents such as calamine lotion are used to reduce itching. The use of aciclovir

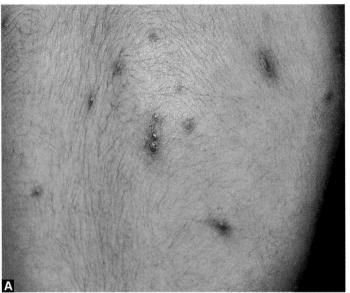
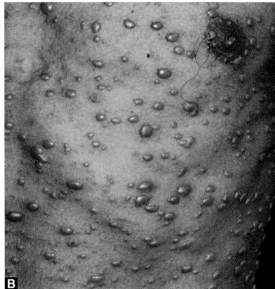

Fig. 4.11A and B: Vesicles on an erythematous base, also termed as the "dewdrop on a rose petal" appearance seen in varicella

Table 4.4	Summary of management of varicella

Prevention
- Varicella virus vaccine
- Varicella-zoster immune globulin

Initially for symptomatic infection
- Antihistamines:
  - Diphenhydramine: 25–50 mg qid; elixir–12.5 mg/5 mL, 5 mg/kg daily in four divided doses
  - Hydroxyzine: 10–25 mg qid; syrup–10 mg/5 mL, 2 mg/kg daily in four divided doses
- Oatmeal bath
- Calamine lotion

Alternative for adults, severe infection, immunosuppression
- Aciclovir: 20 mg/kg (800 mg max) orally qid for 5 days or 10 mg/kg intravenously every 8 h

Table 4.5	Antiviral drug therapy		
Drug	*Dose*		*Duration*
Varicella (chickenpox): Uncomplicated cases[Q]			
Aciclovir	800 mg po 5×/d		7–10 days
Valaciclovir	1,000 mg po TDS		
Famciclovir	500 mg po TDS		
Varicella (chickenpox): Severe or complicated cases			
Aciclovir	10–15 mg/kg IV q8h; may switch to oral acyclovir, famciclovir, or valaciclovir (as dosed above for uncomplicated cases) if no evidence of visceral involvement		7–10 days
Foscarnet	90 mg/kg IV 12 h		14–28 days

po—per oral

in immunologically normal children generally is not indicated unless rare visceral involvement is present, such as varicella pneumonia. An overview is given in Table 4.4.

If oral antiviral drugs are to be administered, Table 4.5 provides a correct dose drug regimen.

Varicella in Pregnancy

1st and 2nd trimesters: In 25–50% of cases, transplacental transfer of VZV to fetus with risk of *varicella embryopathy syndrome*.[Q]

3rd trimester: *Congenital varicella* with poor prognosis.[Q]

Therapy: Pregnant patients with varicella should receive both varicella-zoster immune globulin and antiviral therapy (aciclovir).[Q]

Zoster (Herpes Zoster, Shingles)

This is a segmental (dermatomal) painful skin disease which is caused by reactivation of VZV.
- 10 to 20% of individuals develop herpes zoster during their lifetime.
- Two-thirds of these individuals are older than 50.
- The frequency of second attacks may be 5%.

Pathogenesis

Following the initial varicella infection, VZV persists lifelong in the sensory ganglia of the spinal chord and cranial nerves. When reactivated, it follows the associated nerves into the skin; thus both the peripheral nerve and the skin of its dermatome involved (Fig. 4.12).

Clinical Features

Prodromal phase: Dysesthesias or pain in distribution of the affected nerve may last up to **7 days**.

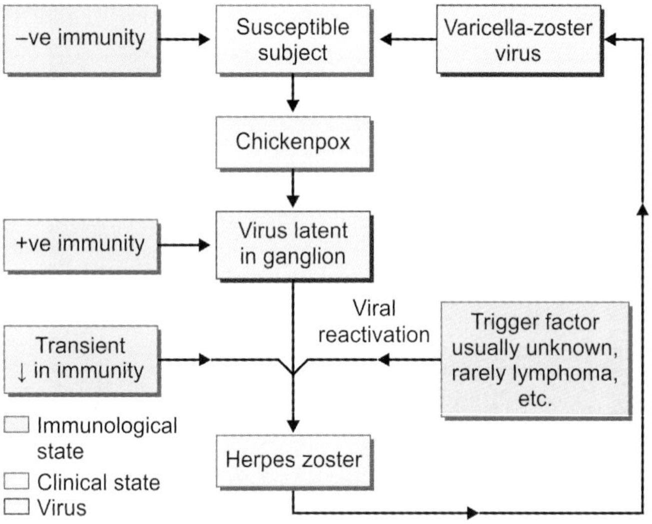

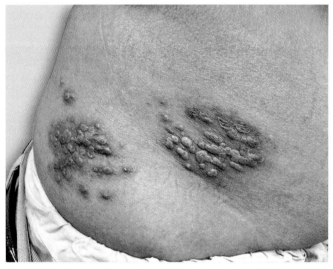

Fig. 4.12: Pathogenesis of herpes zoster

Most common site—thoracic dermatome[Q]:

Eruption of grouped vesicles and then pustules on an erythematous base occasionally hemorrhagic or necrotic; also lasts about **7 days**. Always spares the midline and involves the dermatome (Fig. 4.13).

Healing with drying, crusting, and usually some scarring; also **7 days**.

Complications

Ocular involvement: When 1st branch of trigeminal nerve (ophthalmic nerve) is involved, 50% have ocular involvement. Vesicles on the tip of the nose (Hutchinson sign)[Q] indicate nasociliary nerve involvement and greater likelihood of eye involvement (Fig. 4.14).

Otic involvement: Ramsay Hunt syndrome[Q] is seen with involvement of both 7th and 8th cranial nerves, leading to triad[Q] of ipsilateral facial palsy, ear pain and vesicles on ear and face, along with hearing loss and vertigo (Fig. 4.15).

Post-herpetic neuralgia: Pain in the involved dermatome that lasts more than 3 months[Q]; the most dreaded complication of zoster.

Treatment

Aciclovir, at a dosage of 10 mg/kg every 8 hours intravenously or 800 mg five times daily orally for 7 to 10 days, halts the progression of herpes zoster in immunocompromised patients and is most effective when started within 3 days[Q] of the beginning of the eruption (Table 4.6).

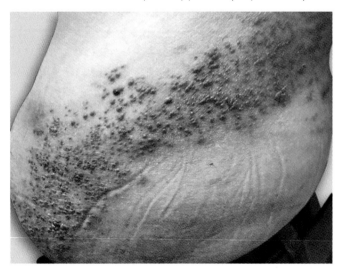

Fig. 4.13A: Grouped vesicles, which were preceded by lancinating pain and the patient was referred to a surgeon for suspected renal colic before the eruption appeared (Herpes zoster)

Fig. 4.13B: Herpes zoster affecting the thoracic dermatome. Grouped, erythematous vesicles are seen in a 'zosteriform' distribution

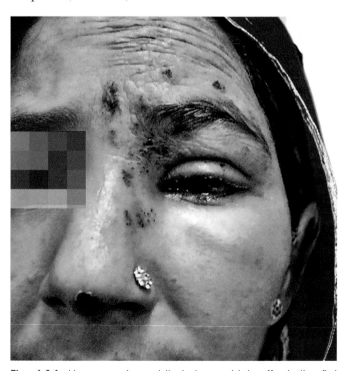

Fig. 4.14: Herpes zoster ophthalmicus, which affects the first branch of the fifth cranial nerve

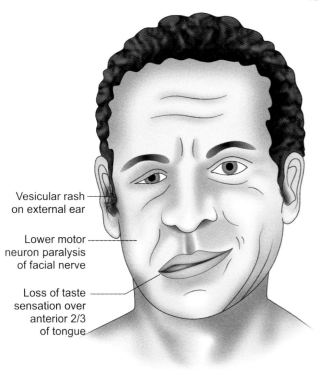

Vesicular rash on external ear

Lower motor neuron paralysis of facial nerve

Loss of taste sensation over anterior 2/3 of tongue

Fig. 4.15: Ramsay Hunt syndrome

Table 4.6	Management of herpes zoster[Q]

Prevention
- Zoster vaccine live OKA/Merck

Initial

Antivirals[a]
- Aciclovir: 800 mg five times daily for 7 days, 10 mg/kg IV every 8 h for 5–7 days
- Valaciclovir: 1 g tid for 8 days
- Famciclovir: 500 mg tid for 7 days

Compresses
- Aluminum acetate

Pain medication
- Analgesics
- Amitriptyline: 25–100 mg at bedtime
- Gabapentin: 100–300 mg tid

Alternative (resistance)
- Foscarnet 40 mg/kg every 8 h for 10 days

[a]Treatment is optional in individuals with (1) mild and pain; (2) eruption >72 h; (3) *less* than 50 years of age.

Advantages of oral therapy

1. Less cutaneous and visceral dissemination
2. Cessation of new vesicle formation
3. Reduced pain.

The modest benefit of aciclovir, valaciclovir, and famciclovir for the otherwise healthy patients may not justify the expense, except in severe infections and in

patients more than 50 years of age, to reduce postherpetic neuralgia.

PHN

- Amitriptyline at a dosage of 50 to 100 mg daily.
- Gabapentin 100 to 300 mg three times daily, may be helpful in managing postherpetic neuralgia once it occurs. Pregabalin (150–600 mg) can also be given.
- Capsaicin analgesic cream 0.075% used topically three or four times daily on affected skin, can also provide pain relief.

PAPILLOMAVIRUSES

Human Papillomaviruses

These are possibly the most common viral infections seen in clinical practice. They cause warts which can have numerous subtypes and viral subtypes as listed in Table 4.7.

Most warts resolve spontaneously in the healthy as the immune response overcomes the infection. This happens within 6 months in some 30% of patients, and within 2 years in 65%. Some warts, like mosaic warts, are difficult to treat.

Clinical Features

- The common wart or verruca vulgaris (means common) is a flesh-colored firm papule or nodule that has a corrugated or hyperkeratotic surface (Fig. 4.16A and B). These warts can spread in a linear fashion by trauma (pseudo Koebner's phenomenon).[Q] Characteristic findings are loss of skin markings[Q] and

Table 4.7	Common types of warts and their HPV
Clinical types	*HPV types/oncogenic potential*
Common, filiform, and plantar mosaic warts[Q]	1, **2,** 3, 4, 7, 54
Plane warts, sometimes in epidermodysplasia Verruciformis[*][Q]	**3, 10,** 28
Plantar warts[Q]	**1, 2,** 4, 60, 63
Condylomata acuminata[Q]	**6, 11** /No less often 16, 18, 31, 33/Yes
Bowenoid papulosis[‡][Q]	**16, 18/**Yes
Focal epithelial hyperplasia (Heck disease)	13, 32
Macular and slightly raised lesions in epidermodysplasia verruciformis	**5, 8,** 14, 17, 20, 38/Yes
Respiratory laryngeal papillomatosis	6, 11

[*]Multifocal pigmented macules or papules on the genital skin and mucosa.
[‡]In childhood, patients develop multiple warts and large flat lesions resembling tinea versicolor.

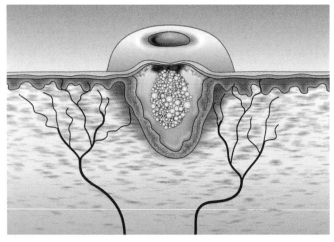

Fig. 4.16A: A wart has a vascular supply thus, on paring the wart with a blade, it bleeds once the vasculature is encountered

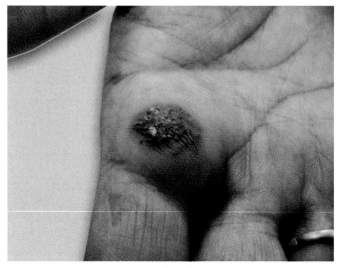

Fig. 4.16C: Punctate 'blackening' that precedes resolution of warts

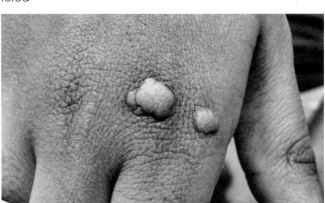

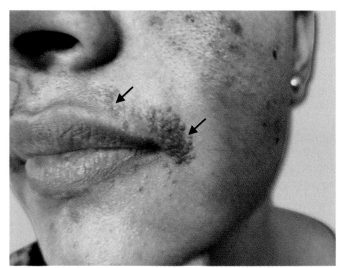

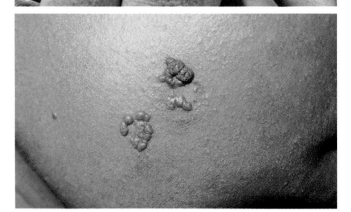

Fig. 4.16B: Common warts on the hand and the face

intralesional hemorrhagic dots or streaks. This is as most warts have a rich vascular supply (Fig. 4.16A). Resolution is preceded by punctate blackening caused by capillary thrombosis (Fig. 4.16C).

- A flat wart is usually missed as it is hardly raised and has a flesh-colored or reddish-brown color which merges with dark skin type (Fig. 4.16D). They become inflamed as a result of an immunological reaction, just before they resolve spontaneously. Frequently spread by autoinoculation, especially on face of men (less often legs of women) by shaving.

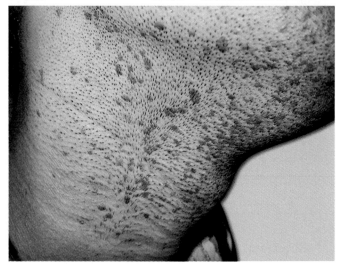

Fig. 4.16D: Plane warts on the face and neck

- A plantar wart may occur as a single, painful papule on the plantar aspect of the foot. There is a callus formation over the lesion and this has to be removed to reveal the wart. Multiple plantar warts may

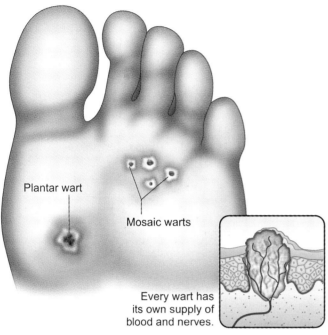

Plantar wart

Mosaic warts

Every wart has its own supply of blood and nerves.

Fig. 4.17A: A depiction of plantar warts

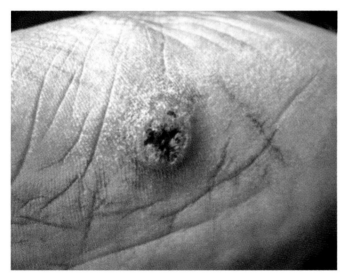

Fig. 4.17B: Plantar wart: Characteristic punctate bleeding is seen after paring. Note the loss of skin markings

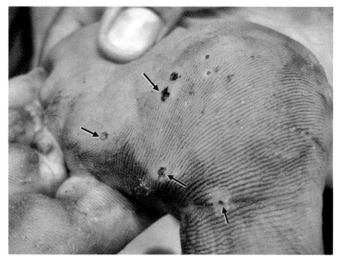

Fig. 4.17C: Multiple discrete plantar warts

coalesce (Fig. 4.17A and B) in a mosaic configuration or may remain discrete (Fig. 4.17C). May become quite large and, when therapy-resistant, may evolve into verrucous squamous cell carcinoma (epithelioma cuniculatum).[Q]

Differential Diagnosis

Clavus or corn is also located at site of pressure, usually over bony prominence; they have a central plug but no punctate hemorrhage (Fig. 4.17D).[Q]

Venereal/genital warts (condylomata acuminata) usually are soft, moist papule and plaque that may be sessile or pedunculated. They may also have a verrucous surface that is often cauliflower-like. Soaking the genital area for 5 minutes with 3 to 5% acetic acid (white vinegar) causes warts to turn white. This is called the aceto-whitening test.[Q]

Diagnosis

It is usually clinical, while paring reveals punctate bleeding unlike callus. A biopsy, if done, reveals vacuolated keratinocytes (koilocytes)[Q] (Fig. 4.17E).

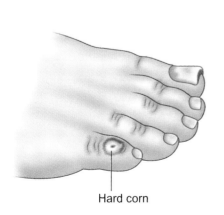

Hard corn

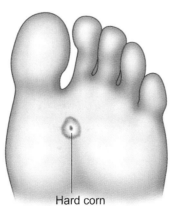

Hard corn

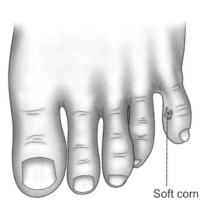

Soft corn

Fig. 4.17D: Types of corn

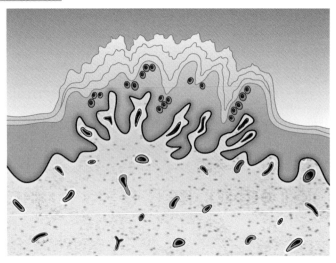

Fig. 4.17E: Wart: Thickened epidermis, with overlying hyperkeratosis. Vacuolated keratinocytes are present in the granular cell layer

Treatment

Treatment of warts is nonspecific, destructive, and usually painful. The goal is destruction of the keratinocytes that are infected with HPV. This may be accomplished with a variety of physical, chemical, or biologic modalities (*see* below). It must be remembered that all forms of therapy have at least a 50% recurrence rate.

The viral and host factors that influence persistence, regression, latency, and reactivation of warts are poorly understood. Serum antibodies to warts have been detected. More importantly, cell-mediated immunity appears to contribute to the regression of warts; in immunodeficient hosts (e.g. those with organ transplants or epidermodysplasia verruciformis), warts may reactivate or persist (Table 4.8).

Table 4.8	Various treatment options for warts
Common warts	• Cryotherapy • Salicylic acid plus occlusion with tape; • Imiquimod
Plantar warts	• Salicylic acid plus occlusion with tape; • Laser destruction with CO_2 (risk of painful scars) or dye laser, or photodynamic therapy
Plane warts	• Topical retinoids • Tretinoin 0.1% cream
Condylomata acuminata	• 50–85% trichloroacetic acid tincture weekly • 25% podophyllin resin • Imiquimod cream—genital warts: Once daily for 3 days/week for 16 weeks
Recalcitrant warts	• Topical 5-fluorouracil • Bleomycin intralesionally • Interferon topically, intralesionally, and systemically
Warts in pregnancy[Q]	70–90% trichloroacetic acid cryotherapy surgical excision

PICORNAVIRUS INFECTIONS

Hand-Foot-and-Mouth Disease

Etiology

Coxsackievirus A[Q] (types 5, 9, 10, 16) and B (types 2 and 5), as well as enterovirus 71.

Epidemiology

Usually children are affected; more common in summer.

Clinical Features

Incubation period 5–8 days. Typical **triad**[Q] (Fig. 4.18):
1. Ulcerative stomatitis, especially on hard palate (lips, tonsils, and pharynx spared).

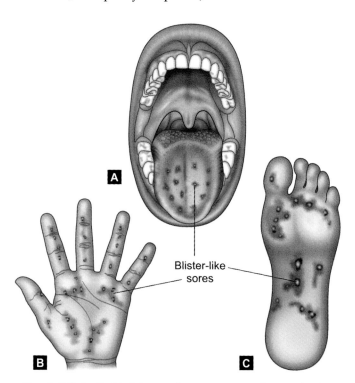

Fig. 4.18A to C: Vesicles on the mucosa, palms and soles

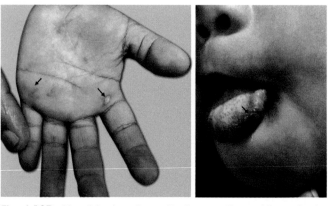

Fig. 4.18D: Hand-foot-and-mouth disease: Gray-white vesicular lesions seen on palms. Discrete erosions seen on the tongue in a 3-year-old child with HFMD

2. Small papules or papulovesicles on the hands and feet, including palms and soles.
3. Less often diffuse exanthem.

Patients generally well; no serious complications.

Herpangina

Etiology

Coxsackievirus A (types 1–6, 8, 10 and 22); also some coxsackievirus B and echoviruses.

Epidemiology

Usually children are affected; more common in summer.

Clinical Features

Incubation period 3–4 days. Patients are ill with sudden fever (up to 40.5°C), malaise, headache, myalgias, sore throat. Lasts around 4 days.

Oral lesions: Characteristic tiny (1–2 mm) ulcerations on hard palate; rapidly ulcerate; often linear. Heal within a week.

VIRAL EXANTHEM

An exanthem is a local or widespread skin eruption usually in response to a viral infection. It can also be in response to bacterial illnesses, toxins produced by pathogens, or drug ingestion. The term *exanthem* actually refers to lesions found on the skin while *enanthem* refers to those on the mucosa. Some causative infectious agents can be potentially harmful to specific patient populations, such as pregnant women or the immunocompromised patient. Here we will focus on the viral exanthems.

A classification of exanthem has been given below which lists the exanthem numerically (Table 4.9).

Here it must be remembered that the most common viral rash is the enteroviral rash that can be of numerous types and is aptly named the "one exanthem, many possible viral causes."[Q] As the exanthems can encompass a wide spectrum of disorders, an overview of the salient types is given as a ready reckoner in Flowchart 4.1 and Figs 4.19 to 4.23.

Parvovirus Infections

Parvovirus B19 is the prototype infection for the adage, *"One virus, many exanthems."*[Q] B19 may be associated with a variety of purpuric or petechial exanthems, including PPGSS (Fig. 4.23) and more generalized presentations. In one outbreak of petechial rashes, B19 was confirmed in 76% of 17 children, and the *petechiae* were widely distributed, often with *accentuation* in the axillary and inguinal regions as well as the distal extremities. Some authors have suggested the terminology parvovirus B19-associated purpuric-petechial eruption for these polymorphous presentations that appear to correspond to the viremic phase of primary infection.

Enteroviral Exanthems

Enteroviruses, subgroup of the picornaviruses, may cause a variety of clinical syndromes with associated exanthems. Human enteroviruses are small, single-stranded RNA viruses that include echovirus (31 serotypes), coxsackievirus A (23 types), coxsackievirus B (six types), enteroviruses 68 through 71 (four types), and polioviruses (three types).

The majority of enterovirus infections seen in practice are benign and manifested by fever alone or distinct syndromes, including *hand-foot-and-mouth* disease (HFMD), *herpangina, hemorrhagic conjunctivitis*, and *pleurodynia*. However, severe or life-threatening infections may also result from enteroviral infection, including meningitis, encephalitis, myocarditis, neonatal sepsis, and polio. Infections in neonates are often disseminated and may be difficult to differentiate from bacterial processes.

Table 4.9	An elucidation of the common exanthems[Q]		
Numerical designation	Name (s)	Agents (s)	Comment
1.	Measles, rubeola	Measles virus (paramyxovirus)	Declining incidence with vaccination; occasional epidemics of imported cases and cases in unimmunized individuals
2.	Scarlet fever, scarlatina	GABHS	Toxin-mediated
3.	German measles, rubella	Rubella virus (togavirus)	Rare with vaccination
4.	Filatov-Dukes disease	Enterovirus	No longer considered a distinct entity
5.	Erythema infectiosum, fifth disease, slapped cheek disease	Parvovirus B19*	Patients not contagious once rash is present
6.	Exanthem subitum, roseola infantum, sixth disease	HHV-6 and HHV-7	Diffuse rash appears after abrupt defervescence

*Parvovirus infections commonly cause petechial rash (please see text).

Flowchart 4.1: An overview of common exanthem with relevant mimickers

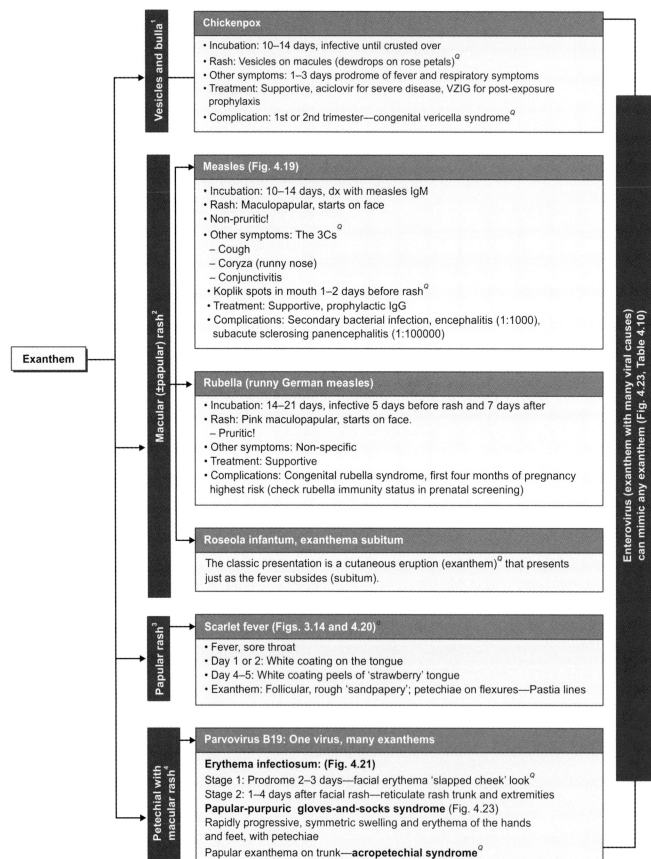

Exanthem

Vesicles and bulla [1]

Chickenpox

- Incubation: 10–14 days, infective until crusted over
- Rash: Vesicles on macules (dewdrops on rose petals) [Q]
- Other symptoms: 1–3 days prodrome of fever and respiratory symptoms
- Treatment: Supportive, aciclovir for severe disease, VZIG for post-exposure prophylaxis
- Complication: 1st or 2nd trimester—congenital vericella syndrome [Q]

Macular (±papular) rash [2]

Measles (Fig. 4.19)

- Incubation: 10–14 days, dx with measles IgM
- Rash: Maculopapular, starts on face
- Non-pruritic!
- Other symptoms: The 3Cs [Q]
  - Cough
  - Coryza (runny nose)
  - Conjunctivitis
- Koplik spots in mouth 1–2 days before rash [Q]
- Treatment: Supportive, prophylactic IgG
- Complications: Secondary bacterial infection, encephalitis (1:1000), subacute sclerosing panencephalitis (1:100000)

Rubella (runny German measles)

- Incubation: 14–21 days, infective 5 days before rash and 7 days after
- Rash: Pink maculopapular, starts on face.
  - Pruritic!
- Other symptoms: Non-specific
- Treatment: Supportive
- Complications: Congenital rubella syndrome, first four months of pregnancy highest risk (check rubella immunity status in prenatal screening)

Roseola infantum, exanthema subitum

The classic presentation is a cutaneous eruption (exanthem) [Q] that presents just as the fever subsides (subitum).

Papular rash [3]

Scarlet fever (Figs. 3.14 and 4.20) [Q]

- Fever, sore throat
- Day 1 or 2: White coating on the tongue
- Day 4–5: White coating peels of 'strawberry' tongue
- Exanthem: Follicular, rough 'sandpapery'; petechiae on flexures—Pastia lines

Petechial with macular rash [4]

Parvovirus B19: One virus, many exanthems

Erythema infectiosum: (Fig. 4.21)
Stage 1: Prodrome 2–3 days—facial erythema 'slapped cheek' look [Q]
Stage 2: 1–4 days after facial rash—reticulate rash trunk and extremities
Papular-purpuric gloves-and-socks syndrome (Fig. 4.23)
Rapidly progressive, symmetric swelling and erythema of the hands and feet, with petechiae

Papular exanthema on trunk—**acropetechial syndrome** [Q]

Enterovirus (exanthem with many viral causes) can mimic any exanthem (Fig. 4.23, Table 4.10)

Other causes of exanthem: [1]Linear IgA disease, SSSS, Stevens-Johnson syndrome. [2]Drug rash, Kawasaki disease. [3]Kawasaki disease. [4]Henoch-Schnolein purpura, meningococcal septicemia

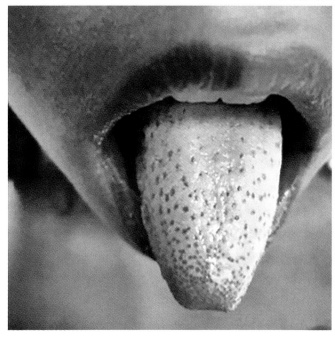

Fig. 4.20B: Strawberry tongue: Seen as bright red erythema with prominent papillae (scarlet fever)

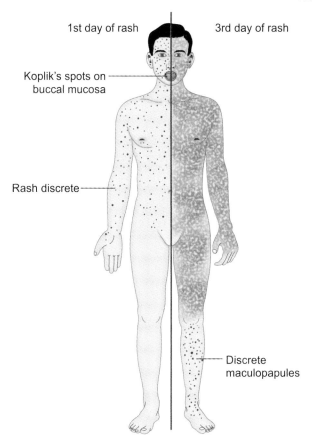

Fig. 4.19: Schematic time lag distribution of measles (rubeola) rash

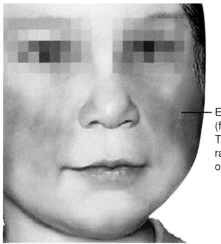

Erythema infectiosum (fifth disease): The erythema, or rash, first appears on the cheeks

Fig. 4.21: Symmetrical erythema on the cheeks of a child with fever: Erythema infectiosum

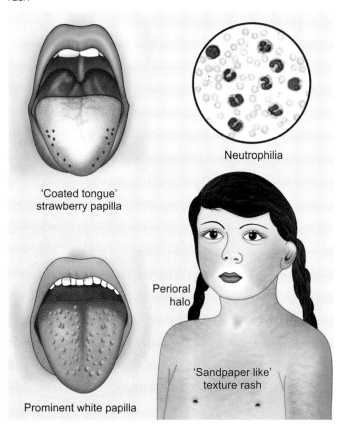

Fig. 4.20A: An artistic depiction of the salient features of scarlet fever

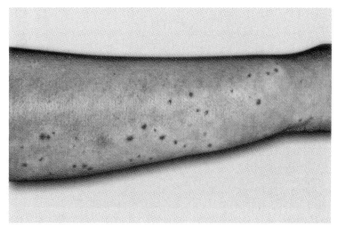

Fig. 4.22: A rash with multiple erythematous papules with a perilesional halo (eruptive pseudoangiomatosis)

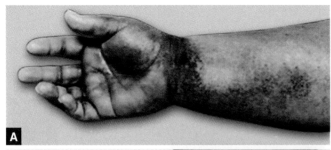

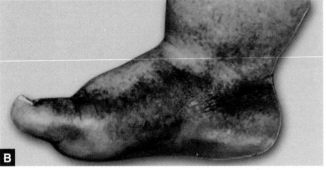

Fig. 4.23A and B: Symmetrical acral erythematous rash that has admixed petechial lesions (papular-purpuric gloves-and-socks syndrome)

Spread of enteroviruses occurs person-to-person via the fecal–oral route and occasionally common source exposure (i.e. swimming pool water). Enteroviral infections tend to predominate during the summer and fall, although sporadic cases may be seen throughout the year.

In case of enteroviral exanthems, each type of exanthem has been associated with many subtypes of coxsackievirus or echovirus (one exanthem, many possible viral causes). A list of common exanthems associated is given in Table 4.10.

Nonspecific exanthems resulting from nonpolio enteroviruses are common and may present as macular and papular nonpruritic eruptions with or without petechiae (Fig. 4.24A to C). When a petechial component is present, the clinical presentation may be confused with that of more serious infections such as meningococcemia. This diagnostic confusion may be exacerbated by the concomitant presence of aseptic meningitis, which may accompany enterovirus, coxsackievirus, or echovirus infections.

Other exanthem patterns may include urticarial, scarlatiniform, zosteriform, and vesicular forms.

Gianotti-Crosti Syndrome

Gianotti-Crosti syndrome or papular acrodermatitis of childhood[Q] is a common viral exanthem, most common in children between 1 and 6 years of age.

Pathophysiology

The cause of Gianotti-Crosti syndrome is unknown. Several viruses have been implicated, including hepatitis B, Epstein-Barr virus, cytomegalovirus, coxsackievirus, adenovirus, respiratory syncytial virus, parainfluenza virus, parvovirus B19, rotavirus, and HHV-6.

Clinical Presentation

There is a prodrome of upper respiratory symptoms, fever, and lymphadenopathy. A few days later, edematous, erythematous, monomorphous papules and papulovesicles appear. As the name acrodermatitis implies, lesions typically occur on the acral surfaces (face, extensor surfaces of extremities; Fig. 4.25A and B). The buttocks may be involved, but the trunk is almost always spared.

Special Considerations

It was once suggested that all patients with Gianotti-Crosti syndrome be tested for hepatitis screen patients

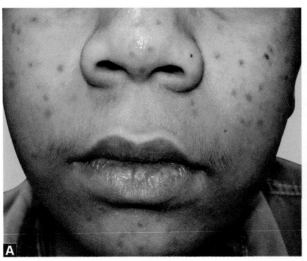
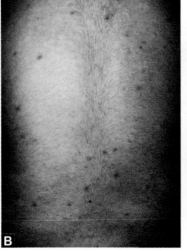
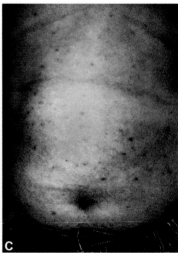

Fig. 4.24A to C: A child who had fever, mild URTI followed by a rash that was largely macular involving the face and trunk. This probably is the commonest cause of a generalized viral rash with fever in children. As a large number of viruses are listed under the enterovirus family, it is also known as the "*one exanthem, with many possible causes*" (enteroviral exanthem)

Table 4.10 Various enteroviral eruptions

Exanthem	Comment
Hand-foot-and-mouth disease	Most common; atypical form with high numbers of vesicles on extremities, palms, soles, face and buttocks may occur, especially in association with epidemics of coxsackievirus A6 infection or B, enterovirus 71
Herpangina	Oral lesions and fever; (coxsackievirus A or B)
Eczema coxsackium	Accentuation of erosions and vesicles in areas of skin previously or currently affected with AD
Hemorrhagic conjunctivitis	Eyelid edema, lacrimation, pain; (coxsackievirus A24 and enterovirus 70)
Nonspecific exanthem	Any enterovirus
Gianotti-Crosti syndrome	Coxsackievirus A or B
Henoch-Schönlein purpura	Coxsackievirus B1
Still-like disease	Coxsackievirus B4
Zoster-like eruption	Echovirus 6
EI-like eruption	Echovirus 12
Congenital skin lesions	Coxsackievirus B3
Eruptive pseudoangiomatosis	Echovirus
AGEP	Coxsackievirus B4
Nail matrix arrest	Patients with preceding hand-foot-and-mouth disease

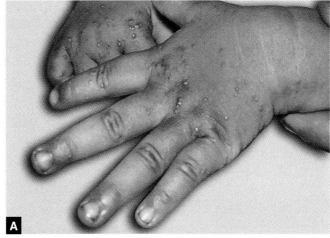
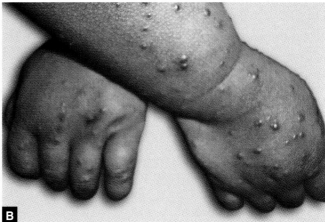

Fig. 4.25A and B: A child with erythematous, monomorphous papules and papulovesicles on the acral surfaces. This is a relapsing, itchy disorder that causes a lot of distress to the parents of the children, but resolutes with time (Gianotti-Crosti syndrome)

for any potential risk factors and examine for jaundice, hepatosplenomegaly, and lymphadenopathy. In the absence of risk factors or symptoms, serum studies are not indicated.

Referral and Consultation

If hepatitis is detected, referral to appropriate specialists is recommended.

Patient Education and Follow-up

It can take 8 to 12 weeks for the exanthem to completely resolve, and patients without hepatitis recover fully. If topical corticosteroids are prescribed, counsel patients on the proper usage, risks, and side effects. Post-inflammatory hypopigmentation can last several months, but will fade on its own.

Fungal Infections

We will be discussing fungal infections under the following subtopics (as below), though the main focus will be on superficial fungal infections:
- Dermatophytes
- Molds
- Yeasts
- Subcutaneous mycoses
- Systemic mycoses

DERMATOPHYTOSIS

Dermatophytes live as parasites in tissue containing keratin. They can be divided into:
1. Anthropophilic: Found in humans.
2. Zoophilic: Found in animals.
3. Geophilic: Found in soil.

The clinical presentation is determined by the nature of the dermatophyte, by the tissue it invades, and by the degree of host response. Dermatophytes invade keratin only, and the inflammation they cause is due to metabolic products of the fungus or delayed hypersensitivity.

The clinical infection usually starts from an inoculation site and spreads peripherally thus forming annular lesions with an active border. The most common cause of superficial fungal infections is *Trichophyton rubrum*.[Q] In India,[Q] though *Trichophyton interdigitale* is now the commonest cause of superficial dermatophytosis.[Q] Zoophilic and geophilic infections always elicit a more intense immune response and thus appear more inflammatory.

Three genera of dermatophyte fungi cause tinea infections (ringworm):
1. *Trichophyton*: Skin, hair and nail infections.[Q]
2. *Microsporum*: Skin and hair.[Q]
3. *Epidermophyton*: Skin and nails.[Q]

The names of the various dermatophyte infections begin with '*tinea*', which is a Latin term for 'worm'. The second word in the name is the Latin term for the affected body site (Fig. 5.1).
- Tinea capitis—scalp
- Tinea barbae—beard
- Tinea faciei—face
- Tinea corporis—trunk and extremities
- Tinea manuum—hands
- Tinea cruris—groin
- Tinea pedis—feet
- Tinea unguium (onychomycosis)—nails

Tinea versicolor is the only exception; its name derives from the several shades of color that lesions may have in this disease.

Investigation

Taking specimen: Disinfect site to reduce contamination. Use a sterile instrument (scalpel blade, curette, scissors) to obtain tissue from border zone between normal and involved tissue (where concentration of organisms is usually highest).
- *Microscopic examination*: Hyphae or spores are identified after dissolving the keratin in a 10–15%[Q] solution of potassium hydroxide (KOH examination). Dyes (chlorazol black E) or fluorochromes (for fluorescent microscopy) can be added. Examination is made at 200–400×.
- *Culture*: Many standard culture media are available; usually two cultures are made, one on a media containing cycloheximide[Q] (for dermatophytes) and

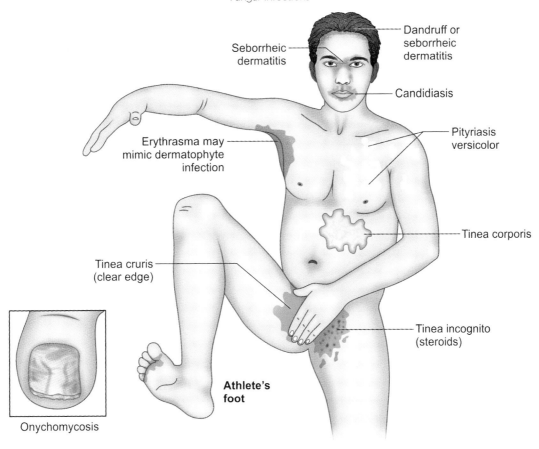

Fig. 5.1: An overview of various sites affected with superficial fungal infection

one without (yeasts and molds). Hairs can be placed directly on the culture media; fragments from the underside of the nail should be used.

- *Wood's light examination* in which a UVA lamp (365 nm)[Q] is used to elicit fluorescence (green) of hair in some dermatophyte infections (e.g. *Microsporum canis* and *T. schoenleinii*).[Q] It is useful for screening in a school outbreak. As a thumb rule, endothrix infections are Wood's light negative.[Q] The Wood's lamp, however, has become much less useful because most cases of tinea capitis are now caused by non- fluorescing *T. tonsurans*.[Q]

> Wood's light (blacklight) is of no help in diagnosing dermatophytic infection of the skin.

Tinea Capitis

Infection of the scalp by dermatophytes with hair shaft involvement.

The most common causes worldwide are *Trichophyton tonsurans* and *Microsporum canis*.

Pathogenesis

After an incubation period of 3 weeks, fungal hyphae grow into the hair shaft and follicle. This growth causes broken hair, scaling, and a host of inflammatory

responses. In case of endothrix, the infection does not spread beyond the Adamson's fringe (Fig. 5. 2).[Q]

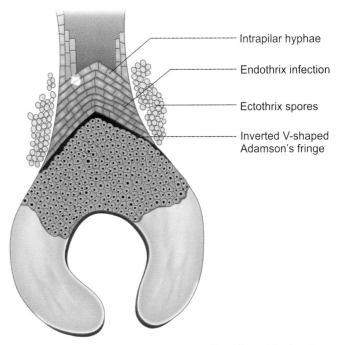

Intrapilar hyphae

Endothrix infection

Ectothrix spores

Inverted V-shaped Adamson's fringe

Fig. 5.2: A depiction of the two types of invasion of the hyphae in tinea capitis, i.e. ectothrix and endothrix. (**Note:** The endothrix infection does not spread beyond the Adamson's fringe)

The infection spreads centrifugally for 8 to 10 weeks, involving an area of scalp up to 7 cm in diameter. Spontaneous cure can occur or persistence depending on the host immune response.

Clinical Features

There are two types of infections depending on the location of spores on the hair shaft (as below). If the spores coat the outer surface of the hair, it is called **ectothrix,** while if it invades the hair shaft, it is called **endothrix** (Fig. 5.3). The clinical types are gray patch, black dot, kerion, and seborrheic dermatitis like (Box 5.1).

Species causing endothrix = TVS—tonsurans, violaceum, schoenleinii.

Box 5.1	Overview of tinea capitis[Q]	
Clinical types	**Species**
Noninflammatory infection (*gray patch*)/gray patch tinea capitis	M. audonii M. ferrugineum.
Noninflammatory (*black dot pattern*)	Trichophyton tonsurans Trichophyton violaceum
Inflammatory tinea capitis (*kerion/agminate folliculitis*)	Trichophyton tonsurans
Kerion	Trichophyton verrucosum or Trichophyton mentagrophytes
Seborrheic dermatitis type	Trichophyton tonsurans
Favus	Trichophyton schoenleinii

Ectothrix infection: Spores coat outer surface of hair.[Q] Areas of hair loss with stubble of varying size (Fig. 5.3). Hairs may fluoresce under Wood's light. The species that cause fluorescence are depicted in Fig. 5.3. Scarring is rare.

Epidemic tinea capitis is the most common form of ectothrix; caused by *Microsporum canis, Microsporum audouinii,* or *Microsporum gypseum.* Responsible for **epidemics** among schoolchildren.[Q] Usually, multiple round areas of hair loss; **inflammation varies** (marked with *Microsporum canis*), while *Microsporum audouinii* produces fine scales with little erythema—also called the '**gray patch**' type of tinea capitis (Fig. 5.4).

Endothrix infection: Spores grow into the hair shaft, making it more breakable. Thus, hairs usually end at skin surface, leaving **black dots** (*Trichophyton tonsurans* or *Trichophyton violaceum*).[Q] Other variants include, diffuse alopecia, seborrheic dermatitis like and even gray patch.

Kerion: Intense inflammatory reaction to zoophilic fungus in previously unexposed host, such as young farmers with first exposure to milking cattle; usually *Trichophyton verrucosum* or *Trichophyton mentagrophytes.*[Q] Erythematous boggy swelling studded with pustules and easily plucked hair, relatively less pain (kerion is Greek for honeycomb). Heals with scarring[Q] (Fig. 5.5A to D).

Favus: Infection with *Trichophyton schoenleinii*;[Q] relatively common in Middle East, South Africa, and Greenland, otherwise rare. Foul smell (mouse urine). Marked inflammation, large (1–2 cm) adherent C-shaped crusts (scutulae)[Q] that may cover entire scalp, heal with scarring (scarring alopecia).

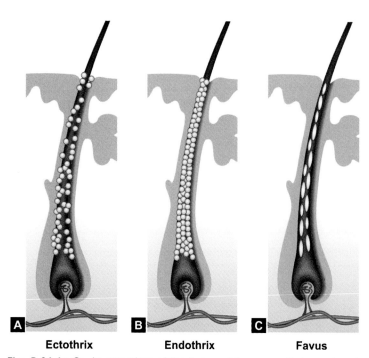

○	Arthroconidia
⬭	Hyphae and air spaces

Ectothrix	**Endothrix**
M. canis*	T. tonsurans
M. audouinii*	T. violaceum
M. ferrugineum*	T. soudanense
M. distortum*	T. gourvilli
M. gypseum	T. yaoundei
T. rubrum (rarely affects the scalp)	T. rubrum (rarely affects scalp)
Favus	
T. schoenleinii**	

*Displays **yellow** fluorescence with Wood's lamp examination
Displays **blue-white fluorescence with Wood's lamp examination

Ectothrix   **Endothrix**   **Favus**

Fig. 5.3A to C: An overview of the types of tinea capitis based on invasion of the hair shaft and the causative organism

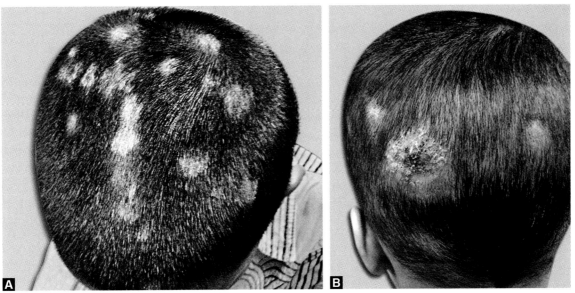

Fig. 5.4A and B: (A) A case of gray patch tinea capitis; (B) A 6-year-old boy with patchy circular alopecia and scaling suggestive of gray patch tinea capitis. The scales represent the fungal arthrospores

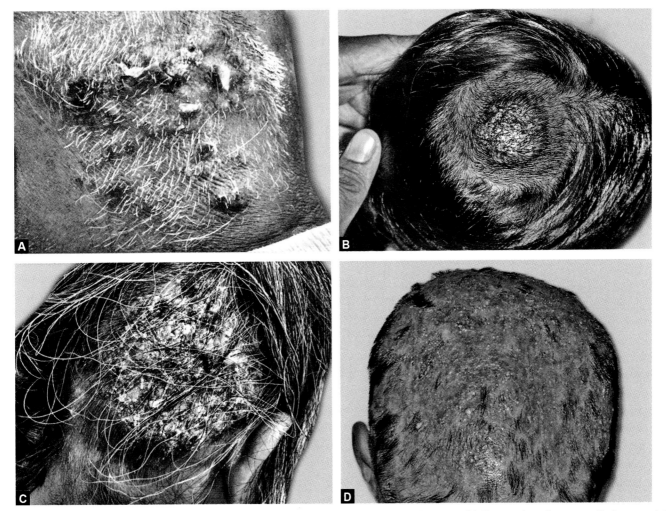

Fig. 5.5A to D: Various types of inflammatory tinea capitis including kerion. (A) A case of inflammatory tinea capitis in an adult patient who was treated with antibiotics and after an unsuccessful course was diagnosed as tinea capitis and treated successfully with griseofulvin; (B) Inflamed, boggy, tender areas of alopecia in a case of kerion; (C) An inflammatory tinea capitis in a lady working in a cowshed, a case of zoophilic tinea capitis; (D) Agminate folliculitis: A rare case with pustules all over the scalp with alopecia and was misdiagnosed and treated as a case of bacterial folliculitis

Differential Diagnosis

1. **Alopecia areata:** Presents with alopecia, but there is no significant scale.
2. **Seborrheic dermatitis:** Presents with mild pruritus, localized or diffuse scale on the scalp; typically there is no significant hair loss.
3. **Psoriasis:** Presents with red, localized or diffuse silvery scaly plaques on the scalp. Similar plaques on the elbows and knees or elsewhere on the body are usually seen.
4. **Bacterial infections and tumors:** These may closely resemble a kerion. However, tumors are rare in children and when they do occur, they should be biopsied to confirm the diagnosis.

Therapy

Oral griseofulvin has been the gold standard of therapy for the past 45 years based on its cost and efficacy, and it is the preferred antifungal medication for a kerion infection.[Q] It should be taken with a fatty meal[Q] or with whole milk or ice-cream to improve absorption.

A recent meta-analysis suggested that **Terbinafine** is more effective in *Trichophyton* infections, but griseofulvin is more effective in *Microsporum* infections.

In addition, 2% ketoconazole (Nizoral) shampoo and 1% or 2.5% selenium sulfide (Selsun) shampoo should be used 2 to 3 times a week for 5 to 10 minutes during therapy to reduce surface fungal colony counts. Solo topical therapy is not given in tinea of scalp and is used only as adjunct.[Q]

It is important to clean combs, brushes, and hats to prevent reinfection. Reinfection can also occur, if household contacts or pets remain infected.[Q]

The use of oral steroids for a kerion infection remains controversial. However, if significant hair loss is noted, they should be considered, as the inflammation that occurs with a kerion can result in scarring alopecia.

With treatment, tinea capitis is cured in 1 to 3 months; if not treated, the inflammatory tinea capitis is self-limiting, with resolution within a few months. In others, the disease lasts for years, with resolution at puberty.

An overview of drugs used for T. capitis is given in Table 5.1.

Tinea Barbae

Dermatophyte infection in beard region of men.

Pathogenesis

Similar to kerion; *Trichophyton verrucosum* or *Trichophyton mentagrophytes*.

Clinical Features

Patients usually farmers with close animal contact. Develop erythematous plaques with follicular pustules,

Table 5.1   Therapy of T. capitis

Drug	Dosage	Duration
Griseofulvin microsize Available in 250 or 500 mg tablets or 125 mg/5 mL oral suspension	• 10–20 mg/kg/day, single or divided doses is more commonly used • Max daily 1 gm	• 4–8 weeks • May need up to 12 weeks, if not cleared
Griseofulvin ultramicrosize Available in 125 and 250 mg (tablets)	• 10–15 mg/kg/ day is more commonly used • Maximum dose is 750 mg/day	Same as above
Terbinafine 250 mg (tablet)	• <20 kg: 62.5 mg daily • 20–40 kg: 125 mg daily • >40 kg: 250 mg daily	2–4 weeks, up to 8 weeks for *Microsporum* infections
Terbinafine (Oral granules sprinkled into nonacid foods such as pudding) 125 mg in a packet 187.5 mg in packet	• 125 mg daily for body weight less than 25 kg • 187.5 mg daily for body weight 25–35 kg • 250 mg daily for body weight greater than 35 kg	6 weeks
Itraconazole 100 mg capsule	• <20 kg: 5 mg/kg daily • 20–40 kg: 100 mg daily • >40 kg: 200 mg daily	2–6 weeks
Fluconazole 50, 100, 200 mg tablets or oral powder for suspension	5–6 mg/kg/day	3–6 weeks

Except for griseofulvin and terbinafine granules none of the rest is approved for use in T. capitis.

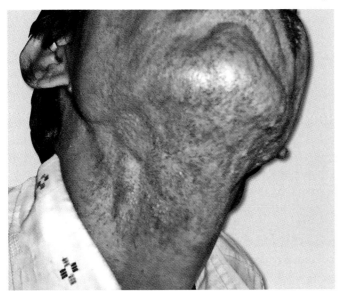

Fig. 5.6: A superficial pattern of tinea barbae in a 23-year-old male lesions resemble tinea corporis

drainage and crusts (Fig. 5.6) which is surprisingly painless. Heals with scarring.

Differential Diagnosis

Staphylococcal infection with multiple furuncles (sycosis barbae); usually painful.

Therapy

Topical therapy ineffective; systemic antifungal agents for 1–2 months (as for T. capitis).

Tinea Corporis

Dermatophyte infection of the skin of the trunk and extremities, excluding the palms, soles, and inguinal region.

Tinea corporis is caused most frequently by the anthropophilic fungi, *Trichophyton rubrum*Q or *Trichophyton mentagrophytes* var *mentagrophytes*, or the zoophilic fungus, *M. canis*. In India, now the more common species is *Trichophyton interdigitale*.

Clinical Features

Tinea corporis presents initially as a red, scaly papule that spreads outward, eventually developing into an annular plaque with a scaly, slightly raised, well-demarcated border. The center of the lesion may partially clear resulting in a 'ring' or 'annular' appearance (Fig. 5.7).

The histology in classical cases reveals hyphae in the stratum corneum (Fig. 5.8).

Less common presentations include:

- *Majocchi granuloma*: In rare instances, tinea corporis does not remain confined to the stratum corneum. Dermal invasion by hyphae following the hair follicle

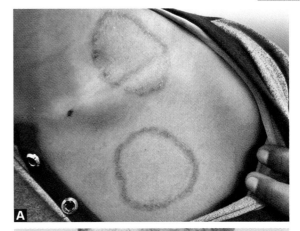
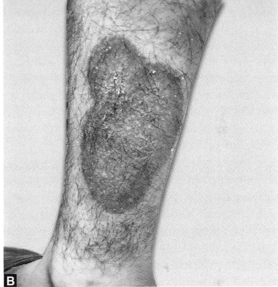

Fig. 5.7A and B: (A) Classical annular rash of tinea corporis; (B) Annular plaque of tinea corporis modified by topical steroid mimicking 'psoriasis'

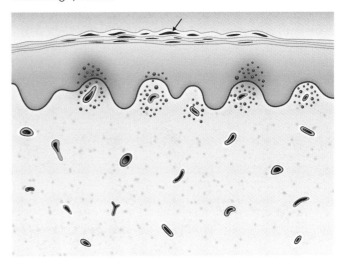

Fig. 5.8: Histology of tinea corporis with hyphae in the stratum corneum with mild inflammation in the dermis

root can produce Majocchi granuloma, which presents as perifollicular granulomatous papules or pustules typically on the shins or arms (Fig. 5.9).

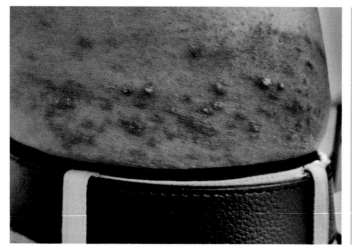 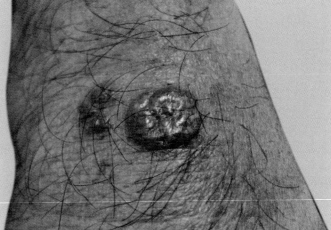

Fig. 5.9: Majocchi granuloma with perifollicular papules and plaques

- *Tinea incognito*: This is an atypical presentation of tinea corporis that can occur when a dermatophyte infection has been treated with potent topical steroids or systemic steroids. It is characterized by dermal papules or kerion-like lesions with no inflammation, scaling, or pruritus (Fig. 5.10).[Q]
- *Tinea profunda* results from an excessive inflammatory response to a dermatophyte (analogous to a kerion on the scalp).
- *Tinea imbricata* resulting[Q] from *T. concentricum*,[Q] an anthropophilic dermatophyte found in southern Asia.
- *Tinea atypica*: This term is used for cases that are modified by therapy and do not look like the classical tinea corporis. In Indian skin, they are pigmented and can have a lichenified look (Fig. 5.11).

Differential Diagnosis

Nummular eczema: Discoid patch with vesicles, oozing and itching. Usually, multiple and symmetrical.

Pityriasis rosea: Scaly plaques, trunk, symmetrical, generalized.

Psoriasis: Scaly plaques, silvery scales, positive grattage test.

Treatment

Topical antifungal medications are effective for isolated lesions of tinea corporis. Topical antifungal medications should be applied at least 1 to 2 cm beyond the visible advancing edge of the lesions and treatment should be continued for 1 to 2 weeks after the lesions resolve. The systemic therapy is given in Table 5.2.

Tinea Faciale

This is now a common issue in India where steroid abuse is common and hence, due to the atypical morphology, is often misdiagnosed fungal infection.

Clinical Features

Tinea faciale appears as an erythematous, usually asymmetric, eruption on the face. An annular pattern is frequently not evident, but an serpiginous outline is seen (Fig. 5.12A and B).

> The finding of sharp serpiginous borders is diagnostic of tinea facie.

Differential Diagnosis

SD: The lesions in seborrheic dermatitis are usually symmetric and are not well demarcated.

Photodermatitis: Rashes resulting from sunlight (photodermatitis) are distinguished by their distribution, which usually is symmetric, sparing areas that are relatively protected from the sun, such as the eyelids and under the chin.

Tinea Manuum

Tinea manuum is a dermatophyte infection that affects the palmar aspect of the hands (Fig. 5.13). It is more common in men and is rare in children.

Etiology

T. rubrum, *Trichophyton mentagrophytes*, and *Epidermophyton floccosum* are the species that commonly cause tinea manuum.

Clinical Types

Tinea manuum can present with *two patterns*, inflammatory and non-inflammatory.

Tinea on the palms presents with diffuse, fine scale (Fig. 5.13). It is frequently associated with the moccasin type of tinea pedis. It is unilateral in about 50% of the cases. In some cases, there is a concomitant fungal infection of the fingernails. The association with bilateral T. pedis is known as the 'one hand, two feet disease'.[Q]

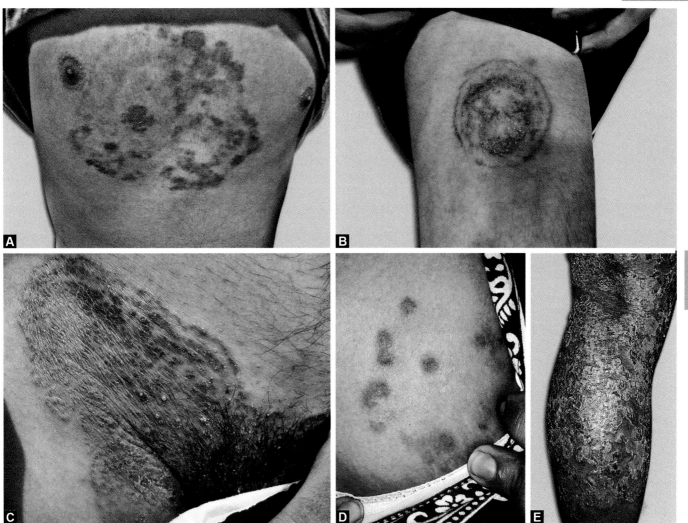

Fig. 5.10A to E: Tinea incognito. These represent various spectrums of steroid modified tinea which is the cause of most so-called 'resistant' cases. (A) Multiple rings with little itching; (B) A case of tinea with multiple rings and follicular lesions which is a classic manifestation of tinea incognito with a Mojocchi granuloma. (C and D) Cases with steroid abuse leading to red papules and pustules. (E) Diffuse scaly plaque—a case of atypical tinea corporis

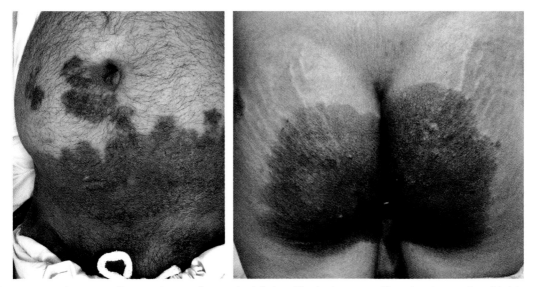

Fig. 5.11: Tinea corporis presenting as hyperpigmented lichenified plaques with raised margins, highly suggestive of *T. rubrum* infection. This presentation is suggestive of chronicity of infection and these patients need for longer duration of antifungal therapy

Table 5.2	Therapy of tinea corporis				
	Griseofulvin	*Fluconazole*	*Terbinafine*	*Itraconazole*	*Ketoconazole*
Tinea corporis	500–1000 mg/day (microsize) or 375–500 mg/d (ultramicrosize) × 2–4 weeks	150 mg/week 2–4 weeks	250 mg daily × 2–3 weeks (3–6 weeks)*	• 200 mg/day × 1 week *or* • 100 mg/day × 2–4 weeks (3–6 weeks)** • 200 mg bd × 7 d	200–400 mg/day for 2 weeks
Tinea corporis (children)	15–20 mg/kg/day (microsize suspension) × 2–4 weeks	6 mg/kg/week × 2–4 weeks	125 mg (<20–40 kg) *or* 250 mg (>40 kg) × 1 week	3–5 mg/kg/day (maximum 200 mg) × 1 week	Not recommended

*In India, terbinafine is increasingly showing non-responsiveness. **The longer duration is a India-specific recommendation.

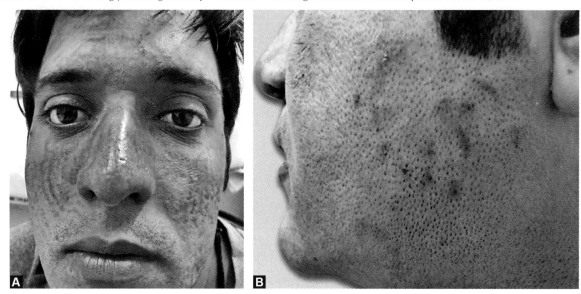

Fig. 5.12A and B: Tinea faciale: (A) Note that the classical annular morphology can be seen; (B) But occasionally a serpiginous outline is more common

Differential Diagnosis

Chronic contact dermatitis: Usually involves both palms, and the border is generally not well demarcated.

Psoriasis: The plaques are sharply demarcated, also they are bilateral, and are more elevated and erythematous.

Treatment

The treatment is same as that for T. pedis (Table 5.3).

Tinea Pedis

Dermatophyte infection of feet and toes.

Pathogenesis

Most common agents are *Trichophyton rubrum*, *Trichophyton mentagrophytes*, and *Epidermophyton floccosum*.Q

Source

Infections are favored by poor hygiene, increased sweating, occlusive footwear; perhaps by impaired peripheral circulation. Swimming pools, community showers, and saunas are likely sources of infection.

Clinical Features

Pattern varies greatly with causative dermatophyte:

1. *Hyperkeratotic/moccasin type*: Also known as moccasin type; diffuse fine scale (Fig. 5.14), rarely symptomatic, often overlooked or mistaken for palmoplantar keratoderma. First noticed with nail involvement. Classically, the skin markings of the soles are affected by the scaling. Usually caused by *Trichophyton rubrum*.

2. *Chronic interdigitale type*: Typically involves space between more lateral toes; macerated epidermis is white and fissured (Fig. 5.15). May spread to soles, and rarely top of foot. Usually caused by *Trichophyton mentagrophytes* var. *interdigitale*.

3. *Dyshidrotic type*: Recurrent attacks of pruritic vesicles and pustules, identical to dyshidrotic dermatitis. Same principle as fungal id reaction, but organisms (usually *Trichophyton mentagrophytes* var. *interdigitale*)

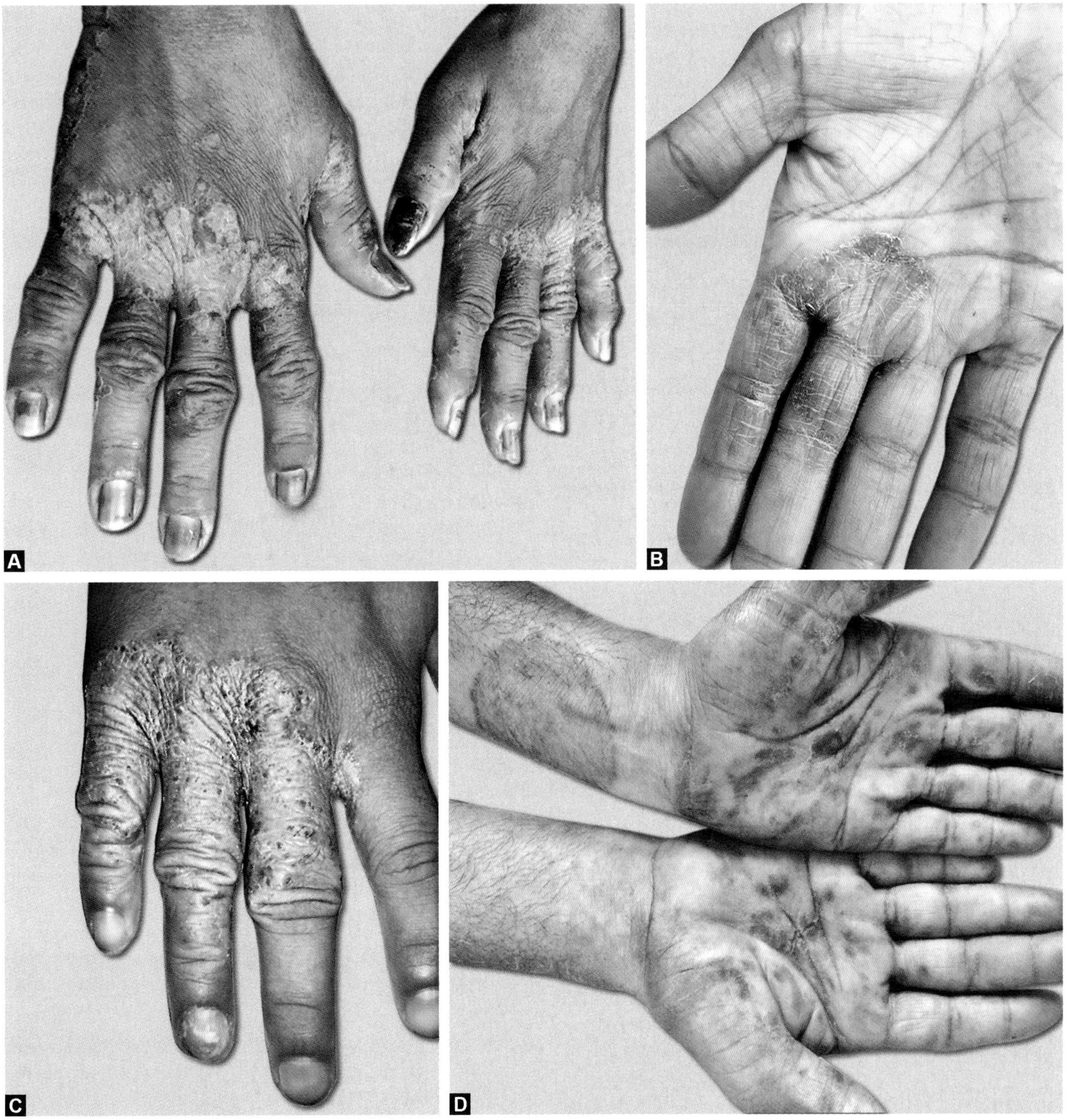

Fig. 5.13A to D: Tinea manuum: (A) Inflammatory tinea corporis on dorsa of hands of a 30-year-old female. Always examine nails and palms in such a case to look for presence of fungus there. Also note that lesions on dorsa of hands are included in corporis and not manuum. (B) A case of tinea manuum present on palmar aspect of right hand characterized by an erythematous scaly plaque with prominent borders. Sometimes vesicles may be seen on the margins of lesion which eventually desquamate to leave behind scaling. (C) A case of tinea manuum with concomitant involvement of nails and dorsa of hands. Patient should be prescribed longer treatment course as for tinea unguium. (D) An unusual case of tinea manuum presenting with hyperkeratotic bilateral symmetrical scaly plaques. It could be mistaken for a form of hand dermatitis but the concomitant presence of tinea corporis on forearm (as seen in picture) and a history of nonresponse to topical steroid therapy are important pointers to diagnosis. Though asymmetry is a feature of tinea, sometimes bilateral lesions may be present

can be found. Vesicles and pustules on the instep of the feet should lead to a suspicion of this type of

tinea pedis (Fig. 5.16). A KOH preparation of the roof of the vesicle or pustule reveals fungal hyphae.

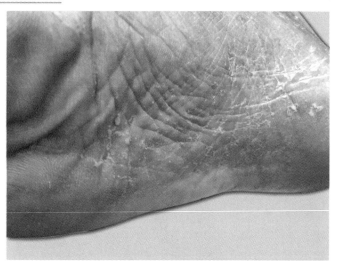

Fig. 5.14: Moccasin type of tinea pedis note the scaling on the soles that involve the skin dermatoglyphics

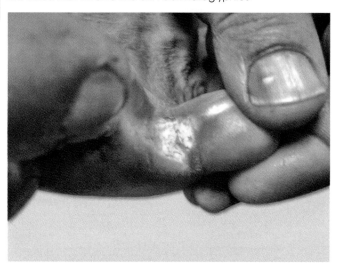

Fig. 5.15: Interdigitale tinea pedis

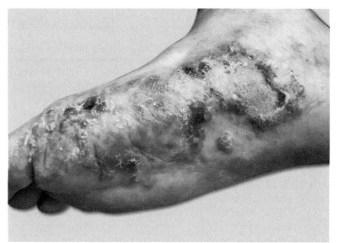

Fig. 5.16: Vesicles and bulla on the instep 'dyshidrotic type' of tinea pedis

Complications

Gram-negative toe web infections, entry site for erysipelas, predisposing factor for postcoronary bypass cellulitis.

Treatment

Topical antifungal agents; in severe cases, systemic antifungal agents for 1–3 months (Table 5.3). Treatment of associated onychomycosis and continued prophylactic use of topical agents are essential to reduce the relapse rate. In the case of macerated forms, keep area dry, wear absorbent socks, use sandals in summer. Shoes should be disinfected with antifungal sprays to reduce likelihood of reinfection.

Tinea Cruris

Tinea cruris (jock itch) or *dhobi* itch^Q is a dermatophyte infection of the inguinal and perianal areas. It is three times more prevalent in men than in women. Obesity and activities that cause increased sweating are risk factors.

Pathophysiology

Tinea cruris is usually caused by *T. rubrum*, *T. mentagrophytes*, and *E. floccosum*. Sweating and tight or damp clothing produces maceration of the skin allowing the dermatophytes to easily penetrate into the epidermis.

Autoinoculation commonly occurs from tinea pedis or tinea unguium. The organisms may also be transmitted from fomites such as towels and sheets.

Clinical Features

Patients present with pruritic, semicircular plaques with sharply defined scaly borders in the inguinal folds and the upper inner thighs (Fig. 5.17). The penis and scrotum are not involved in contrast to candidiasis that can involve the penis and scrotum.

Differential Diagnosis

Candidiasis: Bright, intensely erythematous (beefy red) eruption with satellite papules and pustules. The scrotum is often affected.

Intertrigo: Simple irritant dermatitis, most often found in obese patients in whom moisture accumulates between skin folds in the inguinal area.

Erythrasma: This is an uncommon disease of intertriginous skin caused by *Corynebacterium minutissimum*.^Q It is a velvety patch with fine scale that, under Wood's light examination, fluoresces a diagnostic coral pink.

Psoriasis and seborrheic dermatitis can also affect the groin.

Treatment

Most cases of tinea cruris can be successfully treated with topical antifungal medications, preferably a cream or lotion. Absorbent powders, such as miconazole

Table 5.3 Treatment of T. pedis/manuum

	Griseofulvin	Fluconazole	Terbinafine	Itraconazole	Ketoconazole
Tinea pedis/ manuum	750–1000 mg/day (microsize) *or* 500–750 mg/d (ultramicrosize) × 6–12 weeks	150–200 mg/week × 4–6 weeks	250 mg daily × 2 weeks	200–400 mg/day 1–2 weeks	Not recommended
Tinea pedis/ manuum (children)	15–20 mg/kg/day (microsize suspension) × 4 weeks	6 mg/kg/week × 4–6 weeks	125 mg (<20–40 kg) *or* 250 mg (>40 kg) × 2 weeks	3–5 mg/kg/day (maximum 200 mg) × 1 week	Not recommended

*In India, terbinafine is increasingly showing non-responsiveness largely.

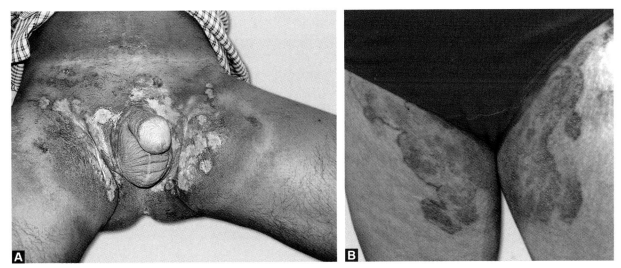

Fig. 5.17A and B: (A) A case of recalcitrant tinea cruris in a patient. Note the lichenified look and the sparing of the scrotum. This 'look' is classic example of *T. rubrum* infections and these infections are chronic in nature as the organism tends to subvert the Th1 response and the increased Th2 response leads to persistence of infection. The scratching due to the Th2 response causes the lichenified look. (B) A case of tinea cruris presenting with an erythematous plaque with red-brown less scaly center. Red papules at the margins and within the plaque are suggestive of dermal nodules seen in chronic infection with *T. rubrum*

powder, are very helpful treatment adjuncts and can help prevent recurrences. Systemic therapy is same as that for T. corporis (as above). Coexisting tinea pedis and tinea unguium should be treated to prevent reinfection. Men should be instructed to wear loose-fitting pants and boxer shorts.

Onychomycosis (Tinea Unguium)

Onychomycosis is a very common nail disorder and accounts for about 50% of nail diseases. The infection of nail fold and nail plate can be due to **dermatophytes** (*Trichophyton rubrum, Trichophyton mentagrophytes, Epidermophyton floccosum*) as well as **molds** (*Hendersonula toruloidea, Scopulariopsis brevicaulis*), and **yeasts** (*Candida albicans*, other *Candida* species).

Clinical Features

The initial findings are white/yellow or orange/brown streaks or patches under the nail plate. As the infection progresses, subungual hyperkeratosis, onycholysis (separation of the nail plate from the nail bed), and a thickened nail plate may develop.^{Q}

The classification is given below (Fig. 5.18):

- *Distal subungual:*^{Q} Nails are dystrophic and thickened (Fig. 5.18A). Here the nail plate invasion originates below the distal edge of the nail. Color changes are present (white, yellow, orange, or brown).
- *White superficial:*^{Q} Nail plate invasion starts with penetration of the upper nail plate surface. Nail plate appears white, and chalky (Fig. 5.18B). The two main types are patchy and transverse (striate).
- *Proximal subungual:*^{Q} Proximal portion of nail appears white, but not crumbly or chalky (Fig. 5.18C).
- *Totally dystrophic onychomycosis:*^{Q} Here the nail invasion is so advanced that the original site of

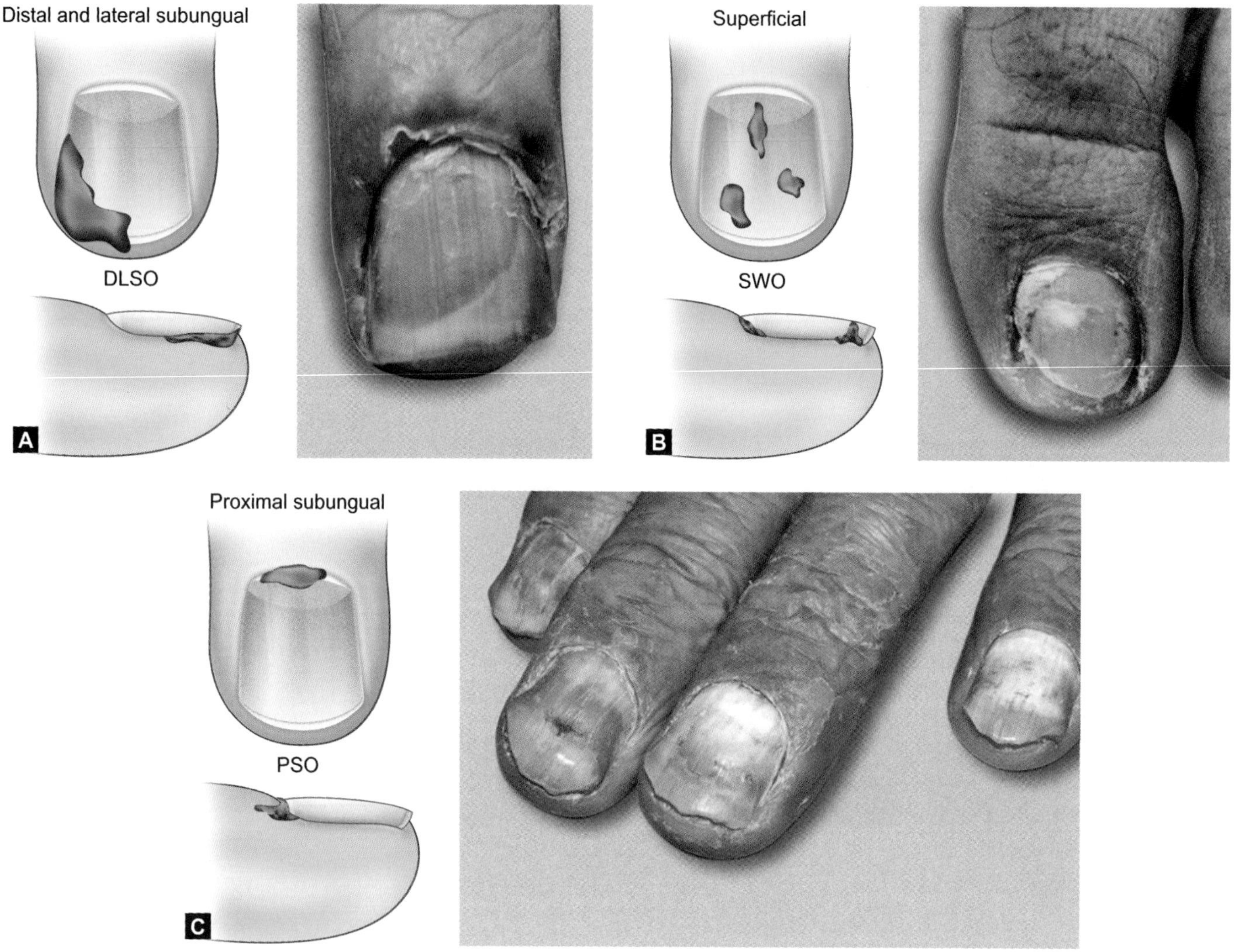

Distal and lateral subungual

DLSO

A

Superficial

SWO

B

Proximal subungual

PSO

C

Fig. 5.18A to C: (A) Distal and lateral subungual onychomycosis; (B) Superficial onychomycosis; (C) Proximal subungual onychomycosis with distal onychomycosis

invasion of the nail plate cannot be seen and the whole plate is largely destroyed (Fig. 5.18D).

- *Endonyx onychomycosis:*[Q] Here the fungi invade the upper and medial aspect of the nail plate (Fig. 5.18E).
- *Candida:* Mild cases may produce nothing more than diffuse leukonychia (white spot[s] under the nail plate). Severe cases may present with a yellow-brown discoloration, with a thick nail bed and lateral and proximal nail fold swelling. Onycholysis is common and subungual hyper-keratosis can occur (Fig. 5.19).

Investigation

KOH smear of nail dipping and scraped subungual debris shows hypae. A fungal culture is the least sensitive, but most specific, method for demonstrating a fungal infection. The most sensitive method to detect fungus is to clip the distal portion of the nail plate, place it in formalin, and send it for histopathologic examination with PAS staining.

Treatment

It takes 4 to 6 months for a fingernail and 12 to 18 months for the great toenail to grow out completely. As a result, patients will not see a completely normal nail plate until that length of time has passed. The first sign that treatment is working will be a transition to normal nail plate growth from the proximal nail fold, which, for the fingernails, can usually be seen within a few months of starting treatment. *Asymptomatic* onychomycosis of toenails needs *no treatment.* An overview of the treatment protocol is given in Fig. 5.20 and Box 5.2.

Onychomycosis is recurrent in 10 to 53% of previously 'cured' patients. Some studies have shown that there is a lower recurrence rate in patients initially treated with oral terbinafine (12%) than in those treated with itraconazole (36%).

Patients should continue to use antifungal creams on their feet, or powders inside their shoes, at least 3 times a week after treatment with oral medications is completed. Proximal subungual onychomycosis should

Totally dystrophic

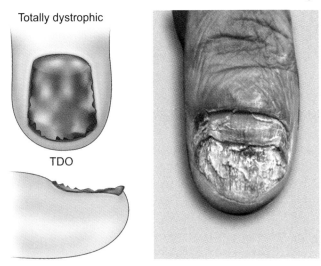

TDO

Fig. 5.18D: Total dystrophic onychomycosis

Endonyx

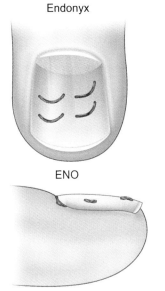

ENO

Fig. 5.18E: Endonyx onychomycosis

prompt investigation for immunosuppression, specifically HIV infection.[Q] Candidal onychomycosis is usually considered a sign of immunosuppression.

The systemic agents used to treat onychomycosis are given in Box 5.2.

| **Box 5.2** | Therapy for onychomycosis |

Initial
- Terbinafine: 6 weeks for fingernails, 12 weeks for toenails
  - <20 kg: 62.5 mg *daily*
  - 20–40 kg: 125 mg *daily*
  - >40 kg: 250 mg *daily*

Alternative
- Itraconazole: 2 pulses for fingernails, 3 pulses for toenails[Q]
  - <20 kg: 5 mg/kg *daily* for 1 week/month
  - 20–40 kg: 100 mg *daily* for 1 week/month
  - >40–50 kg: 200 mg *daily* for 1 week/month
  - >50 kg: 200 mg *bid* for 1 week/month

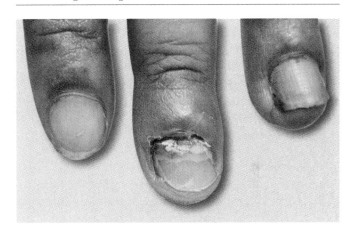

Fig. 5.19: Candidiasis due to paronychia with involvement of proximal nail (candidal onychomycosis)

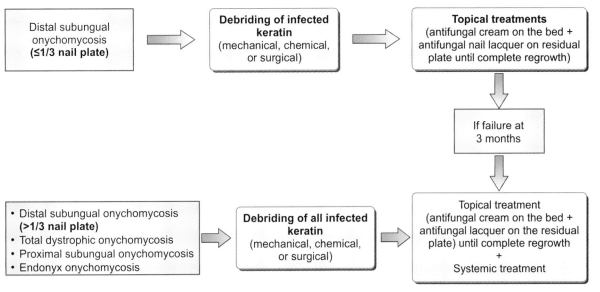

Fig. 5.20: A protocol for treatment of onychomycosis

Topical medications for onychomycosis are often unable to fully penetrate the nail plate, and, therefore, complete fungal eradication with these medications alone is difficult. The various agents used include ciclopirox solution 8% in a nail lacquer formulation (daily). Amorolofine nail lacquer is worth a trial and is applied once or twice a week for 6 months; it is effective against stubborn molds such as *Hendersonula* and *Scopulariopsis*. Lately efinaconazole 10% solution has successfully been tried in DLSO.

SUPERFICIAL YEAST INFECTIONS

Tinea Versicolor

Tinea versicolor (pityriasis versicolor) is a common fungal infection caused by *Malassezia*,[Q] a lipophilic, **dimorphic** yeast.[Q] It is more prevalent in young adults and is seen in the summer months and in tropical areas and is not infectious.

Pathophysiology

Tinea versicolor is caused by *Malassezia furfur*[Q] and *Malassezia globosa*,[Q] which are saprophytes that normally colonize the skin. After converting to their mycelial form, they spread into the superficial epidermis, resulting in the appearance of the rash. In humans, the seborrheic areas (scalp, face, back, and trunk) are always colonized by one or several species of the *Malassezia* genus (Fig. 5.21).

Clinical Features

Patients usually present during the summer months with a history of asymptomatic, hypopigmented or hyperpigmented, scaly areas on the trunk.[Q] The patient's chief complaint is usually cosmetic, because these lesions do not tan with sun exposure.

Macules with a fine powdery scale are seen on the upper arms, upper chest (Fig. 5.22), back, and occasionally on the face (children). The initial lesions are 3 to 5 mm, oval or round macules. Over the course of time, they may coalesce and cover more extensive areas of the body creating large irregularly shaped patches. The color of lesions varies from white to reddish-brown to tan-colored. Hypopigmentation is very conspicuous in dark-skinned individuals and the hypopigmentation may last for weeks or months until the area has repigmented through sunlight exposure.

Investigation

If a Wood's light examination is performed, the lesions will appear hypopigmented but not chalk white, as in vitiligo.[Q] Sometimes the scale fluoresces pale yellow or orange, but this finding is not always seen.

The organisms are seen in the stratum corneum (Fig. 5.23).

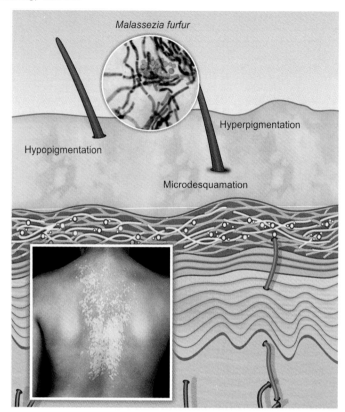

Fig. 5.21: A figurative depiction of the infections caused by *Malassezia* (pityriasis versicolor)

KOH examination of infected scale shows numerous strands of fungal hyphae (mycelia) and numerous spores commonly referred to as **'spaghetti and meatballs'**.[Q]

Differential Diagnosis

1. *Seborrheic dermatitis:* Presents with scaly, pink patches on the central trunk; usually the scalp and central face are involved. KOH examination is negative.
2. *Pityriasis rosea:* Presents initially with a pink herald patch with a very fine peripheral scale (collarette scale). Approximately 1 week later, multiple similar but smaller lesions develop on the chest and back, usually in a 'Christmas tree' pattern.[Q] KOH examination is negative.
3. *Vitiligo:* Presents with macular areas of complete pigment loss, with no scale or other surface changes.

Treatment (Box 5.3)

- 2.5% selenium sulfide lotion and 2% ketoconazole shampoo are cost-effective first-line treatments. *Ketoconazole* shampoo lather should be applied to damp skin of all involved areas and left on for 5 minutes, and then showered off. Selenium sulfide lotion should be applied to involved areas and left on for 10 minutes, and then showered off and reapplied in the same manner for 7 days. In warmer humid weather, the application of these medications may need to be repeated biweekly or monthly to prevent recurrence.

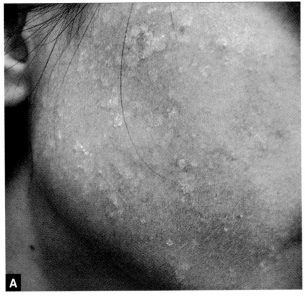 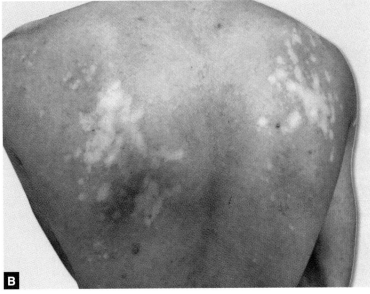

Fig. 5.22A and B: (A) Pityriasis versicolor: Multiple scaly macules on the face of an adult female; (B) Depigmented well-circumscribed macules coalescing at places over the back of a 25-year-old male

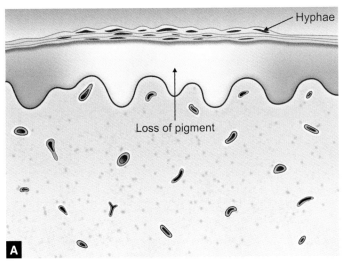 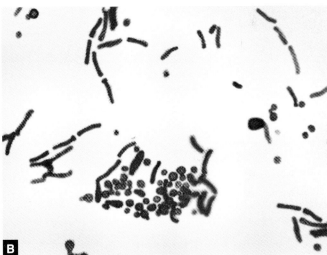

Fig. 5.23A and B: Histology of tinea versicolor. (A) The organism has a classic spaghetti and meatball appearance (B)

- Clotrimazole, miconazole, and ketoconazole creams are inexpensive treatment options. The creams are applied nightly for 2 to 3 weeks and then repeated on once a month basis to prevent recurrences.
- Oral antifungals could be used for extensive cases in adults that do not respond to topical treatments (Box 5.3). Oral fluconazole is the cheapest therapy and in adults a single 200–300 mg dose, which may be repeated. Efficacy is enhanced, if the patient "works up" a sweat 2 hours after ingesting the fluconazole, thereby delivering the drug, which is concentrated in sweat, to the stratum corneum. For recurrent disease, this regimen can be repeated every 3 months for 1 year. Intraconazole is effective in a total dose of 800–1000 mg.

Oral terbinafine and griseofulvin are *not* effective therapies.[Q]

Box 5.3	Therapy of pityriasis versicolor
Topical agents	• Apply 2.5% selenium sulfide lotion and 2% ketoconazole shampoo Rinse after 10 minutes Repeat this 3 days in a row, then for 4 weeks, then monthly to prevents recurrence
Systemic agents	• Ketoconazole 200 mg daily for 7 to 10 days • Itraconazole 200 mg daily for 5 days or 100 mg daily for 10 days • Fluconazole 300 mg as a pulse 1 day a week for 2 to 4 weeks

Clinical improvement is not evident until 3 to 4 weeks after treatment. Patients should be advised that pigmentation changes will resolve slowly over several weeks with the aid of exposure to sunlight.

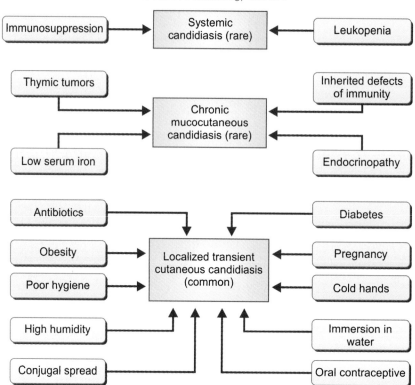

Fig. 5.23C: Factors that predispose to candidiasis

CANDIDIASIS

Introduction

C. albicans is often present as part of the normal flora in the mouth, gastrointestinal tract, and vagina. In certain scenarios, it can become a pathogen, especially in the vaginal tract and intertriginous areas. Risk factors for superficial candidiasis[Q] include infancy, pregnancy, aging, occlusion of epithelial surfaces (dentures, occlusive dressings), maceration, immunodeficiency, diabetes, obesity, and use of medications such as oral glucocorticoids and antibiotics[Q] (Fig. 5.23C).

Pathogenesis

Candida is a **dimorphic** yeast that has the ability to transform from a budding yeast phase to an invasive mycelia growth phase, which is necessary for tissue infection (Fig. 5.24). The most common cause of superficial candidiasis is *C. albicans*.[Q] Occasionally, other species such as *Candida glabrata*, *C. tropicalis*, *C. krusei*, and *C. parapsilosis* can be pathogenic.

Clinical Features

Various sites can be involved as shown in Fig. 5.25 and discussed below.

Oral Candidiasis

Though there are many forms, the classic variant is the acute pseudomembranous candidiasis (thrush) (Fig. 5.26). Here one or more whitish adherent plaques appear on

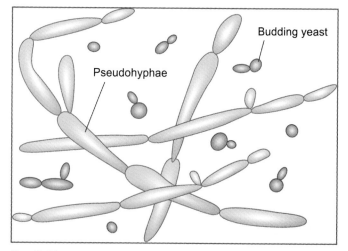

Fig. 5.24: A depiction of the pseudohyphae which are non-septate (candidiasis)

the mucous membranes which when wiped off, they leave an erythematous base. Under dentures, candidiasis will produce sore red areas. The predisposing factors include:

1. Dentures
2. Steroids
3. Antibiotics
4. Immunosuppression

Angular stomatitis (cheilitis):[Q] Usually in denture wearers may be candidal but in most cases represents a combination of fungal and bacterial infection, e.g. *C. albicans* and *Staphylococcus aureus* (Fig. 5.27).

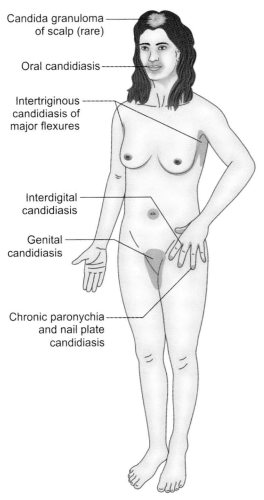

Candida granuloma of scalp (rare)

Oral candidiasis

Intertriginous candidiasis of major flexures

Interdigital candidiasis

Genital candidiasis

Chronic paronychia and nail plate candidiasis

Fig. 5.25: Depiction of the sites of involvement in candidiasis

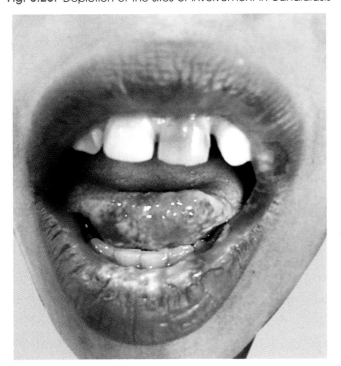

Fig. 5.26: Pseudomembranous candidiasis: White deposits present on the labial mucosa and tongue which on removal leaves an erythematous mucosal surface

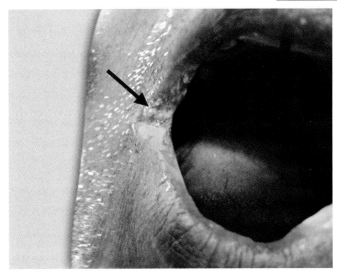

Fig. 5.27: A case of angular cheilitis—the skin folds at the angles of the mouth are red and eroded

Other variants

Acute atrophic candidiasis:[Q] Often painful, flat erythematous areas; typically involves tongue and is secondary to long-term antibiotic usage.

Chronic hyperplastic candidiasis:[Q] Thick persistent white plaques, usually in men; not easily removed; chronic atrophic candidiasis affects denture wearers; atrophic dusky erythematous area confined to area under denture (Fig. 5.28).

Median rhomboid glossitis:[Q] Erythematous rhomboid patch without papillae on the midline of the dorsal surface of the tongue.

Treatment

* Fluconazole: Fluconazole (200 mg/day × 7 days for adults)
  Fluconazole oral suspension 2–3 mg/kg daily for children
* Itraconazole: 100 mg of itraconazole administered twice daily (200 mg/day) for 14 days.
* Clotrimazole: Children and adults are effectively treated by clotrimazole oral paint
* Amphotericin B (80 mg/mL) may be used as a rinse.
* Gentian violet solution 1 to 2% may be tried in difficult or recurrent cases.

Candidal Intertrigo

A moist glazed area of erythema and maceration appears in a body fold; the edge shows soggy scaling and outlying satellite papulopustules. These changes are most common under the breasts, and in the armpits and groin, but can also occur between the fingers of those whose hands are often in water (Fig. 5.29A and B).

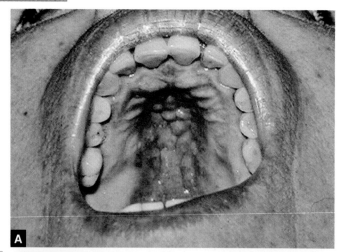

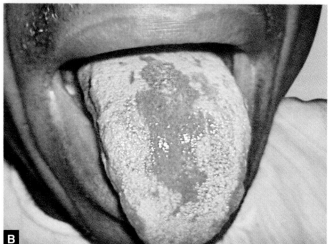

Fig. 5.28A and B: (A) Denture stomatitis also known as chronic erythematous candidiasis; (B) The central part of the tongue shows atrophic erythematous candidiasis

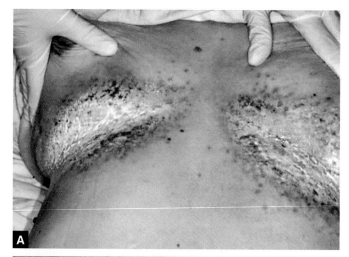

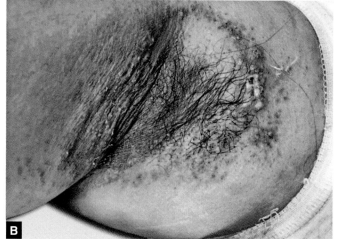

Fig. 5.29A and B: (A) Intertrigo with central maceration and peripheral pustules (candidiasis); (B) Pinpoint pustules seen at the advancing border are an important clue for diagnosing candidal intertrigo

Treatment

Fluconazole

- 50 to 100 mg daily for 14 days
- 150 mg weekly for 2–4 weeks

Itraconazole

- 200 mg twice daily for 14 days

Genital Candidiasis

Most commonly presents as a sore itchy vulvovaginitis, with white curdy plaques adherent to the inflamed mucous membranes, and a whitish discharge^Q (Fig. 5.30). The eruption may extend to the groin folds. Conjugal spread is common; in males similar changes occur under the foreskin and in the groin. Diabetes, pregnancy and antibiotic therapy are common predisposing factors.

In males, there are pustules on a red base with fissuring of the prepucial skin (Fig. 5.31).

Treatment: Apart from topical agents, clotrimazole 1% or miconazole 2%, systemic antifungal agents.

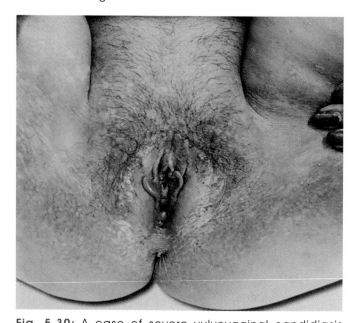

Fig. 5.30: A case of severe vulvovaginal candidiasis characterized by extensive vulvar erythema, edema, excoriation, and whitish deposits on the vulva with discharge

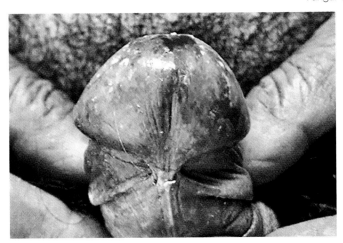

Fig. 5.31: A case of candidal balanitis, with multiple pustules on an erythematous base

Fluconazole 150 mg can be given either as a single dose or in case of RVVC (recurrent vulvovaginal candidiasis) 100, 150, or 200 mg oral dose of fluconazole every third day for a total of three doses (days 1, 4, and 7).

Paronychia

Acute paronychia is usually bacterial, but in chronic paronychia *Candida* may be the sole pathogen, or be found with other opportunists such as *Proteus* or *Pseudomonas* sp.

Acute paronychia is painful, red, and swollen, and may be accompanied by an abscess or cellulitis. The proximal and sometimes the lateral nail folds of one or more fingers become bolstered and red. Although any finger may be involved with paronychia, the second and third digits are the most commonly affected.

Chronic paronychia is characterized by loss of the cuticle, slight tenderness, swelling, erythema, and sometimes, separation of the nail fold from the plate. A purulent or 'cheesy' discharge and deformity of the nail plate are frequently seen. The cuticles are lost and small amount of pus can be expressed. The adjacent nail plate becomes ridged and discolored. Predisposing factors include wetwork, poor peripheral circulation and vulval candidiasis.

For chronic paronychia, a candidal origin can be confirmed, if the pus under the cuticle is examined under KOH, but culture, if taken, often reveals mixed flora, including bacteria and Candida species.

Treatment: Successful treatment of a chronic paronychia often requires weeks to months, and nails will grow out normally within 3 to 6 months of the paronychia healing.
- Avoid trauma, water, and irritants
- An imidazole, such as ketoconazole, sertaconazole, clotrimazole, miconazole, or ciclopirox olamine, should be applied several times a day. If there is associated pain or edema, use a combined steroid-antifungal ointment.

- Amphotericin B lotion or cream or 1% alcoholic solution of gentian violet may also be used.
- Fluconazole (200 mg/day) for 1 to 4 weeks may sometimes control chronic inflammation.

Treatment for acute paronychia is as under:
- Cephalexin: 25–50 mg/kg daily in oral suspension, 500 mg bid.
- Erythromycin: 30–50 mg/kg daily in oral suspension, 500 mg bid.
- Dicloxacillin: 500 mg bid.

Chronic Mucocutaneous Candidiasis

Persistent candidiasis, affecting most or all of the areas, starts in infancy. Patients have persistent cutaneous, mucosal, and nail infections, usually with *Candida albicans*. Candida granulomas may appear on the scalp. Several different forms have been described including those with autosomal recessive and dominant inheritance patterns.

In Candida endocrinopathy syndrome, chronic candidiasis occurs with one or more endocrine defects, the most common of which are hypoparathyroidism,[Q] and Addison's disease. A few late-onset cases have underlying thymic tumors.

DEEP FUNGAL INFECTIONS

This includes subcutaneous and systemic mycosis. Subcutaneous mycoses are caused by inoculation of naturally occurring fungi to the deeper tissues by a penetrating injury. They mostly occur in tropical countries and treatment is generally unsatisfactory.

Classification

i. Mycetoma
ii. Chromoblastomycosis
iii. Sporotrichosis
iv. Zygomycosis (phycomycosis)
   Entomophthoromycosis (conidiobolomycosis, basidiobolomycosis)
   Mucormycosis
v. Hyalohyphomycosis
vi. Phaeohyphomycosis

Mycetoma

Chronic soft tissue infection caused by a wide variety of fungi and bacteria; placed under fungal infections for convenience. Also called Madura foot (from the Indian state of Madura).

Pathogenesis

The list of causative agents is long. All cause disease in the same way—they are inoculated into the skin via an injury and then proliferate in the subcutaneous tissue, extending to fascia, muscles, and bones.

Two types:[Q]

Eumycetoma: Caused by fungi in the genera *Aspergillus, Exophiala, Madurella, Pseudallescheria,* and others.[Q]

Actinomycetoma: Caused by bacteria in the genera *Actinomadura, Actinomyces, Nocardia,* and *Streptomyces.*[Q] (*SAN: Streptomyces, Actinomadura, Actinomyces and Nocardia*).

Clinical Features

Initial finding is a soft tissue swelling, usually involving the foot. The condition progresses to involve deeper structures with formation of abscesses and draining sinuses with discharge of colored granules (Fig. 5.32) (colonies of organisms).

Investigation

The granules have different colors (white, yellow, black), which give clues to the organisms; microscopic examination and culture needed to confirm diagnosis.

Therapy

Culture-directed antibiotic or antifungal therapy, the latter usually with amphotericin B. The bacterial forms are relatively therapy-responsive; the eumycetomas are often resistant and amputation is the most reasonable approach.

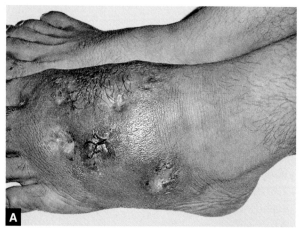

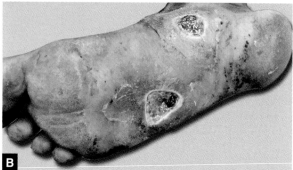

Fig. 5.32A and B: (A) A case of eumycetoma with chronic swelling of the dorsum of foot, fumefaction and sinuses; (B) A case of eumycetoma with visible black grains (*Courtesy:* Dr. Ramya, RML Hospital)

Sporotrichosis

Subcutaneous and occasionally systemic mycosis caused by *Sporothrix schenckii.*[Q]

Pathogenesis

The fungus is inoculated through injuries, usually from wood or plants;[Q] a classic injury is from a rose thorn. Common in farmers and gardeners.

Clinical Features (Fig. 5.33)

Lymphangitic sporotrichosis: Verrucous papules and plaques develop following inoculation. Then spread with firm subcutaneous nodules appearing along the path of lymphatic drainage.[Q]

Fixed sporotrichosis: In this form, many spores are inoculated by abrasion.

Systemic sporotrichosis: Rare; involves lungs, muscles, bones, and even CNS.

Investigation

Occasionally, cigar-shaped yeasts[Q] can be seen on biopsy with periodic acid-Schiff (PAS) stain;[Q] *Sporothrix schenckii* is dimorphic; culture at 25°C reveals a mold and at 37°C, a yeast. Biopsy findings classically shows asteroid bodies[Q] (Fig. 5.34).

Therapy

Itraconazole 400–600 mg per oral daily for 6–8 weeks. With systemic involvement, amphotericin B also is a possibility. Potassium iodide preparations are also used.

Localized lesions can be treated with either cryotherapy or hyperthermia to speed healing.

Chromoblastomycosis

Chronic infection, usually involving foot or leg, following inoculation injury with soil-borne fungi.

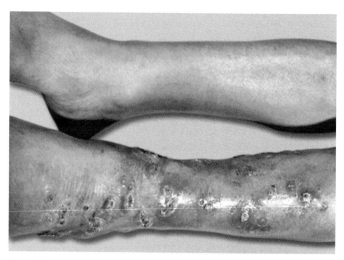

Fig. 5.33A: Erythematous crusted plaques over right lower limb, arranged linearly (sporotrichosis)

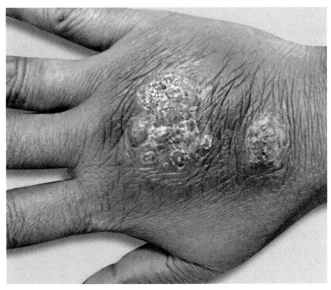

Fig. 5.33B: A 'fixed' plaque with ulceration on the dorsum of the hand. A case of fixed sporotrichosis

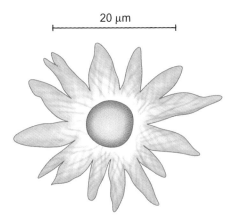

Fig. 5.34: Asteroid body (sporotrichosis)

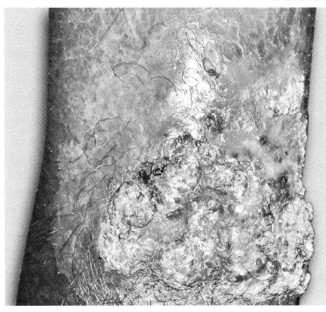

Fig. 5.35: Chromoblastomycosis: Verrucous cauliflower-like growth on the limbs

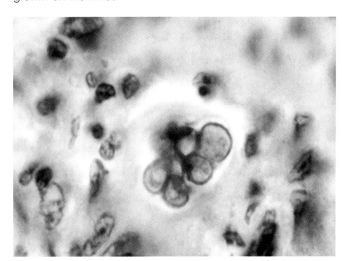

Fig. 5.36: **Medlar bodies** seen in chromoblastomycosis

Causative Agents

Many dematiaceous fungi including *Phialophora verrucosa*, *Fonsecaea pedrosoi*, *Fonsecaea compacta*, *Cladosporium carrionii*, *Rhinocladiella aquaspersa*.

Clinical Features

The lesion is characterized by development of verrucous nodules and plaques at the site of injury (mossy foot) (Fig. 5.35).

Investigation

Histology reveals subcutaneous granulomas containing small (5–15 µm) brown bodies that divide by equatorial splitting, not budding. They have many names: Copper pennies, sclerotic bodies, Medlar bodies[Q] (Fig. 5.36).

Therapy

Small lesions should be excised.

Systemic antifungal therapy is difficult; itraconazole and voriconazole are least toxic. Amphotericin B intralesional is a useful adjunct. Cryotherapy and hyperthermia may also be of supplemental value.

Zygomycosis (Mucormycosis)

Fungi of the Zygomycetes class (Mucor, Rhizomucor, Rhizopus, and others).

Clinical Features

Seen in immunosuppressed or diabetic patients; cutaneous inoculation or sinus infections which can extend to the CNS.

- *Rhinocerebral* disease may manifest as unilateral, retro-orbital headache, facial pain, numbness, fever, hyposmia, and nasal stuffiness, which progresses to black discharge (Fig. 5.37A and B). Initially, mucormycosis may mimic sinusitis. Late symptoms that indicate invasion of the orbital nerves and

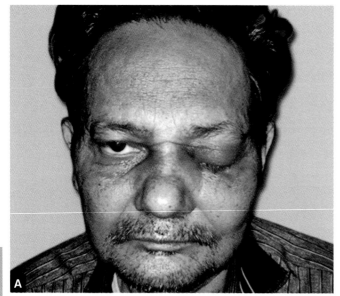
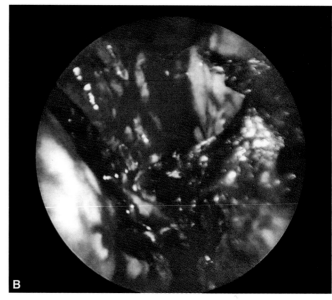

Fig. 5.37A and B: (A) A patient showing the drooping of eyelids because of complete ophthalmoplegia due to mucormycosis; (B) Nasal endoscopic picture showing black necrotic crusts in the nasal cavity (mucormycosis) (*Courtesy*: Dr Pooja Arora)

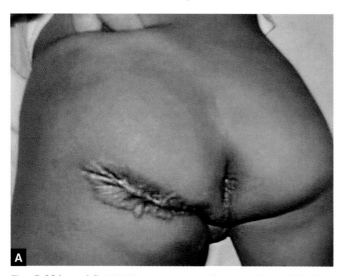
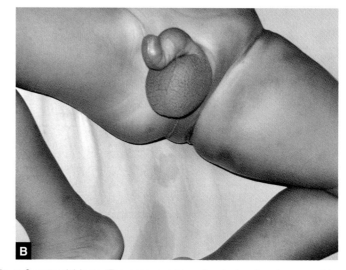

Fig. 5.38A and B: (A) Woody hard swelling over the left buttock in a 2-year-old boy. (The scar overlying the lesion is subsequent to inappropriate incision and drainage); (B) Swelling of the scrotum and shaft of penis resembling 'saxophone' penis (zygomycosis) (*Courtesy*: Dr Pooja Arora)

vessels include diplopia and visual loss. Orbital swelling and facial cellulitis are progressive.

- Other variants are *pulmonary* and *cutaneous* variants.

Treatment: Amphotericin B plus debridement.

Subcutaneous Zygomycosis
(Basidiobolus and Conidiobolus)

Subcutaneous granulomas in non-immunosuppressed children; Indonesia, India and Africa.

Clinical Features

Basidiobolomycosis affects the limb or limb girdle area of children. Rarely other parts of the body may be involved. The disease presents as a single painless, subcutaneous swelling with a hard consistency that does not pit on pressure[Q] (Fig. 5.38A and B). The smooth edge can be raised up by inserting the fingers underneath.

Conidiobolomycosis (Fig. 5.39) causes subcutaneous inflammation of the submucosa in the central facial region. It is mainly seen in young adults. The disease starts from the inferior turbinates and spreads to involve the facial tissues. Nasal obstruction occurs first followed by infiltration and thickening of the skin over the nose with subsequent deformity.

Treatment

Itraconazole is the treatment of choice and is used in a dose of 300 mg/day. Saturated solution of potassium iodide may be used in doses similar to sporotrichosis.

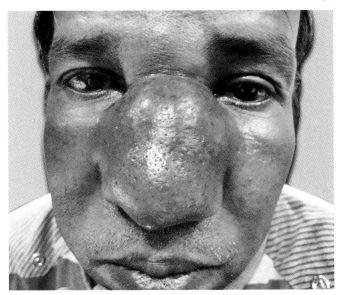

Fig. 5.39: Conidiobolomycosis

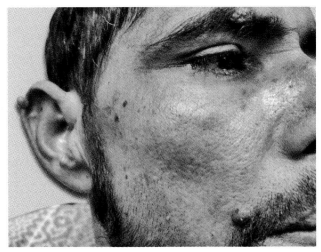

Fig. 5.40: Molluscoid papulo-nodules on the face, ear and over the eyebrow (cryptococcosis)

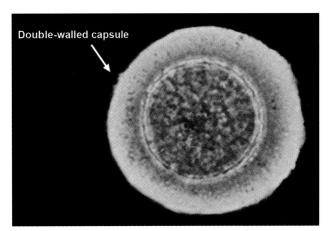

Fig. 5.41: Double-walled yeast cell of cryptococcosis

Cotrimoxazole has been shown to be effective in conidiobolomycosis and may be added to first-line treatment.

SYSTEMIC MYCOSIS

The systemic mycoses are caused by dimorphic fungi that live as a yeast or a mold, depending on environmental conditions. They often cause asymptomatic infections in healthy individuals, but are frequently more aggressive in weakened individuals. Risk factors include HIV/AIDS, cancer chemotherapy, solid organ transplantation, and long-term intensive care treatment. This is an elaborate topic that is not within the purview of this book, thus only a few important infections are being discussed below.

Cryptococcosis

Pathogenesis

Cryptococcus neoformans is presumably spread from bird droppings. Initial infection is via the lungs; dissemination seen only in immunosuppressed individuals.

Clinical Features

CNS is the main organ of involvement and can present as chronic meningitis or may simulate a brain tumor. This may be accompanied by fever.

Cutaneous lesions (that occur due to dissemination) may occur before or after the appearance of CNS or pulmonary symptoms. Skin is involved in 10% of cases. The presentation is variable and can range from multiple papulo-nodules (around the nose and mouth) to ulcers (punched out with rolled edge) and abscesses, molluscum contagiosum-like lesions (Fig. 5.40). Most frequent type of cutaneous lesions are subcutaneous erythema nodosum-like swellings.

Encapsulated budding cells (5–15 μm) can be seen in tissue sections or in direct microscopy of CSF or pus. PAS stain can be used to visualize the yeast form, whereas mucicarmine or alcian blue stain helps to visualize the capsule (Fig. 5.41). India ink preparations can also be used.

Therapy

Previous mainstays of therapy were amphotericin B and flucytosine. Fluconazole appears effective for meningitis; voriconazole also shows promise.

Histoplasmosis

Epidemiology

Histoplasma capsulatum var. *capsulatum* is the most common cause.

Pathogenesis

Primary infection is in the lungs. Reactivation occurs after many years, causing chronic pulmonary disease. An aggressive course may be seen in children or in HIV/AIDS with widespread involvement (Fig. 5.42).

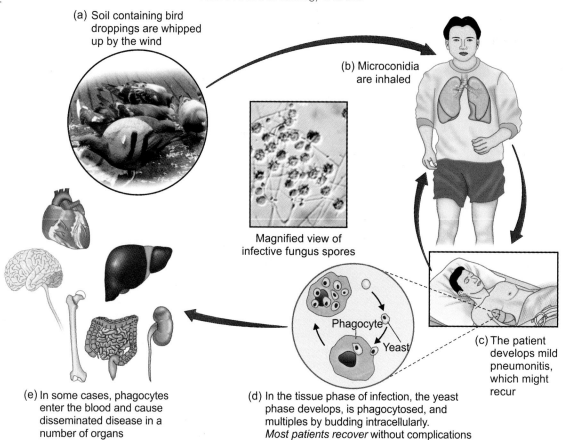

(a) Soil containing bird droppings are whipped up by the wind

(b) Microconidia are inhaled

Magnified view of infective fungus spores

Phagocyte

Yeast

(c) The patient develops mild pneumonitis, which might recur

(e) In some cases, phagocytes enter the blood and cause disseminated disease in a number of organs

(d) In the tissue phase of infection, the yeast phase develops, is phagocytosed, and multiples by budding intracellularly. *Most patients recover* without complications

Fig. 5.42: Overview of pathogenesis of histoplasmosis

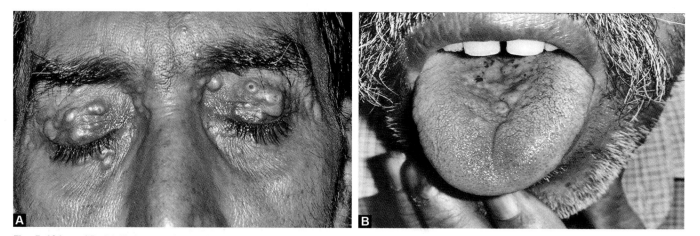

Fig. 5.43A and B: Multiple papules and nodules in a case of histoplasmosis in an HIV patient. The patient was put on amphotericin B but died after 2 weeks due to pulmonary complications

Clinical Features

Skin involvement is uncommon in disseminated disease; less than 10% have papules or nodules following hematogenous seeding (Fig. 5.43A and B). Oral infiltrates and ulcers are more common. Major systemic problems are hepatosplenomegaly, bone marrow infiltrates with pancytopenia, endocarditis, and meningitis.

Therapy

Itraconazole and ketoconazole are used for non-life-threatening cases. In immunosuppressed patients, initial control must be obtained with amphotericin B. In HIV/AIDS, once the infection is under control, then lifelong prophylaxis with itraconazole is needed.

Mycobacterial Infections: Tuberculosis

Chapter Outline

Mycobacteria are small, non-motile, slightly curved acid-fast rods. *Mycobacterium tuberculosis* causes almost 95% of human tuberculosis; *Mycobacterium bovis* is responsible for the rest.[Q]

Epidemiology

The male-to-female ratio is 1.5:1 in India. The men are more likely to have verrucous or ulcerative forms of cutaneous TB, while women have more of lupus vulgaris or scrofuloderma. While lupus vulgaris is more common in elderly, children frequently have scrofuloderma.

The commonest cutaneous TB is lupus vulgaris[Q] (57.5%) followed by scrofuloderma (35.4%), verrucous tuberculosis (4.5%) and ulcerative tuberculosis (2.6%).[Q]

Classification

There are numerous classification systems, but the easiest system depends on pathogenesis and the immune status of the individual (Table 6.1).

Primary infections are those where there is no previous immunity, and the tuberculin test is negative.

Secondary infections are those with pre-existing immunity, and the tuberculin test is positive.

The mode of causation can be either external (exogenous) or internal (endogenous). The latter can be either by direct contact or hematogenous.

Diagnostic Approach

- **Microscopic examination:** Staining with Ziehl-Neelsen stain or auramine fluorescence staining can be used to examine tissue sections or bodily fluids.

Table 6.1	Classification of cutaneous TB (immunity)
Primary	TB chancre (immunity –)
Secondary	***Exogenous:*** TB verrucosa cutis (immunity +)
	Endogenous: Scrofuloderma (contiguous) (immunity +)
	TB cutis orificialis (autoinoculation) (immunity –)
	Lupus vulgaris (hematogenous) (immunity +)
	*Gumma (hematogenous) (immunity –)
	**Miliary (lung) (immunity –)
Tuberculid[Q]	• Lichen scrofulosorum (immunity +)
	• Papulonecrotic tuberculid (immunity +)
	• Erythema induratum (immunity +)

*Tuberculous gumma—firm subcutaneous nodule or fluctuant swelling that often ulcerates.
**Miliary TB—small erythematous papules that develop central crusting and may resemble a viral exanthem or pityriasis lichenoides et varioliformis acuta (PLEVA).

Rapid, but only sensitive when large numbers of organisms are present (10^3–10^4/mL).[Q] Thus, in skin, useful for primary infections, gumma and scrofuloderma.

- **Culture:** Both species grow slowly on special media (Löwenstein-Jensen)[Q] under anaerobic conditions. Initial growth takes 3–10 weeks, followed by differentiation and determination of drug sensitivity (total of 2–3 months). BACTEC method with radiometric measurement of metabolites takes 7–10 days.[Q]

- **Other possibilities:** PCR for *Mycobacterium tuberculosis* DNA in skin biopsies; this technique has become important because it is difficult to culture the organisms in skin.

6

Box 6.1   Diagnostic criteria for skin TB

Absolute criteria
1. Recovery of bacilli from the lesion
2. Successful guinea pig innoculation
3. Positive culture or PCR isolation

Relative criteria
1. Clinical signs and symptoms
2. Presence of active systemic TB elsewhere in the body
3. Histopathology (tuberculoid pathology)
4. Positive tuberculin test/gamma interferon test
5. Therapeutic response to ATT in 6–8 weeks time.[Q]

- **IGRA:** The QuantiFERON®-TB Gold (In-Tube) test directly measures IFN-γ levels and is considered to be better than the conventional tuberculin test, for the following reasons:[Q]
  a. Requires a single patient visit.
  b. Results can be available within 24 hours.
  c. Prior BCG vaccination does not cause a false-positive result.
  d. Does not boost responses measured by subsequent tests.

For skin TB, a modified criterion is used for diagnosis as in most cases, culture and AB isolation are inconclusive (Box 6.1).

Treatment

Cutaneous tuberculosis should be treated with ATT, like any other systemic tuberculosis. The therapy for

Table 6.2	Overview of TB therapy guidelines under RNTCP[Q]	
Category	*Patient*	*Regimen†*
New	• Sputum smear-positive • Sputum smear-negative	• *Intensive phase* (IP) $2H_3R_3Z_3E_3$ • *Continuation phase* (CP) $4H_3R_3$
Previously treated	• Smear-positive relapse • Smear-positive failure • Smear-positive treatment after default • *Others**	• *Intensive phase* (IP) $2H_3R_3Z_3E_3S_3/1H_3R_3Z_3E_3$ • *Continuation phase* (CP) $5H_3R_3E_3$

*In rare and exceptional cases, patients who are sputum smear-negative or who have *extrapulmonary disease* can have recurrence or non-response.

†The number before the letters refers to the number of months of treatment. The subscript after the letters refers to the number of doses per week. The dosage strengths are as follows: Isoniazid (H) 600 mg, rifampicin (R) 450 mg, pyrazinamide (Z) 1500 mg, ethambutol (E) 1200 mg, streptomycin (S) 750 mg. Patients who weight 60 kg or more receive additional rifampicin 150 mg. Patients who are more than 50 years old receive streptomycin 500 mg.

cutaneous TB in India under the National Guidelines (http://www.tbcindia.org) is part of the extrapulmonary TB spectrum and is given in Table 6.2. Skin TB comes in the first category and four drugs are administered (HRZE) for 2 months followed by two drugs (HR) for 4 months (Table 6.2).

CLINICAL FORMS OF CUTANEOUS TUBERCULOSIS

Primary Cutaneous Tuberculosis
(Inoculation Tuberculosis)

Lesion resulting from direct introduction of *Mycobacterium tuberculosis* or *Mycobacterium bovis* into skin of previously unexposed host.

Epidemiology: Uncommon; most patients are children.

Clinical Features

- At first, small papules develop at inoculation site; they expand into a painless ulcer several centimeters across (primary lesion—analogous to tubercle in lung) (Fig. 6.1).
- After 3–8 weeks, regional lymphadenopathy appears (primary complex—analogous to Ghon complex).[Q] Healing within a year, usually with scarring.

TB Cutis Orificialis
Clinical Features

Patients with a high load of *Mycobacterium tuberculosis* and poor resistance develop mucosal lesions with ragged, painful oral ulcers. Prognosis is not good.

Tuberculosis Verrucosa Cutis

This is defined as a verrucous (wart-like) form of reinfection tuberculosis.

Pathogenesis

It occurs when the skin of a previously infected or BCG-immunized host, possessing a moderate or high degree

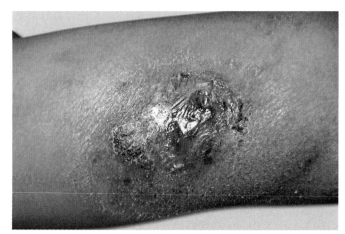

Fig. 6.1: A chronic relatively painless ulcer with associated lymph node enlargement in a child (TB chancre)

of immunity, is subjected to exogenous reinfection. Reinoculation occurs at sites of minor abrasions or wounds.

Occupation: It is commonly seen in physicians, pathologists, medical students, laboratory attendants, veterinarians, farmers,[Q] and butchers (tuberculous cattle). Historically, it was described after injuries during autopsies—known as prosector's wart.[Q]

Clinical Course

The main features are depicted in Box 6.2 and Fig. 6.2.

Scrofuloderma

Subcutaneous tuberculosis with development of cold abscesses and contiguous spread to skin.[Q]

Pathogenesis

The tuberculous foci are commonly in the lymph nodes (cervical lymph nodes most common),[Q] bones and joints, and epididymis. It originates as a tuberculous process of the subcutaneous tissues leading to the formation of cold abscesses and then secondary breakdown of the overlying skin. Scrofuloderma is the most common form of skin TB in children.[Q]

Clinical Course (Box 6.3)

An overview is given below and a set of images are given in Fig. 6.3A to C.

Differential diagnosis: Syphilitic gumma, deep fungal infections, acne conglobata, acne inversa.

Box 6.2	Overview of TBVC[Q]

Site: Hands and fingers, lower extremities
1. Initial lesion: Painless, dusky red, firm papule or papulo-pustule.
2. Expands peripherally and is surrounded by inflammatory halo.
3. It develops into a polycyclic, serpiginous, or annular plaque with a warty, advancing border and central area of atrophy
4. Pus and keratinous material may be expressed from the fissures in the warty areas.
5. Lymphadenopathy is rare
6. Paucibacillary, AFB (–ve)

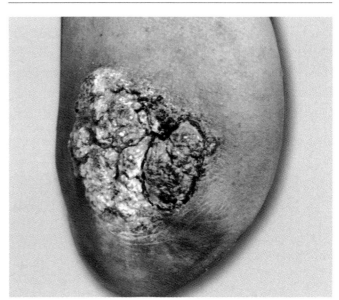

Fig. 6.2: Chronic verrucous growth with fissuring in a case of TBVC

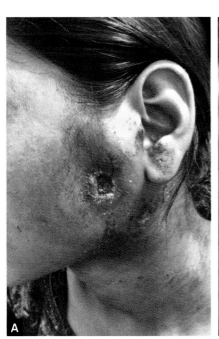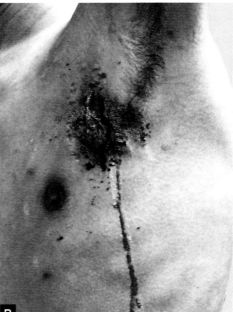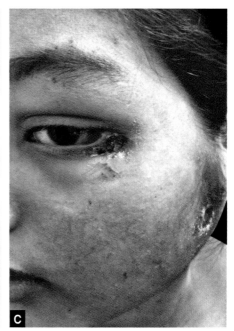

Fig. 6.3A to C: Scrofuloderma: (A) Chronic discharging sinus with underlying regional lymphadenopathy. (B and C) A female patient with discharging sinus on the cervical, preauricular and infraorbital area: Multifocal scrofuloderma

Box 6.3	Overview of scrofuloderma[Q]

1. Initial lesion: Firm, subcutaneous or deep cutaneous swelling or nodule.
2. Freely movable initially but soon attaches firmly to the skin and later ulcerates.
3. The ulcers have a bluish, undermined edges.
4. Watery, purulent, or caseous discharge may exude from the sinuses.
5. Lesions heal with cord-like scarring.
6. Mulibacillary, AFB(++)

Lupus Vulgaris

It is a reinfection tuberculosis of the skin and is seen in previously sensitized individuals with high immunity.[Q]

Epidemiology

Most frequent types of cutaneous tuberculosis in adults:[Q]
- Two-thirds of patients with lupus have visceral foci of tuberculosis.

- Almost 40% have tuberculous adenitis or involvement of the mucous membranes.
- 10 to 20% have pulmonary, bone, or joint tuberculosis.

Clinical Course

Site: Lower extremities, especially the buttocks, are the primary site of involvement (India).[Q] Also seen on the face (nose and cheeks, followed by the ears), the extensor surfaces of the extremities.

When one presses on a lupus nodule with a sound (blunt object), it break through the nodule with little pain 'sound phenomenon'.[Q]

The overview is given in Box 6.4 and a set of images are depicted in Fig. 6.4A to D.

Tuberculids

Symmetrical, generalized exanthem in the skin of a tuberculous patient, which is due to an allergic or hypersensitivity reaction to the tubercle bacillus or one of its constituent parts. The diagnosis is based on the following features (Box 6.5).

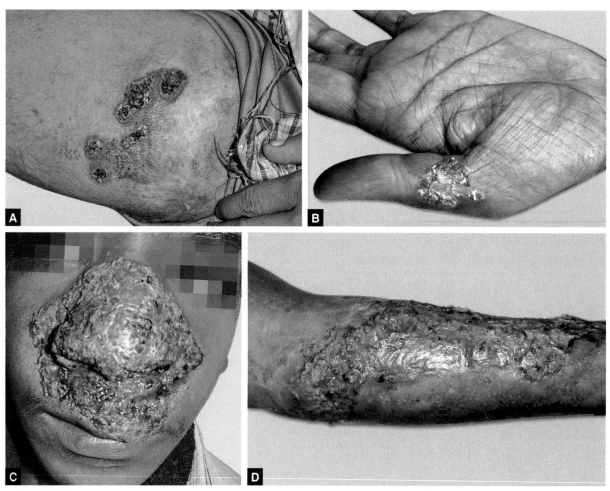

Fig. 6.4A to D: (A) A case of lupus vulgaris with a plaque showing activity at one edge and healing at the other edge; (B) A chronic scaly plaque on the thumb that was treated as a case of contact dermatitis; (C) Large plaque with hypertrophy and areas of ulceration on the nose in a child; (D) Chronic serpiginous non-healing ulcer diagnosed as a case of pyoderma gangrenosum (ulcerative lupus vulgaris)

| Box 6.4 | Overview of lupus vulgaris[Q] |

1. Earliest lesion appears as small, brownish red papules of soft gelatinous consistency.
2. The lesions have an advancing serpiginous edge with scarring in centre.
3. As the lesions enlarge, caseation necrosis proceeds, resulting in softening of the lesions.
4. On diascopy,[Q] the characteristic translucent, apple jelly[Q] colored lupoid infiltrates can be seen.
5. Paucibacillary, AFB(–ve).

| Box 6.5 | Diagnosis of tuberculid[Q] (Darier, 1896) |

Diagnostic criteria

1. Positive tuberculin skin test
2. Tuberculous involvement of lymph nodes or internal viscera or both.
3. Absence of tubercle bacilli from skin biopsy and culture.
4. Skin lesions that heal on remission of the tuberculous infection.

The common tuberculids are:[Q]
- Lichen scrofulosorum (most common)[Q]
- Papulonecrotic tuberculid
- Erythema induratum
- DNA PCR has shown *M. tuberculosis* in these disorders

Clinical Features

- *Lichen scrofulosorum*: Sites of predilection are the sides of the trunk. Lesions are arranged parallel to the skin relaxation lines. Eruption is asymptomatic.

  The rash is composed of symmetrically arranged groups of tiny papules (Fig. 6.5). The primary lesion is a white, pale-yellow, brown, pale-red, or skin-colored follicular or perifollicular soft papule with a fine scale on its summit. The lesions may form annular patches.
- *Papulonecrotic tuberculid*: Girls and young women (more susceptible).

  Typically, symmetrical, loosely disseminated, grouped eruptions of papulonecrotic lesions arise in crops on the extensor surfaces of the extremeties, lower trunk and buttock (Fig. 6.6). The eruption tends to worsen in the winter and fade in the summer months.
- *Erythema induratum*: This is a form of panniculitis. The classic feature is of subcutaneous nodules that may ulcerate and the commonest site is the posterior calves (Fig. 6.7).

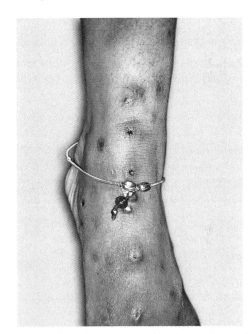

Fig. 6.6A: Lower limb shows symmetrical papules and nodules with central crusting—papulonecrotic tuberculid

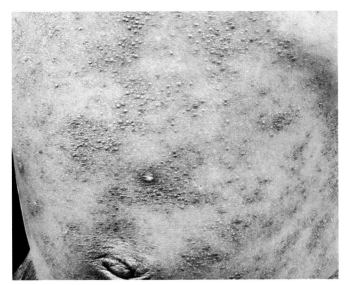

Fig. 6.5: Perifollicular grouped papules seen over the trunk in a 10-year-old boy with 'lichen scrofulosorum'

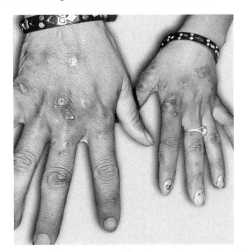

Fig. 6.6B: Hand shows symmetrical papules and nodules with central crusting in a case of papulonecrotic tuberculid

Table 6.3	An overview of atypical mycobacteriosis[Q]

Organism	Mode of infection	Clinical morphology
M. marinum (Others: *M. kansasii, M. simiae*) *Slow grower, photochromogen*	History of trauma and water or fish/seafood-related hobbies	Site: Hand • Verrucous papules or nodules (*swimming pool granuloma*);[Q] • Sometimes associated with sporotrichoid—lymphangitic spread
M. ulcerans (Others: *M. tuberculosis, M. avium, M. haemophilum, M. bovis*) *Slow grower, nonchromogen*	Infection occurs in wet, marshy or swampy areas. Most commonly occurs in children and young adults	**Buruli ulcer** (*M. ulcerans*)[Q]: The ulcer is deeply undermined, and necrotic fat is exposed. It may destroy nerves and blood vessels
M. avium-intracellulare *Slow grower, nonchromogen*	HIV/AIDS Pneumonia, osteomyelitis, and lymphadenopathy	More likely to cause localized disease such as soft tissue abscesses or lymphadenitis Rarely cutaneous papules and nodules
M. scrofulaceum (Others: *M. szulgai, M. gordonae, M. xenopi*) *Slow grower, scotochromogen*	It presents as lymphadenitis in young children of 1 to 3 years	**Submandibular and submaxillary** nodes are typically involved[Q]
M. fortuitum complex (Others: *M. abscessus, M. chelonae, M. fortuitum*) *Rapid grower*	Route of infection by contamination of various materials, including surgical supplies	Primary cutaneous inoculation occurs through skin injuries (puncture wound or surgical procedure), in all age group, without immunosuppression. Also called injection abscess[Q]

Slow growers: 2–3 *weeks*; Rapid growers: 3–5 *days*
Photochromogens: Capable of yellow pigment formation upon exposure to light.
Scotochromogens: Capable of yellow pigment production without light exposure.

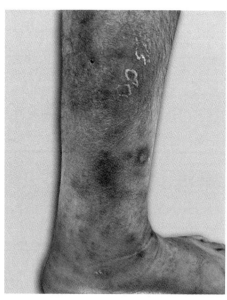

Fig. 6.7: A female patient with recurrent nodules on the calves—erythema induratum

ATYPICAL TUBERCULOSIS

In contrast to *M. tuberculosis*, atypical mycobacteria, is acquired from environmental sources (water, soil). The following features define their clinical features:

• They are usually commensals or saprophytes than pathogenetic.

• An immunosuppressed state of the host or damage to particular organ facilitates these infections.

• Infection with atypical mycobacteria run a more benign and limited course than *M. tuberculosis*.

• They are less responsive to antituberculous drugs, but may be sensitive to other chemotherapeutic drugs. The therapy is based on local expertise and includes doxycycline, rifampicin, macrolides, rifampicin and ethambutol in various combinations.

An overview of mode of infection and clinical features is given in Table 6.3.

Leprosy

INTRODUCTION

Leprosy, also known as Hansen's disease, is a chronic, infectious, granulomatous disease caused by *Mycobacterium leprae* with spectral clinical presentation determined by the immune status of the host.

Mycobacterium leprae is an acid- and alcohol-fast, Gram-positive bacilli, measuring nearly 5 × 0.5 μm in size. The *acid-fastness* is due to the presence of *mycolic acid* in the cell wall of the bacteria.[Q]

ETIOPATHOGENESIS

- *M. leprae* replicate by binary fission in **11–13 days** (generation time) and can survive outside the human body for 3–9 days.
- Incubation period is believed to be between 2 and 5 years.[Q]
- Route of infection is primarily through *respiratory tract*[Q] but percutaneous infection may also be important. Man is the only known natural reservoir of *M. leprae*.[Q]
- The attack rate among household contacts of lepromatous cases varies from 4.4 to 12%.
- The relative risk for a household contact of a patient to have the leprosy is 8–10 for lepromatous disease and 2–4 for the tuberculoid forms.
- HLA DR2 and DR3 alleles are associated with tuberculoid disease, while HLA DR1[Q] is linked to lepromatous leprosy.

- The characteristic *virulence factor* of *M. leprae* is phenolic glycolipid I,[Q] a prominent surface lipid, specific of this bacillus and is also used for serological diagnosis of leprosy.[Q]
- Target organ of *M. leprae* is Schwann cells of peripheral nerves and nerves are involved in 100% of cases.[Q] Systemic involvement is seen in highly bacillated forms. Since *M. leprae* prefers cooler areas of the body, more commonly involved sites include skin, peripheral nerves, anterior eye, lymphoid organs, liver, upper respiratory tract, testes, kidneys, etc.
- The warmer areas of the body and some internal organs are not involved and are called *sanctuary* sites or *immune zones* of leprosy (Scalp, axillae, groin, transverse band of skin over lumbosacral area, midline of back and perineum, CNS, uterus, ovary, lower respiratory tract).[Q]

Epidemiology

- Leprosy is known since ancient times and has been a cause of significant physical/emotional morbidity and social stigma for the sufferers of the disease.
- It is known to occur at all ages ranging from early infancy to very old age, youngest patient being a **3-month**-old baby.
- Although, its prevalence has markedly reduced, it remains a major public health problem.
- The important epidemiological indicators have been detailed in Table 7.1.

Table 7.1 Epidemiological indicators of leprosy[Q]

Prevalence	Total number of cases of leprosy in a defined population at a specified time.
Incidence	Number of newly detected cases over a defined time
Annual new case detection rate	New cases recorded in an area per one lakh population
Deformity rate	Percentage of patients with deformities amongst newly detected cases in a period of one year
Criteria for leprosy elimination	Achievement of prevalence rate below 1 case per 10000 population[Q]

Table 7.2 Leprosy statistics 2015–2016

Indicator	World total	India
Prevalence rate (/10,000)	1.72	0.88
Incidence	214783	135485
No. of cases with Gr 2 disability	12819	5095

- Leprosy was eliminated from India in December 2005.[Q] The current global and Indian statistics are listed in Table 7.2.
- The most common type is the paucibacillary (PB) type (indeterminate Hansen's disease).[Q]

CLASSIFICATION

The clinical presentation of leprosy varies from mild to very severe, from a single cutaneous/neural lesion to the multiple systemic involvement, determined mainly by the host immunity. Various classification schemes have been proposed to explain the wide range of manifestations. The common ones include the following.

Ridley and Jopling Classification (1966)

- Based on *clinical, bacteriological, histological* and *immunological* criteria,[Q] it has been divided into five groups, which include 2 polar (stable) forms and 3 nonpolar (unstable) forms (Fig. 7.1):
  1. Tuberculoid type (TT)—stable
  2. Borderline tuberculoid (BT)
  3. Borderline borderline (BB)
  4. Borderline lepromatous (BL)
  5. Lepromatous leprosy type (LL)—stable
- The polar forms including TT group signify good host immunity, whereas LL patients are least immune. The borderline ones (BT, BB, BL) are unstable forms and can either upgrade or downgrade, depending upon host immune status and/or treatment. BB is the most unstable form of leprosy.[Q]
- It is a complex classification and is meant primarily for research purposes.

New IAL Classification (1981)

- The New Indian Association of Leprologists (IAL) classification is a simple clinico-bacteriological classification which has the following five classes:
  1. Lepromatous (L)
  2. Tuberculoid (T)
  3. Polyneuritic/pure neuritic (P)
  4. Borderline (B)
  5. Indeterminate (I)

WHO Classification (1988)[Q]

This is the most important classification for the treating physician. It divides the patients into paucibacillary (PB) and multibacillary (MB), based upon three criteria,

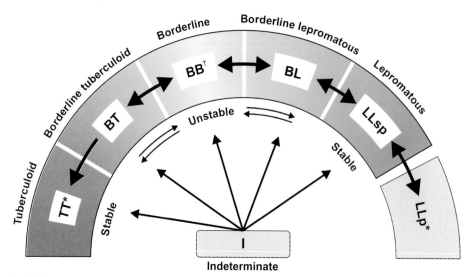

*Immunologically stable (if BT upgrades to TT, it is called TTs [subpolar]). †BB is the most unstable and inconsistent form and is thus rarely seen. The indeterminate form has not been described in the R-J classification

Fig. 7.1: Diagrammatic depiction of the relationship between various leprosy types according to the Ridley-Jopling classification

Table 7.3	WHO classification of leprosy (1988)		
S. no.	Characteristics	PB (paucibacillary)	MB (multibacillary)
1.	**Skin lesions**	1–5 lesions	6 and above
2.	**Peripheral nerve involvement**	No nerve/only one nerve with or without 1 to 5 lesions	More than one nerve irrespective of number of skin lesions
3.	**Skin smear**	Negative at all sites	Positive at any site

Note: If skin smear is positive irrespective of number of skin and nerve lesions, the disease is classified as MB leprosy, but if skin smear is negative, it is classified on the basis of the number of skin and nerve lesions.

as explained in Table 7.3. Amongst these, *SSS* is the *gold standard* criterion.^{Q}

Similar classification has also been proposed by the National Leprosy Eradication Program (NLEP), India (2009).

CLINICAL FEATURES AND IMMUNOLOGY

Leprosy has a wide range of clinical presentations with diverse signs and symptoms, complications and variable prognosis. The type of presentation is determined by interaction between the three processes:
- Multiplication and dissemination of *M. leprae*
- The patient immune response

The complications of peripheral nerve damage are a result of the first two processes.

It should be appreciated that though the disease has an immunological basis (Fig. 7.2), patients of leprosy have a specific diminution of immune status only towards *M. leprae* and are otherwise immunologically normal. The majority (95%) of those exposed do not develop the disease. Out of the rest (5%), 75% heal on their own, while of the remaining, the majority develop indeterminate lesions. Indeterminate leprosy often

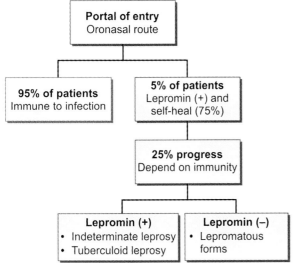

Fig. 7.2: Natural course of infection in leprosy

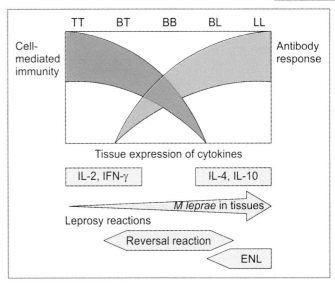

Fig. 7.3: Immunology of leprosy and leprosy reactions

heals spontaneously, but it may progress into the spectrum of determinate leprosy. The determinate types include the various types of PB or MB leprosy.

The varying clinical forms of leprosy are determined by the underlying immunological response to *M. leprae* (Fig. 7.3). At one pole, patients with tuberculoid leprosy **(TT)** have a high cellular immune response to the *Mycobacterium*, which limits the disease to a few well-defined skin patches or nerve trunks. Immune deviation is evident since skin and nerve lesions in tuberculoid leprosy are infiltrated by **Th1-like** T cells, which produce abundant interferon γ, TNF-α, and interleukins 2 and 15.

At the other pole, lepromatous leprosy **(LL)** is characterized by the absence of specific cellular immunity. There is uncontrolled proliferation of leprosy bacilli with many lesions and extensive infiltration of the skin and nerves. The dermis contains foamy macrophages filled with many bacteria, but a few CD4+ and CD8+ T lymphocytes and no organized granulomas. The lepromatous pole has **Th2-like** cytokines interleukins 4 and 10.

Most patients have the intermediate forms of borderline tuberculoid (BT), mid-borderline (BB), and borderline lepromatous (BL) leprosy but these are clinically unstable.

Type 1 leprosy reactions or reversal reactions are caused by spontaneous increase in T cell reactivity to mycobacterial antigens. Reversal reactions are associated with the infiltration of interferon γ producing CD4+ lymphocytes in skin lesions and nerves, resulting in edema and painful inflammation. Type 2 reaction or erythema nodosum leprosum (ENL) is a systemic inflammatory response to the deposition of extravascular immune complexes leading to neutrophil infiltration and activation of complement in many organs.

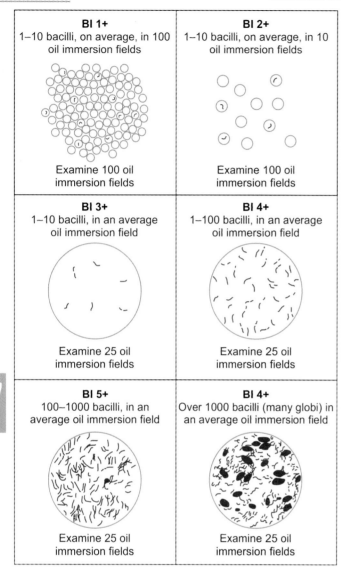

BI 1+
1–10 bacilli, on average, in 100 oil immersion fields

Examine 100 oil immersion fields

BI 2+
1–10 bacilli, on average, in 10 oil immersion fields

Examine 100 oil immersion fields

BI 3+
1–10 bacilli, in an average oil immersion field

Examine 25 oil immersion fields

BI 4+
1–100 bacilli, in an average oil immersion field

Examine 25 oil immersion fields

BI 5+
100–1000 bacilli, in an average oil immersion field

Examine 25 oil immersion fields

BI 4+
Over 1000 bacilli (many globi) in an average oil immersion field

Examine 25 oil immersion fields

Fig. 7.4: Calculation of BI in leprosy

CARDINAL SIGNS OF LEPROSY

- A case of leprosy is defined as an individual who has at least one of the three cardinal signs:[Q]
  1. Hypopigmented or erythematous skin lesions with definite loss/impairment of sensations.
  2. Involvement of peripheral nerves, as demonstrated by definite thickening with sensory impairment.
  3. Slit skin smear positive for acid-fast bacilli (Fig. 7.4).
     BI: Bacteriological Index: Live + dead bacilli (falls by 1 log/year). Used for classification.[Q]
     MI: Morphological Index: Live bacilli (becomes zero in 6 weeks of therapy). Used for monitoring therapy.[Q]

The WHO has modified these criteria for field workers by removing the last criterion and now any one of the first two is enough for diagnosing leprosy.

CLINICAL TYPES OF LEPROSY

The diagnosis of leprosy is usually a correlation of clinical signs along with the use of accessory tools such as slit smear and biopsy. The clinical diagnosis cannot be always perfect as the clinical features are a continuum of changes. Some general principles can help, which are given below. As an overview, the clinical features correlate with the immunity.

- *Higher the immunity*: Lesser the lesions (skin and nerve), asymmetrical, more nerve damage, less AFB, positive lepromin.
- *Lower the immunity*: More the lesion number (skin and nerve), papules, nodules, symmetrical, more AFB, less nerve damage, negative lepromin.

1. **Higher immunity (I, TT and BT):**
   - There are a few countable lesions which are asymmetrically distributed.
   - Plaques with well-defined and regular borders are characteristic.
   - Anesthesia, hair loss and hypo/anhidrosis are seen. (This is as the high immunity destroys the bacilli which reside in the nerve.)[Q]
   - A few asymmetrical nerve enlargements are seen.
   As a corollary, AFB are scant and the lepromin test is positive.

2. **Lower immunity (BL and LL):**
   - There is symmetrical distribution of numerous lesions.
   - Macules-papules that have ill-defined borders.
   - Hypo/normoesthetic lesions.
   - Multiple symmetrical nerve enlargement is seen.
   - As a corollary, AFB are numerous and the lepromin test is negative.

3. **Mid-immune (BB):** Features of both the spectrums are present and as it is immunologically unstable, they are prone to reactions. The instability makes this the rarest type.

While we discuss the various types for a ready reckoner, Table 7.4 provides a summary of the types.

Indeterminate Leprosy

- Most common type in India.
- Patient is usually a child.
- One or more hypopigmented faintly erythematous macules. Normoesthesia, no nerve enlargement. Commonly seen on face and extensor aspects of limbs (Fig. 7.5).[Q] Hair growth and sweating is generally not affected.
- Lepromin test: (+/−).
- Slit smear for AFB (−).
- Biopsy: Mild periappendegeal and perivascular infiltrate.

Table 7.4	Overview of salient features of leprosy types					
		Tuberculoid leprosy (TT)	*Borderline tuberculoid (BT)*	*Borderline-borderline (BB)*	*Borderline lepromatous (BL)*	*Lepromatous leprosy (LL)*
Cutaneous lesion	**Morphology number**	Plaques 'Saucer-right way up'[Q] Well defined/regular border dry surface <3 number	Plaques 'Satellite lesions'[Q] Well- to ill-defined/regular to irregular borders 3–10 number	• Macules • Plaques • Papules 'Punched out'[Q] 'Swiss cheese'[Q] 'Geographic' lesions[Q]	Papules 'Inverted saucer'	• Madarosis[Q] • Macules • Papules • Nodules • Leonine facies[Q] • Epistaxis and nasal stiffness[Q]
	Appendages	Complete loss	Reduced	Variable	Normal	Normal
	Sensory loss	Anesthetic	Hypoesthetic	Hypo-/normoesthesia	Hypo-/normoesthesia	Normoesthesia
Nerve		Nerve to patch	Numerous Asymmetrical	Numerous Symmetrical	Numerous Symmetrical	Numerous Symmetrical
Lepromin		3+	2+	(–)[Q]	(–)	(–)
BI		0–1+	2–3+	4–5+	5–6+	6+/globi[Q]
Histopathology		Compact granuloma Hugging the epidermis	Less compact Grenz zone appears[Q]	Diffuse epitheloid Granuloma Langhans (–)[Q] giant cell	'Onion peeling of nerve'[Q]	Foamy granuloma Marked Grenz zone[Q]

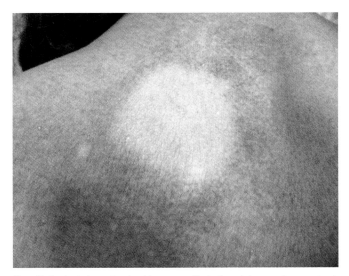

Fig. 7.5: Indeterminate Hansen: Ill-defined hypopigmented, normoesthetic macule is seen on the back

Polyneuritic Leprosy

- It is characterized by primary involvement of nerves in the absence of any active or previously active skin lesions and/or history of previous treatment.[Q]
- Presents as single or multiple asymmetrical nerve enlargement with associated sensory and/or motor defects.
- It is commonly seen in India and Nepal, where it makes up to 5–10% of all leprosy patients.
- In the absence of typical cutaneous lesions, diagnosis can be challenging. NCV testing, nerve FNAC and/or cutaneous sensory nerve twig biopsy demonstrating typical leprosy infiltrate or AFB, can be done. SSS is negative.[Q]
- As per the WHO classification, a patient with >1 nerve involvement has MB leprosy.[Q]

Tuberculoid Type (TT)

- This is a benign and stable form of leprosy.
- The number of skin lesions varies from single to three and may appear on any body part.
- The typical TT lesions appear as a well-defined erythematous large plaque with either uniformly raised or sharp outer edges that slope towards the center of lesions looking like a 'saucer right way up'.[Q]

> The border of the plaque or both borders of the margin are sharply marginated (Fig. 7.6A and B).

- The lesions are almost completely anesthetic, hairless and anhidrotic (no sweating) (Fig. 7.6C).
- Lesions may be associated with a grossly thickened nerve in the vicinity of the lesion (feeder nerve).

Borderline Leprosy

- It is a large group that falls between the tuberculoid and lepromatous poles. It is known as 'dimorphous leprosy' as lesions in one patient may have features of both tuberculoid and lepromatous leprosy.

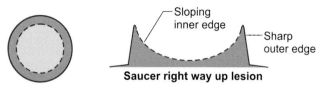

Fig. 7.6A: A depiction of the morphology of TT leprosy

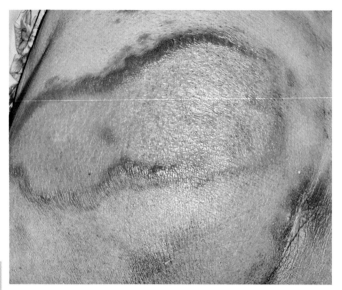

Fig. 7.6B: A well-defined 'annular' plaque with both the borders of the plaque having a well-defined configuration—the so-called **'saucer right way up'** appearance (TT leprosy)

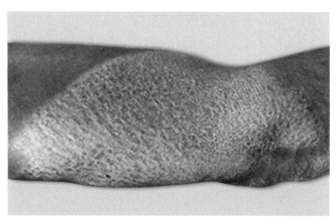

Fig. 7.6C: TT leprosy: Well-defined, hypopigmented, anesthetic, dry, scaly, hairless plaque with sharply raised border seen over the right elbow

- Lesions are generally multiple but countable, with variable morphology. They show variable loss of sensation, hair and sweating.
- Multiple but asymmetrically thickened peripheral nerve trunks are typically noticed.

BT Spectrum

- Solitary or a few well-defined asymmetrically distributed lesions either in the form of hypopigmented macules, or erythematous plaques of variable size.

- They has a dry surface with some scaling and variable degree of hairloss.
- The lesions may have pseudopod-like[Q] extensions and a few smaller 'satellite lesions'[Q] may be present in the periphery of the plaques appearing to branch out of the mother plaque, indicating spread of the disease and lowered immune status than in TT spectrum of leprosy (Fig. 7.7).

The lesions have a clearly-defined, outer border which merges into a flat vague border.

- Nerve thickening in the vicinity of the lesion.
- Moderate to marked sensory loss may be present.
- SSS is 1+ to 2+ or may be negative Lepromin test is positive.

BB Spectrum

- The lesions are an admixture of TT and LL types. The lesions may be macules, plaques or papules or a combination of these types.
- Multiple, bilaterally present, asymmetrically distributed lesions of variable size with sloping outer edges and central punched out area, or a Swiss-cheese appearance[Q] (Fig. 7.8A and B). Also seen are geographic lesions[Q] where the lesions are characterized by streaming, irregular borders and satellites which represent an infiltration around immune areas (Fig. 7.8C).
- Slight hypoesthesia may be present along with asymmetrical nerve thickening.
- The SSS is (3–4+).
- Lepromin is negative

BL Spectrum

In BL disease, there is maximum damage as the bacillary load is high and the inherent immunological instability predisposes the patient to reactions.
- More numerous, bilateral, tending to symmetry, less defined lesions with slight anesthesia, diffuse infiltration may be seen at certain areas. Patchy glove and stocking anesthesia may be present.
- The lesions are mostly small macules (Fig. 7.9A), papules and nodules (Fig. 7.9B).
- Centrally infiltrated plaques with sloping ill-defined borders are also typical, giving 'inverted saucer' appearance (Fig. 7.9C).
- Widespread asymmetrical nerve enlargement. SSS (3–5++). Lepromin test is negative.

Lepromatous Leprosy (LL)

This pole has the least immunity to the bacterium and thus, severe manifestations.
- Multiple, bilaterally symmetrical, uncountable lesions are seen. These are ill-defined, hypopigmented,

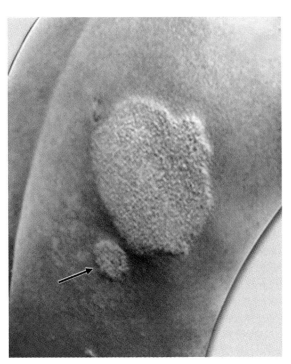
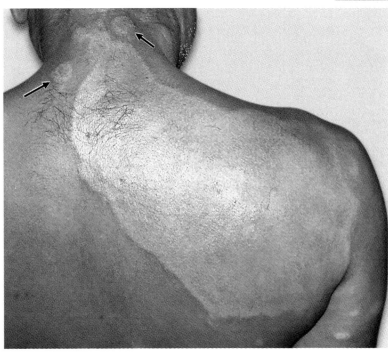

Fig. 7.7: BT Hansen: Well-defined, large, hypopigmented to erythematous, hypoesthetic plaque with downward sloping edges seen over the back. A smaller **satellite lesion** is also seen in the periphery of lesion

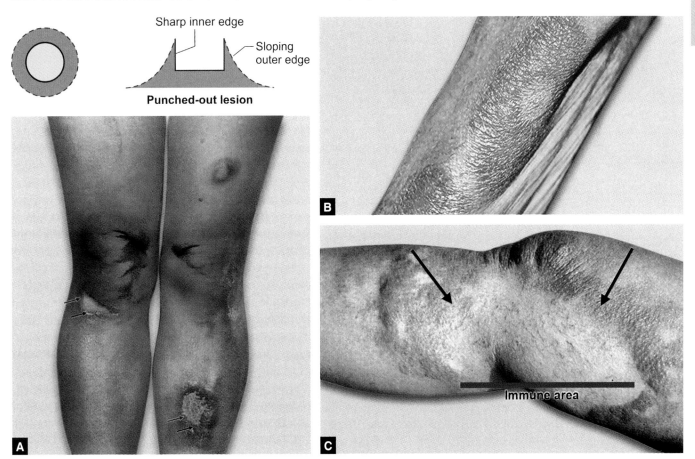

Fig. 7.8A to C: (A) BB leprosy with an 'ill-defined' outer border (lepromatous type) (red line) and a 'well-defined' inner border (tuberculoid type) (blue line)—the so-called **'Swiss cheese'** or **'dimorphic' lesion;** (B) BB Hansen: Well-defined, large irregularly shaped, erythematous, slightly hypoesthetic punched out plaques with central raised edge and outwards sloping margins **(punched-out lesion)** are seen over the right upper arm; (C) A large lesion has formed consequent to infiltration around an 'immune area' forming a **'geographic lesion'.** The immune area is consequent to healing of a preceding lesion

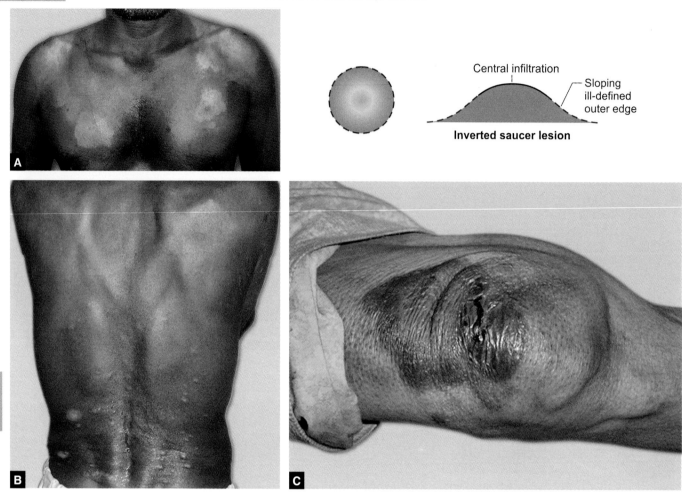

Fig. 7.9A to C: (A) BL leprosy: Multiple irregularly shaped, hypopigmented, slightly hypoesthetic to normoesthetic macules of variable sizes, tending to be symmetrical present over the upper chest; (B) Multiple papules, macules and nodules seen on the trunk in a case of BL leprosy; (C) The outer border is ill-defined and the center of the lesion is raised giving the **'inverted saucer appearance'** (BL leprosy)

shiny macules/plaques/nodules present on infiltrated skin.

- Typical leonine facies[Q]: Oil-smeared appearance, gross infiltration of forehead, earlobes, and malar eminences, loss of lateral third of eyebrows (madarosis), saddle nose, drooping ear lobules (Fig. 7.10).
- Nasal stuffiness and epistaxis may be seen.[Q] Larynx involvement may cause hoarseness of voice. Eye involvement includes iris pearls[Q] and blindness.
- Multiple symmetrically thickened nerves present along with patchy glove and stocking anesthesia.[Q] As a result, multiple sensory and motor complications develop including trophic ulcers, claw hands, etc. This produces disabilities, deformities and social stigmatization.
- In males, the testicular sensation may be lost and gynecomastia[Q] may result from the testicular damage-induced hypoandrogenic state. Lymphadenopathy, hepatomegaly and other systemic involvement may be seen.

- The musculoskeletal system involvement may produce resorption of digits, periostitis, cyst formation, tarsal disintegration, atrophy of the anterior nasal spine and of the maxillary alveolar process.

Special Variants

Lucio Leprosy[Q]

Described in Mexico.

Clinical features: Diffuse non-nodular lesions. Shiny thickened skin, loss of body and facial hair, puffy hands, chronic edema and ulceration of legs. Widespread sensory loss. Eyes have a shiny, thickened upper eyelids with a sleepy look.

Develop peculiar form of lepra reaction called Lucio phenomenon.

Histoid Leprosy (Variant of LL)[Q]

Type of lepromatous leprosy but with better CMI.

Usually seen in patients whose disease is relapsing due to:

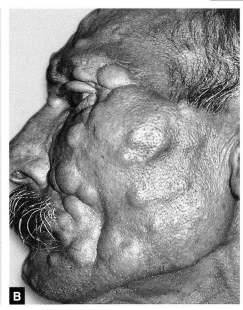

Fig. 7.10A and B: LL leprosy: (A) Facial infiltration with depressed nasal bridge and corneal opacity, madarosis and (B) large nodules in another patient

    i. Stoppage of treatment.   ii. Drug resistance.
Or even *de novo*

Skin lesions: Firm, erythematous, round to oval, shiny, succulent nodules, appearing classically on uninfiltrated normal skin (Fig. 7.11).

Slit smear: AFB seen of slit smear long, lying singly or in parallel bundles (histoid habitus).[Q]

NERVE INVOLVEMENT

- Leprosy is primarily a disease of nerves and the mycobacteria thrive best in the lower temperature of Schwann cells, also called 'biological refrigerator' for leprosy.
- Nerve involvement is the major cause of morbidity in leprosy, seen in form of nerve thickening, beading/nodularity or nerve abscess or neuritis. It results from cell-mediated immune damage, infiltration of nerves with lepra bacilli as well as from reactionary episodes. Nerves that are superficial are easily damaged, especially where they pass through a tight tunnel.
- The immunologically unstable borderline leprosy undergoes reactions that account for maximum nerve damage in these patients.
- Sensory component of the nerves is damaged first (The earliest sensation to be lost is the cold followed by warm sensation, touch and pain),[Q] but eventually autonomic as well as motor functions are deranged. Vibration and proprioception are not affected.[Q]
- Commonly involved peripheral nerves include posterior tibial nerve, ulnar nerve (most common low palsy),[Q] lateral popliteal nerve, radial cutaneous nerve, and sural nerve.
- Of the cranial nerves, facial and trigeminal nerves are most commonly affected.[Q]

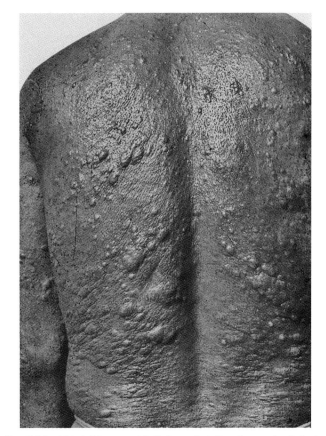

Fig. 7.11: Histoid Hansen: Multiple well-defined succulent, fleshy skin-colored normoesthetic nodules scattered all over the back, both arms, and forearms. There may be history of incomplete therapy or dapsone monotherapy in the past

DEFORMITIES AND DISABILITIES

Mainly caused due to nerve damage and add to morbidity caused by the disease. Risk is highest in highly bacillated lepromatous leprosy and borderline

Table 7.5	Common deformities in leprosy[Q]
Partial claw hand	Ulnar nerve
Complete claw hand	Combined ulnar and median nerve
Wrist drop	Radial nerve
Foot drop	Lateral popliteal nerve
Claw toes	Posterior tibial nerve
Lagophthalmos	Facial nerve
Keratitis/conjunctivitis	Trigeminal nerve

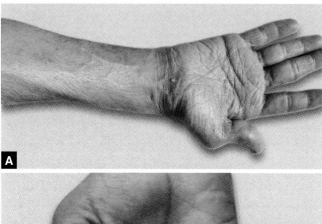
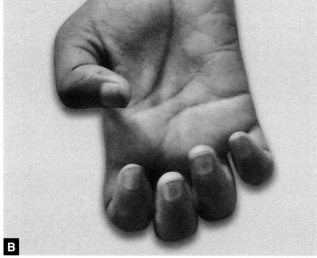

Fig. 7.12A and B: (A) Combined ulnar and median nerve palsy; (B) Complete claw hand due to wasting of both the thenar and hypothenar eminences

leprosy due to reactions. The common deformities seen in leprosy are listed in Table 7.5 and Fig. 7.12.

WHO grading of the disabilities is detailed in Table 7.6.

LEPRA REACTIONS

The leprosy reactions are immunologically mediated acute or subacute events, which affect various organs and are the main complication of the disease, leading to morbidity as well as mortality. Although they are more common in the non-polar unstable subgroups, they can happen in any type of leprosy, except the indeterminate one. Two distinct types of lepra reactions are recognized:

1. **Type I lepra reaction (upgrading/reversal reaction)**[Q]
   * It is a delayed type hypersensitivity (type IV)[Q] reaction.
   * It is predominantly seen in immunologically unstable borderline leprosy patients (BT, BB, BL)
   * Typically presents after starting leprosy treatment (first 6 months) but may appear before or after completion of therapy.
   * Existing lesions of leprosy become inflamed, i.e. erythematous, edematous, painful and tender. Crops of new inflamed lesions may appear on previously uninvolved skin[Q] (Fig. 7.13A to C).
   * Nerves may become inflamed **(neuritis)** and cause pain as well as sensorimotor deterioration. Rarely nerve abscesses may form.
   * Systemic features like fever and malaise are either absent or mild.

2. **Type II lepra reaction—erythema nodosum leprosum (ENL)**[Q] (Fig. 7.14A to C)
   * It is an immune complex mediated (type III) reaction. TNF-α plays a central role.[Q]
   * It is seen in heavily bacillated groups of BL and LL patients.

Table 7.6	Disability grading for leprosy			
Examination of parts	WHO disability grades	Sensory testing (ST)	Voluntary muscle testing (VMT)	
Hands	0	Sensation present	Muscle power normal (S)	
	1	Sensation absent	Muscle power normal (S)	
	2	Sensation absent	Muscle power weak or paralysed (W/P)	
Feet	0	Sensation present	Muscle power normal (S)	
	1	Sensation absent	Muscle power normal (S)	
	2	Sensation absent	Muscle power weak or paralysed (W/P)	
Eye		*Vision*	*Lid gap*	*Blinking*
	0	Normal	No lid gap	Present
	2	Cannot count fingers at 6 meters	Gap between eyelids present/ red eye/corneal ulcer or opacity	Absent

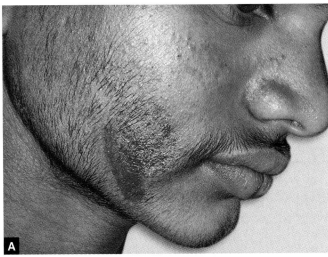

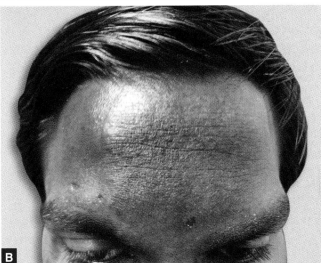

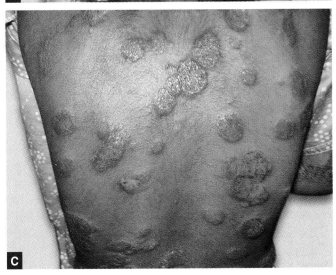

Fig. 7.13A to C: Type I lepra reaction: (A) Erythematous, edematous, raised plaque present over the right cheek. On palpation, the plaque is warm and tender along with tenderness of the feeder nerve; (B) Similar erythematous, edematous, raised plaques present over forehead, which are warm and tender on palpation. Bilateral supraorbital and supratrochlear nerves were enlarged and tender in this case; (C) A case of Type I reaction where all the lesions become inflamed and tender

- It occurs mostly during the course of the antileprosy treatment.
- The leprosy lesions remain unchanged while new ENL lesions (erythematous, tender, evanescent subcutaneous nodules) develop over various areas including face, trunk. These subside in 48–72 hours but recur in crops.
- It is a multi-system disease with associated iridocyclitis, epididymoorchitis, neuritis, glomerulonephritis, etc.
- Systemic symptoms like fever, malaise and joint pains can be very severe and debilitating.

DIAGNOSIS

The diagnosis of leprosy is mainly a clinical one, especially based upon the cardinal signs. However, investigations might be needed to confirm diagnosis and monitor treatment.

Slit skin smear: Done from 3 sites (ear lobule, eyebrow and lesional) and stained with modified ZN stain. Presence of AFB confirms the diagnosis and classification of disease, thus deciding treatment. SSS of LL leprosy shows bacilli stacked in clumps, called globi (6+).[Q]

Histopathology: Well-defined epithelioid cell granulomas with perineural inflammation are seen in tuberculoid leprosy, whereas, ill-defined collection of bacilli filled foamy macrophages (Virchow cells)[Q] with clear zone between it and epidermis (Grenz zone)[Q] are seen in the lepromatous spectrum. Caseous necrosis in granulomas is seen only in nerves.[Q]

Lepromin test[Q]: Intradermal injection of lepromin detects the host immunity to bacilli. A positive test is seen in the tuberculoid spectrum, whereas lepromin negativity is seen in the lepromatous end. It is not a diagnostic test and is used mainly to *classify*, and *prognosticate*.

TREATMENT[Q]

- The standard treatment regimen for adults with MB leprosy is:
  - Rifampicin: 600 mg once a month
  - Clofazimine: 300 mg once a month, and 50 mg daily
  - Dapsone: 100 mg daily
  - Duration: 12 months
- The standard adult treatment regimen for PB leprosy is:
  - Rifampicin: 600 mg once a month
  - Dapsone: 100 mg daily
  - Duration: 6 months.
- Ideally, the entire course of PB MDT should be completed in 9 months and MB MDT in 18 months. The drugs have a color code for adult and children. (Figs 7.15 and 7.16).

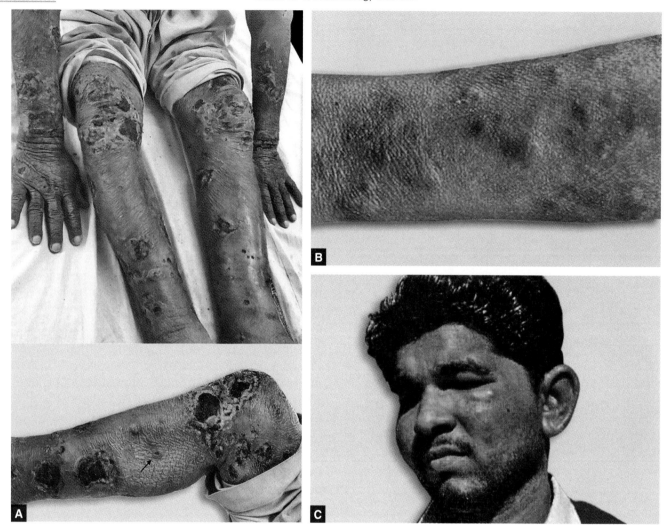

Fig. 7.14A to C: Type II lepra reaction: Erythema nodosum leprosum (ENL) and necroticans: (A) Multiple ulcers with central eschar present over both arms, forearms. Margins of the ulcers are punched out with erythematous to yellowish pus exuding floor. Pedal and hand edema is seen in both hands and feet; (B) Ill-defined erythematous tender subcutaneous nodules; (C) Tender (evanescent) nodules in ENL on the face

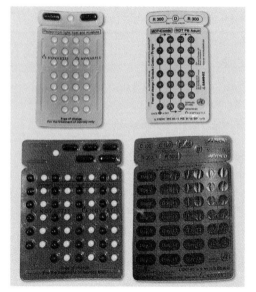

Fig. 7.15: Color-coded treatment packs of leprosy for **adults** (green color for paucibacillary, red color for multibacillary)

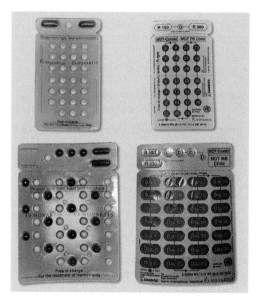

Fig. 7.16: Color-coded treatment packs of leprosy for **children** (blue color for paucibacillary, orange color for multibacillary)

Rifampicin: 4 days after 1 dose—viable bacilli are killed.
Newer drugs:
- Ofloxacin 400 mg, 22 doses—viable bacilli are killed.
- Minocycline 100 mg, 56 doses—viable bacilli are killed.
- Clarithromycin 500 mg, 56 doses—viable bacilli are killed.

Treatment of Lepra Reactions

- **Type I lepra reaction:**
  - Continue MDT
  - Rest and splinting of affected area or limb will lessen the pain.
  - Mild reactions may require only anti-inflammatory agents like NSAIDs.
  - In case of severe reaction and/or neuritis, systemic steroids are indicated. WHO recommends a 12-week course of systemic steroids for both types I and II lepra reaction.
  - Indian studies show that 20 weeks is an ideal duration.
  - Steroids work in nerve abscess also but severe/nonresponsive cases may require drainage.
  - *Other drugs*: Methotrexate, cyclosporine, azathioprine, mycophenolate mofetil.
  - *DOC*—systemic steroids (both severe reaction and neuritis)
  - Clofazimine and thalidomide have *no role* in the treatment.[Q]
- **Type II lepra reaction:**
  - Continue MDT
  - Rest and NSAIDs
  - DOC—systemic steroids are indicated in severe cases and in those with systemic involvement; dose and course similar to that for type I reaction.

Table 7.7	Important side effects of drugs used in treatment of leprosy	
Drug	*Side effects*	*Pregnancy category*
Dapsone	Hemolytic anemia (hydroxylamine metabolite), Dapsone hypersensitivity syndrome, methemoglobinemia, peripheral motor neuropathy	C
Rifampicin	Exfoliative dermatitis, hepatitis, flu-like syndrome	C
Clofazimine	Reddish brown pigmentation of skin, xerosis	C
Thalidomide	Teratogenicity (phocomelia), peripheral sensorimotor neuropathy, insomnia, constipation	X

  - Dose of clofazimine can be increased up to 100 mg three times a day.
  - Thalidomide (100–400 mg/day)[Q] is extremely effective in *steroid non-responsive* or *chronic cases* but it is not recommended by WHO due to its teratogenicity.

Other drugs: Chloroquine, colchicine, pentoxifylline, zinc, leukotriene inhibitors (montelukast, zafirlukast), thalidomide derivatives (revimid, actimid),[Q] infliximab.

The main side effects of these drugs have been listed in Table 7.7. Multidrug therapy is safe in pregnant women and should be continued throughout the pregnancy.

Miscellaneous Parasitic Disorders

This chapter will cover in brief the various disorders that can be seen in practice and caused by various parasites including protozoa, worms and arthropods. Of these, the common afflictions include arthoprod bites, leishmaniasis and certain disorders caused by worms.

LEISHMANIASIS

Leishmaniasis is caused by a protozoal parasite with over 20 Leishmania subspecies and is transmitted to humans by the bite of infected female phlebotomine sandflies. Over 90 sandfly species are known to transmit Leishmania parasites. (Phlebotomus in Old Word, Lutzomyia in New World.)[Q]

The species are identified on the basis of geographic distribution and disease forms. A simplified scheme is given in Table 8.1.

There are three main forms of the disease:

1. *Visceral leishmaniasis (VL),*[Q] also known as kala-azar, is fatal, if left untreated in over 95% of cases. It is characterized by irregular bouts of fever, weight loss, enlargement of the spleen and liver, and anemia. It is highly endemic in the Indian subcontinent and in East Africa.
2. *Cutaneous leishmaniasis (CL)*[Q] is the most common form of leishmaniasis and causes skin lesions, mainly ulcers, on exposed parts of the body, leaving lifelong scars and serious disability.
3. *Mucocutaneous leishmaniasis* leads to partial or total destruction of mucous membranes of the nose, mouth and throat. Almost 90% of mucocutaneous leishmaniasis cases occur in Bolivia, Brazil and Peru.[Q]

Epidemiology

In South-East Asia, visceral leishmaniasis is the main form of the disease. Transmission generally occurs in rural areas with a heavy annual rainfall, a mean humidity above 70%, a temperature range of 15–38°C, abundant vegetation, subsoil water and alluvial soil.

The disease is most common in agricultural villages where houses are frequently constructed with mud walls and earthen floors, and cattle and other livestock live close to humans. People are considered to be the sole reservoir of the Leishmania parasites in this region.[Q]

Diagnosis

This depends on clinical features, smear or scraping and biopsy. Microscopic examination reveals intense lymphocytic infiltrate. Giemsa stain may make it easier to find the intracellular parasites (2–5 μm). Speciation is based on the polymerase chain reaction (PCR).

Acute Cutaneous Leishmaniasis
(Old World—Cutaneous Leishmaniasis)

Synonym: These are named after the cities where one can become infected: Baghdad boil, Aleppo boil, Jericho boil, or simply oriental boil.[Q]

Cutaneous infection with *Leishmania tropica complex*. Sandflies are low-flying (3 meters) nocturnal insects, hence those staying at upper stories have less risk.

Table 8.1	Species causing leishmaniasis
Complex	*Disease*
Leishmania tropica	Old World—cutaneous leishmaniasis
Leishmania mexicona	New World—cutaneous leishmaniasis
Leishmania viannia (brasiliensis)	New World—cutaneous and mucocutaneous leishmaniasis
Leishmania donovani	Visceral leishmaniasis

Types

a. **Moist or rural type:** The incubation period is relatively short (1–4 weeks). This type is contracted from rodent reservoirs such as gerbils via the sandfly vector.

This is a slowly growing, indurated, indolent papule, which enlarges in a few months to form a nodule that may ulcerate in a few weeks to form an ulcer (Fig. 8.1). Spontaneous healing may take as long as 6 months, leaving a characteristic scar.

b. **Dry or urban type:** This has a longer incubation period (2–8 months or longer), develops much more slowly, and heals more slowly than the rural type. In both types, the ulcer or crust forms on a bed of edematous tissue (Fig. 8.2A to C).

c. **Ethiopian:** More chronic and less severe (*Leishmania aethiopica*) but may lead to diffuse cutaneous leishmaniasis.

Leishmaniasis Recidivans

A form of either wet or dry leishmaniasis, characterized by chronic course, central healing, and development of serpiginous lupoid nodules at the periphery.

Diffuse Cutaneous Leishmaniasis

Rare form in patients who are relatively anergic and develop disseminated disease, with both local and hematogenous spread to produce nodular lesions resembling lepromatous leprosy, as well as mucosal disease. Also called anergic cutaneous leishmaniasis. Caused by *Leishmania aethiopica*^Q and several New World species.

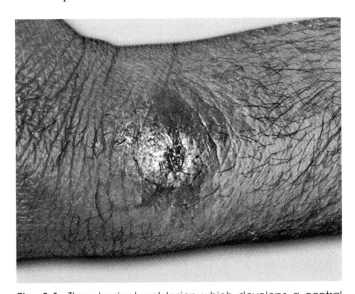

Fig. 8.1: The classical wet lesion which develops a central ulceration in due course of time. The lesion may look like a furuncle or a boil at this stage but is not as tender and does not discharge as much pus as a boil would on rupture (*Courtesy:* Dr Khalid Mahmood, UK)

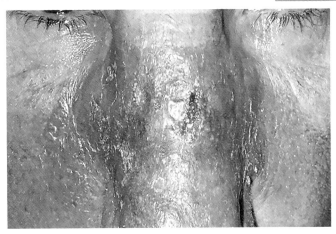

Fig. 8.2A: Dry type: Some lesions especially those due to *L. tropica* may follow a chronic course. They may start as an indurated plaque that may not ulcerate for many months or may only develop a small ulceration (*Courtesy:* Dr Khalid Mahmood, UK)

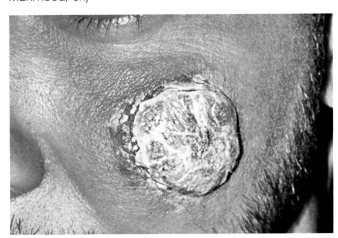

Fig. 8.2B: Depending upon the host immune response, some lesions may develop into large crusted nodules and on removing the crust frank ulceration may be visible (*Courtesy:* Dr Khalid Mahmood, UK)

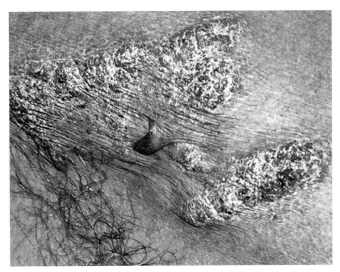

Fig. 8.2C: Cutaneous tuberculosis like lesions: Chronic lesions may resemble cutaneous tuberculosis especially lupus vulgaris (*Courtesy:* Dr Khalid Mahmood, UK)

Mucocutaneous Leishmaniasis

This usually occurs in the New World from *L. brasiliensis*, less often in the Old World through *L. aethiopica*. There is marked mucosal damage following hematogenous or lymphatic spread (not local advancement to mucosa) with high morbidity.

Therapy of Cutaneous Leishmaniasis

Spontaneous healing is the rule, so often no therapy is needed for acute cutaneous leishmaniasis. An overview of treatment is given below.

Local therapy

- 15% paromomycin[Q] and 12% methylbenzethonium chloride ointment twice daily for 20 days.[Q]
- Thermotherapy: 1–3 sessions with localized heat (50°C for 30 s).
- Intralesional antimonials[Q]: 1–5 mL per session every 3–7 days (1–5 infiltrations).

Systemic therapy

- Ketoconazole: Adult dose, 600 mg oral daily for 28 days.
- Sodium stibogluconate[Q]: 20 mg/kg/day intramuscularly or intravenously for 20 days.
- Amphotericin B deoxycholate: 0.7 mg/kg/day, by infusion, for 25–30 doses.
- Liposomal amphotericin B: 2–3 mg/kg/day, by infusion, up to 20–40 mg/kg total dose.

Post-Kala-Azar Dermal Leishmaniasis (PKDL)

Post-kala-azar dermal leishmaniasis (PKDL) is a sequel of visceral leishmaniasis that appears as macular, papular or nodular rash usually on face, upper arms, trunks and other parts of the body. It occurs mainly in East Africa and on the Indian subcontinent, where up to 50%, and 5–10% (India)[Q] of patients with kala-azar, develop this condition.

It usually appears 6 months to 1 or more years[Q] after kala-azar has apparently been cured.

Clinical Presentation

Most patients on the Indian subcontinent have a polymorphic presentation (Fig. 8.3A) comprising macular, papular or nodular lesions.

Site: The lesions have a predilection for the area around the chin and mouth (Fig. 8.3B).

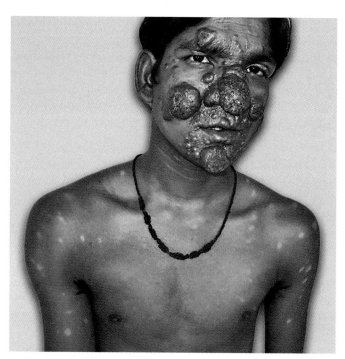

Fig. 8.3A: Polymorphic lesions with nodular, papular lesions on the face and macular lesions on the trunk (PKDL)

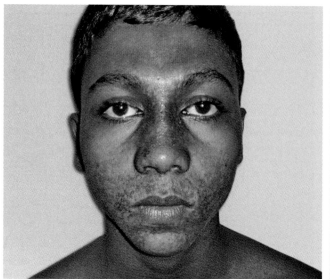 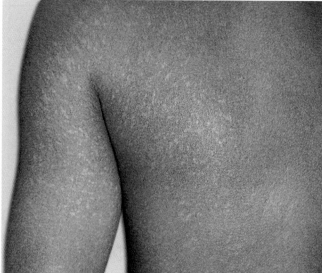

Fig. 8.3B: Macular lesions with a perioral accentuation and involvement of the back

This presentation can be subdivided into different forms:

- Monomorphic (macular and nodular)
- Polymorphic or mixed (both macules and indurated lesions such as papules are present)
- Rare presentations (e.g. erythrodermic).

Diagnosis

PKDL should be suspected in patients in endemic areas who present with a skin rash combined with previous or concomitant visceral leishmaniasis. The diagnosis can be made using clinical criteria or by identifying the parasite, or both.

Clinical diagnosis is made by assessing the presence of the typical *rash*, its *distribution*, whether the patient has a history of *visceral leishmaniasis*, or because PKDL can occur without previous visceral leishmaniasis, whether the patient lives in an endemic area or has recently travelled to one. In a setting where diagnostic methods are limited, diagnosis will often be based on these clinical criteria and history (Fig. 8.4).

- Slit-skin smears or samples obtained by biopsy can be used to identify parasites to confirm the diagnosis of PKDL. Nodular lesions are more likely to show amastigotes (LD bodies).[Q]
- Skin biopsies may also be examined by histopathology and immunohistochemistry.
- Serological tests, such as the direct agglutination test, enzyme-linked immunosorbent assay (ELISA) and the rK39 rapid diagnostic ELISA,[Q] are usually positive.

These tests are of limited value because a positive result may be caused by antibodies persisting after a past episode of visceral leishmaniasis. Their use is when other diseases (e.g. leprosy) are considered in the differential diagnosis, or if a history of visceral leishmaniasis is uncertain.

The rK39 rapid diagnostic ELISA can be used as strong evidence for past visceral leishmaniasis and is more sensitive in the Indian subcontinent.

- Species-specific polymerase chain reaction (PCR) may be used on skin biopsy samples or slit-skin specimens.

Treatment

In the Indian subcontinent, all cases are treated as they are considered as chronic cases (given the long interval after VL). While the skin lesions return to normal, repigmentation may take time and cannot be taken as a parameter for cure.

The therapy is given in Table 8.2 and the preferred drug is miltefosine (first oral drug for PKDL).[Q]

The criteria of cure are given in Box 8.1.

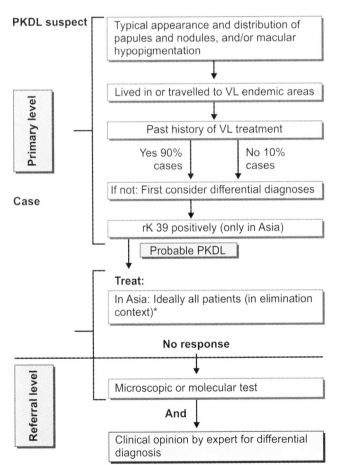

Fig. 8.4: Algorithm for diagnosing and treating post-kala-azar dermal leishmaniasis (PKDL)

Table 8.2	Treatment of PKDL in Bangladesh, India, Nepal
Miltefosine for 4 weeks*	Adults (>12 years) weighing more than 25 kg: **50 mg BD** Adults (>12 years) weighing more than 25 kg: **50 mg OD** Children (2–11 years): **2.5 mg/kg** once daily
Amphotericin B deoxycholate**	1 mg/kg/day by infusion, up to 60–80 doses over 4 months (20 days on, 20 days off)
Liposomal amphotericin B	5 mg/kg/day by infusion two times per week for 3 weeks for a a total dose of 30 mg/kg

*Precautions with miltefosine: Pregnant women should not be treated with miltefosine. Women of reproductive age and their partners should be counselled appropriately about the need to use effective contraception during the 12-week course of miltefosine treatment and for 2 months after completing treatment.

**Amphotericin B: The second-line drug amphotericin B is recommended in the following cases:
- Patient not responding to the first-line of drug or the drug was discontinued due to toxic effect.
- Women during pregnancy.
- Women who are breastfeeding their babies.
- Children less than two years of age.
- PKDL patient with liver or kidney disease.

Clinical cure

Demonstrated of clinical cure of papular and nodular lesions, and complete resolution of macular lesion or repigmentation of macular lesions at 12-month follow-up visit.

Parasitological cure

At the end of treatment and at subsequent follow-up visits, parasites should no longer be present.

WORMS

Cutaneous Larva Migrans

Synonym: Creeping eruption.

Definition

Infestation of human skin by larva that are unable to complete their life cycle in the skin.

Ancylostoma, *Strongyloides*, and *Necator* are commonly implicated.[Q] The larval worms are deposited in moist soil via stool. They enter their accidental host via the skin, and wander about creating complex burrowing patterns. In the case of *Strongyloides stercoralis*, if the larva mature rapidly in the bowel, they can penetrate the perianal skin causing larva currens.

Clinical Features

After a few hours, the entry site begins to itch and a red papule develops. After a few days, the larva begins to migrate in the skin, creating bizarre erythematous curved lines (Fig. 8.5).

It is seen in patients who go barefoot on the beach, children playing in sandboxes, carpenters and plumbers working under homes, and gardeners. The most common sites involved are the feet, buttocks, genitals, and hands.[Q]

The larval migration begin 4 days after inoculation and progress at the rate of about 2 cm/day. If the progress of the disease is not interrupted by treatment, the larvae usually die in 2–8 weeks, with resolution of the eruption.

Treatment

Apart from spontaneous resolution which can occur in the case of nonhuman worms, the therapeutic agents include:

- Topical thiabendazole
- Ivermectin 200 μg/kg, generally given as a single 12 mg dose and repeated the next day or
- Albendazole 400 mg/day for 3 days

Criteria for successful therapy are relief of symptoms and cessation of tract extension, which usually occurs within 1 week.

Miscellaneous Disorders

Myiasis

Many different fly larvae (maggots) can invade human flesh and usually affect a chronic ulcer or wound. Most maggots only eat necrotic debris, although some attack healthy tissue. They can migrate below the skin surface (myiasis migrans).[Q]

Enterobiasis

Worldwide infection caused by *Enterobius vermicularis*, the pinworm. Most common in young children; frequently brought home from day nurseries or kindergarten.

Symptoms are pruritus ani,[Q] worse at night and complications include chronic urticaria, vulvovaginitis (direct spread).

Therapy is mebendazole 100 mg or albendazole 400 mg in single dose; perhaps repeated in 2 weeks.

Onchocerciasis

This is seen in equatorial Africa as well as Central and South America. It is one of the leading causes of preventable blindness in the world (river blindness)[Q].

Onchocerca volvulus[Q] is transferred from human-to-human by black flies (*Simulium* spp.).[Q] Larvae reach the subcutis, where they grow in a fibrous capsule. They then release microfilariae, which can be transmitted by another black fly bite, but move through the lymphatics eliciting an aggressive immune response, especially when they die and release antigens from *Wolbachia* symbiotic bacteria.

Clinical features: They cause urticaria, intensely pruritic papules, erysipelas and lymphadenopathy,

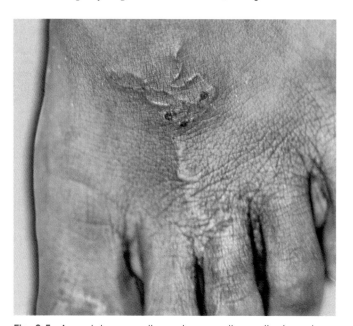

Fig. 8.5: A serpiginous, erythematous eruption on the lower legs: 'Cutaneous larva migrans'

leading to hypopigmentation and skin atrophy (*leopard skin*).[Q] They also cause intense inflammatory eye disease with scarring.[Q]

Therapy: The treatment of choice is ivermectin 150 μg/kg[Q] in a single dose. It does not kill the worms but prevents them from breeding. Doxycycline kills symbiotic Wolbachia bacteria, reducing the inflammatory reaction.

Schistosomiasis

This common disease is seen following contact with contaminated water, wherein the cercariae of the genus *Schistosoma* once again penetrate the skin, and pass through the veins and lymphatics to the urogenital veins where they develop into mature worms.

Clinical features: Initial infection is characterized by symptoms of fever, urticaria, and eosinophilia (Kata-Yama fever).[Q] Later, there are chronic anogenital warty papules, nodules, and fistulas with slowly healing ulcers that can evolve into squamous cell carcinoma.

Therapy: Praziquantel is the treatment of choice; either 40 mg/kg in a single dose or 20 mg/kg q8h × 3d.

Cercarial Dermatitis (Swimmer's Itch)[Q]

There are many non-human flukes involving, for example, water birds. When humans swim in shallow infested water, the cercariae may penetrate their skin, causing pruritic red papules and nodules. The animal parasites cannot complete their life cycle in humans, so there is no risk of internal involvement.

ARTHROPODS

Papular Urticaria/Insect Bite Reactions

This is a generic term that signifies a host reaction to insect bites and can range from just itching to intense reaction. Acute skin reactions appear as hives or papular urticaria, and more chronic reactions appear as inflammatory papules. Insects that sting (usually when threatened) include bees, wasps, and fire ants. Insects that bite (usually out of hunger) include mosquitoes, fleas, flies, bedbugs, and lice. Spiders, ticks, and chiggers are other arthropods can sometimes attack human skin.

- The most commonly identified causes are insects that live on cats and dogs, particularly the human flea (*Pulex irritans*) and mites.
- Bed bugs seem to be resurging in developed countries, possibly due to international travel and changes in pest control practices. The two main species of bed bugs are *Cimex lectularius* and *Cimex*

hemipterus, which are found in temperate areas and tropical zones, respectively.
- Other causes include mosquitoes and various other insects including blister beetles.

Clinical Features

The clinical morphology depends on the type of causative factor and is known as papular urticaria.

This is a misnomer as it is not urticaria. This is a common condition of childhood characterized by a chronic or recurrent papular eruption caused by hypersensitivity to a variety of bites, including those of mosquitoes, fleas, bed bugs, and mites[Q] (Fig. 8.6). It is often pruritic and uncomfortable, and the resultant scratching may result in open erosions and secondary bacterial superinfection.

- Not all persons dwelling in the same household are affected.
- The two prerequisites required are a biting insect and a host who is allergic to the bite.
- Both these have interindividual variation
- Sometimes, a central punctum can be identified in the papule which is diagnostic (Fig. 8.6).

- **Fleas (pulicosis):** Fleas are small, brown insects about 2.5 mm long, flat from side-to-side, with long hind legs. They slip into clothing or jump actively when disturbed. They are capable of jumping 50 cm high or wide.
  Clinical features: Flea bites are usually multiple and linear—breakfast, lunch, and dinner. They bite about the legs and waist and may be troublesome in houses where there are dogs or cats. The lesions are often grouped and may be arranged in zigzag lines. Hypersensitivity reactions may appear as papular urticaria, nodules, or bullae (Fig. 8.7). A typical feature of flea bites is that when a new bite occurs, the older lesions also begin to itch again.

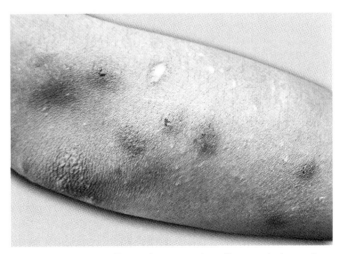

Fig. 8.6: Multiple erythematous papules with a central punctum which is the site of the insect bite

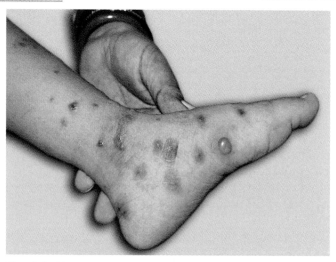

Fig. 8.7: Hypersensitivity reactions to fleas manifesting as an admixture of papule, urticarial lesions and bullae

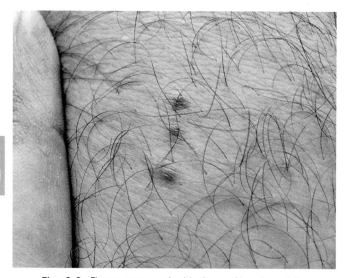

Fig. 8.8: Three aggregated lesions of bedbug bite

- **Bedbugs (cimicosis):** Bedbugs are usually transported passively, mainly in clothing and luggage, so history of recent travel is important. They can also be transported in old furniture, e.g. mattresses and sofas. Less commonly, they spread actively from room-to-room in communities, mainly through electric wiring or ventilation ducts.
Clinical features: Because bedbugs feed at night and inject an anesthetic when biting, the initial bite is not felt. Symptom onset, caused by an allergic reaction to saliva, can be delayed with reactions to bites taking several days to manifest up.

It is common for bedbugs to inflict a series of bites in a row (Fig. 8.8) (breakfast, lunch, and dinner).[Q] Bites may mimic urticaria, and patients with papular urticaria commonly have antibodies to bedbug antigens. Unilateral eyelid swelling has been described as a common sign of bedbug bites in children. Bullous and urticarial reactions also occur.

- **Mites:** Trombiculidae mites are scattered around the world. They are sometimes known as harvest mites because they so often infect grains, but they are also seen in gardens and forested areas. They are indiscriminate, attacking birds, mammals, and humans. In East Asia, they transmit *Rickettsia tsutsugamushi*,[Q] the causative agent of scrub typhus. *Clinical features:* They generally bite at sites where their progress is restricted by tight clothing, and then fall off again. They are seen typically on the legs just above the *sock line* or on the trunk just above the *belt line*. They cause pruritic urticarial papules, which itch for about a week and may persist for 2 weeks.
- **Mosquito:** Moisture, warmth, CO_2, estrogens, and lactic acid in sweat attract mosquitoes. Drinking alcohol also stimulates mosquito attraction.

Mosquito bites are a common cause of papular urticaria. More severe local reactions are seen in young children, individuals with immunodeficiency, and those with new exposure to indigenous mosquitoes.

- **Blister beetle:** Members of the family Staphylinidae (genus *Paederus*) contain a different vesicant, pederin. None of the beetles bites or stings; rather, they exude their blistering fluid, if they are brushed against, pressed, or crushed on the skin. Many blister beetles are attracted at night by fluorescent lighting.
Clinical features: 'Blister beetle dermatitis' is consequent to exposure to cantharidin[Q] (or another vesicant, pederin,[Q] found in the genus *Paederus*) and may mimic shingles, herpes infection, allergic contact dermatitis or impetigo (Fig. 8.9A).

Slight burning and tingling of the skin occur within minutes, followed by the formation of bullae, often arranged linearly. 'Kissing lesions'[Q] are observed when the blister beetle's excretion is deposited in the flexures of the elbows or other folds (Fig. 8.9B).

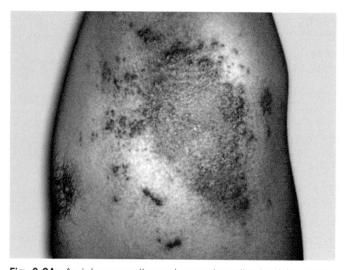

Fig. 8.9A: An intense erythematous rash on the trunk in a case of *Paederus dermatitis*

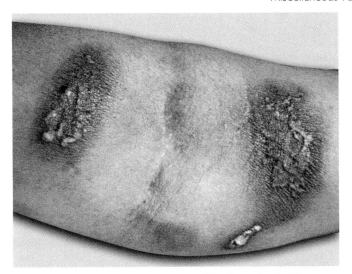

Fig. 8.9B: A case of *Paederus dermatitis* with a classic **'kissing or mirror lesion'** consequent to the contact of the flexural surface

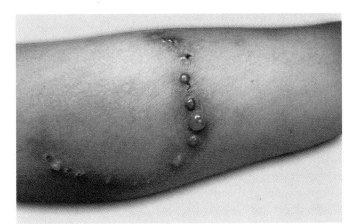

Fig. 8.9C: Linear vesicular eruption due to rove beetles (dermatitis linearis)

In many tropical and subtropical habitats, rove beetles (genus *Paederus*) produce a patchy or linear, erythematous vesicular eruption (dermatitis linearis)

(Fig. 8.9C). It occurs frequently during the rainy season and appears predominantly on the neck and exposed parts.

Treatment

One of the most challenging aspects of papular urticaria is convincing parents that the lesions are related to a bite reaction and identifying and eradicating the source of the offending insect as in most cases the adults in the family are unaffected.

Symptomatic therapy for itching

- Topical steroids (e.g. clobetasol 0.05% cream bid × 2 weeks).
- Antihistamines: The local application is of topical steroids and antihistamines.

Though the most important aspect involves separation of the insect from the host, an overview of the measures is given in Table 8.3.

TICK-INDUCED DISORDERS

The European wood tick (*Ixodes ricinus*)[Q] is a significant carrier of diseases. The significant diseases spread are:

- Borrelia burgdorferi[Q]
- Arbovirus that causes tick-borne meningoencephalitis.
- Rickettsial infections
- Kyasanur Forest disease (KFD)[Q]
- Crimean-Congo hemorrhagic fever (CCHF)

Distribution of Important Tick Vectors in India

India contributes a huge share in world's livestock industry with approximately 199 million cattle and 105 million buffaloes, most of which are suffering from multi-species tick infestations. Around 106 species have been found in India, but a few have been established as vectors of diseases. The genera Rhipicephalus and Hyalomma are most widely distributed in India.

Table 8.3	Overview of measures to identify and treat common arthropods	
Fleas and mites	• Look for fleas in pets, their bedding and soft furnishings. • Mites are only visible under a microscope.	Camphor and menthol preparations, topical corticosteroids, and topical anesthetics can be of benefit.
Bedbugs	• Have the appearance of a collection of **apple seeds** • They can be found in almost any place in the bedroom where they will not be disturbed.	Eradication is required by: a. Vacuuming of exposed hiding locations b. Washing all linens in hot water and drying on low heat c. Use of mattress and box spring encasements d. Pesticide spraying e. Ivermectin: 200 µg/kg of oral ivermectin
Mosquitoes	The best option is to use a insect repellant 'advanced odomos cream' applied at 10 mg/cm² concentration provides a 100% protection from Anopheles mosquitoes for up to 11 h and about 6 h protection against '*Aedes aegypti*'.	Insect repellents a. DEET (N, N-diethyl-3-methylbenzamide, previously called N,N-diethyl-m-toluamide). b. Neem oil>Citronella candles c. Permethrin, marketed in a 0.5% spray on clothes

Rickettsial Diseases

Rickettsiae are small, nonflagellated, Gram-negative pleomorphic coccobacilli bacteria, and mostly are obligate intracellular parasites. An overview of the common disorders is given in Box 8.2.

- They are primary parasites of lice, fleas, ticks and mites in which they are found in the alimentary canal.
- They are spread by the bites of blood sucking arthropods and cause widespread infection in endothelial cells, which may result in vascular infarcts, extravascular fluid loss and disseminated intravascular coagulation.

Epidemiology

Rickettsiae live within the gut of arthropods and are transferred to humans by bites. Often the natural host is a rodent; the human is an incidental host. After an infection, there is long-standing immunity.

Distribution

Rickettsial infections are prevalent throughout the world except in Antarctica. In India, most cases are reported from Jammu and Kashmir, Himachal Pradesh, Uttarakhand, Rajasthan, Assam, West Bengal, Maharashtra, Kerala and Tamil Nadu.

Clinical Features

Headache, nausea, chills, and high fever 1–3 weeks after bite. RMSF is usually transmitted via a tick bite, although up to one-third of patients with proven RMSF do not recall a recent tick bite or recent tick contact

- Headache is a very prominent feature, may be severe, and is usually accompanied by severe myalgias.
- Children may also have prominent abdominal pain that may be mistaken for other intra-abdominal processes, like appendicitis.
  a. *Tick typhus*: Typical is a necrotic papule at the site of bite **(eschar—the 'tache noire')**. This is seen in 80% of cases and the onset of fever coincides with this ulcer which is 2–5 mm in diameter, has a black necrotic center and a red areola.

Classic **triad** *of rickettsial pox consists of fever, eschar, and rash.*

Box 8.2	Overview of rickettsial infections[Q]	
Organism	*Disease*	*Vector*
Rickettsia rickettsii	Rocky mountain spotted fever	Ticks
Rickettsia prowazekii	Endemic typhus	Lice
Rickettsia typhi	Epidemic typhus	Lice, fleas
Rickettsia conorii	Mediterranean tick bite fever	Ticks
Rickettsia akari	Rickettsial pox	Mites

b. *Rocky mountain spotted fever* (*RMSF*) may have lymphadenopathy; typically absent in typhus. In RMSF, first lesions are on palms and soles.
  c. *Rash*: Four days later, a pink maculopapular eruption develops first on the ankles, wrists, palms, and soles, and then rapidly generalizes, involving the face, palms and soles.

- Epidemic typhus may also have a *thrombotic vasculitis*. In severe cases may be hemorrhagic; rarely more severe reactions such as digital necrosis and pneumonia have been described.

Investigation

- The classic Weil-Felix test[Q] is first positive after 2 weeks and does not help identify the species of rickettsia.
- Microimmunofluorescence or immunoblot tests are usually used; the same immunofluorescence antibodies can be applied to skin biopsies.
- PCR can be used.

Differential diagnosis: Exanthems are not clinically specific; history and presence of eschar help.

Treatment

- Doxycycline 100 mg bid for 5–7 days for mild disease; severely ill patients should be hospitalized for IV medications.
- *Alternative treatments*: Chloramphenicol is also effective and has been recommended for Rocky mountain spotted fever in pregnant women and children aged 8 years and under.

Borreliosis

Synonyms: Lyme borreliosis or Lyme disease.[Q]

Infection with *Borrelia burgdorferi* transferred by ticks. Stage I and stage II represent early disease; stage III, late.

The natural hosts are ticks; in endemic areas, over 90% may be infected. In 50% of cases, not noticed as the bites are painless. The risk of infection is estimated at 1–5/100 bites, depending on the endemicity of the disease.

Transmission in the first 36 hours is rare, as the organism must be activated in the tick following attachment.

Clinical Features

The course of the disease is depicted in Fig. 8.10.

Stage I: *Erythema chronicum migrans* (*ECM*): Red papule develops on trunk or limb at site of bite. Slowly a spreading annular erythema evolves as the papule fades (Fig. 8.11A). The center sometimes becomes intensely erythematous and indurated, vesicular, or necrotic (Fig. 8.11B). It should be at least 5 cm in diameter.

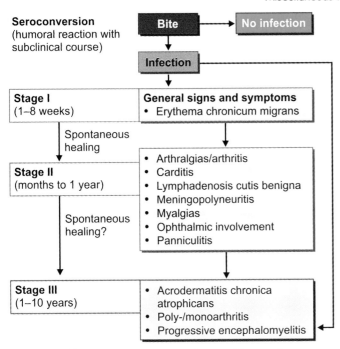

Fig. 8.10: An overview of the stages of Lyme disease

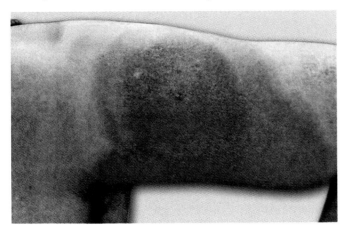

Fig. 8.11A: Annular erythematous patch with smooth surface present over left upper arm measuring 7 × 8 cm with a papule in the center of the lesion (erythema chronicum migrans)

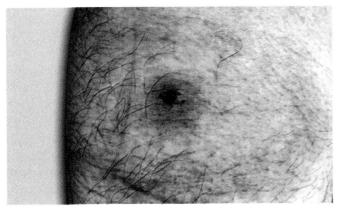

Fig. 8.11B: A large annular ring of erythema around a central necrotic area (erythema chronicum migrans)

Stage II: This stage occurs due to hematogenous spread of *B. burgdorferi* to many sites within days or weeks after the onset of EM characterized by secondary annular lesions similar to EM but smaller in size and multiple in number.

Early edematous stage with lymphocytic infiltrate, usually on ear lobe, nipple, or cheek (children); evolves into solid red-brown tumor with smooth surface, 1–2 cm large over months to a year.

Systemic features are depicted in Fig 8.10.

Stage III
- *Acrodermatitis chronica atrophicans*: Most dramatic change with development of very atrophic skin (cigarette paper skin) over the distal extremities (ankles, knees). Initially puffy vague erythema which over years becomes atrophic with loss of subcutaneous fat so that underlying vessels can be easily visualized.
- *Juxta-articular nodules*: Fibrous proliferations over the elbows and knees; when the lesion is linear extending down the forearm, known as ulnar streak.

Investigation

Serological studies include ELISA and Western blot demonstration of antibodies; in stage I, 20–50% (usually IgM); stage II 70–90% (initially IgM, then IgG); stage III 100%.

Treatment

The stage-wise therapy:

Stage I: Doxycycline 100 mg p.o. bid for 14–21 days.

Stage II: Doxycycline 100 mg p.o. bid for 14–21 days OR ceftriaxone 2 g IV daily for 14 days.

Stage III: Ceftriaxone 2 g IV daily for 14 days.

Kyasanur Forest Disease

Kyasanur Forest disease (KFD) is a zoonotic viral hemorrhagic fever and has been endemic to Karnataka[Q] state, India. Outbreaks of KFD were reported in new areas of Wayanad and Malappuram districts of Kerala, India during 2014–2015.

Seasonal outbreaks are expected to occur during the months of January to June.

The vector is the tick specifically *Haemaphysalis spinigera* and *H. turturis*.

Clinical Features

The classic symptoms are fever, headache, gastrointestinal symptoms and bleeding. It is associated with monkey deaths in the area.

Investigation

IgM, ELISA, RT PCR and viral isolation.

Treatment

Therapy is primarily supportive and may require ICU care.

Common Infestations

Infestations are defined as the presence of animal parasites on or in the body and is more common in tropical countries. Though we have discussed a wide-spectrum of protozoan and insect infections in Chapter 8 and listed in Table 9.1, here we will focus on two main types of infestations—pediculosis and scabies.

PEDICULOSIS

Lice (Pediculus spp.) are blood-sucking, wingless, ectoparasitic insects that infest their victims for long periods of time with a high degree of host specificity.

Three varieties of the flattened, six legged (3 pairs)^Q Anoplura insects infest humans: *Pediculus humanus* var. *capitis* (head louse),^{Q} *P. humanus* var. *corporis* (body louse), and *Phthirus pubis* (pubic or crab louse).^{Q} A depiction of the different types of pediculosis infestation is given in Fig. 9.1.

Lice can also transmit a number of important diseases:
1. Epidemic typhus (*Rickettsia prowazekii*).
2. Relapsing fever (*Borrelia recurrentis*).
3. Trench fever (*Bartonella quintana*).

Pediculosis Capitis

Synonyms: Head lice.
Infestation with *Pediculus humanus capitis*.

Epidemiology

Often seen in epidemics among kindergarten and grade schoolchildren; also common in homeless people. About 10% of children in schools have head lice with most of them having a few or no symptoms. Infestations peak between the ages of 4 and 11, and are more common in girls than boys.

Pathogenesis

Lice live on the scalp and suck blood there. They firmly attach their eggs (nits) to the hair shaft just at the skin surface.

A typical infested scalp will carry about **10 adult lice**,^{Q} which measure some 1–3 mm in length and are greyish, and often rather hard to find. An adult female louse lives for about 1 month and during that time lays 5–10 eggs per day of an average size of 0.8 mm (Fig. 9.2A).

Clinical Features

The main symptom is itching, although this may take several months to develop after the first infestation. Subsequent infestations produce itching more rapidly, suggesting that this is due to a delayed-type hyper-sensitivity reaction to the saliva of the lice.^{Q}

Pruritic eruption on back of *scalp* and *nape* (Fig. 9.1B and 9.2B);^{Q} often with excoriations and secondary infections **(lice dermatitis)**. The hairs may become matted from repeated scratching **(plica polonica)**^{Q} and the secondary infection leads to enlarged lymph nodes.

Table 9.1	An overview of the infestations that can affect humans
Insects	
Anoplura	**Lice** infestations
Hymenoptera	Bee and wasp stings, ant bites
Diptera	Mosquito and midge bites, myiasis
Hemiptera	**Bedbugs**
Aphaniptera	Human and animal fleas
Blisters	Paederus dermatitis
Mites	
Sarcoptes scabei	Human and animal scabies
Demodex folliculorum	Normal inhabitant of facial hair follicles
House dust mite	Atopic eczema
Cheyletiella	Papular urticaria
Ticks	Tick bites. Vector of rickettsial infections and erythema migrans

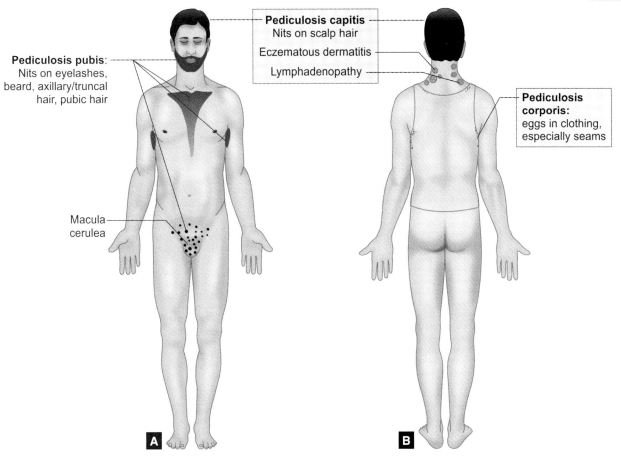

Pediculosis pubis:
Nits on eyelashes, beard, axillary/truncal hair, pubic hair

Pediculosis capitis
Nits on scalp hair

Eczematous dermatitis

Lymphadenopathy

Pediculosis corporis:
eggs in clothing, especially seams

Macula cerulea

A

B

Fig. 9.1: A depiction of the sites affected by pediculosis

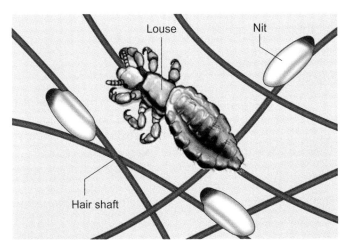

Louse

Nit

Hair shaft

Fig. 9.2A: A depiction of adult louse with nits which are attached to the hair shaft

> In patients with persistent dermatitis of the nape pediculosis capitis is a commonly ignored cause.

Diagnosis: Look for nits on the hair shafts, as well as for lice on the scalp.

Differential Diagnosis

Hair casts look similar to nits, but form an encompassing cylinder, whereas the nits are attached at an angle. Also casts can be moved along the hair shaft.

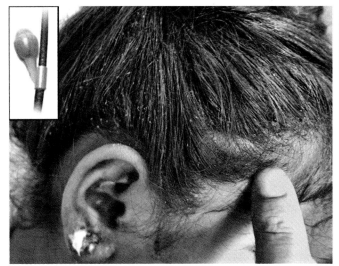

Fig. 9.2B: Nits on the scalp hair. The concomitant itching lead to secondary infection in and around the ear. Inset shows a nit

Piedra is an uncommon condition and consists of clumps of bacteria or fungi.

Therapy

- The finding of living moving lice means that the infestation is current and active, and needs treatment. Empty egg cases signify only that there has been an infestation in the past, but suggest the need for periodic re-inspection.

- Though ova close to the scalp are viable, and nits noted along the distal hair shaft are empty egg cases, but in humid climates, viable ova may be present along the entire length of the hair shaft. It should be remembered that viable nits are deposited on hair close to the scalp (usually within **1 to 2 mm**), and most nits that are further out than **5 to 7 mm**[Q] are no longer viable.

- All agents should be applied twice, 7–14 days apart. The second application is needed to kill young nymphs that hatch after the first application, usually 6–10 days after being laid. Recommendations vary regarding length of application, including overnight use, but all appear effective when used for 10–30 minutes and rinsed.

The general measures are listed in the Box 9.1 and details of active therapy follows:

1. **Dimethicone** is a non-neurotoxic agent that coats the lice and probably suffocates them. It is rubbed into dry hair and scalp and left for 8 hours. This is then repeated 1 week later. Cure rates of 70% or more are reported and it is non-irritant and well tolerated.

2. **Pyrethrins** and the synthetic **permethrin 1%** lotion have fair action and a reasonable resistance profile.
   - Applying to dry hair lessens dilution of the medication.
   - Product labelling states the medication should be applied for 10 min, then rinsed off, but longer applications may be required.
   - Shampooing should not take place for 24 hours afterward.
   - Although permethrin is both pediculicidal and ovicidal, many physicians recommend a second treatment 7 to 10 days after the initial therapy.[Q]

Box 9.1 | General treatment measures for pediculosis capitis

1. Family members and close contacts should be examined, and those with evidence of infestation should also be treated.
2. Play areas and furniture can be vacuumed, and bedding, clothing, and headgear should be machine washed in hot water and dried on a high-heat setting.[Q]
3. Items that cannot be washed may be dry-cleaned or placed in sealed plastic bags for 2 weeks.
4. Hats, combs, brushes, grooming aids, towels, school lockers and hooks, and other items that come into contact with the head or head coverings should not be shared.
5. Combs and brushes may be coated with the pediculicide for 15 minutes or soaked in alcohol for 1 hour followed by washing in hot soapy water. Alternatively, these items can be discarded and replaced with new ones.

- This agent is FDA approved for children as young as 2 months of age and is recommended as a first-line therapy.[Q]

3. **Ivermectin 0.5% lotion** is approved in children 6 months of age and older and is derived from the fermentation of the bacteria *Streptomyces avermitilis*. It is applied to dry hair and rinsed after 10 minutes.

4. **Lindane** (gamma benzene hexachloride) is still widely used, but relatively ineffective for this indication and with marked resistance.

5. Systemic **ivermectin**[Q] therapy can be given, if the topical therapies fail, 200 µg/kg (single dose, followed by a second dose in 7 days, if persistent infestation is present), similar to its use in scabies.

6. **Removal of nits:** The nits are always a problem; many schools have rules banning children returning as long as nits are present.
   - Best solutions following treatment are soaking with vinegar and water (50:50) and using a fine-toothed nit comb.
   - Wet combing with a fine toothed comb every 3 days for 14 days is a good alternative to the treatments mentioned above.
   - Shampoo or conditioner acts as a lubricant and helps with combing, but occasionally the hair has to be clipped short.
   - Pillow cases, towels, hats and scarves should be laundered or dry-cleaned.

Pediculosis Corporis

Infestation with *Pediculus humanus corporis*.

Epidemiology

Pediculosis corporis is primarily a disease of the unwashed, and is thus a water-washed disease.[Q] It is common in homeless people and during wars and other disasters. It is also called the Vagabond disease.[Q]

Pathogenesis

The lice feed on the body, but live in the clothing and tend to lay their eggs along the seams.[Q] They are slightly larger than a body louse (*Pediculus humanus corporis*) and jump onto the body only to feed.

Clinical Features (Fig. 9.1)

Presents with marked pruritus, lack of personal hygiene, and secondarily infected, excoriated dermatitis on trunk (vagabond skin). The skin becomes generally thickened, eczematized and pigmented; lymphadenopathy is common. Look for the lice and nits on the *clothing*, not on the skin.

Differential Diagnosis

In scabies, characteristic burrows are seen.

Body louse infestation is differentiated from scabies by the lack of involvement of the hands and feet, although infestation by both lice and scabies is common, and a given patient may have lice, scabies, and flea infestation.

Other causes of chronic itchy erythroderma include eczema and lymphomas, but these are ruled out by the finding of lice and nits.

Therapy

Lice may live in clothing for 1 month[Q] without a blood meal. Thus the various general options include:
1. Disinfection of clothing and bedding[Q] (boiling, hot ironing, fumigation).
   * Clothing placed in a dryer for 30 min at 65°C is a reliable method of disinfection.
   * Pressing clothing with an iron, especially the seams, is also effective.
   * Treating the clothes is more important
2. Attempt to change living conditions.
3. Same pediculicides as for *Pediculus humanus capitis* can be used, but are of *less importance* here.
   * Permethrin spray or 1% malathion powder can be used to treat clothing and reduce the risk of reinfestation.
4. In mass epidemics, usually insecticidal dusting powders employed.

Pediculosis Pubis

Infestation with *Phthirus pubis*.

Pubic lice (crabs) are broader than scalp and body lice, and their second and third pairs of legs are well adapted to cling onto hair[Q] (Fig. 9.3). They are usually spread by *sexual contact*, and most commonly infest young adults.

Epidemiology: Usually transmitted by sexual contacts.

Clinical Features

* Patients usually identify moving lice on their pubic hairs (crabs).
* Also complain of pruritus. Itching, especially at night, is the most common presenting symptom, take 1 to 3 weeks to develop after the first infestation.
* Nits usually on pubic hair, but occasionally elsewhere (axillary or body hairs; eyelashes, eyebrows). The nits look like a black speck (Figs 9.4 and 9.5A and B).

The shiny translucent nits are less obvious than those of head lice.
* Louse feces are often visible as rust-colored speckles on the skin, hair and underwear.
* The feeding sites turn into distinctive blue-gray hemorrhagic macules (Fig. 9.5C) (*maculae ceruleae* or *taches bleuâtres*).[Q] These are located chiefly on the sides of the trunk and the inner aspects of the thighs.

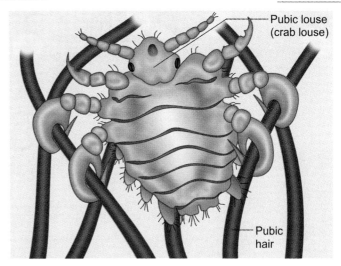

Fig. 9.3: A depiction of a pubic louse

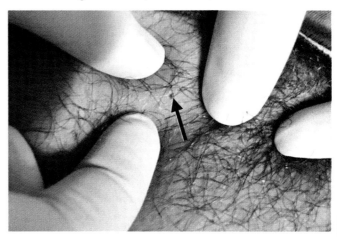

Fig. 9.4: Pediculosis pubis, note the louse which looks like a pigmented speck, patients complain of a creeping sensation that helps to localize the louse

These blue gray macules are consequent to altered blood at the site of bites.

Diagnostic approach: Identification of lice or nits.

Therapy

Consider whether the pubic lice infestation has been acquired via sexual or non-sexual contact. If acquired via sexual contact, screening for other sexually transmitted infections and contact tracing is advisable.

1. **Permethrin cream** or lindane lotion or shampoo is applied and repeated in 1 week.
   * The preparation should be applied for **12 hours or overnight**, and apart from the pubic area, also to all surfaces of the body, including the perianal area, limbs, scalp, neck, ears and face (especially the eyebrows and the beard, if present).
   * The infected sexual partners should also be treated. Any close contacts over the previous **three months** should be examined for pubic lice.
   * Shaving the area is not necessary.

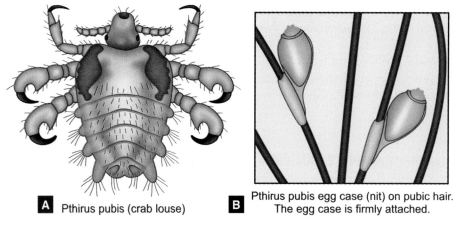

A Pthirus pubis (crab louse)

B Pthirus pubis egg case (nit) on pubic hair. The egg case is firmly attached.

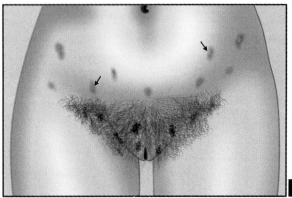
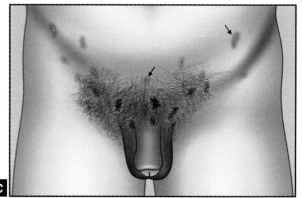

C

Fig. 9.5A to C: Depiction of (A) Adult louse; (B) Nits on pubic hair; (C) Maculae ceruleae (arrow)

2. **Ivermectin** p.o. is also effective for resistant cases.
3. Infestation of the eyelashes is particularly hard to treat, as this area is so sensitive that the mechanical removal of lice and eggs can be painful.
   - Applying a thick layer of petrolatum twice a day for 2 weeks has been recommended.
   - An inert occlusive ophthalmic ointment (e.g. simple eye ointment BP) twice a day for at least three weeks.
4. If pubic lice infestation is unresponsive to initial insecticide treatment, repeat the previous treatment with the correct technique (rather than switching to a different treatment).

   If insecticide resistance is suspected, switch to the alternative insecticide (malathion or permethrin).
5. *Cotrimoxazole*^{Q}: It is given in pediculosis as an antibiotic that kills the commensal flora in the gut of the lice.

SCABIES

This is an intensely pruritic infestation due to the mite *Sarcoptes scabiei*.

The discovery in 1687 of the 'itch mite' made this parasite one of the first causes of human disease to be identified.

Epidemiology: Worldwide distribution. In the past, it typically appeared in cycles (7-year itch),^{Q} but this is no longer the case. In recent years, epidemics in homes for the elderly have become a problem.

Pathogenesis

Sarcoptes scabiei^Q is a mite that lives only on humans. It does not transfer any disease. Transfer is by close personal contact.
- The impregnated female burrows into the stratum corneum,^{Q} where she lays two or three eggs daily for as long as 30 days (Fig. 9.6).
- The number of adult mites varies from case-to-case—from less than 10 (average 10–15) ^{Q} in a clean adult to many more in an unwashed child.

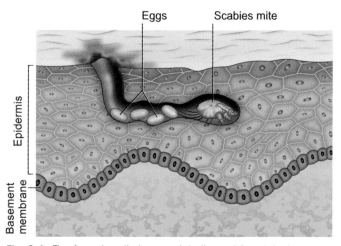

Fig. 9.6: The female mite burrows into the epidermis laying eggs (2–3 /day) for 30 days

- Once on the skin, the fertilized female mites can move over the surface at up to 2 cm a minute, but can burrow through the stratum corneum at only about 2 mm/day. They produce two or three oval eggs each day, which turn into sexually mature mites in 2–3 weeks.

(2 cm/min; 2 mm/day; 2–3 eggs/day; 2–3 weeks)

Each egg produces a larva, which leaves the burrow and molts to produce a nymph. Several further moltings result in a mature mite, which then mates. After mating, the male dies, and the female completes the life cycle by burrowing back into the stratum corneum.

The first infestation remains asymptomatic for a period of 4–5 weeks,[Q] until an immune response develops and pruritus results. Upon re-infestation, the symptoms appear in a matter of days.

The itching and inflammation are thought to be a result of a hypersensitivity reaction by the host to the foreign material (i.e. mites, eggs, and feces) in the skin.[Q] This may account for the persistence of the itching for 1 to 2 weeks after successful treatment; it may take that long for the stratum corneum to turn over and to shed the foreign material, and for the hypersensitivity reaction to subside.

Clinical Features

The clinical features of the infestations can have myriad manifestations with various types of lesions in a single patient (Fig. 9.7):

> Always think of scabies when a patient complains of night-time pruritus[Q] or when multiple family members are itching.

1. **Burrows:** Fine slightly raised, sometimes erythematous, irregular lines with a terminal swelling where the female mite can be found. Typical sites (Figs 9.8 and 9.9) include interdigital spaces, sides of the hands and feet, flexural surface of the wrist, anterior axillary line, penis, and nipples. These sites can be joined by an imaginary circle, referred to as the circle of Hebra.[Q] The lesions often get secondarily infected (Fig. 9.10A) and can develop secondary eczema (Fig. 9.10B), also there is risk of post-streptococcal glomerulonephritis infection of lesions.[Q]

2. **Intense pruritus:** A few skin diseases itch as much as scabies; usually worst at night. For about 4–6 weeks after a first infestation, there may be no itching,[Q] but thereafter itching tends to progressively increase. But in a second attack of scabies, itching starts within a

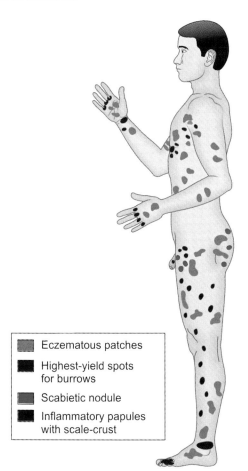

Eczematous patches

Highest-yield spots for burrows

Scabietic nodule

Inflammatory papules with scale-crust

Fig. 9.7: Range of cutaneous lesions in scabies. Crusted scabies may show prominent hyperkeratosis of acral sites

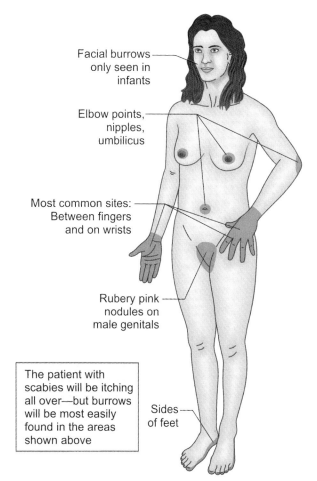

Facial burrows only seen in infants

Elbow points, nipples, umbilicus

Most common sites: Between fingers and on wrists

Rubery pink nodules on male genitals

The patient with scabies will be itching all over—but burrows will be most easily found in the areas shown above

Sides of feet

Fig. 9.8: Distribution of burrows in a scabies patient

day or two, because these patients already have immunity to produce the itchy allergic reactions. Norweigian scabies often does not itch.[Q]

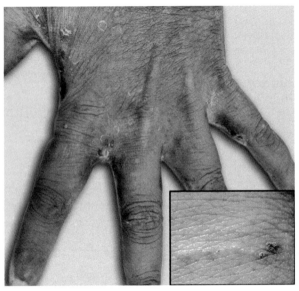

Fig. 9.9: Burrows seen as small irregular tracks in the finger web space in a patient with scabies (inset shows a burrow, the raised vesicle at the end is the location of the mite)

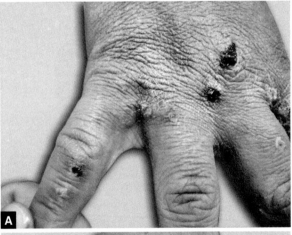

A

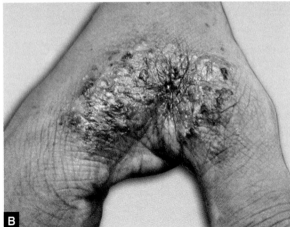

B

Fig. 9.10A and B: (A) A case of scabies, with interdigital area involvement with secondary infection; (B) Scabies with secondary eczema

3. **Dermatitis:** Immune reaction (type IV) to mites leads to both pruritus and diffuse exanthem. Typical sites are thighs, buttocks, and trunk.
4. Relapse of the disease after adequate treatment is common and can be put down to re-infestation from undetected and untreated contacts.

Variants

- **Scabies incognito:** Patients with meticulous personal hygiene (scabies of the clean) or those using topical corticosteroids may completely mask the findings of scabies.[Q]
- **Nodular scabies:** Persistent papules usually in infants, favoring the groin, axillae, and genitalia. Occasionally seen in adults once again genitalia[Q] most common (Figs 9.11 and 9.12). The persistent nodules (Fig. 9.13) on biopsy show a lymphocytic infiltrate. They remain for months after elimination of all mites and are blamed on 'antigen persistence'.

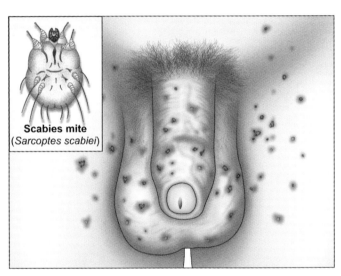

Scabies mite
(*Sarcoptes scabiei*)

Fig. 9.11: Inflammatory excoriated papules (note penile involvement)

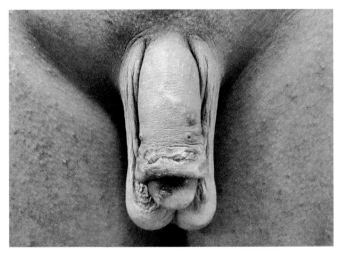

Fig. 9.12: Papules and a few excoriated nodules seen over the shaft of penis and scrotum in patient with scabies

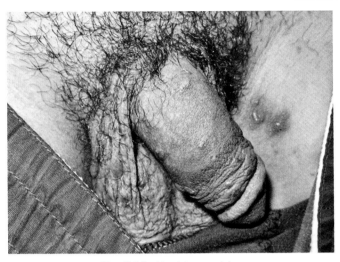

Fig. 9.13: Nodular scabies

- **Crusted scabies (Norwegian scabies):**[Q] Massive scabies infestation with crusted hyperkeratotic, psoriasiform lesions, as well as subungual lesions. Most infectious form of scabies.[Q]

It most commonly arises in patients with the following:
  - Dementia
  - Down's syndrome
  - HIV[Q]
  - Other conditions associated with neurological impairment
  - Immunosuppression

- **Animal scabies:** There are over 40 different forms of animal scabies, including those involving cats, dogs, and birds. These mites cannot reproduce on humans. They tend to bite at sites of contact (hands, arms, face, if sleeping with pet). They cannot proliferate on the accidental host but cause intensive self-limited pruritic reactions without any incubation period, and then die. It is a frequent cause of recurrent scabies.[Q]

- **Infantile scabies:** Only in infancy does scabies affect the face and palms and soles (Fig. 9.14). Also *vesiculobullous* and pustular bullous lesions might be seen.[Q]

Diagnostic Approach

Identification of mite; look at ends of burrows (dermatoscopy can help; hang glider sign);[Q] unroof with fine scalpel and examine under microscope.

Suspect scabies in any unexplained pruritic disease which is worse at night or also present in family members or other contacts.

Infantile scabies to be differentiated from congenital syphilis based on presence of itching and positive family history.

Therapy

Treatment should be started, if the diagnosis seems likely on clinical grounds, even if the presence of mites cannot be confirmed microscopically. Treat all members

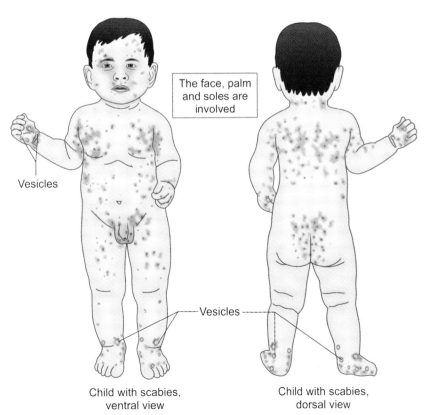

The face, palm and soles are involved

Vesicles

Vesicles

Child with scabies, ventral view

Child with scabies, dorsal view

Fig. 9.14: A depiction of the distribution of scabies in an infant

Table 9.2	Therapeutic agents for scabies	
Permethrin 5% cream	Apply from neck down; rinse in 8–14 hours	Not for use under 2 months of age; may repeat in 1 week, if necessary; treat scalp in infants
Sulfur 6% ointment	Apply from neck down for 3 consecutive nights; rinse 24 hours after last application	Older therapy; malodorous; compounded in petrolatum; safe in infants, pregnant females
Crotamiton cream	Apply from neck down for 2 consecutive nights; rinse 48 hours after last application	High failure rate; may require up to 5 applications
Benzyl benzoate	Apply nightly or every other night for 3 applications	
Ivermectin	200 µg/kg per dose given orally for 2 doses, 2 weeks apart	Consider for severe infestations, crusted scabies, immunocompromised patients, scabies epidemics; should not be used under 5 years of age

of the family and sexual contacts too, whether they are itching or not.

General Measures

- Clothing, bed linens, and towels should be machine washed in hot water and dried using a high-heat setting. Clothing or other items (i.e. stuffed animals) that cannot be washed may be dry-cleaned or stored in bags for 3 days to 1 week, because the mite will die when separated from the human host.
- All contacts need to be managed in exactly the same way as the patient, however, for most only one treatment is needed. Only symptomatic contacts require two treatments.

Specific Measures

An overview of the therapy options are given in Table 9.2 and discussed in the following text.

1. **Permethrin 5%** cream has the best safety record and the least reports of resistance. It should be viewed as the agent of choice.[Q]
   - The treatment should be applied to the scalp, neck, face and ears as well as to the rest of the skin. Areas that must be included are the genitals, soles of the feet, gluteal fold and the skin under the free edge of the nails.
   - The face and scalp should only be treated, if they are affected, which is uncommon in adults and older children.
   - Apply at night, wash in morning; repeat after 1 week. Bedding and clothing should be washed

in hot cycle of washing machine; under normal conditions no other precautions are needed.

2. **Lindane lotion** is the worldwide standard, but not as effective as permethrin. It should be used in the same way. Lindane should *not* be used in *pregnancy* or in *infants*. It is potentially neurotoxic and there are several alternatives.

3. **Ivermectin:** For resistant cases, epidemics or crusted scabies, ivermectin 200 µg/kg by mouth µg/kg p.o. administered on days 1 and 14 is highly effective.

4. **Infantile scabies:** For children up to 2 years old, permethrin 5% is used, but it is licensed for use *over* the age of *2 months*. A safer alternative is 6% precipitated sulfurin petrolatum.[Q]

5. **Pregnancy:** Permethrin is probably safe in pregnancy and in nursing mothers as little is absorbed, and any that is absorbed is rapidly detoxified and eliminated.

6. Treat secondary infection, if present with a systemic antibiotic, e.g. flucloxacillin, or erythromycin, if the patient is allergic to penicillin.

7. Residual itching may last for several days, or even a few weeks, but this does not need further applications of the scabicide. Rely instead on calamine lotion or crotamiton.

DEMODICOSIS

Demodex folliculorum and *Demodex brevis* are 0.3 mm mites that favor the sebum-rich facial area of older individuals. They cause a rosacea-like eruption with pruritic follicular papules, often asymmetrically distributed. Infection is treated with permethrin or crotamiton.

Inflammatory Disorders

Psoriasis

INTRODUCTION

Psoriasis is a common, chronic, inflammatory disease that can result in decreased quality of life. Psoriasis is characterized by increased epidermal proliferation (regular acanthosis) resulting in an accumulation of stratum corneum (scale). Celsus gave a convincing account of psoriasis vulgaris almost 2000 years ago. About **2–3%** of the population have psoriasis and **10%** of these individuals will develop psoriatic arthritis. Of this group, in 3–5% of them, it is severe (Box 10.1).

PATHOGENESIS

1. **Genetics:** A child with one affected parent has a 14% chance of developing the disease, and this rises to 41%, if both parents are affected. There are two peaks of onset of psoriasis (Fig. 10.1A). Type I has onset in the second and third decades and a more common family history of psoriasis. Type II has onset in late adulthood in patients without obvious family

history. Early onset psoriasis shows a genetic linkage with a psoriasis susceptibility locus (PSOR-1) located on 6p21 within the major histocompatibility complex Class I (MHC-I) region. The HLA-Cw6^Q allele at this site, which affects immune function, particularly confers a risk of developing psoriasis.

2. **Hyperproliferation:** The growth fraction of epidermal basal cells is increased sevenfold compared with normal skin. The cell turnover time decreases from 30 to 5 days (Fig. 10.1B), similarly the cell cycle time reduces from 311 to 36 hours.^{Q}

3. **Inflammation:** The importance of T lymphocytes is shown by their presence early in the development of psoriatic plaques and the response of the disease to treatment such as ciclosporin.
   - Release of **interleukin-12** causes differentiation to type 1 helper cells **(Th1)**.
   - **Interleukin-23** determines the formation of **type 17** helper cells.
   - In the dermis, Th1 cells release γ-interferon and TNF-α, and Th17 cells release interleukin-17 and 22.
   - Neutrophils are drawn to the epidermis by these chemokines, particularly IL-8, producing the characteristic pustules of severe psoriasis.

   Thus it seems likely that psoriasis is a disturbance in keratinocyte proliferation that can be elicited indirectly by Th1/Th17 cells, IL-23 and TNF, or directly by physical stimuli (Fig. 10.2).^{Q} Why this process happens in localized often symmetrical areas remains a mystery.

   Psoriatic keratinocytes contain high levels of the antimicrobial peptides IL-37 (cathelicidin), β defensin and psoriasin (S100A7), which may account for the surprisingly low incidence of bacterial skin infection.

Box 10.1 | **Overview of psoriasis (mnemonic)**

P Pink bleeding: Auspitz sign/physical injury (Koebner phenomenon)^Q

S Silver scale/sharp margins

O Onycholysis/oil drop sign^Q

R Rete ridges with regular elongation

I Non-itching (itching* ranges from mild to severe)

A Arthritis/abscess (Munro)

S *S. corneum* (Munro) and *S. spinosum* (Kogoj) with neutrophils^Q

I Immunological (Th1)

S *S. granulosum* absent

*Itching (psoriasis is derived from the Greek word for 'itching') ranges from mild to severe.

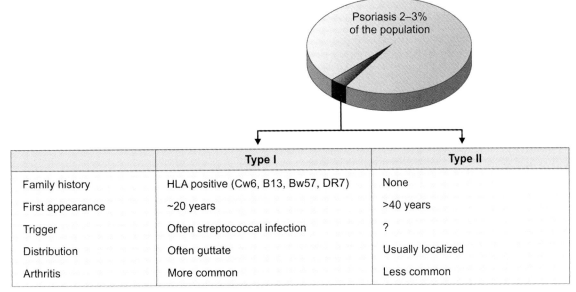

	Type I	Type II
Family history	HLA positive (Cw6, B13, Bw57, DR7)	None
First appearance	~20 years	>40 years
Trigger	Often streptococcal infection	?
Distribution	Often guttate	Usually localized
Arthritis	More common	Less common

Fig. 10.1A: Subtypes of psoriasis[Q]

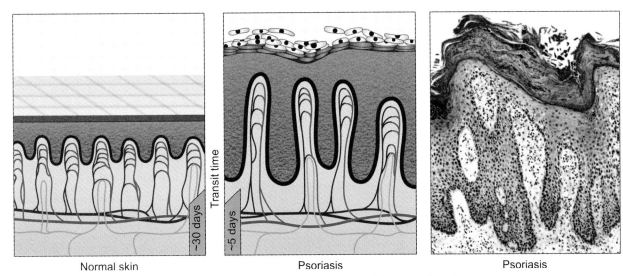

Normal skin   Psoriasis   Psoriasis

Fig. 10.1B: A depiction of the *normal* epidermis and *hyperproliferative* psoriasis skin

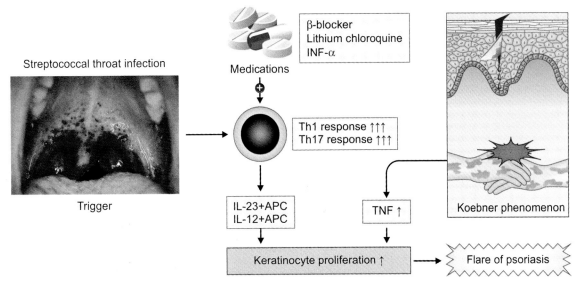

Fig. 10.2: Overview of pathogenesis of psoriasis

4. Psoriasis is also now appreciated to be an intimate part of the metabolic syndrome, associated with hypertension, diabetes mellitus, and coronary artery disease. The persistent immune stimulation may thus have wide-reaching effects.

TRIGGERING FACTORS

An overview of triggering factors is given in Box 10.2, but a few important factors are:

- The sudden appearance of multiple small (guttate) lesions of psoriasis in a generalized distribution is often preceded by a streptococcal throat infection.[Q]
- In patients with severe sudden onset or rapidly worsening large-plaque psoriasis, a predisposing human immunodeficiency virus (HIV) infection should be considered.

Box 10.2	Trigger factors for psoriasis[Q]
Trauma	Koebner phenomenon
Infection	• β-hemolytic streptococci: Guttate psoriasis
	• *Staphylococcus aureus* and certain streptococci can act as superantigens
	• HIV infection often worsens psoriasis, or precipitates explosive forms
Hormonal	Improves in pregnancy only to relapse postpartum
Sunlight	Improves but in 10% worsens
Drugs	• Antimalarials, β-blockers, NSAID and lithium may worsen psoriasis
	• It may 'rebound' after withdrawal of treatment with systemic steroids or potent topical steroids.
Alcohol/smoking	Aggravates
Season	Worse in winter (lack of sun and humidity)

HISTOLOGY

The appearance of psoriasis depends on the stage of the lesion and type of lesion. Early guttate lesions demonstrate no acanthosis. Established plaques demonstrate a characteristic pattern of regular acanthosis. Pustular psoriasis may never demonstrate acanthosis. Acral and intertriginous lesions of psoriasis commonly demonstrate a background of spongiosis.

The main changes are the following (Fig. 10.3A and B):[Q]

1. *Parakeratosis*: Parakeratosis (nuclei retained in the horny layer).
2. *Hypogranulosis*: Decreased to absent granular layer.
3. *Abscess*: Epidermal polymorphonuclear leukocyte infiltrates and microabscesses (described originally by Munro). A similar collection in the S. *granulosum* is called spongiform pustule of Kogoj (this is more diagnostic[Q] than Munro abscess).
4. *Irregular thickening*: Irregular thickening of the epidermis over the rete ridges, but thinning over dermal papillae. Bleeding may occur when scale is scratched off (Auspitz sign).[Q]
5. Dilated tortuous capillaries
6. T lymphocytes

CLINICAL TYPES

1. **Plaque-type psoriasis vulgaris** accounts for 90% of all cases. The primary lesion is a scaly, red- to salmon-pink-colored papule that expands to form a plaque. It is usually covered by a white or silvery scale (Fig. 10.4A) that, when removed, may show pinpoint bleeding (Auspitz sign)[Q] (Fig. 10.4B).

Plaque-type psoriasis is classically an extensor disease often involving the knees, elbows, gluteal cleft, lumbosacral region, and the umbilicus (sites of trauma).

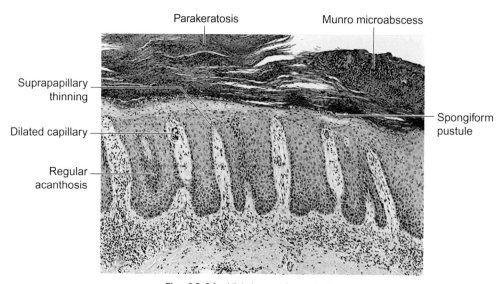

Fig. 10.3A: Histology of psoriasis

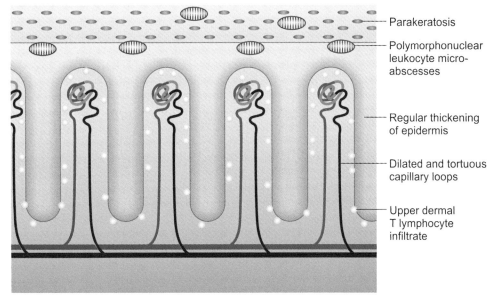

Parakeratosis

Polymorphonuclear leukocyte micro-abscesses

Regular thickening of epidermis

Dilated and tortuous capillary loops

Upper dermal T lymphocyte infiltrate

Fig. 10.3B: A depiction of the histology of psoriasis

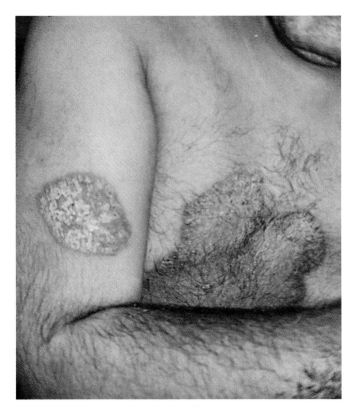

Fig. 10.4A: A case of psoriasis with an erythematous plaque with silver white scaling

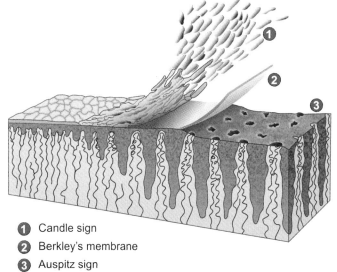

1 Candle sign
2 Berkley's membrane
3 Auspitz sign

Fig. 10.4B: Steps of **Grattage test** and demonstration of **Auspitz sign** while using a blunt object the scales in a case of plaque psoriasis come off like 'candle wax'[Q] if progressively removed a red membrane is revealed called the Berkley membrane and removal of that leads to pinpoint bleeding called the Auspitz sign

Psoriasis may involve the scalp where it classically extends beyond the hair margin (Fig. 10.5). Scalp psoriasis has a clear edge, typically with some areas unaffected, in contrast to dandruff that affects the whole scalp. Psoriasis does not cause alopecia, nor does it involve the oral mucosa.[Q]

2. **Inverse psoriasis** presents with thin pink plaques with minimal scale in the axillae (Fig. 10.6), inguinal and inframammary area, and body folds of the trunk.[Q] It may occur in conjunction with typical plaque psoriasis or it may be the only manifestation of psoriasis. The area must be made less moist (careful drying with hair dryer, weight loss); then the lesions usually respond well to vitamin D analogs in a gel base.

3. **Guttate psoriasis** (rain drop-like) occurs in less than 2% of cases, but it is a common subtype in children and is preceded by streptococcal sore throat.[Q] It is characterized by small 'droplet-like' thin pink to salmon-colored papules and plaques surmounted by a fine white scale.

10

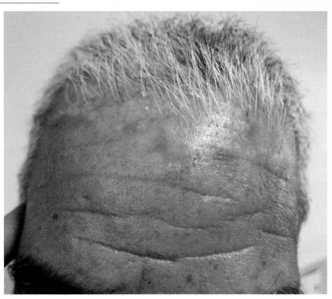

Fig. 10.5: A patient with scalp psoriasis which extends beyond the frontal hair margin, unlike seborrheic dermatitis

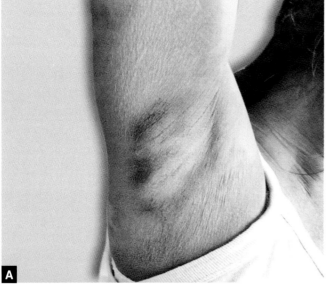

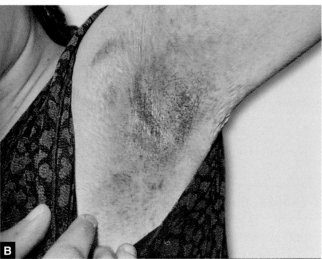

Fig. 10.6A and B: The psoriasis plaque here lacks the scaling that is seen in classic plaque psoriasis (inverse psoriasis)

4. **Pustular psoriasis** (von Zumbusch)[Q] is an acute variant of the disease that presents with small, monomorphic sterile pustules surmounting painful, inflamed, erythematous papules (Figs 10.7 and 10.8). The lesions can coalesce to form 'lakes of pus'.[Q] Fever, systemic symptoms, and an elevated white blood cell count often accompany generalized pustular psoriasis.

- An acral variant has been described around the nails (acrodermatitis continua) as also a variant localized to the palms and soles (palmoplantar pustulosis).
- Pustular psoriasis in pregnancy begins in the last trimester and involves the flexures and this is referred to as impetigo herpetiformis.[Q]
- Some common aggravating factors include hypocalcemia and sudden withdrawal of steroids.[Q]

> The pustules can be localized, or generalized when the trigger is systemic, such as when systemic corticosteroids are used to treat psoriasis and then stopped. This risk is just one reason why corticosteroids are not routinely used systemically in psoriasis.

5. **Erythrodermic psoriasis** is a skin reaction pattern of total (>90%) body redness and desquamation of the skin[Q] (Fig. 10.9).

There is loss of margins of the lesions and they spread rapidly to involving the entire body.

The massive shedding of skin that occurs during an erythrodermic flare of psoriasis can result in infection, hypothermia, protein loss, hypoalbuminuria, dehydration, and electrolyte disturbances. The main problems that can ensue include:

- Increased fluid loss through the skin
- Increased protein loss
- Mild heart failure, as 25% of the cardiac output may be diverted to the skin.

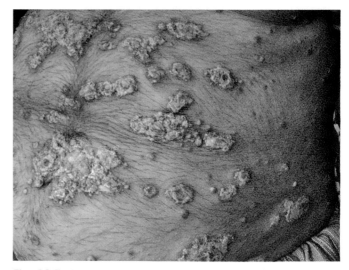

Fig. 10.7: Plaque psoriasis surmounted by pustules in a case of pustular psoriasis

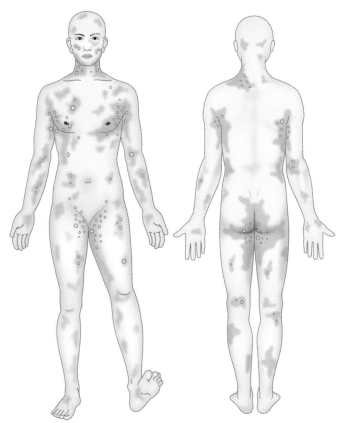

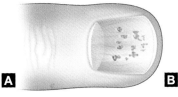

A **Pitting:** Parakeratotic cells fall away, leaving depressions (pits) on the surface of the nail

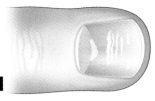

B **Leukonychia:** White spots in the nail plate due to psoriatic parakeratosis in nail plate

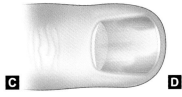
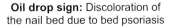

C **Oil drop sign:** Discoloration of the nail bed due to bed psoriasis

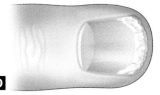

D Nail bed hyperkeratosis

Fig. 10.10A to D: An overview of nail findings in psoriasis

Fig. 10.8: A depiction of pustular psoriasis. Note the pustules aggregated over the body, which coalesce to form 'lake of pus' appearance

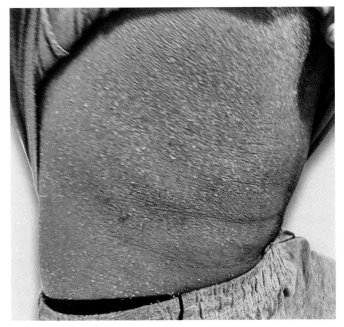

Fig. 10.9: Diffuse erythema and scaling in a case of psoriatic erythroderma

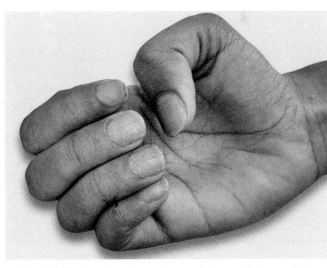

Fig. 10.11: Random, irregular, and deep pits in psoriasis

6. **Psoriatic nails** can be seen in up to 50%^{Q} of patients with psoriasis. It may be the only manifestation of psoriasis. It is recognized that nail disease is more closely linked with psoriatic joint disease. Up to 90%^{Q} of patients with psoriatic arthritis have nail disease.

The most common nail defect is pitting^Q and subungual hyperkeratosis^Q (Figs 10.10 and 10.11). The pitting can be remembered by the mnemonic RIDL.

RIDL (random, irregular, deep and large pits) (Fig. 10.11).^{Q}

Psoriasis is characterized by a plaque of psoriasis in the distal nail bed with accumulation of scale, which lifts the plate from the nailbed. This leads to onycholysis (nail plate separation) with red border, oil spots (yellow-orange subungual discoloration) and splinter hemorrhages. The most diagnostic feature is the 'oil drop' sign.^{Q}

- Although the skin feels hot, there is great heat loss from radiation, resulting in hypothermia.

Aggravating factors: Lithium, beta-blockers, NSAIDs, antimalarials, phototoxic reaction, infection.^{Q}

10

7. **Psoriatic arthritis:** Every patient with psoriasis should be specifically screened for joint disease and enthesitis (inflammation of the tendon insertions).

There are 5 main types:
- Asymmetric oligoarthropathy (most common and site is knee joint)[Q]
- Distal interphalangeal (DIP) joint involvement (classic)[Q]
- Rheumatoid pattern (symmetric polyarthropathy)
- Psoriatic arthritis mutilans (most severe form)
- Predominant spondylitis or sacroiliitis.

The criteria used for classification of psoriatic arthritis is called CASPAR criteria.

Methotrexate appears to delay the disease progression, while the TNF antagonists seem to arrest it.

DIFFERENTIAL DIAGNOSIS

Diagnosis is easy as the lesions have the characteristic silvery scale and involve the typical locations. Some variants where the diagnosis may be a problem include:
- Intertriginous areas: They may be confused with tinea cruris, candidiasis, and intertrigo.
- Scalp: Psoriasis of the scalp is most often confused with seborrheic dermatitis, in which the scaling is usually finer, yellower, and more diffuse with indistinct borders.
- Guttate psoriasis on the trunk is sometimes confused with pityriasis rosea or tinea corporis.
- Chronic dermatitis and T cell cutaneous lymphoma can rarely mimic psoriasis.
- Nail involvement may be clinically indistinguishable from onychomycosis.

TREATMENT

The therapy of psoriasis depends on the type and extent of disease. There are four arms of therapy—topical, systemic, phototherapy and biological drugs.

The severity of psoriasis can be scored on the Psoriasis Area and Severity Index (PASI), which quantifies the scaliness, erythema, thickness and extent. Although the maximum score is 72, most dermatologists would interpret a PASI of 12 as severe disease. While very useful and reproducible for clinical research studies, the PASI is cumbersome for routine use in the clinic.

Some other measures of extent of psoriasis are given in Box 10.3.

First-Line Treatment

- Mainly topical, usually prescribed, if less than 5–10% of total body surface area is involved.

Box 10.3	Measures of severity of psoriasis
Handprint	1% of body surface area
PASI	This measures redness, scaling, thickness and area over four body regions. Score range 0–72, but most patients' scores are <10
DLQI	Used to assess how badly the patient's life is being affected
The Rule of Tens	• The body surface area >10% • The PASI >10 • The DLQI >10 • This means that the psoriasis is 'severe' • Active therapy, possibly systemic, is required

- First-line topical treatments include moderate to potent steroids, vitamin D analogues, retinoids, anthralin **(Ingrams regimen[Q])**, coal tar **(Goeckerman regimen[Q])**, and salicylic acid.
- With topical steroids, a good response is usually noted within several weeks, but tachyphylaxis (loss of effect with continued use of a drug) may develop. Therefore, for long-term use of topical steroids, a good option is to use an **intermittent regimen** (e.g. use the agent for only 2 of every 3 weeks or skipping days when doing well).
- Topical tazarotene is applied at bedtime, often in conjunction with a topical steroid applied in the morning.
- Calcipotriene ointment, cream, and lotion is a vitamin D derivative with antimitotic activity. It is applied twice daily and requires several months of use for full effect.
- If the affected area is >10%, use topical medications as adjuncts to phototherapy or systemic drugs.

A summary of the topical agents is given in Table 10.1.

Second-Line Treatment (Phototherapy)

Phototherapy options include UVB for guttate psoriasis and UVB 311 nm or PUVA for plaque psoriasis.[Q]

PUVA is the least toxic systemic approach.

Third-Line Treatment (Systemic Agents)

Systemic treatment should be considered, if:[Q]
- Psoriatic lesions cover >10% of total body surface area
- Unsuccessful topical therapies
- Psychological distress
- Patients with moderate to severe disease

Table 10.1 Topical agents in psoriasis

Drug class	Salient features	Indications
Topical agents Vitamin D analogues Calcipotriol (calcipotriene), calcitriol and tacalcitol	• Calcipotriol: Reduces scaling, not to be used on the face, up to 15 g/day or 100 g/week[Q] • Tacalcitol ointment: Once daily at bedtime, the maximum amount being 10 g/day.[Q] • Calcipotriene + betamethasone Dipropionate: For use in adults >18 years old for up to 4 weeks	Localised plaque psoriasis
Topical corticosteroids	<50 g/week of a moderately potent topical corticosteroid	Short-term, or intermittent, treatment of psoriasis
Tazarotene	Works slowly and seldom clears psoriasis but reduces the induration, scaling and redness of plaques	Localised psoriasis
Dithranol (anthralin)	• It is irritant, so treatment should start with a weak (0.1%) preparation. • Short contact therapy,[Q] in which dithranol is applied for no longer than 30 minutes	Used for resistant patches
Phototherapy Narrowband UVB (311 nm)[Q]	2–3 times weekly for 8 weeks or until the skin clears	Safest therapy for psoriasis

Table 10.2 A overview of systemic agents and phototherapy for psoriasis

Phototherapy Narrowband UVB (311 nm)[Q]	2–3 times weekly for 8 weeks or until the skin clears.	Safest therapy for psoriasis
Systemic therapy Photochemotherapy (PUVA)	The 8-MOP (crystalline formulation 0.6–0.8 mg/kg body weight or liquid formulation 0.3–0.4 mg/kg) is taken 1–2 h before exposure to UVA tubes two or three times a week Clearance takes 5–10 weeks	Used for chronic plaque psoriasis
Acitretin	10–25 mg/day SE: Xerosis, hyperlipidemia, teratogenicity (avoid conception 2 years[Q] after stopping therapy)	Retinoids and PUVA act synergistically and are often used together in the so-called Re-PUVA regimen. This is used for plaque psoriasis
Methotrexate	7.5–20 mg/week (Weinstein Frost regimen)[Q] • Risk of hepatic fibrosis • Liver biopsy after 1.5–2 gm • Liver biopsy is now being replaced by serial assays of serum procollagen III aminopeptide (PIIINP)[Q]	• Used for plaque and pustular psoriasis. • Methotrexate should not be taken at the same time as retinoids or ciclosporin.
Cyclosporine	The initial daily dose is 3–4 mg/kg/day and not more than 5 mg/kg/day SE: Renal side effects raised cholesterol, triglycerides, hyperkalaemia and hypomagnesemia hirsutism and gingival hyperplasia.[Q]	Short term therapy

The **non-biological agents** are summarized in Table 10.2 and broadly include:
• Cyclosporin, methotrexate and acitretin
  – *Methotrexate*: Drug of choice for chronic plaque and erythrodermic psoriasis.[Q]
  – *Acitretin*: Drug of choice for pustular psoriasis.[Q]
  – *Alitretinoin*: A systemic retinoid, may be helpful for palmoplantar disease.
  – *Cyclosporin*: Is effective as a rapid control agent.[Q]

Biological treatment includes:
• Alefacept, etanercept, infliximab, adalimumab, ustekinumab and secukinumab.[Q]
  – A list of common biological agents are listed in Table 10.3, but it must be emphasized that the ideal biological agent is yet to be discovered and a plethora of drugs are constantly discovered that target the wide array of cytokines.
• *TNF-alpha biological agents*:

Table 10.3 Biologics in psoriasis

Etanercept	**SC** twice weekly	TNF-α
Adalimumab	**SC**, 80 mg followed by 40 mg every 2 weeks	TNF-α
Infliximab	**IV** 5 mg/kg 0, 2, 6 weeks then once in 2 months	TNF-α
Secukinumab	**SC**, dose at 0, 1, 2, 3, 4 weeks (300 mg), then monthly	IL-17A
Ustekinumab	**SC** every 3 months in maintenance phase	IL 12/23

SC: Subcutaneous

- The TNF-α[Q] blocking agents are generally recommended as the first-line biological treatment, with etanercept and adalimumab being favored in stable chronic plaque psoriasis.
- For unstable and general pustular psoriasis, infliximab has the advantage of rapid onset of action and disease control. Infliximab probably works fastest of all the biological agents, but requires intravenous infusions.
- The biggest worry with this class of drugs is the potential for reactivation of tuberculosis.
- *IL-17/IL-12/IL-23 biological agents*: If these fail, an alternative anti-TNF-α, or secukinumab or ustekinumab (a second-line agent) can be used. With these drugs, rapid response rates can be achieved.

A summary of the drugs of choice for various types of psoriasis is given in Table 10.4 as a ready reckoner.

Table 10.4 Treatment of various types of psoriasis[Q]

Stable plaque (localized)	• Local corticosteroid[Q] • Vitamin D analogue • Narrowband UVB phototherapy • Tar
Extensive stable plaque (>30% surface area) recalcitrant to local therapy	• Narrowband UVB • PUVA • PUVA + acitretin • Methotrexate • Cyclosporine • Biologicals
Guttate	• Systemic antibiotic[Q] • Emollients with then UVB • Mild topical steroids
Facial/flexural	• Mild to moderately potent topical corticosteroid • Tacrolimus • Calcitriol
Acute erythrodermic, unstable or generalized pustular	• Acitretin/phototherapy (UVB) • Methotrexate, cyclosporine • Biologic agents
Palmoplantar psoriasis	• Moderately potent or potent local steroid • Retinoids • Methotrexate
Psoriatic arthropathy	Etanercept /methotrexate[Q]
Impetigo herpetiformis	Steroids/cyclosporine[Q]
HIV	Retinoids, NB-UVB[Q]

10

Lichenoid Skin Disorders

LICHEN PLANUS

This is a common inflammatory disease featuring pruritus, distinctive^Q violaceous flat-topped papules^Q and often oral erosions. It is classified by various books as a papulosquamous skin disorder. It affects all age groups but is most common between the ages of 30 and 60. Children and infants are not commonly affected. There are no gender or racial predispositions.

Pathogenesis

- The disorder is primarily a immunological disorder. Activated T lymphocytes are recruited to the dermo-epidermal junction where CD8+ cytotoxic and to a lesser extent CD4+ T cells predominate. The infiltrate of Th1 cells^Q and cytotoxic cells secrete IFN-γ and TNF-α which increase the expression of HLA-DR8 adhesion molecules on keratinocytes causing **basal cell layer** damage and consequent reactive hyperkeratosis (model of T cell-mediated epidermal damage). The antigen for the autoimmune attack is unknown in LP.^{Q}

  (Similar basal keratinocyte apoptosis also occurs in subacute cutaneous lupus erythematosus and erythema multiforme, but elevated intercellular adhesion molecule 1 (ICAM-1) expression is specific to lichen planus.)

- In some countries, especially Italy, association between lichen planus and hepatitis viruses (usually hepatitis C)^Q is seen. IFN therapy for hepatitis can also trigger lichen planus.

- Drug eruptions resembling lichen planus are frequently induced by medications (Box 11.1).

Box 11.1	Common causes of lichenoid drug eruption^Q
• Mepacrine	• Propranolol
• Gold^Q	• Labetalol
• Quinine	• Enalapril
• Thiazide diuretics	• Captopril
• Isoniazid	• Naproxen
• Methyldopa	

Clinical Features

The 5 Ps of LP—Purple, Pruritic, Polygonal, Papules, Planar (flat topped).

Classic lesions are glistening violaceous flat-topped papules (Fig. 11.1A and B), usually 2–10 mm in diameter, that usually heal with hyperpigmentation^Q.

- Fine lacy white markings on top of papules known as **Wickham striae**^{Q} (Fig. 11.2) (seen in 50% of patients)^Q. These striae are most prominent in the oral mucosa. Wickham's striae are more readily visible through a hand-held lens after the application of a drop of oil on the surface of the papule.

- The reason for the violaceous hue is the Tyndall effect.^{Q}

- Scratching and trauma induce new lesions: **Köebner**^{Q} phenomenon.

- Pruritus is usually present and is sometimes intense. The patients rub rather than scratch, so that excoriations are uncommon.^{Q}

- Sites of predilection include inner aspects of wrists,^{Q} ankles, anterior shins, buttocks. On the scalp, it can cause cicatricial alopecia (Fig. 11.3).^{Q}

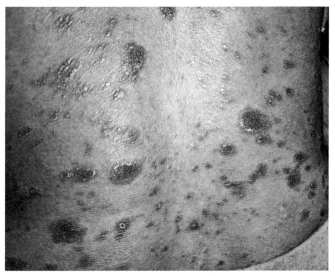

Fig. 11.1A: Purple papules coalescing to form annular plaques in lichen planus

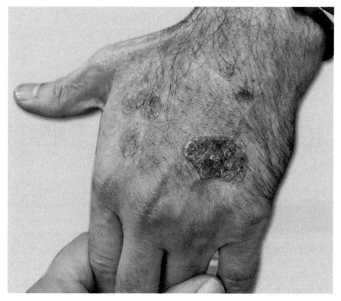

Fig. 11.2: A case of LP with a distinct reticular pattern on the plaque **(Wickham striae)**

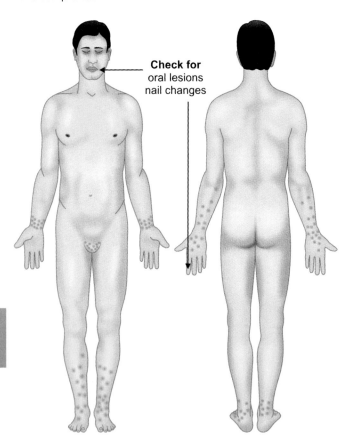

Check for
oral lesions
nail changes

Fig. 11.1B: Depiction of the distribution of lesions in LP

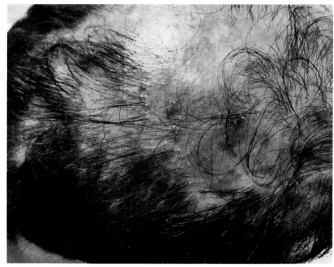

Fig. 11.3: A case of follicular LP on the scalp with consequent cicatricial alopecia

- If the epidermal repair reaction dominates, then the lesions becomes hyperkeratotic (especially when follicular) or even verrucous (on the shins and soles of the feet).
- In oral and genital lesions, the destruction usually dominates over the repair, so the lesions tend to be ulcerated.
- In erosive LP, there is a risk for SCC^Q due to the chronic irritation hence erosive lichen planus must be monitored closely.

Nail: Involvement is seen in 10%^{Q} of patients. The clinical features of lichen planus depend upon which portion of the nail unit is affected. Lichen planus can cause longitudinal ridging of the nail plate, with eventual nail plate thinning. With advanced disease,

Variants

There are numerous variants with varied features (Table 11.1):

- Acute LP can be exanthematous with papular lesions and it is intensely pruritic (Fig. 11.4).
- The papules can appear anywhere on the body and may be follicular, annular (Figs 11.1A and 11.5A and B), or linear.

Table 11.1 Variants of lichen planus

Hypertrophic lichen planus	Verrucous persistent plaques, especially shins and ankles; painful when on soles (Fig. 11.6)
Lichen planopilaris	Hyperkeratotic follicular papules, usually on scalp; infiltrate confined to follicular epithelium; can lead to scarring alopecia (Fig. 11.3)
Linear lichen planus	Linear grouping of lichen planus papules that cannot be explained by Koebner's phenomenon
Erosive lichen planus	Most common on oral mucosa, less often genital mucosa or soles; painful, often chronic erythematous erosions (Fig. 11.7)
Bullous lichen planus	Sometimes ordinary lesions become bullous because of intensity of dermoepidermal junction damage.
Lichen planus pemphigoides:	Combination of lichen planus and bullous pemphigoid. Also triggered by drugs such as captopril, PUVA, and cinnarizine.
Atrophic lichen planus	Atrophic, often hyperpigmented areas
Lichen planus pigmentosus	This is characterized by pigmented macules which show a lichenoid histology

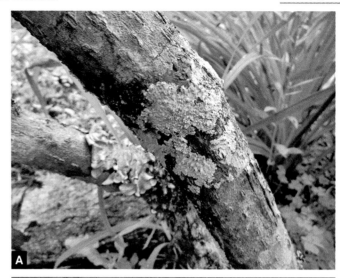

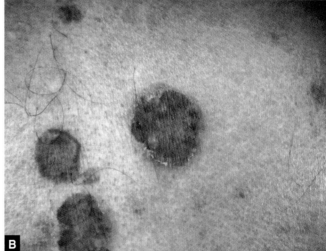

Fig. 11.5A and B: (A) Lichen on a tree which is the origin of the word 'lichen' planus; (B) Annular violaceous plaques of LP

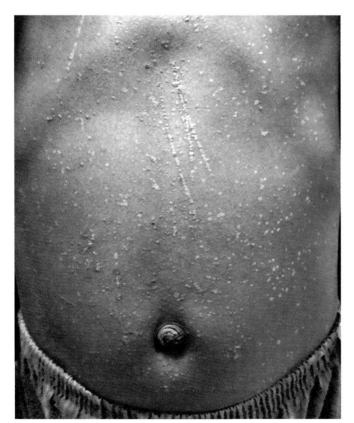

Fig. 11.4: Multiple guttate papules in a child with linear lesions reminiscent of Koebner's phenomenon

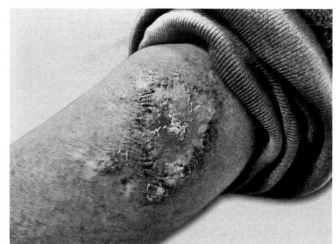

Fig. 11.6: A case of hypertrophic LP

there can be scarring of the matrix that causes pterygium^Q (a wing-like permanent nail dystrophy) and anonychia (Fig. 11.8). Rarely the papules split the nails and give the 'tented nail' or 'pup tent sign'.^{Q}

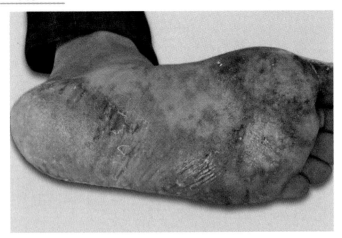

Fig. 11.7: Erosive LP on the soles

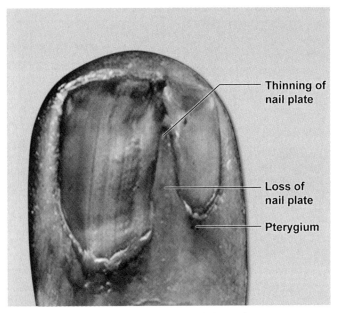

Thinning of nail plate

Loss of nail plate

Pterygium

Fig. 11.8: Nail findings in lichen planus

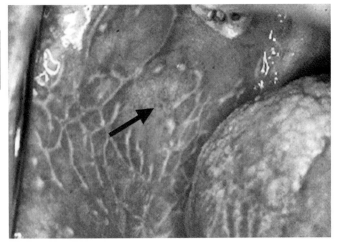

Fig. 11.9: 'Lacy white pattern' (Wickham's striae) seen classically in the oral mucosa

Mucous membrane lesions: Lacy, whitish reticular network (Fig. 11.9), milky-white plaques/papules (Fig. 11.10); increased risk of SCC in erosions and ulcers.

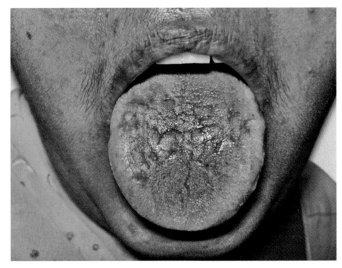

Fig. 11.10: Violaceous plaques on the tongue in case of LP

Patient complains of burning sensation in the oral cavity, on intake of hot and spicy meals.[Q]

Complications

The most distressing problem is permanent loss of nail and hair loss. The ulcerative form of lichen planus in the mouth may lead to squamous cell carcinoma. Ulceration, usually over bony prominences, may be disabling, especially if it is on the soles. Any association with liver disease may be caused by a coexisting hepatitis C infection.

Histology (Fig. 11.11A and B)

1. Compact hyperkeratosis,[Q] usually no parakeratosis except when rubbed or oral mucosal lesions.
2. Hypergranulosis, often wedge-shaped[Q], irregular-acanthosis with 'saw-toothed'[Q] rete ridges.
3. Colloid-bodies/civatte bodies/cytoid bodies[Q]
4. Vacuolization of basal cells.
5. Liquefactive degeneration of basement membrane.
6. Band-like lymphocytic inflammatory infiltrate in the papillary dermis.
7. Max Joseph cleft.[Q] Artifactual finding of subepidermal bullae.
8. Saw toothing of rete ridges.
9. Pigment incontinence.
10. Direct immunofluorescence reveals:
    - Immunoglobulin (mainly IgM), complement, in the DEJ and civatte bodies
    - Fibrin staining about the dermal vessels.

Findings of 4+5 → Pathognomonic HPE of LP.[Q]
Findings of 4+5+6 → Interface dermatitis.[Q]

Differential Diagnosis

- *Classic lesions*: Lichenoid drug eruptions, lichen nitidus, secondary syphilis, pityriasis lichenoides et varioliformis acuta, early pityriasis rubra pilaris.

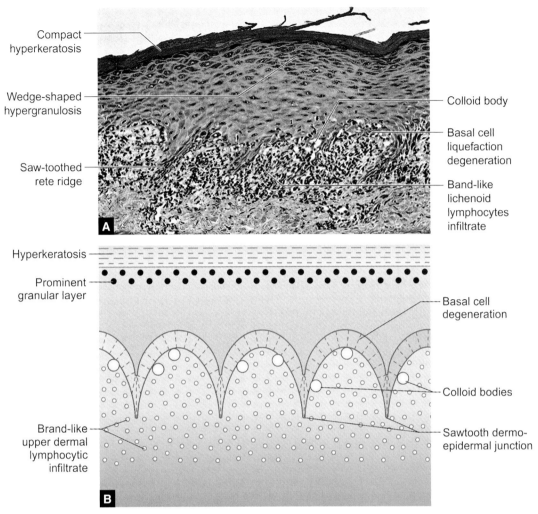

Compact hyperkeratosis

Wedge-shaped hypergranulosis

Saw-toothed rete ridge

Colloid body

Basal cell liquefaction degeneration

Band-like lichenoid lymphocytes infiltrate

Hyperkeratosis

Prominent granular layer

Basal cell degeneration

Colloid bodies

Brand-like upper dermal lymphocytic infiltrate

Sawtooth dermo-epidermal junction

Fig. 11.11A and B: Histology of lichen planus

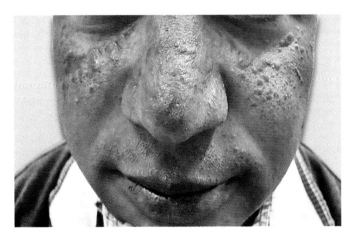

Fig. 11.12: A case of lichenoid eruption on the face

- *Lichenoid drug eruption* (Fig. 11.12):[Q]
  - Generalized
  - Photo distributed (may be)
  - More eczematous
  - Leads to persistent signs of hyperpigmentation
  - Lichenoid drug eruption is more likely to have eosinophils and parakeratosis.

- *Hyperkeratotic lesions*: Lichen simplex chronicus, prurigo nodularis, warts.
- *Linear lesions*: Lichen striatus, linear epidermal nevus, linear psoriasis.
- *Lichen planopilaris*: Early lesions—keratosis pilaris, other follicular keratoses, Darier disease, early pityriasis rubra pilaris. Advanced lesions—lupus erythematosus; other forms of scarring alopecia.
- *Erosive lichen planus*: Oral lesions—lupus erythematosus, autoimmune bullous diseases. Soles—secondary syphilis.
- Occasionally, scale can be present, in which case, the other papulosquamous disorders must be considered, including psoriasis, pityriasis rosea, and discoid lupus erythematosus.

Treatment

- Self-resolving[Q] in up to 2 years.
- Heals with hyperpigmentation.[Q]

In most instances, high-potency topical corticosteroids, perhaps under occlusion are most effective. For erosive lichen planus, either corticosteroid solutions or intralesional injections topical calcineurin inhibitors

11

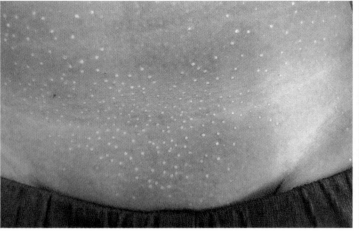
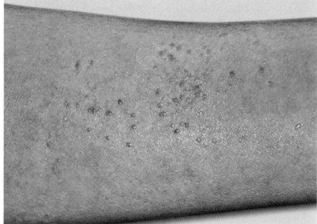

Fig. 11.13: Flat-topped, shiny papules of lichen nitidus

Table 11.2	Therapy of lichen planus
Topical agents	Topical corticosteroids, tacrolimus
Systemic agents	• Steroids • Retinoids (acitretin) • Cyclosporine • Phototherapy

(tacrolimus);[Q] hypertrophic lesions may also do better with intralesional corticosteroids. The basic aim is to suppress the immune response that is autoreactive.

• Systemic corticosteroids are needed for widespread or rapidly spreading disease. Usually 60 mg daily, tapered over 6–8 weeks. Other indications[Q] are nail destruction, painful and erosive oral lichen planus and impending cicatricial alopecia.

Caution: Risk of rebound flare is considerable; it is wise to taper slowly, if medically tolerable.

• Other choices include acitretin, antimalarials, and even cyclosporine as a last resort.

• Bath and cream PUVA are promising alternatives; effective and with much less risk of triggering flare than ordinary PUVA. Phototherapy (e.g. narrow band ultraviolet B [UVB]) can be beneficial for generalized lichen planus and lichenoid drug eruptions.

An overview of the therapy of LP is given in Table 11.2.

LICHEN NITIDUS

Uncommon dermatosis featuring tiny white papules; considered by some as lichen planus variant.

Epidemiology: Either more common or more easily noticed in blacks.

Clinical Features

• Multiple pinhead-sized glistening white papules, favoring forearms, abdomen, penis, and buttocks (Fig. 11.13). May be accompanied by typical lesions of lichen planus.

• Mucosal lesions less common; tiny yellow papules, less often lacy network as in lichen planus.
• Pruritus uncommon.

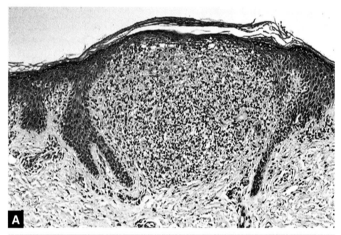
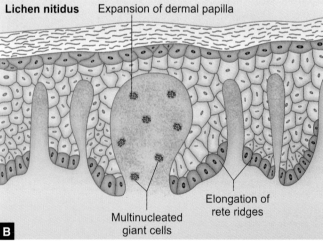

Fig. 11.14A and B: (A) Dense, well-circumscribed subepidermal infiltrate involving superficial dermis. The infiltrate consists of lymphocytes, histiocytes, melanophages, epithelioid cells and multinucleated giant cells. Claw-like acanthotic rete ridges are present at the margin of the inflammatory focus. Some overlying parakeratosis is present; (B) A depiction of the histology showing the rete ridges enclosing the infiltrate

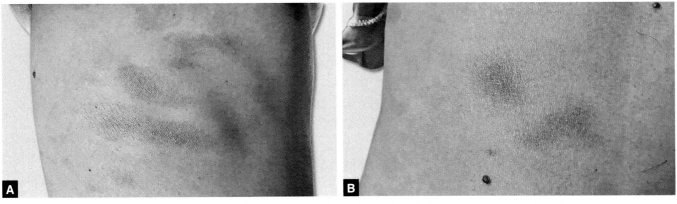

Fig. 11.15A and B: Ashy gray pigmented macules with erythematous halo in erythema dyschromicum perstans

Histology

Small granulomatous infiltrate just beneath the epidermis, involving only 2–3 rete ridges; very early lesions may have minuscule band-like infiltrate. The Bx pattern is called the 'claw clutching the ball'[Q] appearance (Fig. 11.14).

Diagnostic approach: Clinical examination, biopsy.

Differential diagnosis: Lichen planus, sarcoidosis, disseminated granuloma annulare, eruptive xanthomas, plane warts.

Therapy: Nothing standard, spontaneous healing[Q] occurs; if symptomatic, try topical corticosteroids.

ERYTHEMA DYSCHROMICUM PERSTANS

This is also known as ashy dermatosis and presents as a variant seen primarily in patients of pigmented skin and while the inflammatory phase is not recognized, commonly the patients present with post-inflammatory pigmentary changes (Fig. 11.15), with abundant melanin in the dermal macrophages. There is no good treatment.

CHAPTER 12

Miscellaneous Papulosquamous Disorders and Erythroderma

PITYRIASIS ROSEA

Acute self-limited^Q erythematosquamous exanthem with a classical clinical pattern.

Epidemiology: Most patients are young adults; male: female ratio 1:1. More common spring and fall; tends to occur in mini-epidemics.

Pathogenesis: Viral etiology long suspected, herpes virus 6 and human herpes virus 7^Q are commonly implicated.

Clinical Features

Initial lesion is often a large annular patch with collarette scale^Q (herald patch/mother's patch,^{Q} Fig. 12.1); usually on trunk.

After 1–2 weeks, typical exanthem with 1–3 cm patches with fine scale, often arranged along skin folds in a **Christmas-tree pattern**^{Q} on the back (Figs 12.2 and 12.3). In addition, in children, papular or vesicular variants of the disease can occur.

Typically, not found on face or distal extremities. In white individuals, the face and limbs are usually spared, but in black individuals, facial and acral involvement common; known as inverse pityriasis rosea. More chronic, often pruritic, heals with hypopigmentation.

It is almost *never pruritic*^{Q} unless treated with drying agents.

Typically resolves spontaneously over 6–12 weeks.^{Q}

> Look for other causes, if the condition lasts for more than 2–3 months.

Drug induced^Q: *Gold* and *captopril* are the drugs most likely to cause a pityriasis rosea-like drug reaction, but

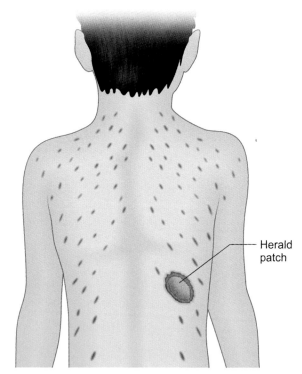

Fig. 12.1: A case of pityriasis rosea with a initial large lesion **'herald patch/mother's patch'**

barbiturates, *penicillamine*, some *antibiotics*, tyrosine *kinase* inhibitors and other drugs can also do so. These drug-induced rashes show an interface dermatitis and eosinophils on histology. A transient pityriasis rosea-like rash has been reported after a number of *vaccinations*.

Differential Diagnosis

Tinea corporis: Patients usually have only a few lesions. If doubt, however, exists a KOH preparation should be done.

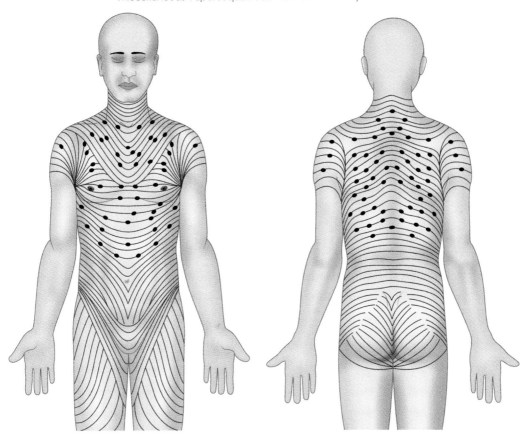

Fig. 12.2: Distribution of lesions on the trunk along the Langer's lines in a 'Christmas tree' distribution

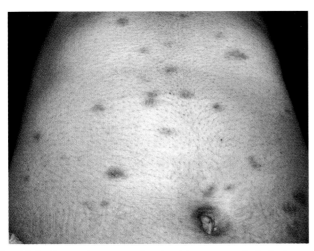

Fig. 12.3: Scaly plaques on the trunk in a case of pityriasis rosea

If patient gives history of tinea corporis spreading rapidly under therapy, suspect pityriasis rosea.

Guttate psoriasis: The lesions have a sudden onset and the scale in psoriasis is thicker and more silvery, and the course is more prolonged.

Drug eruptions: A drug eruption is more brightly erythematous, more confluent, less scaling, and is more itchy than pityriasis rosea.

Secondary syphilis: The most important diagnosis to consider in the differential is secondary syphilis,

particularly if the eruption is atypical—this includes no herald patch, involvement of palms and soles[Q] and constitutional symptoms are present.

In all cases of 'atypical' pityriasis rosea, a serologic test for syphilis should be ordered.

- Herald patch often mistaken for tinea corporis.
- Other differentials include subacute cutaneous lupus erythematosus and pityriasis lichenoides et varioliformis acuta.

Therapy

- Self-resolving disease.[Q]
- The most important step is to lubricate the skin and avoid drying therapies (frequent washing, antibacterial soaps, lotions, alcohol-based products).
- On occasion, topical corticosteroids may be used briefly; low to midpotency in emollient base bid.
- Topical antipruritic agents and systemic antihistamines are rarely needed for the pruritus.
  An overview of therapies is given in Table 12.1.

Table 12.1	Therapy of pityriasis rosea
Topical	Moisturizers, topical steroids
Systemic	UV light (NB UVB)
	Erythromycin 500 mg bid for 2 weeks

REACTIVE ARTHRITIS

This is an uncommon disorder, also known as Reiter syndrome, and the classic *triad*[Q] is arthritis, conjunctivitis and urethritis.

Patients may be ill with fever, chills, and malaise. They may have lumbar or sacral pain. Other features include urethritis or cervicitis (only when *Chlamydia trachomatis* is involved), dysentery (with other triggers), and conjunctivitis or iritis. The conjunctivitis is more common with *Chlamydia trachomatis* triggers and is bilateral. The iritis comes later and is usually unilateral.

Pathogenesis

- Genetic factors are important, most common link is with HLA-B27 positive.[Q]
- Molecular mimicry or bacterial superantigens are involved.
- Signs and symptoms often develop 1–4 weeks after an infection.

Etiology

Postdysentery Reiter syndrome: Causative agents[Q] include *Shigella flexneri, Salmonella typhimurium, Yersinia enterocolitica*, and *Campylobacter jejuni*. The inciting factors are a gastrointestinal infection,[Q] which may or may not be symptomatic.

Posturethritis Reiter syndrome: Causative agent: *Chlamydia trachomatis* (serotypes D-K).[Q] Signs and symptoms start 1–3 weeks after sexual contact, often with a new partner.

HIV-associated Reiter syndrome: In advanced HIV infection, appearance of overlapping features of severe psoriatic arthritis and Reiter syndrome.

Clinical Features

Cardinal features (Figs 12.4 and 12.5)

- *Circinate balanitis*: Annular erosive lesions on glans, often polycyclic with white periphery[Q] (Fig. 12.4C).
- *Keratoderma blennorrhagicum*: Pustular and hyperkeratotic lesions on palms and soles, similar to pustular psoriasis (Fig. 12.4B).[Q]
- *Oral lesions* (much more common than in psoriasis): Erythema and even ulcerations (Fig. 12.4A).
- *Arthritis* (Fig. 12.6): Reactive arthritis or seronegative spondyloarthropathy—asymmetric,[Q] favors lower extremities; rheumatoid factor negative.[Q] The arthritis starts an enthesopathy,[Q] involving tendons at their sites of insertion, most often on the feet (Achilles tendonitis, plantar fasciitis).

Therapy

- In case urethritis is confirmed, then treat with doxycycline 100 mg bid, even empirically.
- NSAIDs are standard for arthritis; if more severe, systemic corticosteroids (prednisolone 60–100 mg daily until improvement, then taper over 2–4 weeks).
- In chronic arthritis, methotrexate (15–25 mg weekly) or TNF antagonists are given.

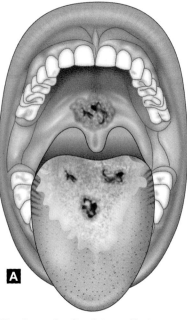

A Erosions of soft palate and/or tongue. Oral ulcers are typically painless.

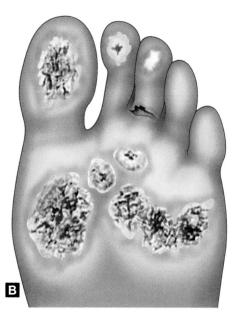

B Keratoderma and/or grouped pustules on plantar surface of foot (keratoderma blennorrhagica)

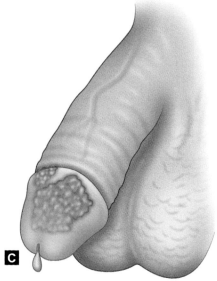

C Urethritis and balanitis circinata

Fig. 12.4A to C: A depiction of the clinical involvement in a case of reactive arthritis

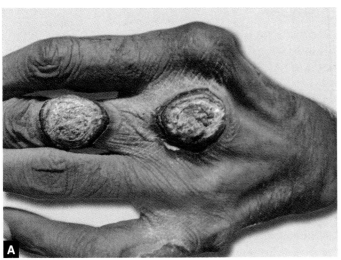 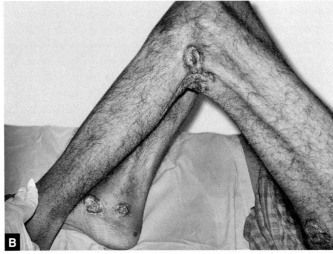

Fig. 12.5A and B: Rupioid-crusted plaques with associated arthritis (reactive arthritis)

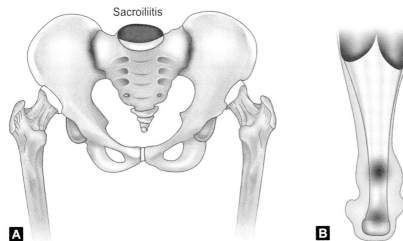

Sacroiliitis

A

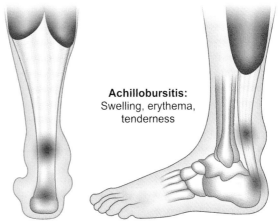

Achillobursitis:
Swelling, erythema,
tenderness

B

Fig. 12.6A and B: Arthritis and enthesopathy (inflammation at the insertion of tendon)

PITYRIASIS LICHENOIDES

Pityriasis Lichenoides Chronica (PLC)

Chronic lichenoid dermatitis with persistent scale.

Pathogenesis: In some instances, evolves out of PLEVA, but also occurs spontaneously.

Clinical features: Polymorphic, flat brown papules, usually on trunk, covered with fine micaceous scale that can be peeled off in one piece (Fig. 12.7). The lesions tend to heal with hypopigmentation (Fig. 12.8). Lesions symmetrical, often following skin lines. Asymptomatic, but lasts for years or decades.

Therapy: Extremely difficult; light is best—either PUVA or NB UVB. Oral antibiotics can also be tried, but less helpful than with PLEVA. Methotrexate not as effective as in PLEVA and not warranted because of chronic course.

Pityriasis Lichenoides et Varioliformis Acuta (PLEVA)

PLEVA, pityriasis lichenoides acuta, Mucha-Habermann disease.

Acute dermatitis with hemorrhagic crusted papules. Most patients are children or young adults.

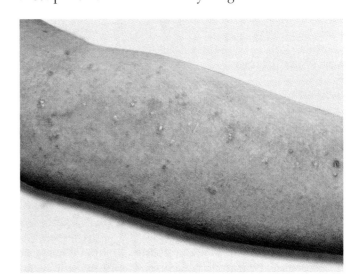

Fig. 12.7: Papules with micaceous scale that can be peeled off (PLC)

12

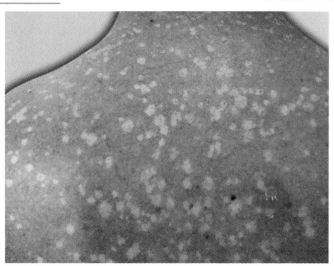

Fig. 12.8: A case of PLC healing with hypopigmentation. Note the active papules with fine scales

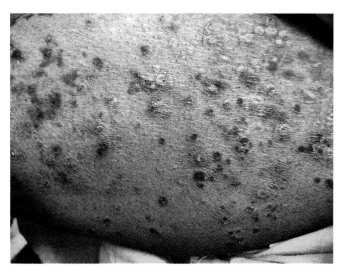

Fig. 12.9: PLEVA with crusted papules that mimic varicella

Clinical features: Sudden appearance of red-brown 0.5–3.0 cm papules that rapidly develop hemorrhagic crusts. Sometimes necrotic, ulcerated, and heal with scars (Fig. 12.9). Rarely associated with systemic signs and symptoms.

> Patients complain that they look terrible but feel fine.

Therapy: Often resolves spontaneously. Systemic antibiotics (erythromycin or tetracycline) frequently tried. If symptomatic, consider systemic corticosteroids or PUVA. Exquisitely sensitive to methotrexate but rarely indicated in young patients.

PITYRIASIS RUBRA PILARIS

This heading describes a group of uncommon skin disorders characterized by fine scaling (pityriasis), redness (rubra) and involvement of hair follicles (pilaris).

Etiology

No cause has been identified for any type. There is epidermal hyperproliferation in lesional skin. The rare familial type has an autosomal dominant inheritance.

Clinical Features

There are many types but the most common variant is the acquired adult type. In this, erythema and scaling of the face and scalp is seen followed by involvement of the trunk. The course of the disease is referred to as the cephalocaudal spread[Q] and the disease spreads to the trunk and limbs and red or orange plaques[Q] grow quickly and merge, so that patients with pityriasis rubra pilaris are often erythrodermic (Fig. 12.10).

Perifollicular papules and keratinous follicular plugs develop at this stage (Fig. 12.11). Small islands of skin may be 'spared' from this general erythema, but even here the follicles may be red and plugged with keratin. This is referred to as 'islands of sparing' (Fig. 12.13).[Q]

The palms and soles become thickened, smooth and yellow. Fissures are common there and this is called the 'PRP sandal'[Q] (Figs 12.12 and 12.13). Equally striking may be the relative sparing of the periareolar and axillary skin. Follicular keratotic papules on knuckles give a nutmeg appearance.[Q]

Nail changes include distal yellow brown discoloration, subungual HK, and nail plate thickening. Nail pitting is not seen.

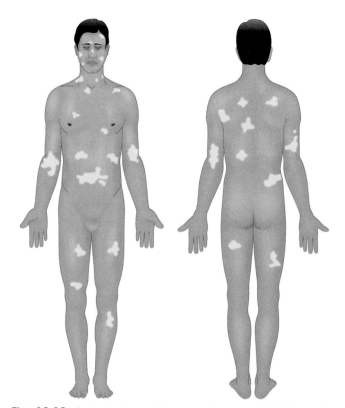

Fig. 12.10: A depiction of the morphology of PRP. Note the **'islands of sparing'** and erythroderma

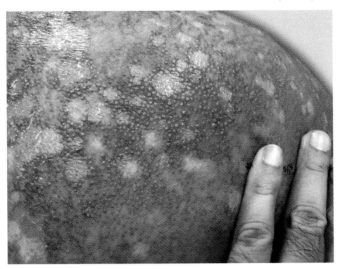

Fig. 12.11: Multiple, follicular, erythematous papules, which have a **nutmeg grater** feel with islands of sparing

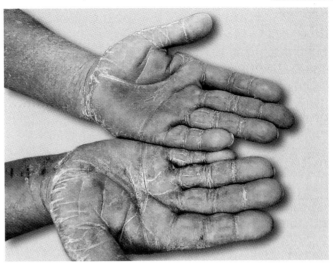

Fig. 12.12: Bilateral involvement of the palms with thickened skin, this is referred to as PRP sandal

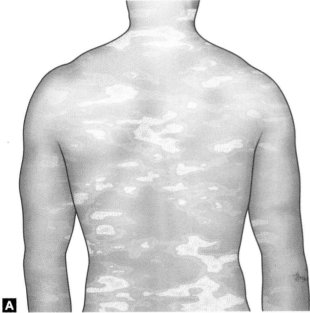

A

Islands of sparing appear as normal area of skin within a sea of redness (erythroderma)

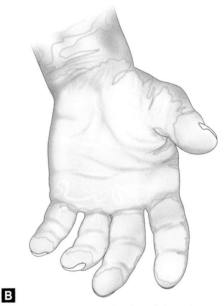

B

Carnauba wax-like thickening of the palms and soles is a common clinical finding in pityriasis rubra pilaris.

Fig. 12.13A and B: A depiction of the erythroderma seen in PRP and involvement of the palms (and soles) called PRP sandal

In children, the disease tends to start on the lower part of the body. Onset is usually between 5 and 10 years of age and it develops slowly in the familial form, and more rapidly in the acquired. A circumscribed juvenile type affects the palms and soles, fronts of the knees and backs of the elbows in younger children.

Differential Diagnosis

Psoriasis is the disorder closest in appearance to pityriasis rubra pilaris, but lacks its slightly orange tinge. The thickening of the palms and soles, the follicular erythema in islands of uninvolved skin, and follicular plugging within the plaques, especially over the knuckles, are features that help to separate them.

Investigation

- A biopsy may help to distinguish psoriasis from pityriasis rubra pilaris. There are no polymorphonuclear leukocyte, microabscesses of Munro, less parakeratosis and broader rete pegs in pityriasis rubra pilaris.
- In the classic lesion, there is alternation of orthokeratosis and parakeratosis in a pattern that resembles vaguely a 'checkerboard'.Q

Treatment

The mainstay of treatment is the use of emollients and keratolytics.

About 50% of patients respond slowly to systemic retinoids such as acitretin (in adults, 25–50 mg/day for 6–8 months). A short burst of systemic corticosteroids may speed improvement. Cyclosporine for 3–4 months or even longer may induce prolonged remissions.

Oral methotrexate in low doses, taken once a week, may also help.

Biological drugs, specifically, TNF antagonists α inhibitors infliximab, etanercept and adalimumab are useful in refractory cases.

PARAPSORIASIS

Synonyms: Chronic digitate dermatitis, parapsoriasis en petites plaques.

It is a chronic superficial scaly dermatosis with distinctive clinical pattern and controversial relationship to large-patch parapsoriasis and mycosis fungoides. There are two suggested variants.

Epidemiology: Most common in adults >50 but seen in all ages; male: female ratio—5:1.

Clinical Features

Sites of predilection include trunk, upper arms, thighs.
- *Small-patch parapsoriasis*: Multiple salmon-colored 1–2 cm macules with fine scale. Oval poorly circumscribed macules with fine (pityriasiform) scale, often following skin lines. Wrinkled appearance but not truly atrophic. Usually yellow-brown, not red. Lesions are chronic; may be present for decades.
- *Large plaque parapsoriasis*: Large erythematous violet atrophic patches often on buttocks or trunk. Usually, <10% surface area is involved (Fig. 12.14).

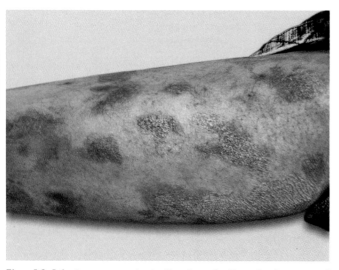

Fig. 12.14: Large psoriasis-like (psoriasiform) plaques of parapsoriasis

Table 12.2 Difference between parapsoriasis and premycosis

Parapsoriasis (benign type)	Premycotic/prelymphomatous eruptions
Smaller plaques	Larger
Yellowish	Not yellow-pink, slightly violet, or brown
Sometimes finger-shaped lesions	Asymmetrical with bizarre outline running around the trunk
No atrophy	Atrophy ± poikiloderma
Responds to UVB	Responds better to PUVA
Remains benign although rarely clears	May progress to a cutaneous T cell lymphoma

Histology

Basal dermatitis with slight spongiosis and mild parakeratosis. Marked interface change suggests large-patch parapsoriasis.

T cell receptor gene rearrangement studies can determine clonality of the T cells within the lymphoid infiltrate, and in combination with immunophenotyping helps to differentiate benign parapsoriasis from premycotic/prelymphomatous eruptions.

Differential Diagnosis

This includes psoriasis, tinea and nummular (discoid) eczema. In contrast to psoriasis and pityriasis rosea, the lesions of parapsoriasis, characteristically, are asymmetrical. Topical steroids can cause atrophy and confusion. It is important to distinguish it from premycotic eruption (Table 12.2).

Therapy

Usually asymptomatic and no treatment required. Topical midpotency corticosteroids can be used for pruritic or inflamed lesions; also emollients containing urea.

Phototherapy is useful; bath PUVA or narrow-band 311 nm irradiation work best.

ERYTHRODERMA/EXFOLIATIVE DERMATITIS

Sometimes the whole skin (>90% BSA)^Q becomes red and scaly (Fig. 12.15). Though numerous conditions can cause this, the best clue to the underlying cause is a history of a previous skin disease. Sometimes, the histology is helpful but often it is non-specific.

Etiology

The main causes are listed in Table 12.3 and the common causes are shown in Fig. 12.16A to D.

Even after extensive evaluation, the cause of erythroderma remains unclear in about 30% of patients.

For a clinician, the single most important question for the patient is: Is there any history of pre-existing skin diseases? (Box 12.1).

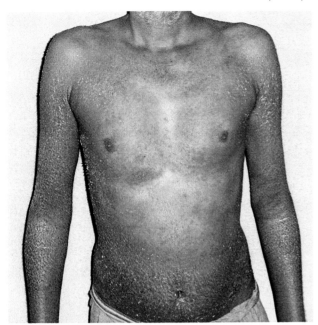

Fig. 12.15: A case of erythroderma with scaling associated with erythema all over the body

Table 12.3	Causes of erythroderma
Pre-existing skin disease	Atopic dermatitis, allergic contact dermatitis, air-borne contact dermatitis, psoriasis, pityriasis rubra pilaris
Drug induced	Allopurinol, antibiotics (e.g. penicillin, sulfonamides), anticonvulsants (e.g. carbamazepine, phenytoin, barbiturates), captopril, NSAIDs, furosemide, thiazides
Bullous skin diseases	Pemphigus foliaceus, bullous pemphigoid
Malignancies	Cutaneous T cell lymphoma, lymphoproliferative malignancies, Sézary syndrome
Erythroderma in the neonatal period or infancy	Ichthyosis (e.g. Netherton's syndrome), severe combined immunodeficiency, infections (e.g. staphylococcus-scalded skin syndrome, candidiasis)

Box 12.1	Underlying causes
• Atopic dermatitis	• Pityriasis rubra pilaris
• Psoriasis	• Cutaneous T cell lymphoma
• Drug reaction	• Allergic contact dermatitis
• ABCD	• Tinea corporis

Clinical Features

Erythroderma is the term used when the skin is red with little or no scaling, while the term **exfoliative dermatitis** is preferred, if scaling predominates. In dark skin, the presence of pigment may mask the erythema, giving a purplish hue. The skin folds are often exaggerated.

- The epidermal barrier is often breached, leading to scaling, desquamation, and then exudation of fluids. A similar process in the gut can cause protein-losing enteropathy.
- Nail changes typical for psoriasis or atopic dermatitis, or islands of sparing, so suggestive of pityriasis rubra pilaris, may provide clues to the underlying diagnosis. Both hair loss and shedding of nails may occur.
- One of the most striking forms of erythroderma is **Sezary syndrome**[Q]—a form of cutaneous T cell lymphoma with marked erythroderma, lymphadenopathy, and circulating atypical T lymphocytes.[Q]
- Lymphadenopathy is also common, reflecting cutaneous secondary infections, immunologic reactions, and in rare cases, cutaneous lymphoma. It may be very difficult to separate dermatopathic lymphadenopathy from a lymphoma.

Investigation

Diagnosis

A diagnostic approach is depicted in Figs 12.17 and 12.18.
- Work-up of an erythrodermic patient requires a complete history and physical examination, with special attention to age-related malignancy screens, and appropriate laboratory and imaging evaluation.
- Skin biopsies rarely help distinguish the multiple causes of erythroderma show spongiosis.
- A complete blood count (CBC) and routine blood chemistry; check electrolytes and serum proteins.
- Check the peripheral blood for atypical lymphocytes (Sezary cells—shows cerebriform nuclei[Q]); generally >20% atypical T cells is taken as diagnostic.
- A large proportion of cases of erythroderma are of unknown trigger, labeled idiopathic, and require periodic evaluation to search for underlying causes.

Complications (Fig. 12.19)

1. Erythroderma is major medical problem; patients suffer from impaired temperature control (too much skin blood flow) with chills, as well as protein loss (scales) and water loss.
2. Problems include edema (ankle, facial), tachycardia, both hyperthermia (increased blood flow) and hypothermia (evaporative cooling).
3. They may develop enteropathy because of the protein loss. 20% have hepatomegaly.
4. Skin infections and septicemia (loss of skin barrier function).
5. Renal failure (loss of fluid and electrolytes).
6. Lymphadenopathy is the most common extracutaneous finding and does not always indicate

12

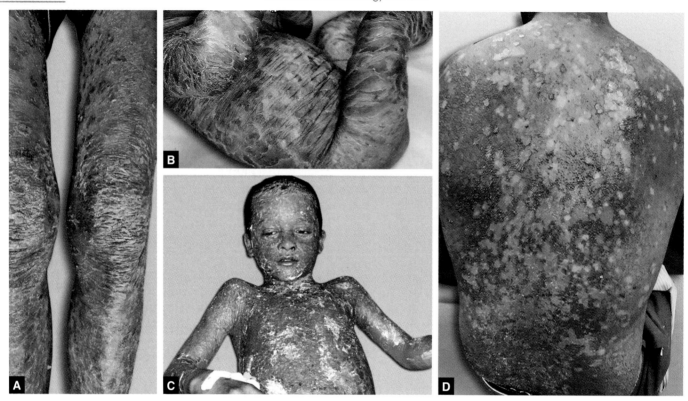

Fig. 12.16A to D: (A) Psoriatic erythroderma in an HIV positive male, with CD4 count of 218; (B) Ichthyosiform erythroderma with large lamellar plate-like scales in a 3-week-old baby. The baby had a history of collodion membrane at birth; (C) Crusted plaques with erosions in a child of pemphigus foliaceus. The patient was being treated as a case of psoriasis by a general practitioner; (D) Diffuse erythema with follicular keratotic lesions of PRP with 'island of sparing'

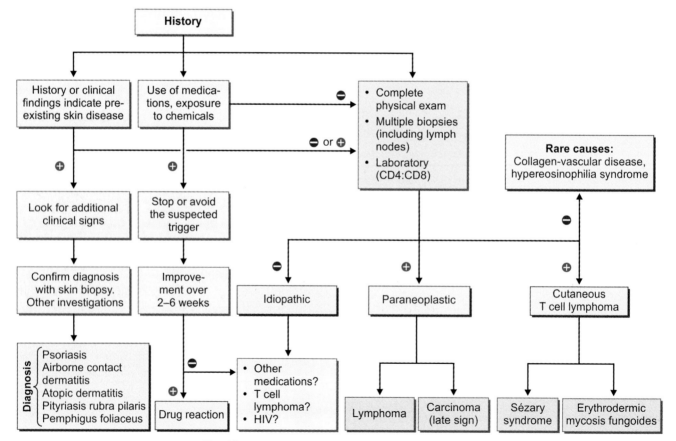

Fig. 12.17: Approach to diagnosis of erythroderma

cutaneous T cell lymphoma. Dermatopathic lymphadenopathy as a response to severe cutaneous disease is a well-established clinicopathologic entity.

A depiction of the common complications is seen in Fig. 12.18.

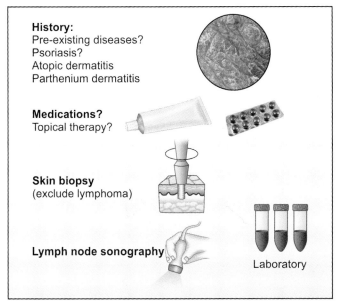

Fig. 12.18: A basic diagnostic approach to erythroderma

Therapy

Some main principles of the treatment of this condition (Fig 12.20) are:

- Identify and treat or withdraw underlying cause (e.g. drugs).
- Supportive care
- Prevention of complications.

> The most important point is to set the skin at rest. An analogy is that erythroderma is a 'broken skin' like a 'broken leg'.

- The patient should be managed in a warm environment to prevent hypothermia, with regular monitoring of core body temperature, blood pressure, pulse, fluid balance and for evidence of sepsis.
- Initially, good supportive care, fluid management, and attention to secondary infections are essential.
- Oral antihistamines are as useful adjunct.
- Systemic *corticosteroids* are sometimes used empirically with an initial dose of 1–3 mg/kg daily of prednisolone tapered rapidly to 0.5 mg/kg daily. They are specially useful, in case *drug-induced* erythroderma is the cause.
- Cyclosporine 4–5 mg/kg daily for 3 months as a last resort.
- Topical treatment should be bland.

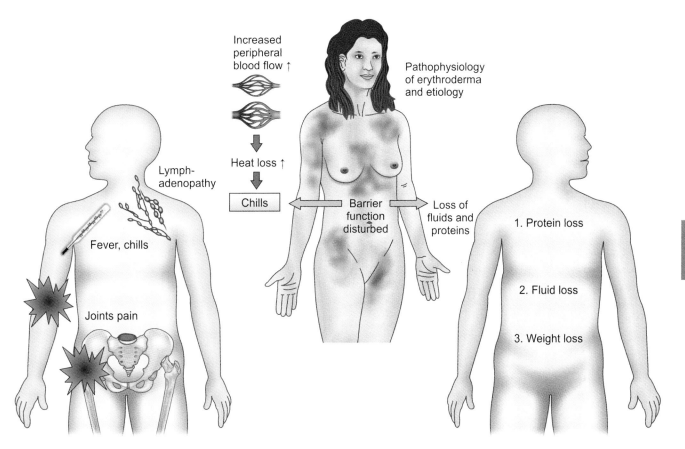

Fig. 12.19: A diagram depicting the main features and complications of erythroderma

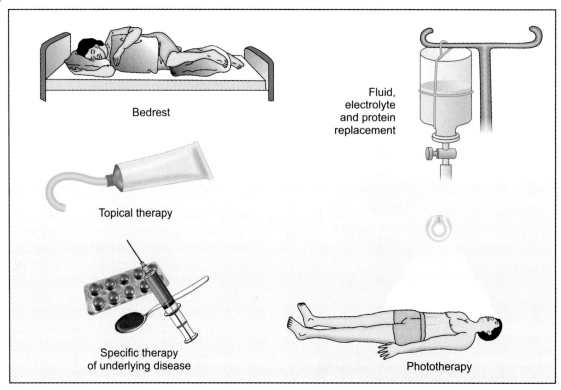

Fig. 12.20: Main principles of therapy of erythroderma

- Once the erythroderma is resolving, primary treatment for the underlying disease can be started.

This includes disease-specific therapy, such as photochemotherapy or methotrexate for psoriasis or T cell lymphoma, or retinoids for pityriasis rubra pilaris.

CHAPTER 13

Eczema and Dermatitis

Chapter Outline

INTRODUCTION

Eczemas are probably the most common skin conditions seen by dermatologists after acne. The word eczema comes from the Greek for **'boiling'**^{Q}—a reference to the tiny vesicles (bubbles) that are often seen in the early acute stages of the disorder, but less often in chronic stages.

While being disparate group of diseases, they have some common features including the presence of itch and in the acute stages, edema (spongiosis) in the epidermis (Fig. 13.1A and B). In early diseases, the stratum corneum remains intact, so the eczema appears as a red smooth edematous plaque. With worsening disease, the edema becomes more severe, tense blisters

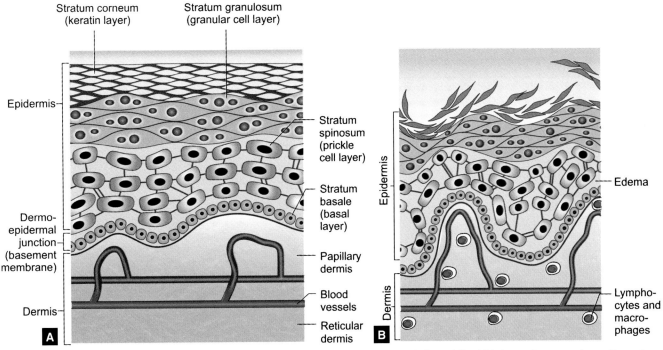

Fig. 13.1A and B: (A) A depiction of the normal histology of the skin; (B) A depiction of the histology of eczematous skin; edema develops between the keratinocytes (spongiosis), the epidermis is thickened (acanthosis) and there are inflammatory cells in the dermis

appear. If less severe or if the eczema becomes chronic, scaling and epithelial disruption occurs, giving chronic eczemas a characteristic appearance. All these are phases of the reaction pattern.

Dermatitis means inflammation of the skin and is, therefore, strictly speaking, a broader term than eczema—which is just one of several possible types of skin inflammation.

Though various classification exist, we will stick to the time honoured, division into exogenous and endogenous types (Table 13.1).

Pathogenesis

Common to all eczemas is an interaction between precipitating factors/antigens, keratinocytes and T lymphocytes. In allergic contact dermatitis (ACD) (Fig. 13.2), the initial exposure to an allergen is followed by the antigen-processing Langerhans and dermal dendritic cells carrying the antigen to the regional lymph nodes and presenting it to naïve T cells. On subsequent exposure, CD8+ cytotoxic T cells are activated and

Table 13.1   Classification of eczema

Exogenous eczema	*Endogenous eczema*
Irritant eczema	Atopic eczema
Allergic contact eczema	Seborrheic eczema
Photoallergic eczema	Asteatotic eczema
ABCD	Discoid eczema
	Pityriasis alba
	Venous eczema
	Juvenile plantar dermatosis
	Lichen simplex chronicus
	Prurigo nodularis

release Th1 cytokines including γ-interferon (IFN-γ). Following IFN-γ exposure, keratinocytes express major histocompatibility complex Class II (MHC-II) molecules and intercellular adhesion molecule 1 (ICAM-1) on their surface. This potent combination of factors leads to keratinocyte apoptosis, spongiosis and further chemokine release which perpetuates the infiltration of inflammatory cells.

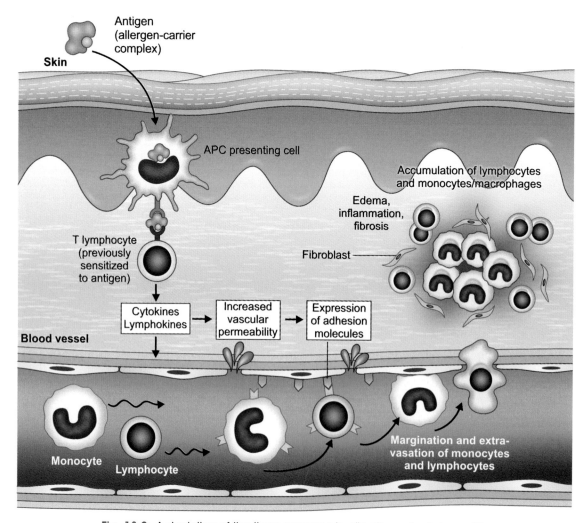

Fig. 13.2: A depiction of the tissue response in allergic contact dermatitis

In *atopic eczema*, skin barrier defects enable allergen penetrations. CD4+ helper T cells predominate, displaying a Th2 profile of cytokine release in acute lesions, but progressing to Th1 with time.

Stages of Eczema

The clinical appearance of the different stages of eczema mirrors their histology. In the acute stage, there is edema in the epidermis (spongiosis) which leads to the formation of intraepidermal vesicles, which may form larger blisters or rupture. The chronic stages of eczema show less spongiosis and vesication but more thickening of the prickle cell layer (acanthosis) and horny layers (hyperkeratosis) (Fig. 13.3).

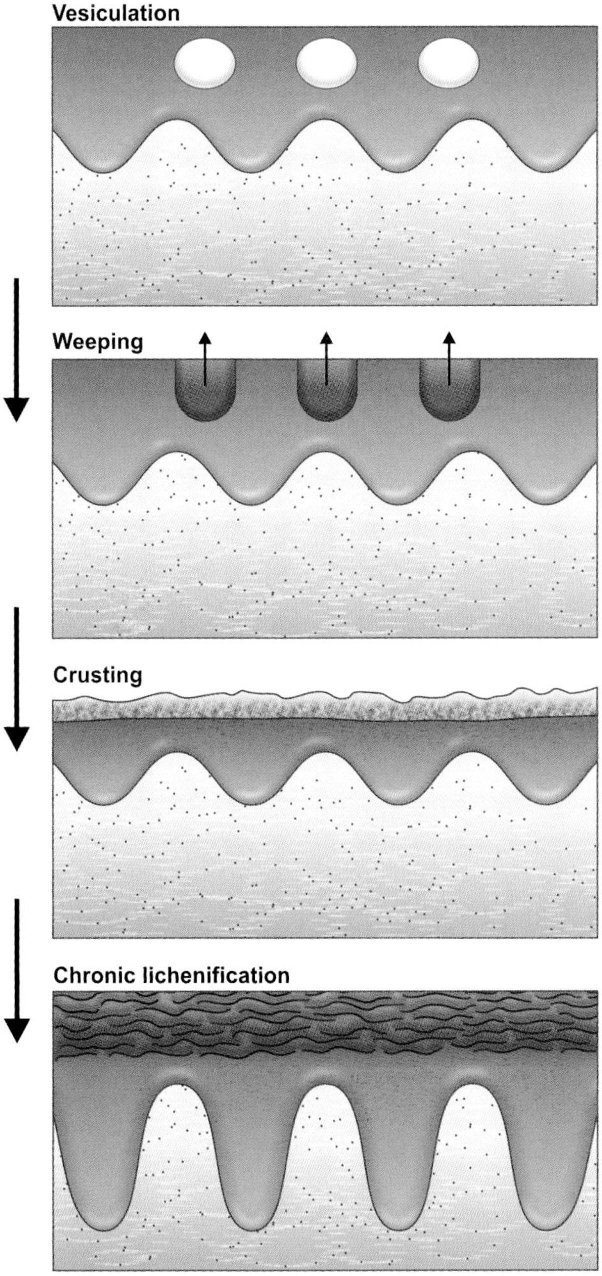

Vesiculation

Weeping

Crusting

Chronic lichenification

Fig. 13.3: A depiction of the stages of eczema

Acute Eczema

Acute eczema is characterized by (Fig. 13.4):
1. Weeping and crusting
2. Blistering—usually with vesicles and in severe cases, large blisters
3. Redness, papules and swelling—usually with an ill-defined border
4. Scaling.

Subacute Eczema

There is erythema and scaling with an indistinct border (Fig. 13.5). The symptoms vary from no itching to intense itching. Subacute eczematous inflammation may be the initial stage or it may follow acute inflammation. If the inciting agent is withdrawn, the condition often resolves.

Chronic Eczema

Chronic eczema has, in addition, the following features (Fig. 13.6):
1. Less vesicular and exudative
2. More scaly, pigmented and thickened
3. More likely to show *lichenification*—a *triad* of thickening of skin, hyperpigmentation and increased skin markings.[Q]
4. Fissuring

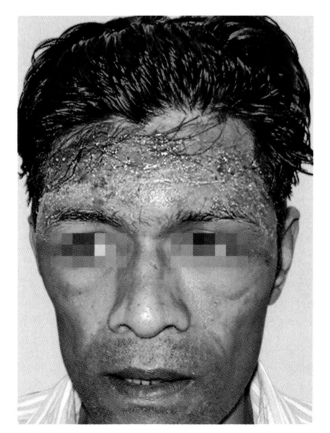

Fig. 13.4: A case of acute eczema in a patient consequent to allergic contact dermatitis to hair dye

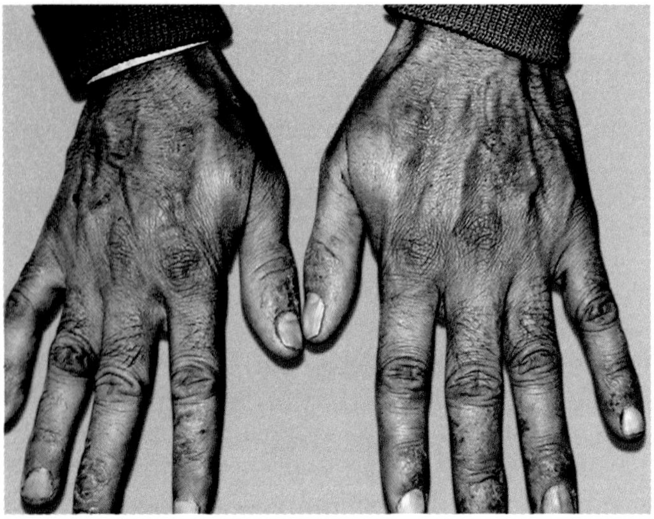

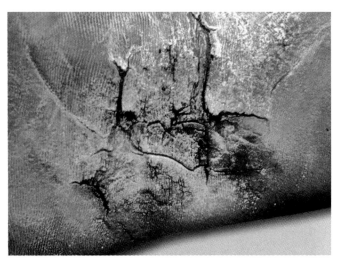

Fig. 13.5: A case of contact dermatitis to cement, a prototype of subacute eczema

Fig. 13.6: A case of hyperkeratotic eczema, a prototype of chronic eczema

Overview of Management of Types of Eczema

A. Acute eczema:

1. This requires rest with liquid applications.
2. The ideal liquid soaks include thrice daily 10-minute soaks in a cool 0.65% aluminum acetate solution or saline followed by a corticosteroid cream. The aluminum acetate solution, saline or water can be applied on cotton gauze, under a polythene covering, and changed twice daily.
3. *Wet wrap dressings:* This is a labor-intensive but highly effective technique, of value in the treatment of troublesome atopic eczema in children. After a bath, a corticosteroid is applied to the skin and then covered with two layers of tubular dressing—the inner layer already soaked in warm water, the outer layer being applied dry. Cotton pyjamas or a T-shirt can be used to cover these, and the dressings can then be left in place for several hours.

The corticosteroid used is one that is rapidly metabolized after systemic absorption like beclomethasone dipropionate ointment diluted to 0.025%, 1% or 2.5% hydrocortisone cream for children and 0.025% or 0.1% triamcinolone cream for adults. Once the condition improves, the frequency of the dressings can be cutdown and a moisturizer can be substituted for the corticosteroid.

B. Subacute eczema: Steroid lotions or creams are the mainstay of treatment; their strength is determined by the severity of the attack. Secondary infection requires systemic antibiotic treatment. Bacitracin, fusidic acid, mupirocin or neomycin can be used, though the last can frequently sensitize.

C. Chronic eczema: This responds best to steroids in an ointment base, but is also often helped by non-steroid applications such as ichthammol and zinc cream or paste.

Bacterial superinfection may need systemic antibiotics but can often be controlled by the incorporation of antibiotics (e.g. fusidic acid, mupirocin) into the steroid formulation. Chronic localized hyperkeratotic eczema of the palms or soles can be helped by salicylic acid (1–6% in emulsifying ointment) or urea preparations.

CONTACT DERMATITIS

This is divided into two types—allergic contact dermatitis (ACD) and irritant contact dermatitis (ICD). The commoner of the two is ICD,[Q] and though there are theoretical differences between the two (Table 13.2), they are often present in the same individual. In fact, there is a wide overlap between various forms of dermatitis (Fig. 13.7).

Irritant Contact Dermatitis

ICD accounts for approximately 80% of all contact dermatitis, while allergic contact dermatitis (ACD) accounts for only 20%.[Q]

ICD can either be very acute, such as when someone spills acid on their skin, or chronic, resulting from

Table 13.2 Difference between ICD and ACD	
Irritant contact dermatitis	*Allergic contact dermatitis*
Non-immunological	Immunological
Dose-dependent	Not dose-dependent
Prior exposure not required	Prior exposure required
Spread to non-exposed sites is not seen	Spread to non-exposed sites is seen
Memory cells not involved	Memory cells involved

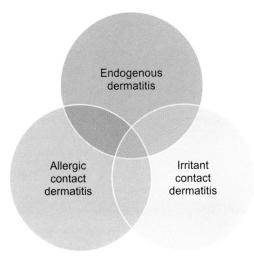

Fig. 13.7: Overlap between various forms of contact eczema

repeated exposures that individually would be harmless. The latter type of irritant disease is known as cumulative irritant dermatitis (Fig. 13.8).

Chronic irritant dermatitis predisposes the patient to allergic contact dermatitis (Fig. 13.9).

Etiology

Strong irritants elicit an acute reaction after brief contact and the diagnosis is then usually obvious. Prolonged exposure, sometimes over years, is needed for weak irritants to cause dermatitis, usually of the hands and forearms. Common agents include water, detergents (housewife eczema),[Q] chemicals, solvents, cutting oils and abrasive dusts. Those with very dry skin and past or present atopic dermatitis are vulnerable.

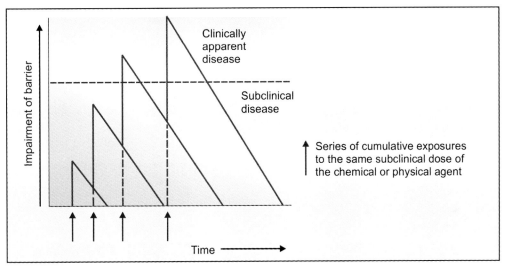

Fig. 13.8: A depiction of the process of cumulative ICD

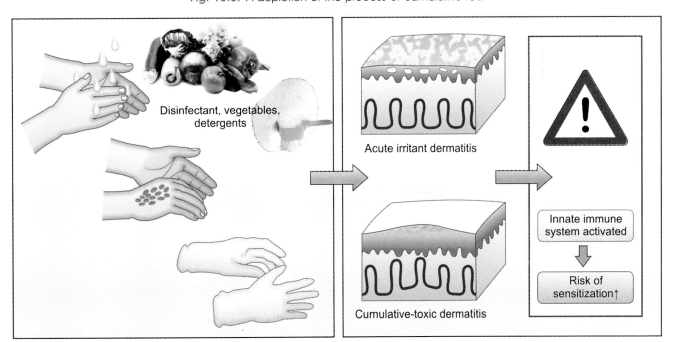

Fig. 13.9: Cumulative irritant contact dermatitis predisposes to allergic contact dermatitis

Clinical Features

The clinical features are remarkably similar to allergic contact dermatitis. ICD never spreads beyond the area of contact, tends to be painful rather than pruritic, and, if the causative agent is strong enough, may form large blisters rather than tiny vesicles.[Q] Acute ICD usually exhibits an 'asymmetrical distribution and sharply demarcated borders' (Fig. 13.10).

Cumulative irritant contact dermatitis is often well demarcated with a glazed appearance. The most common locations are hands, forearms, eyelids, and face (Fig. 13.11) and can have varied morphological appearances (Fig. 13.12A to D).

The groin and buttocks in infants are frequently affected by diaper dermatitis. This condition is an irritant contact dermatitis from moisture and feces. Diaper dermatitis is often complicated by secondary infection with bacteria and yeast (Fig. 13.13).

Diagnosis

Irritant contact dermatitis is a diagnosis of exclusion. The typical patient presents with pruritic or painful dermatitis either immediately after contact with strong irritant approximately 3 months after low-grade irritant exposure.

Treatment

The management of irritant contact dermatitis is twofold:
- Identification and removal of the irritant(s)
- Repair of the normal skin barrier

Other measures include
- Mild soaps and moisturizers should be used.
- For irritant hand dermatitis, vinyl gloves should be worn as a barrier to unavoidable irritant exposures such as dish soap and juice from citrus fruits.
- Cotton gloves over a heavy emollient such as petroleum jelly overnight may also be helpful.
- Each water exposure should be immediately followed by application of an emollient to prevent dehydration of the skin and restore the normal skin barrier.

Allergic Contact Dermatitis

ACD occurs much less frequently than ICD but is of great importance as it can frequently force a worker to change jobs as protective measures often fail to work. When chronic, ICD and ACD can look quite similar clinically; however, vesicles are more common in ACD.

ACD is a delayed (type IV) hypersensitivity reaction[Q] and the most common allergens include:
- Metals[Q] (e.g. nickel 19%; cobalt 8%; chromate 5%)
  Most common cause: Nickel[Q]
- Fragrances (e.g. balsam of Peru 12%; fragrance mix 12%)

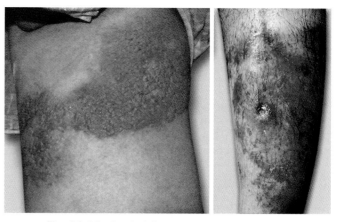

Fig. 13.10: Acute irritant reaction to betadine

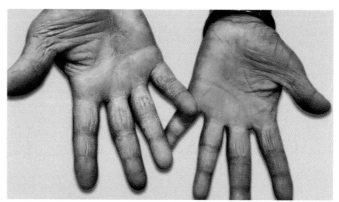

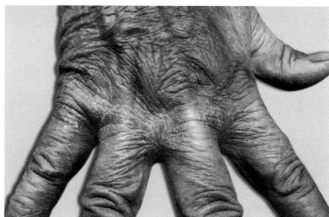

Fig. 13.11: This lady used to wash her hands repeatedly apart from using harsh detergents. The clinical picture is of a 'monomorphic' erythema on the palms and web space—irritant eczema

- Preservatives (e.g. quaternium-15 10%)
- Topical antibiotics (e.g. neomycin 10%; bacitracin 9%).
- Cosmetics (personal care products) contain fragrances and preservatives that cause allergic contact dermatitis is seen on the faces of women due to the use of make-up and moisturizers. This is known as Berloque dermatitis.[Q] Paraphenylenediamine is a dye found in permanent hair coloring. Sensitization to paraphenylenediamine occurs in hairdressers and in patients.

13

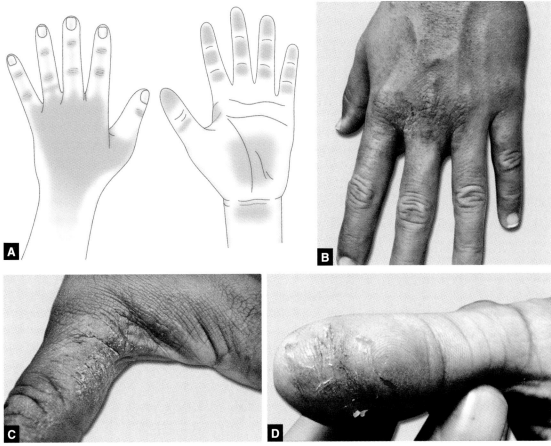

Fig. 13.12A to D: (A) Typical distribution of irritant contact dermatitis on the hands; (B) Affliction of the dorsum of hands (cumulative ICD); (C) Cumulative ICD involving the fingers; (D) A case of cumulative ICD in a housewife localized to the fingertips, primarily due to a combination of detergent use and cutting vegetables

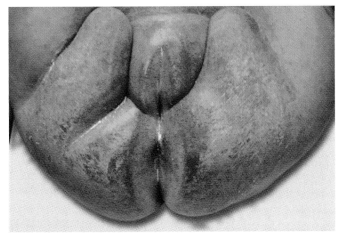

Fig. 13.13: Diaper dermatitis. The most commonly encountered clinical presentation is *erythema of the convex zones.*[Q] The bright red erythema covers the convex areas of the buttocks (in a W shape) and may spread to the pubis and upper thighs. It can become shiny and erosive with a corroded appearance

- Nickel sensitivity is seen most often in women as a result of wearing 'cheap' pierced earrings. It is found in many metal alloys. Although stainless steel contains nickel, it is bound so tightly that it usually does not allow an allergic reaction to occur.

- Rubber compounds are universal and shoes and gloves are the most common sources of ACD and here the reaction is limited to the feet or hands.

Allergic contact dermatitis should be suspected, if:
1. Certain areas are involved (e.g. the eyelids, external auditory meatus, hands or feet, and around gravitational ulcers);
2. There is known contact with the allergens mentioned in Table 13.3;
3. The individual's work carries a high risk (e.g. hairdressing, working in a flower shop, or dentistry).

Clinical Features
- Acute ACD classically presents as papules and vesicles on an erythematous base.
- Chronic ACD may manifest as xerosis, fissuring, and lichenified eczematous plaques.

In general, ACD occurs at the site of contact with the allergen.

Nickel allergy usually results in dermatitis underlying nickel-containing objects (e.g. jewelry-earlobes, neck, wrists; belt buckles[Q]—umbilicus; cell phones—cheeks). However, dermatitis in certain sites, especially the eyelids and face, may result from contact to allergens on the hands (fingernail polish) or scalp (hair products). Figure 13.14 and Table 13.4 list common allergens at selected body sites. A series of images of various causes of allergic contact dermatitis are listed in Figures 13.15A to L).

Table 13.3	Common allergens that cause allergic contact dermatitis
Chrome	Cement[Q]; chromium plating processes; antirust paints; tattoos (green) and some leathers
Nickel	Nickel-plated objects, especially cheap jewellery[Q]
Cobalt	A contaminant of nickel and occurs with it
Colophony	Pine resin, adhesives, printing ink
Paraphenylenediamine (PPD)	Dyes for hair and clothing[Q]
Paraben mix	Preservatives in creams
Cetosteryl alcohol	Emollient, and base for many cosmetics
Formaldehyde	Preservative in some shampoos and cosmetics. Also in pathology laboratories and white shoes
Neomycin	Popular topical antibiotic. Common sensitizer in those with leg ulcers
Epoxy resin	Common in 'two-component' adhesive mixtures (Araldite, M seal)
Balsam of Peru	Perfumes and flavoring agent
Paratertiary butylphenol formaldehyde resin	Used as an adhesive (e.g. in shoes, *Bindi*, wrist watch straps, prostheses, hobbies). Can cause contact leukoderma[Q]
Sesquiterpene lactone mix	Plants, e.g. chrysanthemum, parthenium (India—due to Congress grass)[Q]
Tixocortol-21-pivalate	Topical steroids (hydrocortisone)
Wool alcohols	Ointment base in creams
Thiuram mix	Rubber accelerator

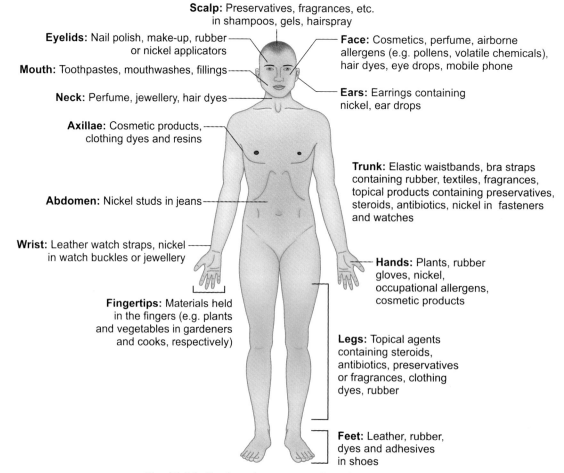

Scalp: Preservatives, fragrances, etc. in shampoos, gels, hairspray

Eyelids: Nail polish, make-up, rubber or nickel applicators

Mouth: Toothpastes, mouthwashes, fillings

Neck: Perfume, jewellery, hair dyes

Axillae: Cosmetic products, clothing dyes and resins

Abdomen: Nickel studs in jeans

Wrist: Leather watch straps, nickel in watch buckles or jewellery

Fingertips: Materials held in the fingers (e.g. plants and vegetables in gardeners and cooks, respectively)

Face: Cosmetics, perfume, airborne allergens (e.g. pollens, volatile chemicals), hair dyes, eye drops, mobile phone

Ears: Earrings containing nickel, ear drops

Trunk: Elastic waistbands, bra straps containing rubber, textiles, fragrances, topical products containing preservatives, steroids, antibiotics, nickel in fasteners and watches

Hands: Plants, rubber gloves, nickel, occupational allergens, cosmetic products

Legs: Topical agents containing steroids, antibiotics, preservatives or fragrances, clothing dyes, rubber

Feet: Leather, rubber, dyes and adhesives in shoes

Fig. 13.14: Region-wise causes of contact dermatitis

Table 13.4 A list of site-dependent causes of ACD

Body site	Allergens
Anywhere	• Topical preparations (bacitracin, neomycin, corticosteroids, preservatives, emulsifiers) • Personal care products (preservatives, emulsifiers)
Face	**Cosmetics and airborne agents** are the most common causes • Cosmetics, personal care products (emulsifiers, preservatives) • Hair products (surfactants, fragrances, preservatives) • Cell phones, eyeglasses, headsets (nickel) • Consort/connubial contact from spouse/partner's products • In India, parthenium is a common cause[Q]
Eyelids	• Cosmetics (emulsifiers, preservatives) • Nail polish (toluene sulfonamide resin) • Artificial nails (acrylates) • Eyelash curlers, tweezers (nickel) • Jewellery (gold—may cause a distant allergic contact dermatitis) • Eye drops (active ingredients, preservatives)
Hands	Commonly seen with **chronic wet exposure** (cement work, machinists, cooks, beauticians) • Gloves (rubber accelerators, leather tanning agents) • Hand soap/sanitizers (fragrance, antibacterial agents, surfactants) • Tools/utensils (rubber, metals) • Occupation-specific chemicals (e.g. hairdressers—hair dye) • Gardeners may react to variety of allergens, such as geraniol in geraniums
Neck, shoulders	• Jewelry (nickel, cobalt, gold) • Hair products (surfactants, fragrances, preservatives)
Flexures	• Seen in the groin and axillae • Patients are sensitized to fragrances or preservatives in personal hygiene items
Legs	• Antibiotics, fragrances, and preservatives
Feet	• Shoes (rubber accelerators, leather tanning agents, glue ingredients)
Under clothing only	• Clothing dye (disperse blue dyes) • Clothing finishes (formaldehyde resins)

A special type of ACD is the *systematized allergic contact dermatitis*. Once topical sensitization has occurred, patients can react dramatically when the same agent, often an antibiotic, is administered systemically. It is seen on the axillae, groin, and buttocks, presumably because of exudation in sweat; this dramatic picture is called baboon syndrome.[Q] Occasionally, a patient may be sensitized to topical antibiotics and then ingests a crossreacting oral antibiotic with generalized distribution (Fig. 13.16).

Diagnosis
The key diagnostic features of ACD are pruritic vesicles or scaly, lichenified plaques that correspond to the area of contact with the allergen. Pruritus should always be present in allergic contact dermatitis.

No standard testing method is available for diagnosing irritant contact dermatitis.

Patch test: This is a test that requires expertise and experience and not all positive reactions are clinically relevant (Box 13.1 and Fig. 13.17).

Box 13.1 Indications of patch testing
• Atopic dermatitis
• Hand dermatitis
• Other dermatoses, e.g. discoid, stasis, seborrheic
• Specific site dermatitis, e.g. eyelids, foot, perineal
• Occupational dermatitis
• Differentiate between ICD and ACD[Q]

• On the first day, allergens are applied to the upper back and taped in place.
• After about 2 days,[Q] the patches are removed and locations are marked and the patch sites are evaluated by the clinician.
• Standard interpretation key:
  – +1 reaction indicates palpable erythema
  – +2 reaction indicates papules and vesicles
  – +3 reaction indicates bullae

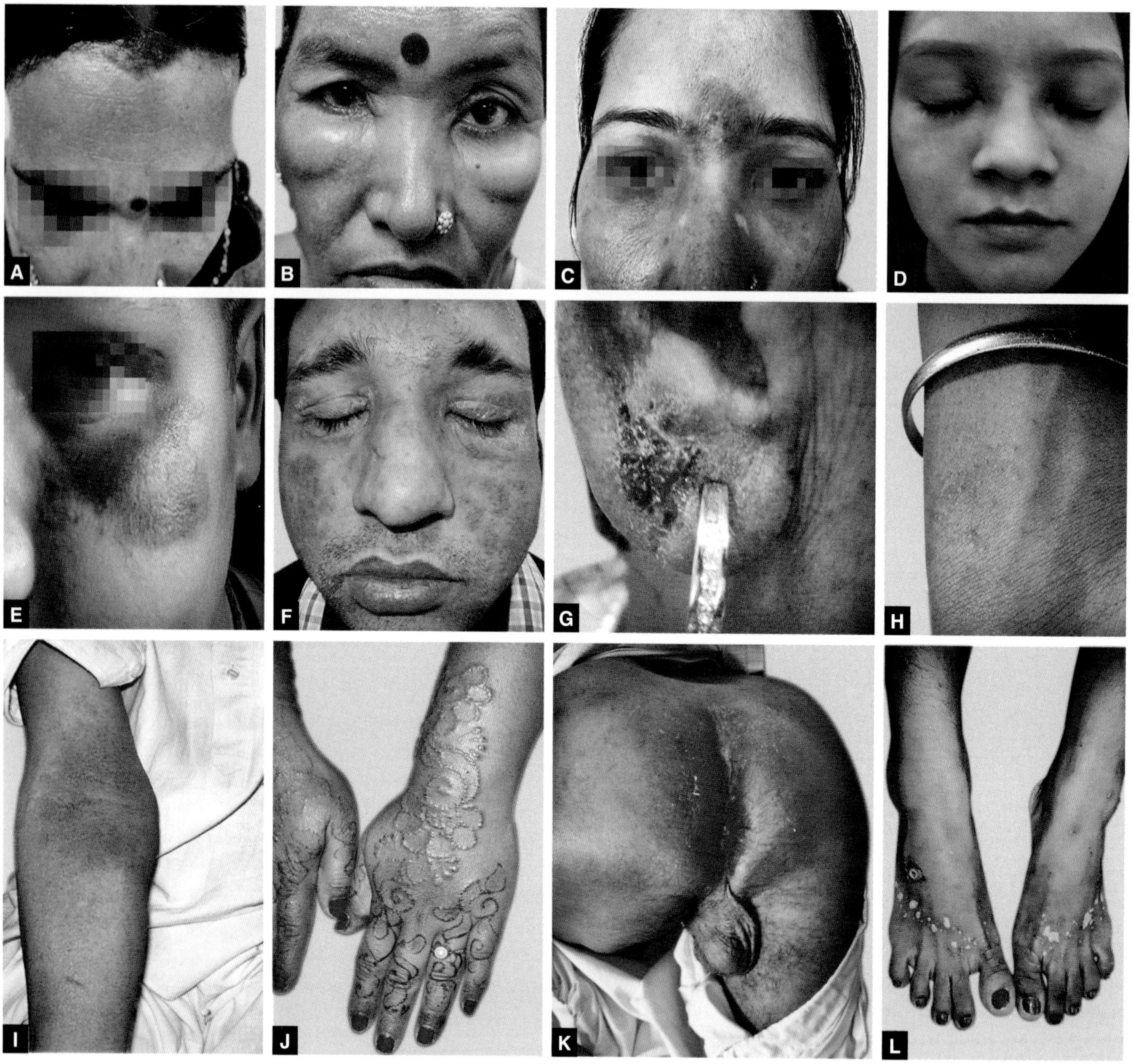

Fig. 13.15A to L: (A) ACD on forehead to sindoor (Kumkum); (B) Acute edematous swelling consequent to PPD; (C) Bindi dermatitis due to PTBP, a compound added to the sticky part of the bindi. The 'adhesive' is the culprit; (D) Contact dermatitis over the face due to BPO gel for acne; (E) Allergic reaction to 'thiomersal' in eye drops; (F) The patient used to drive his bike through a under-construction national highway. The 'dust' with allergens was trapped in his helmet, classic example of 'aeroallergy'; (G) Artificial jewellery is a frequent cause of earlobe dermatitis; (H) Nickle-induced bangle allergy; (I) Intense flexural erythema in a case probably due to 'finishers' of a newly bought shirt; (J) Black henna dermatitis (Dr AK Bajaj); (K) Perianal allergy (*Courtesy*: Dr PK Srivastava, Dr AK Bajaj); (L) Contact leukoderma due to footwear

- They are re-evaluated once again between 3 and 4 days after application.
- After identification of the allergen by patch testing, clinical relevance is determined by evaluating potential exposures to the allergen (identifying the ingredient in the patient's products used in the location of dermatitis).
- The type of response to the antigen applied points to the possible cause being ICD or ACD.

Management

The management of ACD consists of three steps:
- Identification of the allergen through patch testing
- Avoidance of the allergen
- Repair of the normal skin barrier

If the dermatitis clears after avoidance of the allergen, this is good evidence that the allergic reaction is clinically relevant. Improvement of ACD typically

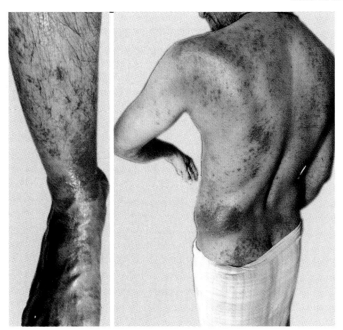

Fig. 13.16: A case of disseminated eczema in a patient who was sensitized to soframycin applied for venous eczema on the lower limb

requires at least 3 weeks and often up to 2 months of allergen avoidance.

Obviously a knowledge of the various allergens and the regional distribution as discussed above is useful. An overview to the diagnosis and treatment is given in Fig. 13.18.

Mid- to high-potency topical corticosteroids applied twice a day are usually sufficient for treatment of ACD. Restoration of the skin barrier includes mild soaps and moisturizers.

Acute, severe, generalized contact dermatitis is treated with a short course of systemic steroids: 40 to 60 mg prednisone daily for a minimum of 5 days and then tapered over the next 5 days.

PARTHENIUM DERMATITIS

This is a special form of plant-induced contact dermatitis of special importance in India.

It is an ACD to *Parthenium hysterophorus*[Q] and is the most common cause of plant dermatitis[Q] in India. Parthenium dermatitis (PD) is caused by airborne dry and friable plant particles, especially trichomes[Q] and sesquiterpenes.[Q]

In India, parthenium hysterophorus is commonly known as 'Congress grass'[Q] or 'Congress weed,' probably referring to the US Congress which allocated the contaminated wheat shipment, containing the herb, for Pune in 1956 (Figs 13.19A and B). Another theory is that the word Congress grass refers to the fact that the Congress government was ruling the state of Maharashtra during that period.

Contact sensitivity to parthenium is everlasting and hence the disease runs a chronic course with exacerbation during summers[Q] initially and some reduction in winters. In southern parts of India, there are often flares in September, October and November which may be owing to increased growth of the plant following monsoons. The seasonal pattern seen initially gradually evolves into a persistent eruption with pruritic lichenified dermatitis over years.

Clinical Features

Males are more commonly affected than females (with male: female ratio being reported between 5.5:1 and 20:1). The difference is related to outdoor exposure and nature of clothing but cannot be completely explained by these alone, as women also work in fields.

The severity varies from brief periods of erythema and itching to persistent erythema, swelling, papules or papulovesicles with itching and burning in moderate

Patch test placement

Positive patch test

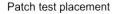

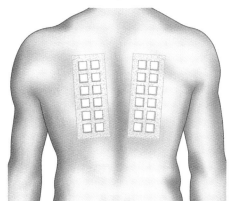

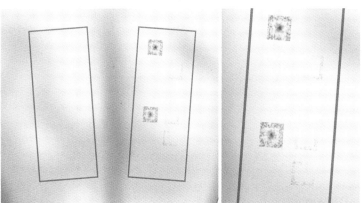

Patch testing is the best method to assess for contact allergies

Evaluation of patch tests at 72 hours shows papular erythema

Fig. 13.17: Patch testing and type IV hypersensitivity for allergic contact dermatitis

13

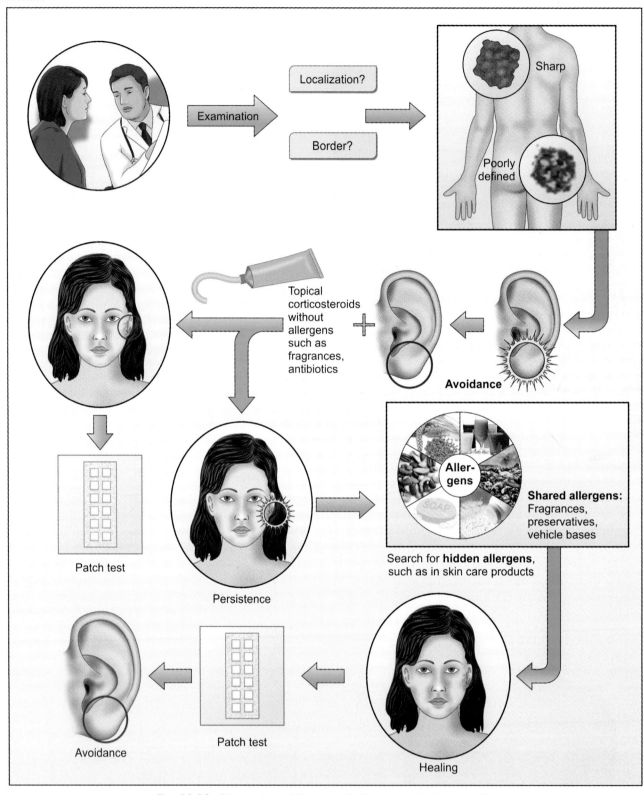

Fig. 13.18: Diagnosis and therapy of allergic contact dermatitis

cases and extensive vesiculation and exudation associated with edema in severe ones.

PD may present with a variety of morphologies.

The classical pattern, also known as *airborne contact dermatitis* (ABCD) pattern,[Q] affects the face, especially eyelids and/or neck, V of chest, cubital and popliteal fossae. The eruption is also termed pseudophoto-dermatitis as the skin of the upper eyelids, the retroauricular and submental areas, which are spared in photodermatitis, are involved in PD (Fig. 13.19C). These patients usually are a common cause of erythroderma in India.

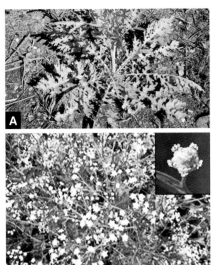
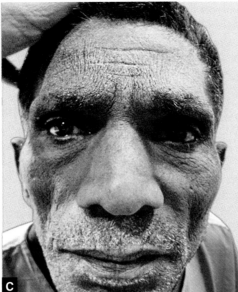
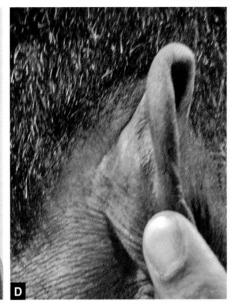

Fig. 13.19A to D: (A) Juvenile plant: Grows like a rosette. Lower leaves are spread on the ground; are relatively large and deeply divided (bipinnatifid or bipinnatisect). Leaves on the upper branches decrease in size and are also less divided; (B) Mature plant with flowering. Each flower-head (capitulum) is borne on a stalk (pedicel) and has five tiny 'petals' (ray florets). They also have numerous tiny white flowers (tubular florets) in the center and are surrounded by two rows of small green bracts (involucre); (C) Parthenium dermatitis involving the folds of the forehead; (D) Involvement of the retroauricular folds

Diagnosis

Patch and Photopatch Test

It is patch testing with addition of UV radiation to include formation of photoallergen.[Q]

The strips of antigen are applied on back, in duplicate. After 2 days, one side is covered and other is exposed to UV-A. The reading is done after further 2 days (total 4). If only exposed sites develop reactions, it confirms the presence of photoallergic contact dermatitis.

Treatment

- Protection from exposure
- Cover as much skin as possible with clothing. *Barrier creams* including coconut oil should be repeatedly applied, with washing off of the area before each application. The clothes must be *dried indoors* to reduce antigen load as pieces of cloth dried outside may have the allergen. The need to take a *bath* after coming indoors and wearing *fresh clothes* must be impressed upon.
- Topical steroids have been used. In severe cases, short course of oral steroids are also given.
- Azathioprine[Q] is used in India. It is especially useful in those patient who have contraindications to oral steroids.

ATOPIC DERMATITIS

Atopic dermatitis (AD) is a very common skin condition that affects approximately 20% of children in developed countries. Ninety percent of patients have onset of disease before age 5 and 65% will have symptoms by 18 months of age.

Diagnosis is clinical and there is no laboratory test for diagnosis of AD.[Q]

Diagnostic criteria, established by Hanifin and Rajka,[Q] and adapted by the UK Working Party in 1994, are based on clinical manifestations (Table 13.5).

Pathogenesis

The etiology of AD is multifactorial, including a combination of genetic susceptibility and environmental triggers and/or exposures.

- Many gene loci have been linked to AD, including genes associated with increased immunoglobulin E (IgE) levels, or T lymphocyte activation.
- Impaired epidermal barrier: Filaggrin,[Q] a protein that is important in the barrier function of the epidermis, is also a factor in the pathogenesis of the disease.

Table 13.5	Criteria for AD (modified Hanifin and Rajka criteria)

Must have:

- *Itchy* skin in the last 12 months[Q]

Plus three or more of the following:

- History of *flexural* involvement
- History of *asthma* and/or hay fever (or in children <4 years, history of atopy in first degree relatives)
- History of a generally *dry skin*
- Visible *flexural* eczema
- Onset in the first *two years* of life

13

- Impaired innate immunity: Atopic patients produce reduced amounts of defensins on their epidermis and in their sweat. Defensins are active against bacteria, fungi, and viruses.
- Patients with AD have increased susceptibility to *Staphylococcus aureus* and other infections such as *Molluscum*, herpes simplex virus (HSV), human papillomavirus (HPV), and *Trichophyton rubrum* and *Malassezia* species. About 90% of AD skin lesions are colonized with microbes, usually *S. aureus*.[Q]
- In *acute AD*, the dermal Th2 immune[Q] response is activated with release of proinflammatory cytokines (e.g. interleukin [IL] 4, 5, 13) which recruit eosinophils, B lymphocytes and induce immunoglobulin E (IgE) production. IgE activates histamine release by mast cells leading to itching.

In the *chronic phase* of AD, eosinophils release IL-12 activating the Th1 immune response[Q] leading to release of α-interferon (IFN-α) by CD4+, and CD8+ T lymphocytes.

Clinical Features

Symptoms

- The cardinal feature of AD is itching;[Q] and scratching may account for most of the clinical picture.
- Affected children may sleep poorly, are hyperactive and sometimes manipulative, using the state of their eczema to get what they want from their parents.

- AD remits spontaneously before the age of 10 years in at least two-thirds of affected children. Eczema and asthma may seesaw, while one improves the other may get worse.
- There is personal or family history[Q] of similar skin condition or other atopic disorders (allergic rhinitis, allergic conjunctivitis, asthma, food allergy, chronic urticaria).

Three classic distributions of atopic dermatitis are recognized: Infantile, childhood, and adult variants (Fig. 13.20).

- **Infants:** After 3 months,[Q] they usually present with itchy[Q] dermatitis involving the cheeks,[Q] trunk, and extensor extremities.[Q] The scalp may also be involved and there is frequent superinfection.
  - The lesions are vesicular and weeping (Fig. 13.21).
  - Up to 90% show marked spontaneous improvement between 2 and 3 years of age.
- **Young children:** Often the atopic child flares again, this time showing involvement of both flexors and extensors.[Q] The sites involved are the posterior neck, flexor extremities (antecubital fossae and popliteal fossae), wrists, hands, ankles, and feet (Fig. 13.22).
  - The lesions are leathery, dry and excoriated.
  - Keratosis pilaris may be present on the extensor arms and thighs.
  - It resolves around puberty.

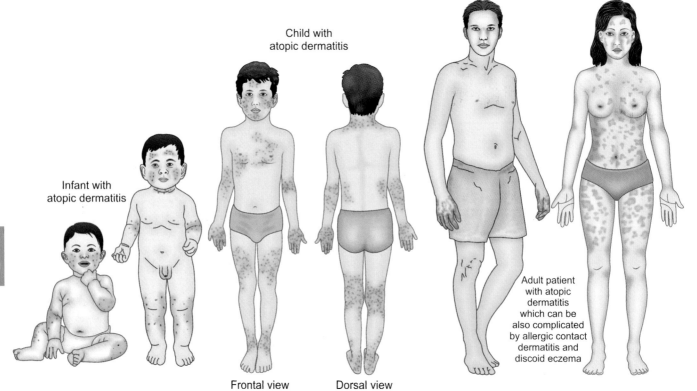

Child with atopic dermatitis

Infant with atopic dermatitis

Adult patient with atopic dermatitis which can be also complicated by allergic contact dermatitis and discoid eczema

Frontal view   Dorsal view

Fig. 13.20: Typical distribution of lesions in atopic dermatitis

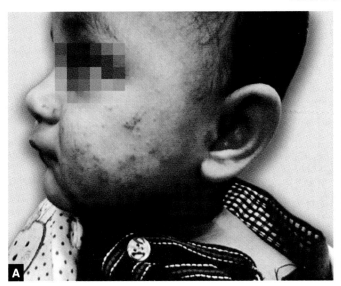

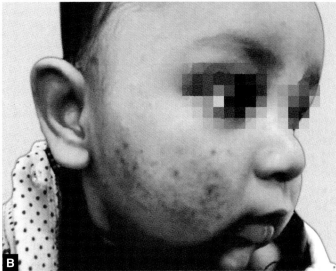

Fig. 13.21A and B: Eczematous papules on the cheek in a child with atopic dermatitis

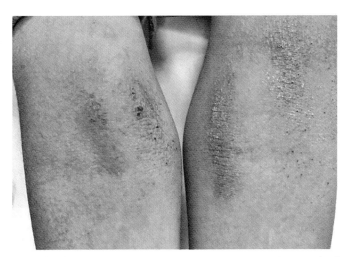

Fig. 13.22: Childhood atopic dermatitis with involvement of the antecubital fossa

- **Older children** and **adults** have posterior neck, flexor[Q] extremities, and hand involvement. Changes of chronic AD, including thickened hyperkeratotic plaques with lichenification and prurigo nodularis, may also be present. Postinflammatory hypopigmentation or hyperpigmentation are common associated findings. Xerosis is a common feature.[Q]
- **Onset of work:** Atopic patients carry a lifelong burden of being more sensitive to irritants. Thus certain *occupations* should be *avoided*, such as beauticians, machinists, or healthcare workers. Instead of developing a proactive hyperkeratotic response, they tend to get cumulative toxic dermatitis. They are also very sensitive to wool.
- **Adults:** Most adults have only a tendency to be more susceptible to irritants, even though the prevalence is <1%, they have localized dermatitis of the hand, eyelid, or neck.

- **Elderly:** There is another peak flare late in life, often with a totally different clinical picture.

  Patients present with pruritus and prurigo nodules. The clinical picture is dominated by single or grouped erythematous papules and nodules with central excoriations. This form is often associated with severe, almost intractable, pruritus and may have eosinophilia.

Morphological Variations

Several regional variants of AD can occur in isolation or together with the classic age-related patterns of involvement (Fig. 13.23). The associated features are depicted in Fig. 13.24. And depictive images are given in Fig. 13.25. It must be emphasized that the associated features are not diagnostic.

Differential Diagnosis

Scabies: The history of other family members with pruritus and a thorough skin examination that reveals burrows, particularly on the hands, are diagnostic of scabies.

Langerhans cell histiocytosis and *immunodeficiency syndromes*, such as Wiskott-Aldrich syndrome, ataxia-telangiectasia, and Swiss-type agammaglobulinemia, seen. These infants have dermatitis that resembles AD, but these conditions are rare, and the patients have pronounced systemic features.

Complications

Bacterial infection: The skin of AD patients is colonized with *Staphylococcus aureus*; their exotoxins act as superantigens which activate the inflammatory process in acute AD.

Eczema herpeticum (Kaposi varicelliform eruption): There is localized or widespread herpes simplex infection of skin affected by AD.[Q]

13

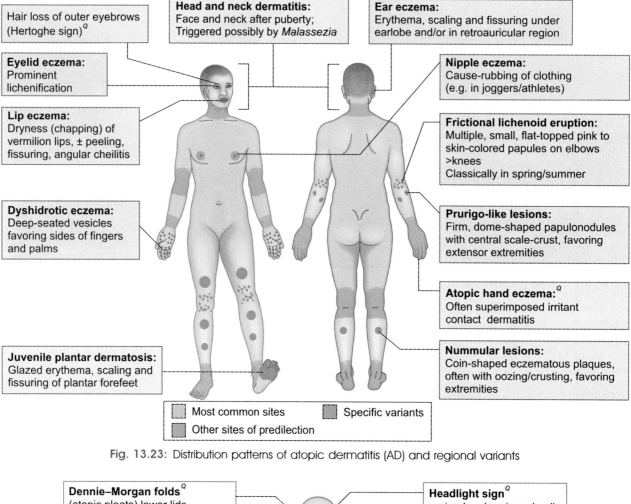

Hair loss of outer eyebrows (Hertoghe sign)[Q]

Head and neck dermatitis: Face and neck after puberty; Triggered possibly by *Malassezia*

Ear eczema: Erythema, scaling and fissuring under earlobe and/or in retroauricular region

Eyelid eczema: Prominent lichenification

Nipple eczema: Cause-rubbing of clothing (e.g. in joggers/athletes)

Lip eczema: Dryness (chapping) of vermilion lips, ± peeling, fissuring, angular cheilitis

Frictional lichenoid eruption: Multiple, small, flat-topped pink to skin-colored papules on elbows >knees Classically in spring/summer

Dyshidrotic eczema: Deep-seated vesicles favoring sides of fingers and palms

Prurigo-like lesions: Firm, dome-shaped papulonodules with central scale-crust, favoring extensor extremities

Atopic hand eczema:[Q] Often superimposed irritant contact dermatitis

Juvenile plantar dermatosis: Glazed erythema, scaling and fissuring of plantar forefeet

Nummular lesions: Coin-shaped eczematous plaques, often with oozing/crusting, favoring extremities

☐ Most common sites   ■ Specific variants
■ Other sites of predilection

Fig. 13.23: Distribution patterns of atopic dermatitis (AD) and regional variants

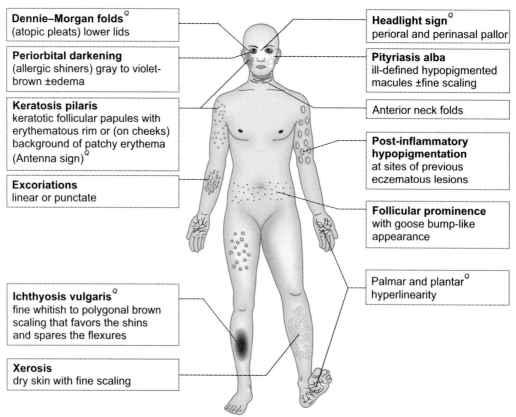

Dennie–Morgan folds[Q] (atopic pleats) lower lids

Headlight sign[Q] perioral and perinasal pallor

Periorbital darkening (allergic shiners) gray to violet-brown ±edema

Pityriasis alba ill-defined hypopigmented macules ±fine scaling

Keratosis pilaris keratotic follicular papules with erythematous rim or (on cheeks) background of patchy erythema (Antenna sign)[Q]

Anterior neck folds

Post-inflammatory hypopigmentation at sites of previous eczematous lesions

Excoriations linear or punctate

Follicular prominence with goose bump-like appearance

Ichthyosis vulgaris[Q] fine whitish to polygonal brown scaling that favors the shins and spares the flexures

Palmar and plantar[Q] hyperlinearity

Xerosis dry skin with fine scaling

Fig. 13.24: Associated features of atopic dermatitis

13

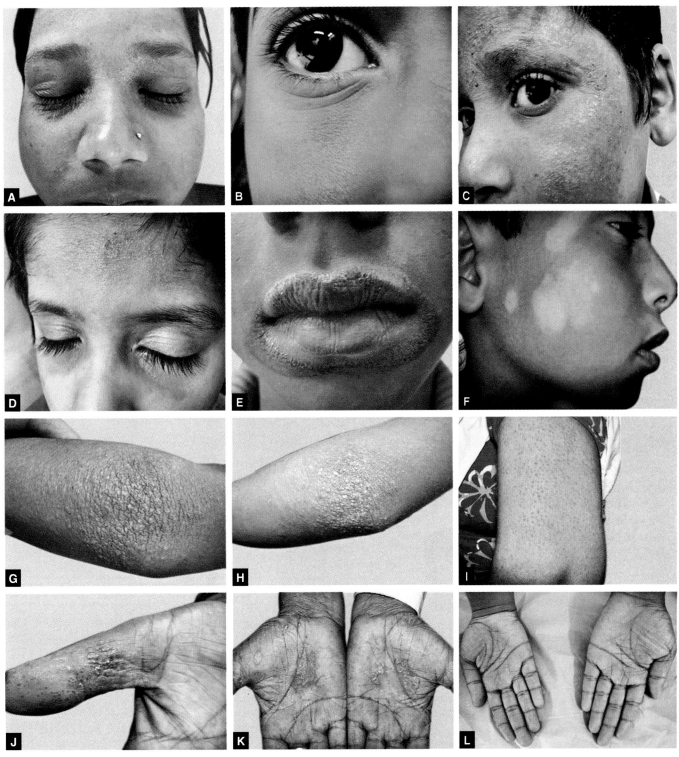

Fig. 13.25A to L: (A) Head and neck dermatitis. Note the marked involvement of periocular area; (B) Dennie-Morgan folds; (C) Marked involvement of forehead, eyes and cheeks; (D) Eyelid eczema; (E) Lip licker's eczema; (F) Pityriasis alba; (G and H) Frictional lichenoid eruption: small, flat-topped, pink to skin-colored papules on elbows more than knees; (I) Follicular papules—keratosis pilaris; (J) Pompholyx; (K) Hyperkeratotic eczema; (L) Hyperlinear palms

Allergic contact dermatitis: This is an often missed diagnosis and can occur even to the patient's own topical treatments (e.g. steroids and/or the preservatives) and should be considered in those with treatment-resistant AD.

Therapy

No disease is more complicated to treat than atopic dermatitis. It is absolutely essential to work with the patient (and the parents). Listen to their observations; make them a part of the treatment team.

Though there is a progressive decrease in severity with time, the disease may persist in adults (Fig. 13.26).

- Prompt and aggressive management of atopic dermatitis may halt the 'atopic march'—progression[Q] to rhinoconjunctivitis and/or asthma.
- Management of AD includes regular moisturizing, control of acute flares with topical corticosteroids and maintaining remission with topical calcineurin inhibitors with avoidance of potential triggers.
- Possible causes for flare-ups of AD include poor treatment compliance, superadded infection or allergic contact dermatitis.

Topical Therapy

1. Routine skin care with emollient creams or ointments; if tolerated, with urea as humectant; bath oils.

    Make sure they are applied when the skin is moist. Prescribe plenty (at least 500 g/week for the whole skin of an adult and 250 g/week for the whole skin of a child and ensure they are used at least 3–4 times a day.

2. Topical anti-inflammatory agents:
    - *Pimecrolimus* (>6 months); *tacrolimus* 0.03% >2 years, 0.1% >15 years. Use bid until response, then taper; can combine with corticosteroids.
    - *Corticosteroids*: Usually class I-II agents suffice; class III-IV reserved for flares, limited time period. In most instances, once daily application is adequate; never more than bid. A method of use of steroids is depicted in Fig. 13.27.
    - *Tars*: Available as creams or mixed as ointments; perhaps for chronic lichenified lesions, such as hands; gels are designed for psoriasis and should not be used in atopic dermatitis.

3. Topical antiseptics, used for baths and topical therapy (bleach bath).

4. Wet wrap therapy[Q] (*see* Page 166).

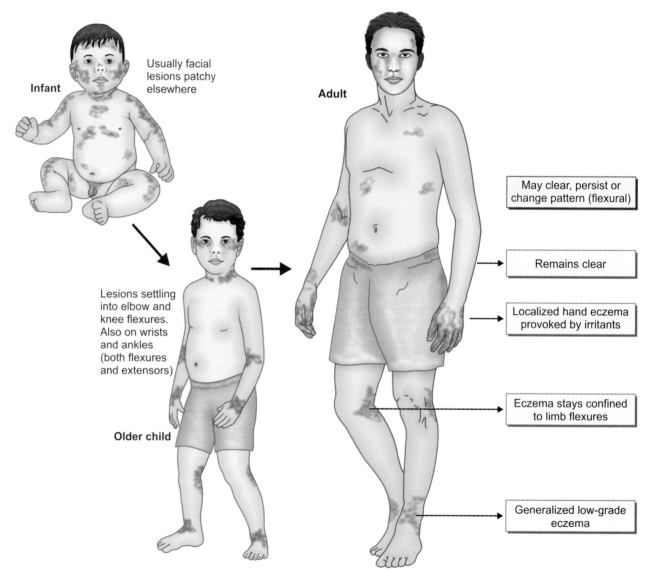

Infant — Usually facial lesions patchy elsewhere

Older child — Lesions settling into elbow and knee flexures. Also on wrists and ankles (both flexures and extensors)

Adult

May clear, persist or change pattern (flexural)

Remains clear

Localized hand eczema provoked by irritants

Eczema stays confined to limb flexures

Generalized low-grade eczema

Fig. 13.26: Course of atopic dermatitis (Pictorial[Q])

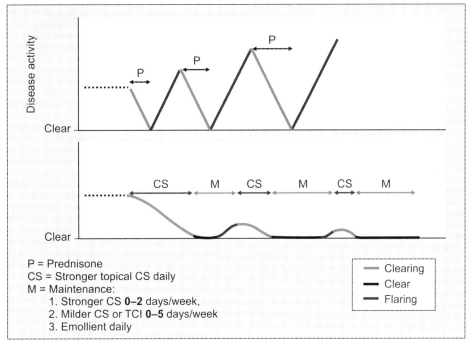

Fig. 13.27: Above panel shows that intermittent use of steroids can lead to worsening of disease. A better approach is a *proactive* therapy where the steroid potency is decreased to enable prolonged remissions of the disease (CS = corticosteroids)

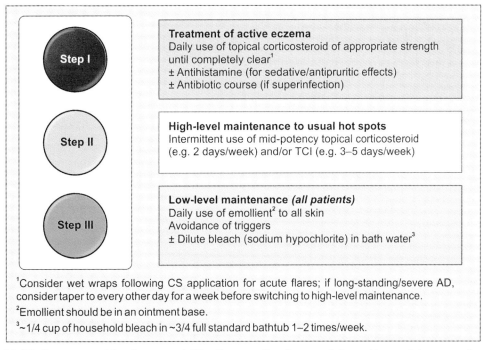

Fig. 13.28: Summary of the therapy of AD with an active therapy followed by maintenance therapy

Systemic Therapy

1. Antihistamines for severe pruritus; in general, the sedating (older) agents work better; some evidence that cetirizine is anti-inflammatory.
2. Cyclosporine for severe refractory disease.
3. Antibiotics for flares; cover for *Staphylococcus aureus*, which is usually involved.
4. Phototherapy: Helpful in patients who report that they tolerate sunlight well.

UVA1 is probably best for acute *flares*;[Q] selective UVB phototherapy (SUP) and **311 nm UVB** best for *chronic disease*.[Q]

5. Avoidance of triggers: Wool clothes, fabric softeners often help, avoid work that requires frequent hand washing.

In essence, the therapy of AD should combine an active arm and a maintenance arm where therapy is directed to the localized areas (Fig. 13.28).

SEBORRHEIC ECZEMA

Seborrheic dermatitis is an extremely common disorder with peaks in infants and the elderly.

Pathogenesis

This condition is not obviously related to seborrhea. It may run in some families, often affecting those with a tendency to dandruff. The success of treatments directed against yeasts has suggested that overgrowth of the *Malassezia* yeast skin[Q] commensals plays an important part in the development of seborrheic eczema.

The immune status plays a key role; there are also neurological factors, as patients with Parkinson disease have severe seborrheic dermatitis.[Q]

HIV patients[Q] have been found to have seborrheic dermatitis more commonly than unaffected population.

Clinical Features

There are three common patterns of this eczema often showing the characteristic greasy yellowish scales.[Q] These patterns are depicted in Fig. 13.29.

1. A red scaly or exudative rash of the scalp, ears, face and eyebrows (Figs 13.30 and 13.31). May be associated with chronic blepharitis[Q] and otitis externa (Figs 13.32 and 13.33).
2. Dry scaly petaloid lesions[Q] of the presternal and interscapular areas (Fig. 13.34). There may also be extensive follicular papules or pustules on the trunk (seborrheic folliculitis or Malassezia folliculitis).
3. Intertriginous lesions of the armpits, umbilicus or groins, or under spectacles or hearing aids.

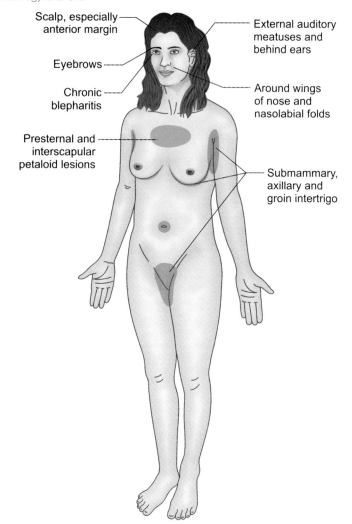

Fig. 13.29: Distribution of seborrheic eczema

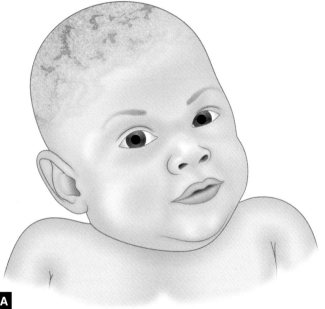

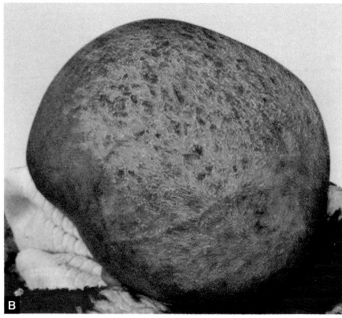

Fig. 13.30A and B: Scalp involvement in infant: (A) In infants, seborrheic dermatitis is referred to as 'cradle cap'[Q] because of the development of greasy crusted patches on the scalp. This common finding in infancy typically improves spontaneously over time; (B) Greasy scales on the scalp in a case of cradle cap

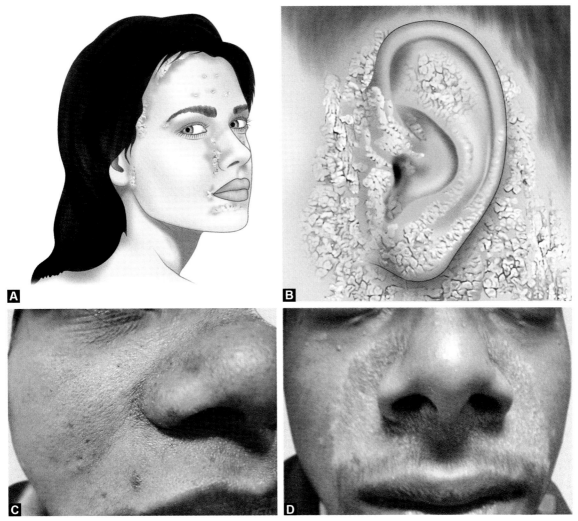

Fig. 13.31A to D: (A and B) Depicts classical morphology of seborrheic dermatitis in adults and manifests with greasy, yellow, scaly patches in the scalp, ears, eyebrow and nasobial folds; (C and D) show facial involvement in seborrheic dermatitis

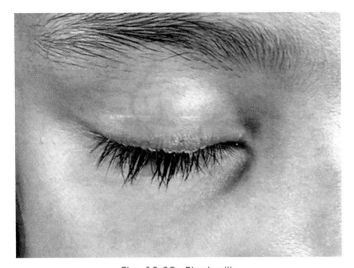

Fig. 13.32: Blepharitis

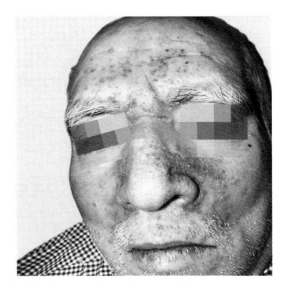

Fig. 13.33: Severe seborrheic dermatitis may be associated with human immunodeficiency virus (HIV) infection

In its mildest form, *dandruff,*[Q] one sees fine, white scale without erythema.

The patches and plaques of seborrheic dermatitis are characterized by indistinct margins, mild to moderate erythema, and yellowish, *greasy scaling*. It is uncommon for hair loss to result from seborrheic dermatitis.

13

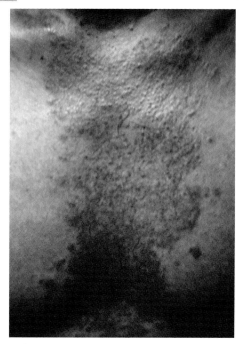

Fig. 13.34: Seborrheic dermatitis affecting the presternal area in a petaloid pattern

Differential Diagnosis

- Seborrheic dermatitis and atopic dermatitis in infancy is often difficult to distinguish; so many clinicians use the term 'infantile eczema.' When the dermatitis involves solely the diaper area and axillae, a diagnosis of seborrheic dermatitis is favored. Lesions on the forearms and shins favor the diagnosis of atopic dermatitis.
- In adults, it overlaps with psoriasis. Concomitant involvement of elbows and knees favors psoriasis.
- Petaloid seborrheic dermatitis resembles pityriasis rosea.
- External ear canal disease is usually misdiagnosed as otomycosis.
- Retroauricular and nasolabial disease mimics allergic contact dermatitis to glass frames.
- Rosacea has inflammatory papules and pustules not seen in seborrheic dermatitis.
- Langerhans cell histiocytosis may appear as a seborrheic dermatitis-like eruption. The occurrence of petechiae and the failure of standard therapy should make one suspect this is cancer and obtain a skin biopsy (Fig. 13.35).

Treatment

- Therapy is suppressive rather than curative and patients should be told about this at the outset.
- High-potency topical steroids should be avoided in prolonged treatment of seborrheic dermatitis, especially the face and intertriginous skin.

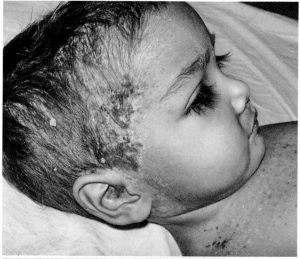

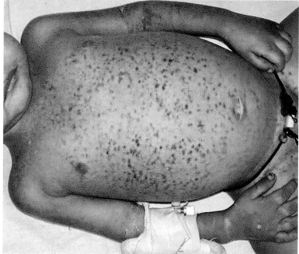

Fig. 13.35: The purpuric lesions interspersed with the scaly papules and enlarged liver and spleen (LCH)

The therapy is based on targeting the yeast and the associated inflammation but is modified by the site of involvement:

- Topical imidazoles: This is the first line of treatment.
- For intertriginous lesions a weak steroid-antifungal combination is often effective.
- For severe and unresponsive cases, a short course of oral itraconazole may be helpful.

An overview is given in the Box 13.2.

Box 13.2	Treatment of seborrheic dermatitis

Initial
- Shampoos—two or three times per week
  - Zinc pyrithione 1%
  - Selenium sulfide 1% or 2.5%
  - Ketoconzale 1% or 2%
- Hydrocortisone cream 1% or 2.5% bid as needed

Alternative
- Tacrolimus ointment 0.1% or pimecrolimus cream

NUMMULAR DERMATITIS/DISCOID ECZEMA

Nummular is a Greek word meaning 'coin'. Nummular dermatitis is a common skin disorder that presents with 'coin-shaped' plaques[Q] on the extremities. It is more common in older individuals and is often associated with dry skin.

Pathogenesis

The pathophysiology of nummular dermatitis is unknown, but thought to be linked to impaired skin barrier function.

A reaction to bacterial antigens is believed to be a trigger as steroid-antiseptic or steroid-antibiotic mixtures do better than either separately.

Other causes include atopy, sensitization to metals and drugs.

Clinical Presentation

The patient typically complains of an itchy rash on the extremities in middle-aged males.

Location is important to the diagnosis. Common affected areas are the distal limbs (lower extremities > upper extremities) and most commonly involves the dorsa of the hands, extensor surfaces of the forearms, upper arms, legs, thighs, and feet. The lesions start as solid plaques that enlarge and develop a peripheral papulovesicular border (Fig. 13.36).

There is often associated pruritus, but this varies greatly, with some patients complaining of almost constant itching and others noticing severe pruritus only at the time of initial outbreak of new lesions.

It may be convenient to recognize the following patterns (Fig. 13.37A to C):

1. Discoid eczema of the *hands* and *forearms*
2. Discoid eczema of the *limbs* and *trunk*
3. *Dry* discoid eczema.

Lesions often have blisters or yellow crusts, suggesting an infectious component, usually *Staphylococcus aureus*.

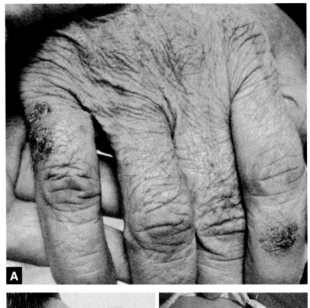

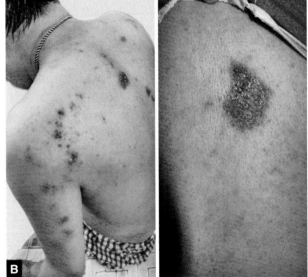

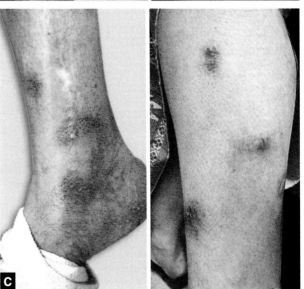

Fig. 13.37A to C: (A) Discoid eczema of the hands; (B) Discoid eczema of limbs and trunk (subacute eczema stage); (C) Dry discoid eczema of the limbs

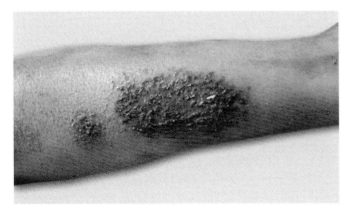

Fig. 13.36: A discoid patch of eczema (acute stage) with peripheral papulovesicles

Diagnosis

The key diagnostic features of nummular dermatitis are pruritic, scaly plaques, with no central clearing, commonly located on the arms and legs. The trunk may also be affected.

Management

Treatment is aimed at:

1. *Rehydration* of the skin, withholding the inciting agent (often hot water showers and harsh soaps).
2. *Repair* of the epidermal lipid barrier
3. Reduction of *inflammation*
5. Treatment of any *infection*

   - The management of nummular dermatitis includes the use of mid- to high-potency topical corticosteroids twice a day, and mild soaps and moisturizers.
   - Traditionally, a range of coaltar pastes or ointments were used in the less acute stages, and sometimes a combination of tar and dilute corticosteroid proved useful in long-term management.
   - Topical immune modulators (tacrolimus and pimecrolimus) also reduce inflammation.
   - When eruptions are generalized and prolonged, phototherapy (generally UVB) may be helpful.
   - Oral antihistamines or sedatives may help reduce itching and improve sleep.
   - Oral antibiotics, such as dicloxacillin, cephalexin, or erythromycin, should be used in cases of secondary infection.

POMPHOLYX/DYSHIDROTIC DERMATITIS

Dyshidrotic dermatitis (sometimes called pompholyx[Q]) is a common pruritic, vesicular skin disorder of the palms and soles. It is characterized by chronic, relapsing eruptions of vesicles[Q] or rarely large bullae.

Etiopathogenesis

The term 'dyshidrosis' (meaning 'difficult sweating') is a misnomer. The condition does not involve dysfunction of sweat glands. The exact cause is unknown.

A few studies have found a link between flares of vesicular palmoplantar dermatitis and oral ingestion of nickel in nickel-allergic patients.

While most cases are idiopathic, possible causes include:

- Atopic diathesis,
- Fungal id reactions,
- Contact dermatitis, and
- Systemic allergic reactions to nickel.

A summary of the factors implicated are given in Table 13.6.

Table 13.6	Causes of pompholyx

- Atopy
- Dermatophytid
- Drug reactions
- Systemic contact dermatitis
- Allergic contact dermatitis (*garlic, compositae plants, balsam of Peru*)
- Metals (*dental metals, orthodontic treatment, Ni, chromium*)
- Ingested metals (*Ni, chromium*)
- Food (*Tuna, coffee, tomato, pineappple, American cheese, milk, egg, wheat, lamb, chocolate and chicken*)

Clinical Presentation

The patient typically complains of pruritic or painful blisters on the palms and soles.[Q] Mostly the lesions are small vesicles, sometimes likened to 'tapioca pudding' (Fig. 13.38) (sago-grain appearance).[Q] The most common locations include lateral fingers, central palms, insteps, and lateral borders of the feet.

Two types have been described: One type is explosive, with eruptions of severe vesiculation (Fig. 13.39) or even

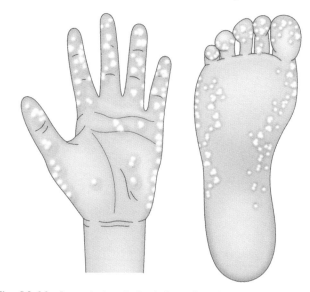

Fig. 13.38: Pompholyx. A depiction of multiple 'sago grain' like vesicles on the sides of fingers[Q]

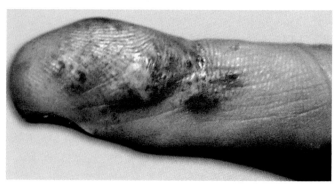

Fig. 13.39: Large vesicles coalescing into a bulla in a case of vesicular hand eczema

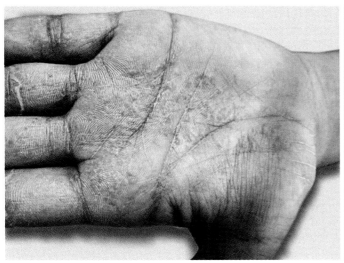
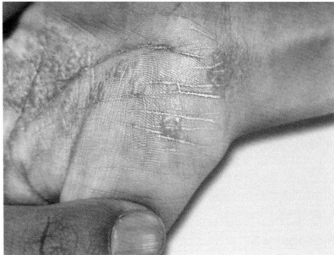

Fig. 13.40: Multiple 'sago grain' like vesicles on the palms

bullous lesions. This type is rare and is representative of the initial descriptions of the dermatosis made in the late nineteenth century.

The more common is the less severe type, with repeated eruptions of tiny, severely pruritic vesicles (Fig. 13.40).

Treatment

Lasting treatment is only when a cause can be found.

Treatment is as for acute eczema of the hands and feet. Appropriate antibiotics should be given for bacterial infections. Saline soaks followed by applications of a very potent corticosteroid cream are often helpful.

LICHEN SIMPLEX CHRONICUS

Lichen simplex chronicus is a term used to describe the clinical appearance of any long-standing, chronically pruritic skin condition. As a primary diagnosis, it exists without a known underlying condition or cause. As a secondary diagnosis, it results after years of scratching due to another condition.

Pathogenesis

The exact pathophysiology is unknown. Chronic rubbing and scratching of the skin leads to thickening of the epidermis and fibrosis of the dermis. Chronic cutaneous nerve stimulation is hypothesized to result in nerve dysfunction in scratch-affected areas.

Clinical Presentation

- The patient typically complains of localized areas of intensely pruritic skin. Sleep is often interrupted. In some cases, the chronic rubbing and scratching becomes a subconscious or compulsive habit.
- The lichenified plaque always occurs within reach of scratching fingers. Common locations for primary

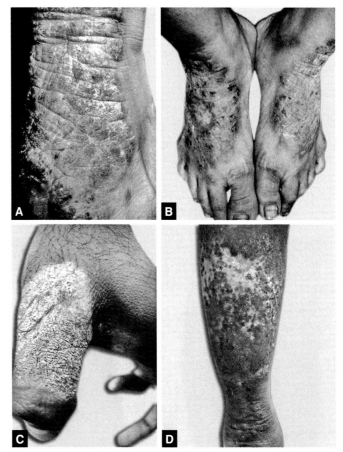

Fig. 13.41A to D: (A) A plaque of lichen simplex chronicus on the back of the foot. Note the thickened and lichenified skin; (B) Bilateral lichen simplex chronicus; (C) An unusual site of lichen simplex chronicus, here the patient used to rub the finger on the side of the office table; (D) A case of lichen simplex chronicus with loss of pigment due to scratching

lichen simplex chronicus include the lateral neck, scrotum/vulva, and dorsal foot. The plaque is typically solitary, well-defined, thick, and lichenified (Fig. 13.41).

13

- Some patients with lichen simplex chronicus have a history of emotional or psychiatric problems. However, for most, it is simply a nervous habit.
- Secondary lichen simplex chronicus occurs at the sites of the underlying skin conditions such as in the antecubital and popliteal fossae in atopic dermatitis.
- Prurigo nodule is a term used for a lichenified papule that has been chronically picked and manipulated (Fig. 13.42). Secondary prurigo nodularis may present with many widespread lichenified papules in patients with generalized pruritus due to systemic diseases such as liver or kidney disease.

Management

The patient must be made to understand that the rash will not clear until even minor scratching and rubbing are stopped, but in most cases, this is a habitual tendency and most patients cannot stop the tendency to scratch. Scratching frequently takes place during sleep, and the affected area may have to be covered to avoid this trauma.

> Goal is to break itch–scratch–itch cycle.

Primary lichen simplex chronicus is typically managed with class 1 or 2 high to superpotent topical corticosteroid ointments or creams twice a day.

Oral antidepressants or antihistamines, especially doxepin, may benefit individuals with nighttime itching and sleep disturbance. It is important that patients become aware of the habit or compulsion to scratch or rub, replacing these activities with pushing on the skin.

Application of ice provides a better alternative. In more severe cases, behavioral therapy may be of benefit.

For generalized prurigo nodularis, ultraviolet light therapy is often very helpful.

PITYRIASIS ALBA

This is a very common and largely idiopathic hypopigmentary condition that appears clinically as white (alba) patches surmounted[Q] by fine, 'bran-like' (*pityron*, Greek for bran) scales.

Though it is seen in children, it is seen more in patients with dry skin and those with atopic dermatitis.[Q]

Clinical Features

The early lesion is a mildly erythematous, slightly scaling patch with an indistinct margin.

This is followed by the subsequent lesion where a 1 to 4 cm white patch with a fine, powdery scale is seen on the face. It can also be seen on the upper arms (Fig. 13.43). This has episodic occurrence with relapses and recurrences.

Differential Diagnosis

- **Tinea versicolor:** Uncommonly adults with tinea versicolor might have a facial involvement, but in children (in whom the disease is much less common), the face is affected in approximately one-third of cases. In a doubtful case, a KOH preparation should be performed on all scaling white spots to rule out tinea versicolor.
- **Vitiligo:** This is characterized by sharp demarcation, complete depigmentation, and lack of scale.

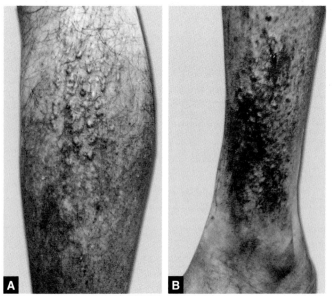

Fig. 13.42A and B: (A) Multiple hyperkeratotic nodules with some showing excoriation on the leg in a male patient; (B) A case of prurigo nodularis with violent bouts of scratching. The patient was found to have an OCD for which he was initiated on pimozide 1 mg BD with a short-course of cyclosporine for prurigo

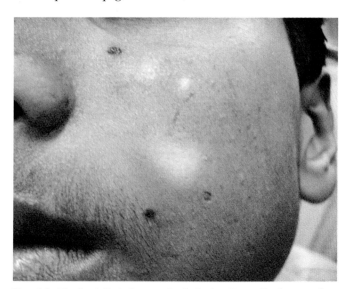

Fig. 13.43: An initial stage of pityriasis alba with fine scaling and an underlying area of hypopigmentation (*pictoral*)[Q]

- **Postinflammatory hypopigmentation:** This is diagnosed by a pre-existing skin lesion and extrafacial distribution of skin lesions.
- **Indeterminate Hansens:** Solitary hypopigmented macule on face, found in younger children, from endemic districts with normal sensation and no minimal scaling.

Therapy

Treatment is not often necessary as spontaneous resolution occurs. Emollients can be used for the dry scaling, and 1% hydrocortisone cream or triamcinolone 0.1% cream can be used for the inflammatory reaction.

ASTEATOTIC ECZEMA

This is a condition that is seen in elderly individuals and they usually have a dry skin and a tendency to chap.[Q] Other contributory factors include the removal of surface lipids by over-washing, the low humidity of winter and central heating, the use of drugs (diuretics, statins and nicotinic acid) hypothyroidism.

Clinical Features

This common and itchy pattern of eczema occurs usually on the legs of elderly patients. A network of fine red superficial fissures creates a 'crazy paving' appearance. The background skin is dry (Fig. 13.44).

Treatment

The condition can be cleared by the use of a mild or moderately potent topical steroid in a greasy base, and use of syndets instead of soaps. Frequent bathing and use of regular soaps should be restricted. Regular use of emollients usually prevents recurrence.

NAPKIN (DIAPER) DERMATITIS

Though there are various types of diaper dermatitis, the most common type is irritant in origin, and is aggravated by the use of waterproof plastic pants. This reaction is consequent to the mixture of fecal enzymes and ammonia produced by urea-splitting bacteria. The overgrowth of yeasts is another aggravating factor.

Clinical Features

The moist, glazed, erythema affects the napkin area generally (Fig. 13.45), with the exception of the skin folds, which tend to be spared. It is now renamed appropriately *irritant diaper dermatitis* (IDD).

Complications

Superinfection with *Candida albicans* is common, and this may lead to small erythematous papules or vesicopustules appearing around the periphery of the main eruption.

Differential Diagnosis

The sparing of the folds helps to distinguish it from infantile seborrheic eczema and candidiasis.

Treatment

The basic regime to be followed in treatment of IDD can be remembered by the *Mnemonic ABCDE:*
A for air or time without diaper
B for barrier cream
C for cleansing/corticosteroids
D for diaper to be used
E for education of the parents.

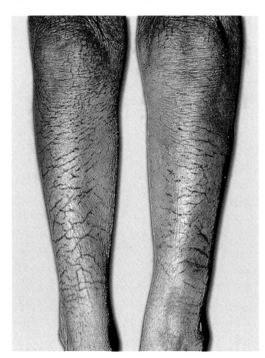

Fig. 13.44: Xerosis with cracked skin (eczema craquelé)

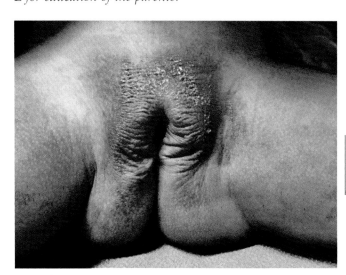

Fig. 13.45: Irritant diaper dermatitis affecting the convex surfaces of labia majora and mons pubis while sparing the vulva and inguinal folds

13

The basic principle is to keep this area clean and dry. Theoretically, the child should be allowed to be free of napkins as much as possible. One option is to use disposable nappies (diapers). The ideal is the superabsorbent type which should be changed regularly. When towelling napkins are used they should be washed thoroughly and changed frequently.

The area should be cleaned at each nappy change with aqueous cream and water. Protective ointments (e.g. zinc oxide 13 % and castor oil ointment), or silicone protective ointments, are often useful, as are topical imidazole preparations that stop yeast growth. Combinations of hydrocortisone with antifungals or antiseptics can be used.

STASIS DERMATITIS

Stasis dermatitis is an eczematous eruption of the lower legs secondary to peripheral venous disease.

Stasis dermatitis occurs as a direct consequence of venous insufficiency (Fig. 13.46). Disturbed function of the one-way valvular system in the deep venous plexus of the legs results in a backflow of blood from the deep venous system to the superficial venous system, with accompanying venous hypertension. This loss of valvular function can result from an age-related

decrease in valve competency. This distends the local capillary bed and widens the endothelial pores, thus allowing fibrinogen molecules to escape into the interstitial fluid, where they form a fibrin sheath around the capillaries. This layer of fibrin presumably forms a pericapillary barrier to the diffusion of oxygen and other nutrients which are essential for the normal vitality of the skin (Fig. 13.46).

Venous incompetence causes increased hydrostatic pressure and capillary damage with extravasation of red blood cells and serum. In some patients, this condition causes an inflammatory eczematous process.

Clinical Features

There is a history of a chronic, pruritic eruption of the lower legs preceded by edema and swelling. Patients with stasis dermatitis have often had thrombophlebitis.
- Varicose veins are often prominent, as is pitting edema of the lower leg. The peripheral pulses are intact.
- The involved skin has brownish hyperpigmentation, dull erythema, petechiae, thickened skin, scaling, or weeping.
- The most common site affected is above the medial malleolus.

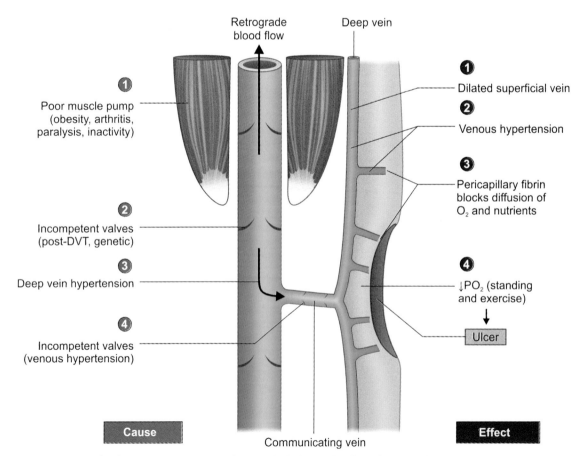

Fig. 13.46: An overview of the factors that determine leg ulcers and venous eczema

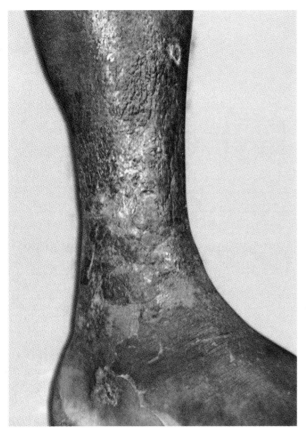

Fig. 13.47: A case of venous eczema with changes of subacute eczema seen on the medial aspect of the limb. Note signs of lipodermatosclerosis

Cardinal signs of stasis dermatitis:
1. Edema
2. Brown pigmentation
3. Petechiae
4. Subacute and chronic dermatitis

Lipodermatosclerosis: Stasis dermatitis can lead to fat necrosis with the end stage being permanent sclerosis (lipodermatosclerosis) with inverted champagne bottle appearance[Q] (Fig. 13.47).

Allergy to topical preparations may occur in 60% of patients with stasis dermatitis. The compromised epidermal barrier from stasis allows sensitization to occur more easily than in normal skin. Contact dermatitis can easily be misdiagnosed as a flare-up of stasis dermatitis. Topical antibiotics are particularly prone to cause ACD.

Treatment

The basic therapy is directed towards prevention of venous stasis and edema. This is done by the use of supportive hose while the patient is ambulatory.

Standing should be restricted, and patients who are obese should be placed on a weight reduction program.

If this approach fails, bed rest with elevation of the legs is required.

The management of the skin as a case of subacute eczema.

13

CHAPTER 14

Urticaria and Reactive Erythemas

Chapter Outline

- Urticaria and Acquired Angioedema
- Hereditary Angioedema
- Erythema Multiforme

- Figurate Erythemas
- Nodose Erythemas

URTICARIA AND ACQUIRED ANGIOEDEMA

Introduction

Urticaria (hives) is characterized by the rapid onset of lesions called wheals[Q] that consist of a central mid-dermal swelling with or without surrounding erythema, with associated pruritus, lasting anywhere from 1 to 24 hours[Q] (Fig. 14.1A). The term urticaria is named after the stinging nettle plant (*Urtica dioica*), which contains histaminic acid (Fig. 14.1B). Associated angioedema can sometimes be seen, characterized by swelling of the deeper dermis and subcutaneous tissue lasting up to 72 hours (Fig. 14.2).

Types

Urticaria can be divided into acute and chronic forms (Table 14.1).

Acute urticaria is defined as urticaria of less than 6 weeks duration,[Q] whereas chronic urticaria lasts more than 6 weeks.[Q]

Only 5% of patients with urticaria will be symptomatic for more than 4 weeks. Recently, episodic (acute intermittent or recurrent activity) has been added to the classification. Patients with chronic urticaria, other than those with an obvious physical cause, have what is often known as chronic spontaneous urticaria.

Chronic spontaneous urticaria (CSU) can be further subdivided depending on the presence (30%) or absence (70%) of histamine-releasing autoantibodies into two subtypes—autoimmune chronic spontaneous urticaria and idiopathic chronic spontaneous urticaria, respectively.

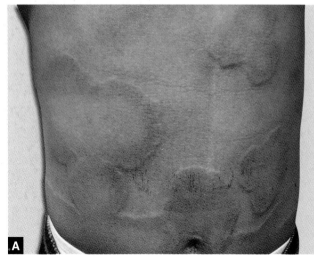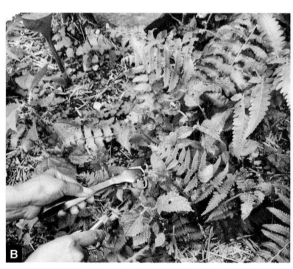

Fig. 14.1A and B: (A) Multiple edematous erythematous wheals on the trunk in urticaria; (B) The stinging nettle plant (*Urtica dioica*), after which the term urticaria has been coined

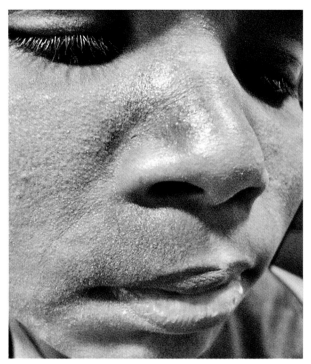

Fig. 14.2: Urticarial wheal with swelling of the lip

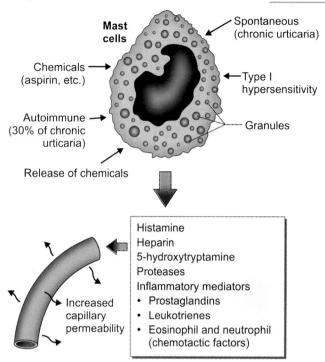

Fig. 14.3: Role of mast cell in urticaria

Table 14.1	A working classification of urticaria
Spontaneous urticaria	**Acute** (up to 6 weeks) **Chronic** (more than 6 weeks—median duration 2–5 years) a. Autoimmune, b. Idiopathic **Episodic** (acute intermittent or recurrent activity)
Physical urticaria	Temperature: Cold > heat urticaria Mechanical stimuli: Dermographism,[Q] delayed pressure urticaria Sweating/exertion: Cholinergic[Q] > adrenergic urticaria, exercise-induced anaphylaxis Others: Solar and aquagenic
Contact urticaria	Immunological and non-immunological
Rare forms	*Schnitzler syndrome*: Defect in inflammasome, with urticarial vasculitis, fever, arthralgias, and IgM gammopathy *Muckle-Wells syndrome*: Familial inflammasome defect with urticaria, fever, deafness, and later renal amyloidosis with nephropathy.

Pathogenesis and Causes

The underlying event leading to urticaria is mast cell degranulation, with release of histamine[Q] and other proinflammatory molecules with numerous stimuli that can lead to mast cell activation through various pathways (Fig. 14.3).

This release can be triggered by allergic, pseudo-allergic, toxic, and physical mechanisms (Fig. 14.4). Urticaria is **allergic** when specific antigens cross-link specific IgE antibodies attached to mast cells. **Pseudoallergic urticaria** describes the release of mast cell mediators after exposure to foods or medications but *without* the presence of specific immunoglobulin (Ig) E *antibodies*. Endogenous or exogenous substances such as opiates, codeine, or complement proteins can alter the sensitivity of mast cells to both stimuli.

Acute urticaria: The most common cause of acute urticaria is viral infections,[Q] particularly of the upper respiratory tract. Other common causes of acute urticaria are listed in Table 14.2. Food-induced type I hypersensitivity reactions are a rare cause of acute urticaria in adults, but are a more common cause in children.

Chronic urticaria: The three most common underlying causes (Table 14.3) of chronic urticaria are:[Q]

• Autoreactivity or expression of circulating mast cell secretagogues including autoantibodies (autoimmune urticaria)
• Chronic infections
• Intolerance to food components (Table 14.3).

Though all the factors listed in Table 14.4 can induce chronic urticaria, they are emphasized here because patients with chronic urticaria are more likely to be subjected to detailed investigations. In the *majority* of patients with chronic urticaria, an underlying disease will not be found. Approximately 35 to 40%[Q] of cases of chronic urticaria are a caused by autoantibodies directed against the IgE receptor of mast cells.

Angioedema occurs with wheals in approximately 40% of cases of urticaria in adults and possibly more frequently in food-induced urticaria.

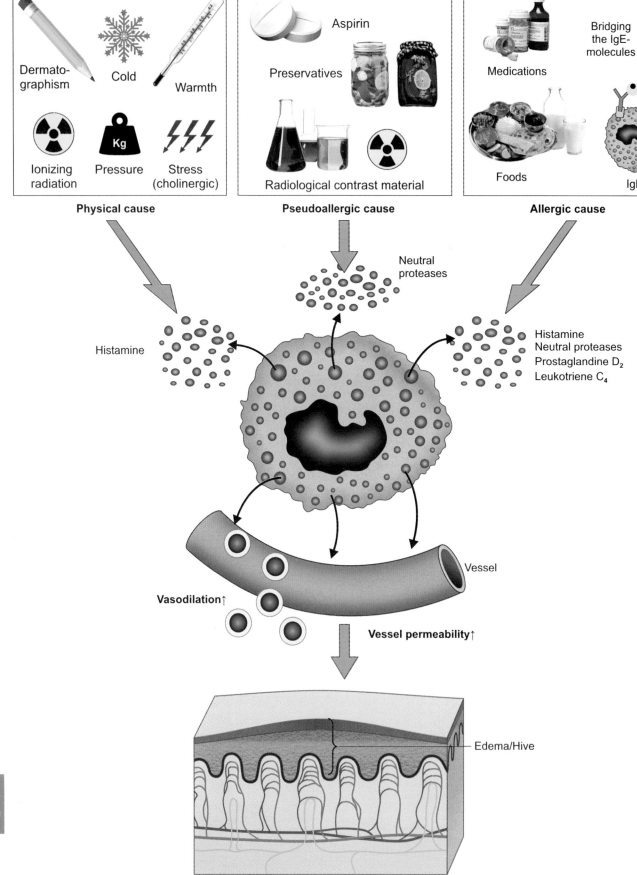

Fig. 14.4: Diagram depicting the various causes of urticaria and angioedema

Table 14.2	Causes of acute urticaria
Infections (~40%)[Q]	Viral respiratory, especially rhinovirus and rotavirus (cause in 80% of children), *Helicobacter pylori*, *Mycoplasma*, hepatitis, mononucleosis, and parasitic helminths
Drugs (~10%)	Beta-lactam antibiotics, nonsteroidal anti-inflammatory drugs (NSAIDs), aspirin, ACE inhibitors, diuretics, opiates, contrast media, and blood
Foods (~1%)	**Adults:** Shellfish, fresh water fish, berries, nuts, peanuts, pork, chocolate, tomatoes, spices, food additives, and alcohol. **Children:** Milk and other dairy products, eggs, wheat, and citrus
Inhalants	Pollens, molds, dust mites, and animal dander
Systemic diseases	Lupus erythematosus, Still's disease, thyroid disease, cryoglobulinemia, mastocytosis, and carcinomas
Emotional stress	

~50% idiopathic

Table 14.3	Possible food allergens that can cause urticaria
Dyes	Quinoline yellow, yellow-orange S, azorubin, amaranth, erythrosine, Ponceau 4R, patent blue, indigo carmine, brilliant black, ferric oxide red, cochineal, tartrazine
Preservatives	Sorbic acid, sodium benzoate, sodium metabisulfite, sodium nitrate
Antioxidants	Butyl hydroxyanisole (BHA), propyl gallate, butyl hydroxytoluol (BHT), tocopherol
Taste enhancers	Monosodium glutamate
Natural substances	Salicylic acid, biogenic amines, p-hydroxy benzoic acid esters, fragrances

Table 14.4	Causes of chronic urticaria
Autoreactivity	Autoimmunity (anti-FcεRI-Ab, anti-IgE-Ab) (40–50%)
Chronic infection	Hepatitis B, *H. pylori*
Intolerance	Foods, drugs, pseudoallergy
Other causes	Type I allergy, internal disease
Idiopathic[Q]	~50%

Clinical Presentation

Spontaneous Urticaria and Angioedema

A detailed history is required, as in most of the cases the lesions may have disappeared by the time of the office visit. It is important to inquire about the location, associated pruritus, and especially the duration of the lesions. Any lesions that last for longer than 24 hours[Q] should raise suspicion of an alternative diagnosis, such as *urticarial vasculitis*.

To determine the underlying cause of urticaria, one should inquire about associated symptoms, including those of upper respiratory infection, sinus infection, autoimmune disease, and *H. pylori* infection. Any symptoms that point to an anaphylaxis-type reaction or to swelling of the throat are important as these are rare, but life-threatening complications. A thorough review of recent medications and foods should be done as these can be triggers for urticaria that usually appears 1 to 2 hours after ingestion.

In cases of chronic urticaria, ask specifically about possible triggers including stress, drugs (analgesics, penicillin, laxatives, oral contraceptives), food components (preservatives, food colorings, foods rich in histamine), and any relation to certain eating situations (certain restaurants); exclude physical triggers (often overlooked by patients, especially when delayed); family history of urticaria or angioedema.

Physical examination

1. *Urticaria*

- Wheals, which are white to pink, pruritic, edematous papules or plaques that may be round annular, or arcuate (Figs 14.1, 14.2 and 14.5). The surface of the lesion is smooth because the pathology is in the dermis, not in the epidermis. Individual wheals have a rapid onset and last less than 24 hours, but the entire episode of urticaria may last much longer.
- Dermographism[Q] can be elicited in many patients with urticaria, including patients who have no visible hives at the time (Fig. 14.6). This 'writing with wheals' reaction represents a wheal and flare

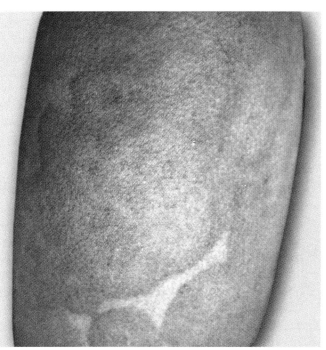

Fig. 14.5: Arcuate wheals in urticaria

14

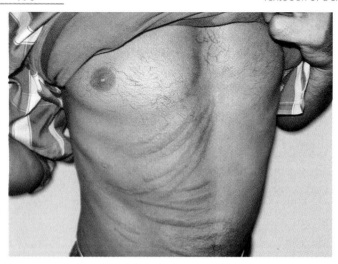

Fig. 14.6: Dermographism

response to scratching the skin. It indicates that the cutaneous mast cells are unstable and are easily provoked to release their histamine content. Many healthy patients develop erythema after stroking the skin, but wheal formation is limited mainly to patients with urticaria.[Q]

2. *Angioedema* presents with a sudden onset of diffuse swelling of the lower dermis and subcutaneous tissues, typically involving the lips, periorbital area, the hands, and the feet.[Q] The tongue, larynx, and the respiratory and gastrointestinal tracts may also be affected. It is also known as angioneurotic edema (Quincke edema).[Q] The swelling may persist for up to 3 days (Fig. 14.2).

   Angioedema without wheals[Q] often has differing underlying causes; therefore, it is important to determine, if the primary lesions are wheals, angioedema, or both (*see* below). Absence of wheals is indicative of hereditary angioedema or more commonly angiotensin-converting enzyme (ACE)[Q] inhibitor consumption (thought to result from the inhibition of kinin degradation).[Q] Hoarseness can be a sign of laryngeal edema that can be a life-threatening complication due to airway compromise. Dyspnea, wheezing, abdominal pain, dizziness, and hypotension are clues to an anaphylaxis-like reaction.

3. *Physical urticarias*: Physical urticarias are conditions in which one specific physical trigger is required to induce urticaria symptoms. Two or more forms of physical urticaria may be present in one patient, and patients with chronic idiopathic urticaria may also have physical urticaria. In some patients, a combination of two or more physical triggers may be required to induce urticaria.

   • *Cold urticaria*: Patients develop wheals in areas exposed to cold. A simple test is to reproduce the reaction by holding an ice cube, in a thin plastic bag. A few cases are associated with the presence of cryoglobulins, cold agglutinins or cryofibrinogens.

   • *Solar urticaria*[Q]: Wheals occur within minutes of sun exposure. Some patients with solar urticaria have erythropoietic protoporphyria.

   • *Heat urticaria*: Direct contact with a warm object elicits urticaria.

   • *Cholinergic urticaria*: Anxiety, heat, sexual excitement or strenuous exercise elicits this characteristic response. The vessels overreact to acetylcholine liberated from sympathetic nerves in the skin. Transient 2–5 mm follicular macules or papules resemble a blush or viral exanthem (Fig. 14.7). Some patients get blotchy patches on their necks.

   The skin findings are not typical of hives, so most patients simply describe an itchy rash,[Q] classically *preceded by sweating*.

   • *Adrenergic urticaria*: Emotional stress triggering urticaria.

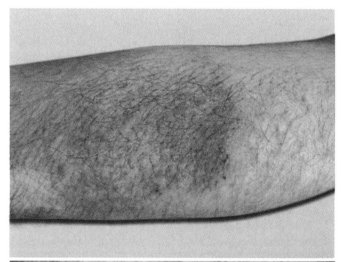

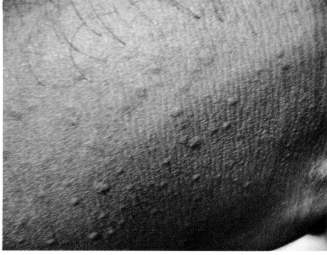

Fig. 14.7: Transient itchy papules associated with sweating in cholinergic urticaria

- *Delayed pressure urticaria*: Sustained pressure causes edema of the underlying skin and subcutaneous tissue 3–6 hours later. The swelling may last up to 48 hours and kinins or prostaglandins[Q] rather than histamine probably mediate it. It occurs particularly on the feet after walking, on the hands after clapping and on the buttocks after sitting.
- *Aquagenic urticaria*: Very rare, caused by contact with water of any temperature.

4. **Contact urticaria**: Contact with chemicals found in foods, plants, and medicines elicits urticaria.

   It is caused by a type I allergy to contact allergens or by an intolerance to substances that come in contact with the skin. Triggers include allergens as well as toxins, pseudoallergens, and mast cell activators (Table 14.5). Most common are arthropod assaults and contact with stinging nettles. Some allergens such as natural latex may cause allergic contact urticaria after sensitization.

5. **Anaphylaxis**: This is the most severe variant of urticaria, in which there is generalized mast cell degranulation leading to vasodilation and bronchoconstriction leading to anaphylactic shock, which is life-threatening. Common allergic triggers are hymenoptera toxin and penicillin.

Course

The course of an urticarial reaction depends on its cause. If the urticaria is allergic, it will continue until the allergen is removed, tolerated or metabolized. Most such patients clear up within a day or two, even if the allergen is not identified.

Contrary to this, only 50% of patients attending hospital clinics with chronic urticaria and angioedema will clear 5 years later. Those with urticarial lesions alone do better, half being clear after 6 months.

Table 14.5	Causes of contact urticaria
Allergic reaction (type I allergen)	**Plants** (latex, cornmeal, pollen, mahogany, teak, roses, wheat flour)
	Animal proteins (fish, milk, meat, silk; saliva, dander, blood)
	Vegetables, spices, and fruits (potato peels, pitted fruits, oranges)
	Medications (bacitracin, cephalosporins, chloramine, chlorhexidine)
	Industrial materials (ammonia, formaldehyde, acrylic acid)
Nonallergic reaction (toxin, pseudoallergen, mast cell secretagogue)	**Food preservatives** (e.g. benzoic acid, sorbic acid)
	Fragrances (cinnamic acid, balsam of Peru)
	Topical antibiotics (bacitracin, neomycin)
	Nettles, insect stings, caterpillar hairs, jellyfish

Differential Diagnosis

Urticarial vasculitis: Presents with wheal-like lesions that last for more than 24 hours and may be accompanied by fever, malaise, and arthritis. These findings should prompt a skin biopsy or specialty referral.

Viral exanthems: May present with urticarial lesions, which can fade quickly, but these lesions typically last for more than 24 hours.

Insect bites: The papular urticarial lesions of insect bites usually have a blanched center and may have a central crust or puncta at the site of the bite. The lesions usually last longer than 24 hours.

Still's disease: Associated with juvenile rheumatoid arthritis; may present transient urticarial lesions that last less than 24 hours. Symptoms of arthritis as well as an exceptionally high ferritin level can help distinguish this rare disease.

Other: Drug reactions such as fixed drug eruption, Stevens-Johnson syndrome, drug rash with eosinophilia and systemic symptoms (DRESS).

A simple enumeration of the common differential diagnosis is given in Box 14.1.

Box 14.1	Differential diagnosis of urticarias
Transient urticaria	Still's disease, erythema marginatum, mastocytosis
Lesions >24 hrs	Drug eruption, viral exanthem, erythema multiforme, Sweets syndrome, urticarial stage of BP, urticarial vasculitis

Investigation

In case of urticaria, *history* is more useful than investigations. The list of causes given in Tables 14.2 to 14.4 can be a sufficiently adequate start to find a possible cause. If the urticaria persists for more than *2–3 months*, a detailed analysis may be warranted.

Some principles that determine the investigation are:

1. Acute urticaria is generally *not* investigated.
2. Acute *recurrent* urticaria is frequently clarified with a history, as a possible trigger (food, medication, activity) can be identified. One should not forget to enquire about mucosal contacts, such as toothpaste, latex condoms, or even semen. Everything that comes in contact with the *mucosa* should be sought for, like drugs (prescription and over-the-counter; asking directly about aspirin and nonsteroidal anti-inflammatory drugs [NSAIDs]), all food-stuffs including spices, drinks and even chewing gum.
3. Chronic urticaria often remains idiopathic.

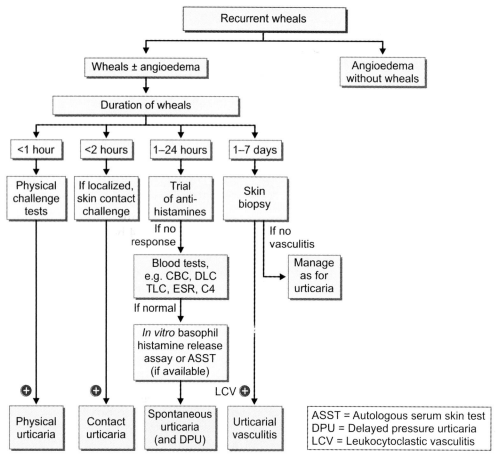

Fig. 14.8: Approach to the diagnosis of chronic urticaria. In a positive ASST, localized wheal and flare response occurs upon intradermal injection of autologous serum, providing evidence of functional histamine-releasing factors in the blood

Tests

- *Thyroid function* and autoantibody testing may be indicated by the history.
- Some specialist centers perform autologous serum intradermal injection to test for the presence of histamine-releasing autoantibodies.
- Patients frequently suspect a food allergy, but this is rarely found in chronic urticaria. Fluoroimmuno-assays have superseded radioallergosorbent tests (RAST) on blood and are safer than prick or oral challenge testing. Their judicious use may be useful in the investigation of some environmental allergens (latex, nuts, fruit, pollen and animal dander). However, cautious interpretation of the results is required, especially in the presence of a raised total IgE.
- A complement (C4) level can screen for acquired or hereditary complement deficiency in patients with angioedema without wheals who are not on angiotensin-converting enzyme (ACE) inhibitors or nonsteroidal anti-inflammatory drugs (NSAIDs).

Chronic urticaria is a frequent and distressing condition. An approach to its diagnosis and differentials is depicted in Fig. 14.8 based on the duration of wheals.

Treatment

If an inciting factor can be identified for urticaria, it should be treated or removed, though this is easier said than done!

An approach to treatment of urticaria is given in Fig. 14.9 and is largely based on the use of antihistamines.

Symptomatic benefit is usually achieved with H_1 antihistamines given on a regular, rather than an intermittent basis.

The nonsedating H_1 antihistamines are the first line of therapy for urticaria with little to choose between loratidine, cetirizine, fexofenadine, levocetirizine, and desloratadine. Multiple experts recommend gradually increasing the dose to up to 4 times the allergic rhinitis dose.

As multiple mediators such as prostaglandins, leukotrienes, and cytokines such as interleukin (IL)-8 or tumor necrosis factor (TNF) are also involved apart from the autoantibodies directed against IgE, antihistamines may have a modest effect in urticraia though most are controlled with combined H_1-H_2 antihistamines.

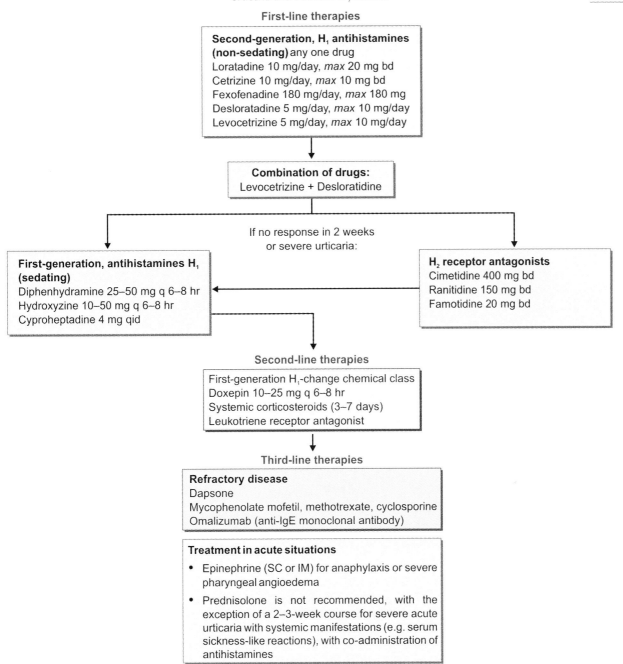

First-line therapies

Second-generation, H₁ antihistamines (non-sedating) any one drug
Loratadine 10 mg/day, *max* 20 mg bd
Cetrizine 10 mg/day, *max* 10 mg bd
Fexofenadine 180 mg/day, *max* 180 mg
Desloratadine 5 mg/day, *max* 10 mg/day
Levocetrizine 5 mg/day, *max* 10 mg/day

Combination of drugs:
Levocetrizine + Desloratidine

If no response in 2 weeks
or severe urticaria:

First-generation, antihistamines H₁ (sedating)
Diphenhydramine 25–50 mg q 6–8 hr
Hydroxyzine 10–50 mg q 6–8 hr
Cyproheptadine 4 mg qid

H₂ receptor antagonists
Cimetidine 400 mg bd
Ranitidine 150 mg bd
Famotidine 20 mg bd

Second-line therapies

First-generation H₁-change chemical class
Doxepin 10–25 mg q 6–8 hr
Systemic corticosteroids (3–7 days)
Leukotriene receptor antagonist

Third-line therapies

Refractory disease
Dapsone
Mycophenolate mofetil, methotrexate, cyclosporine
Omalizumab (anti-IgE monoclonal antibody)

Treatment in acute situations
- Epinephrine (SC or IM) for anaphylaxis or severe pharyngeal angioedema
- Prednisolone is not recommended, with the exception of a 2–3-week course for severe acute urticaria with systemic manifestations (e.g. serum sickness-like reactions), with co-administration of antihistamines

Fig. 14.9: Overview of a step-by-step treatment of urticaria

Addition of an H₂-blocker, leukotriene antagonist, or a sedating H₁-blocker such as hydroxyzine at night can sometimes be beneficial. The tricyclic antidepressant doxepin, in a dose of 25 mg once or twice daily, is also effective and has been shown to have both H₁ and H₂ antihistamine activity. The sedative effects of the older antihistamines (chlorphenamine, hydroxyzine, alimemazine and promethazine) may be especially helpful for relief of nocturnal symptoms.

Chlorphenamine and diphenhydramine are often used during **pregnancy** because of their long record of safety, but hydroxyzine, cetirizine, loratadine and mizolastine should be avoided.

Because only 5% of patients with urticaria will be symptomatic for more than 4 weeks, an effective antihistamine regimen should be continued for **4 to 6 weeks** after controlling symptoms and then gradually tapered off. However, over 50% of patients with chronic urticaria will be symptomatic for over a year, so these patients require long-term treatment.

Signs and symptoms of anaphylaxis or throat angioedema require emergent management with a combination of intramuscular epinephrine,[Q] securing of an airway, vasopressors, and intravenous corticosteroids.

The treatment of physical urticaria is detailed in Table 14.6.

Table 14.6	Treatment of physical urticaria
Cold urticaria	• Warn the patient about sudden exposure to cold (swimming, ice-cream/cold drinks, cold IV infusions); jumping into a cool pool or lake can be fatal. • Oral antibiotics for 3 weeks (penicillin V 500 mg qid or doxycycline 100 mg bid) has about a 40% cure rate. The mechanism is unclear. • Careful conditioning with cold baths or showers may help, but must be continued indefinitely. • Nonsedating antihistamines; sometimes higher dosages are needed
Solar urticaria	Protective clothing, sunscreens and sun blocks, beta-carotene, antihistamines
Cholinergic urticaria	• Avoid heat • Anticholinergics • An antihistamine with a strong cholinergic effect such as cetirizine should be used • Antihistamines
Dermographism	High dose antihistamine

HEREDITARY ANGIOEDEMA

Hereditary angioneurotic edema (HANE).

Types

Defect in C1-esterase inhibitor,[Q] leading to unchecked complement activation and recurrent subcutaneous and mucosal swelling.

Type I (85%): Reduced plasma C1-esterase levels (30% of normal).

Type II (10%): Normal levels of functionally defective inhibitor.

Type III (5%): Inhibitor inactivated by autoantibodies.

Excessive **bradykinin release**[Q] is the main cause of the angioedema, and it causes intense vasodilation[Q] leading to edema in dermis and subcutaneous tissue.

Clinical Features

Recurrent swelling primarily in face and extremities. No urticaria. Nonpruritic.[Q] Rarely, transient or slight erythema before attack. Laryngeal edema can be life-threatening; gastrointestinal wall swelling can be rare cause of acute abdomen.

Investigation

Measure C3, C4; C3 normal, C4 not identifiable;[Q] can be used to monitor treatment. Identify type of esterase defect in cooperation with immunology laboratory.

An approach to the diagnosis of angioedema is given in Fig. 14.10.

Therapy

Acute attack: C1-esterase inhibitor concentrate; if not available, 500–2000 mL fresh or fresh frozen plasma.[Q]

> Systemic corticosteroids, antihistamines, and norepinephrine have no effect.

Prophylaxis: Androgens[Q] (danazol 200–600 mg daily); adjust based on clinical findings and inhibitor levels.

ERYTHEMA MULTIFORME (EM)

It is defined as an acute self-limited inflammatory reaction with typical target or iris-like lesions. As its name suggests, the eruption is characterized clinically by a variety of lesions, including erythematous plaques, blisters, and 'target' lesions.[Q]

Affects young adults (20–40 years of age) with male dominance.

Pathogenesis

The vast bulk of recurrent cases are triggered by herpes simplex virus (HSV) infections.[Q] Immune complexes containing HSV DNA can be found in the lesions. Other triggers include mycoplasma food additives[Q] and only rarely drugs (Box 14.2).

Clinical Features

The classic lesion is a target/iris lesion[Q] (Fig. 14.11) found on the distal extremities.

The rings have three[Q] components (Fig. 14.12):
• Central dark hemorrhagic zone, which becomes blue-violet.
• Intermediate white/edematous area.
• Peripheral erythematous ring.

Classically, the lesions are 1–3 cm in diameter though rarely they may be bullous or urticarial (Fig. 14.13). The lesions heal spontaneously over weeks, sometimes with residual hyperpigmentation. The presence of a prodrome is often emphasized, but the prodrome is caused by the HSV, *Mycoplasma*, or underlying disease requiring drug therapy.

Characteristically, the distribution of the lesions favors the extremities and is strikingly symmetric when erythema multiforme is caused by an infection (Fig. 14.14); the distribution of lesions favors the trunk when caused by a drug.

Differentiating erythema multiforme minor from SJS/ TEN: While target lesions are the classic cutaneous finding, the very name 'erythema multiforme' implies a variable presentation.

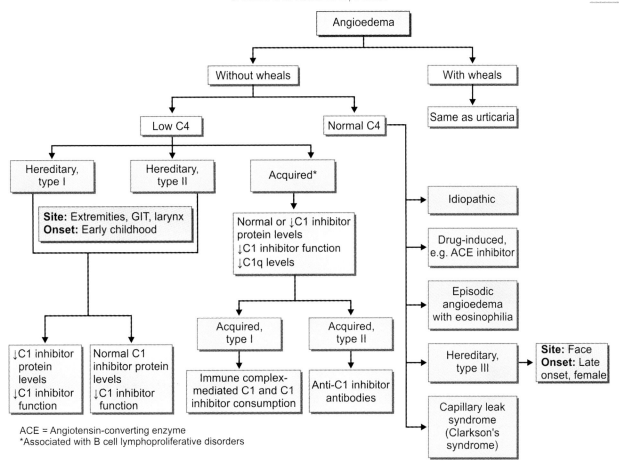

Fig. 14.10: Algorithm for the diagnosis of angioedema. Episodic angioedema with esionphilia as well as weight gain and fever is known as Gleich syndrome. Systemic capillary leak syndrome can lead to life-threatening hypotension and is associated with an IgG monoclonal gammopathy

Box 14.2	Causes of EM

Viral infections: Herpes simplex[Q], Hepatitis A, B and C, Mycoplasma, Orf*

Bacterial infections: *Borrelia burgdorferi, Chlamydia, Lymphogranuloma venereum, Mycobacterium avium, lepra* and *tuberculosis, Mycoplasma pneumoniae, Neisseria meningitidis, Pneumococcus, Proteus, Pseudomonas, Staphylococcus, Streptococcus, Treponema pallidum, Vibrio parahaemolyticus, Yersinia.*

Fungal infections: Coccidiomycosis, histoplasmosis, sporotrichosis, dermatophytes.

Parasitic infestations: Malaria, trichomonas, toxoplasmosis
• Drugs
• Pregnancy
• Malignancy, or its treatment with radiotherapy
• Idiopathic
• Food additives

Others include: Adenovirus, cytomegalovirus (CMV), enterovirus, Epstein-Barr virus, hepatitis, human immunodeficiency virus (HIV), HSV 1 and 2, influenza, molluscum, parvovirus, poliovirus.

A 'classic' target lesion is a round, well-defined pink to red patch/plaque with **three** concentric rings (Fig. 14.12). Commonly, though target lesions are often atypical 'targets' with two, rather than three zones, poorly defined borders, more extensive purpura, bullae, and appear more urticarial than targetoid.

• Classifying the target lesions may help establish the diagnosis, with 'classic' targets more common in EM and 'atypical' targets or targetoid more common in SJS/TEN.

• Oral mucous membrane involvement is common in EM, but is usually mild and limited to a few vesicles or erosions that may or may not be symptomatic. When more extensive mucous membrane involvement is seen, such as widespread vesicles, ulcers, and erosions in multiple sites (e.g. oral, ocular, genital, and perirectal), this is considered a more severe form of the disease (EM major).

• The important thing to note is that patients with classic herpes simplex related EM *rarely* have widespread, severe mucous membrane involvement, and in these patients, it is particularly rare to have ocular lesions.

• Mild pruritus and tenderness have been reported, severe pruritus might incline the clinician toward a diagnosis of urticaria and severe skin tenderness toward a diagnosis of SJS/TEN.

14

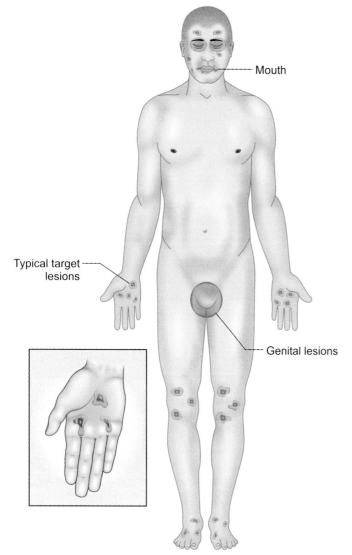

Fig. 14.11: A depiction of the classical sites of involvement of erythema multiforme minor

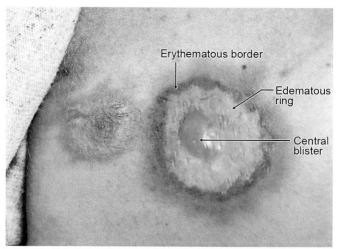

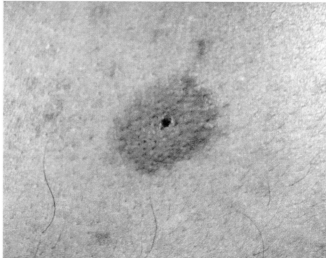

Fig. 14.12: A depiction of the classic zones of EM. Clinically though only two zones are seen

Investigation

The histology of erythema multiforme is distinctive and is characterized by epidermal necrosis and dermal changes, consisting of endothelial swelling, a mixed lymphohistiocytic perivascular infiltrate and papillary dermal edema. The abnormalities may be predominantly epidermal or dermal, or a combination of both.

- History helps rule out a drug reaction.
- A PCR test, Tzanck smear or culture of suspicious prodromal vesicles: HSV.
- Chest X-ray and serological tests: *Mycoplasma pneumoniae.*

A search for other infectious agents, neoplasia, endocrine causes or connective tissue disorder is sometimes necessary, especially when the course is prolonged or recurrent. About 50% of cases have no demonstrable provoking factor.

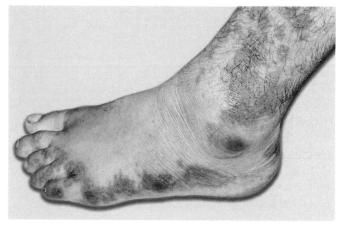

Fig. 14.13: Lesions of EM on the extremities with a central bulla

Therapy

Short course of systemic corticosteroids (prednisolone 60–80 mg for 3–5 days) dramatically shortens course. Topical corticosteroids are less helpful.

If recurrent,[Q] suppressive therapy with antiherpetic medications is most useful. A 6-month trial of

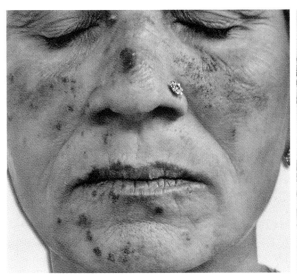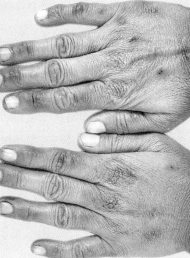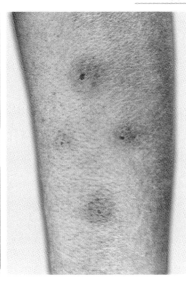

Fig. 14.14: A case with herpes labialis with EM on the face and extremities

continuous treatment with oral valaciclovir 500 mg once daily or famciclovir 250 mg twice daily may prevent attacks, both of herpes simplex and of the recurrent erythema multiforme that follows it.

Erythromycin, azithromycin, or clarithromycin is recommended for *Mycoplasma pneumoniae*.

FIGURATE ERYTHEMAS

There is a long list of diseases that all present with expanding annular or polycyclic erythematous and sometimes scaly lesions. They have no pathogenetic relationship, but instead a wide variety of causes.

Erythema Migrans

This is the most common figurate erythema in Europe, in India it has been reported occasionally and is discussed in Chapter 8.

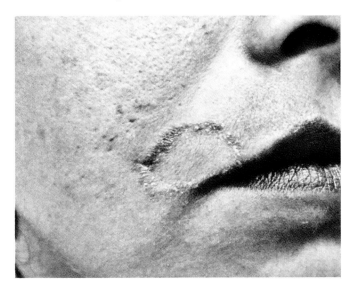

Fig. 14.15: EAC, note the central clearing and peripheral scaling which is on inner border of the trailing edge of the plaque

It is characterized by a slowly expanding erythematosus ring and is caused by *Borrelia burgdoferi*.[Q]

Erythema Annulare Centrifugum

Erythema annulare centrifugum (EAC) is characterized by annular red plaques that expand centrifugally (Fig. 14.15).

Etiology: Causes include infections, tumors, food allergies, and drugs.

There are two forms of the disease:

1. A superficial form with a trailing edge of white scale (Fig. 14.15). (Peripheral scale is found on the trailing edge of the lesion, pointing toward the pale center.)[Q]
2. A deep form with infiltrated borders and no scale.

The most common locations for involvement are the axillae, hips, and thighs. The lesions can be episodic and last for months.

Treatment: The cause remains unknown and treatment is often unsatisfactory. Some investigators believe the condition to be cutaneous response to a distant infection, most often tinea pedis. Azithromycin has been tried successfully.

Erythema Gyratum Repens

Erythema gyratum repens (EGR) most often represents a paraneoplastic figurate erythema. The most common cause of underlying neoplasms is from lung, breast, or esophagus.[Q] The rash can appear either before or after detection of the malignancy.

Clinical features: The rash is striking, characterized gyrate red plaques (Fig. 14.16) that can advance their edges by up to 1 cm per day.

The rash resembles the 'grain of wood'. The skin lesions resolve when the malignancy is treated.

14

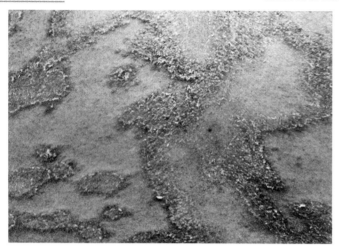

Fig. 14.16: Polycyclic plaque in a case of erythema gyratum repens

Necrolytic Migratory Erythema

This is a paraneoplastic marker, with acral and genital erythematous plaques and erosions with fine scaling. It is associated with glucagonoma.[Q]

Other Gyrate Erythema

- Annular lupus erythematosus and Rowell syndrome (EM-like lupus erythematosus)[Q]
- Annular psoriasis
- Erythema marginatum (rheumatic fever)[Q]

NODOSE ERYTHEMAS

These lesions present as red-brown plaques or nodules. The most common is erythema nodosum, which will be discussed in the next chapter. Another is granuloma faciale, which is rich in eosinophils and has a Grenz zone.[Q] A few other are being discussed below.

Sweet Syndrome[Q]

Also known as acute febrile neutrophilic dermatoses.
- The patients present with fever, elevated erythrocyte sedimentation rate (ESR) and pseudopustular erythematous nodules. Often the trigger is unknown but infections, underlying myeloid leukemia, and drug reactions have been implicated.
- Histology shows an extensive neutrophilic infiltrate with marked edema and sometimes vasculitis.
- The drug of choice is systemic corticosteroids.[Q]

Erythema Elevatum Diutinum[Q]

This is a form of chronic vasculitis, sometimes associated with hematological disorders or HIV. Presents with red-brown nodules on extensor surfaces, especially over joints of hands.

Histopathology shows marked perivascular fibrosis and little active inflammation. Some patients respond to dapsone.

14

Panniculitis and Erythema Nodosum

Panniculitis is an inflammation of the subcutaneous fat, which is conventionally classified into two types—septal and lobular depending on the site of the inflammation within the adipose tissue (Fig. 15.1).

CLASSIFICATION

There are many different ways to classify panniculitis:
1. In order of frequency:
   - Erythema nodosum is the commonest.[Q]
2. Clinically (site):
   - On the shin:[Q] Usually erythema nodosum.
   - On calf, above knee, or not on legs: Consider other possibilities (Fig. 15.2)
3. Histologically (Fig. 15.1):
   - Septal versus lobular
   - With or without vasculitis

A working classification is shown in Table 15.1.

ERYTHEMA NODOSUM

Self-limited **septal** panniculitis with sudden onset of red-brown, bruise-like patches and nodules on shins; usually reactive.

Female: Male ratio 3–5:1.

Etiology

Erythema nodosum has many causes[Q] (Fig. 15.3 and Table 15.2), although in some cases a causal relationship is not clearly established. It is commonly viewed as a type IV delayed hypersensitivity reaction[Q] to various causes (Table 15.2). The absence of prospective studies and the scarcity of large published series, in addition to epidemiological differences according to geographical location, preclude any estimation of the true frequency of the different etiologies, though streptococcal infections and TB are the most common causes worldwide.[Q]

Clinical Features

Prodrome: Fever, chills, perhaps joint pain; varies with trigger.

Skin findings: Usually multiple, bilateral bruise-like tender or painful nodules and plaques covered by a smooth epidermis (Fig. 15.4). Almost always on shin;[Q] rarely thighs, arms, but an occur anywhere there is subcutaneous fat. May be associated with continuing fever, malaise, or arthritis.

> Erythema nodosum never ulcerates.[Q] If a lesion is ulcerated, look for a different diagnosis.

Course: Individual lesions resolve over 2 weeks with new 'crops' appearing for up to 6–8 weeks, if the cause is not removed the condition may persist.

Diagnosis

The etiological workup should be guided by the history, the clinical findings and epidemiological data. A comprehensive history comprises:
- Previous infections, systemic diseases, inflammatory enteropathies, pregnancy;
- Clinical signs: Chronic fever, weight loss, and diarrhea;
- Drugs (oral contraceptives, nonsteroidal anti-inflammatory drugs, antibiotics) and vaccinations.

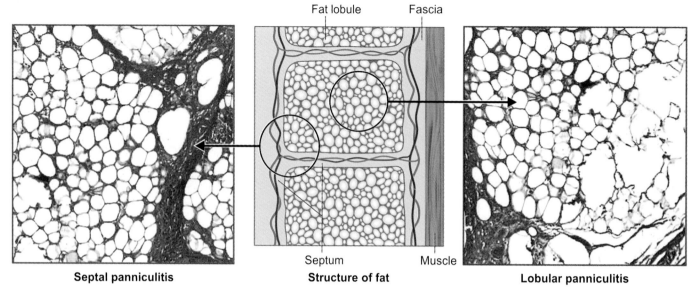

Septal panniculitis   **Structure of fat**   **Lobular panniculitis**

Fig. 15.1: A histological depiction of the two kinds of panniculitis depending on the localization of infiltrate

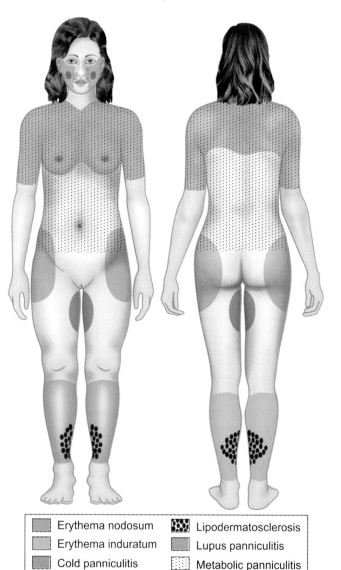

Erythema nodosum	Lipodermatosclerosis
Erythema induratum	Lupus panniculitis
Cold panniculitis	Metabolic panniculitis

Fig. 15.2: Depiction of the localization of the various types of panniculitis

Table 15.1	Classification of panniculitis	
Septal	Without vasculitis[Q]	• Erythema nodosum[Q] • Connective tissue panniculitis
	With vasculitis	• Superficial thrombophlebitis • Polyarteritis nodosa
Lobular	Without vasculitis	• Pancreatic • Lymphoma • Traumatic (cold, injections,[Q] injuries) • Neonatal fat necrosis[Q] • α_1-antitrypsin deficiency • Infectious • Lipoatrophic panniculitis (Rothmann-Makai lipogranu-lomatosis, other variants) • Lupus erythematosus (lupus profundus)[Q] • Sarcoidosis • Weber-Christian disease (idiopathic)
	With vasculitis	Erythema induratum/nodular vasculitis Erythema nodosum leprosum (ENL)

In erythema nodosum precipitated by streptococcal infection, the nodules occur within 3 weeks of pharyngitis. Fever and lower respiratory symptoms may be elicited from patients with pulmonary infections caused by deep fungi or tuberculosis. A history of abdominal pain and diarrhea suggests an inflammatory bowel disorder. Ulcerative colitis is the most common inflammatory bowel disease associated with erythema nodosum. A complete drug history should be elicited, although, with the exception of birth control pills, drugs are uncommon causes. Most cases are of unknown cause and labeled 'idiopathic.'[Q]

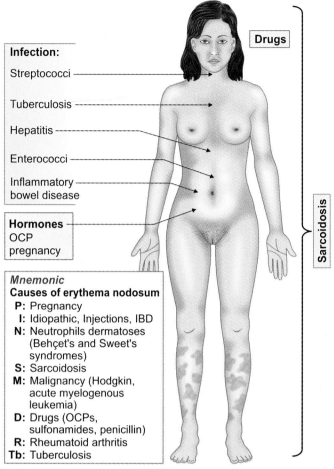

Infection:

Streptococci

Tuberculosis

Hepatitis

Enterococci

Inflammatory bowel disease

Hormones
OCP
pregnancy

Drugs

Sarcoidosis

Mnemonic
Causes of erythema nodosum
 P: Pregnancy
 I: Idiopathic, Injections, IBD
 N: Neutrophils dermatoses (Behçet's and Sweet's syndromes)
 S: Sarcoidosis
 M: Malignancy (Hodgkin, acute myelogenous leukemia)
 D: Drugs (OCPs, sulfonamides, penicillin)
 R: Rheumatoid arthritis
Tb: Tuberculosis

Fig. 15.3: Major causes of erythema nodosum and the sites of primary etiology

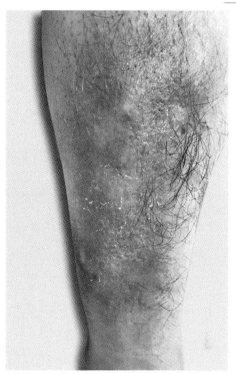

Fig. 15.4: Multiple subcutaneous nodules on the skin with a distinct color variation resembling a bruise that represents the activity of erythema nodosum

A complete *physical examination* should be done.

An investigative protocol is given below but the aim being to rule out other causes of panniculitis as listed in Table 15.2.

Investigation

Table 15.3 describes investigation for erythema nodosum.

Treatment

General Treatment

- *Bed rest* for two weeks is crucial. Hospitalization is not essential, but it is recommended, if the patient is unlikely to adhere to bed rest at home.

Table 15.2	An overview of the common causes of erythema nodosum

Infections	• Bacterial
	  – Streptococcal infections especially of the upper respiratory tract[Q]
	  – Tuberculosis of lung[Q]
	  – Bacterial gastroenteritis: *Yersinia* > *Salmonella, Campylobacter*
	  – Leprosy
	• Viruses (e.g. hepatitis B, Epstein-Barr virus, URTI)
	  – *Mycoplasma*
	  – *Rickettsia*
	  – *Chlamydia*
	  – Fungi (especially coccidioidomycosis—common in USA)

Drugs	Sulfonamides, penicillins, oral contraceptive agents, immunotherapy agents
Systemic disease	Sarcoidosis*, ulcerative colitis, Crohn's disease, Behçet's disease
Pregnancy	—
Malignancy	Hodgkin lymphoma, other lymphomas, leukemias, and following radiation therapy.

*Lofgren's syndrome is an acute, spontaneously resolving form of sarcoidosis characterized by erythema nodosum, fever, hilar lymphadenopathy, polyarthritis, and uveitis.[Q]

Table 15.3	Investigation for erythema nodosum
Basic work-up	Complete blood count, erythrocyte sedimentation rate, C-reactive protein and transaminase levels
Intensive work-up	• Chest X-ray • Tuberculin skin test or IGRA • Viral hepatitis panel • Anti-streptolysin O and/or anti-DNAse B titers • If diarrhea, check fecal WBC and stool culture for bacteria, ova and parasites. Stool for occult blood • Malignancy workup as indicated by history and physical exam

- During the painful phase of the disease, *analgesics* can be prescribed:
  - Paracetamol, 1 to 3 g/24 hr, allowing at least four hours between doses;
  - Acetylsalicylic acid, 2 to 4 g/24 hr for one to two weeks.
- *Nonsteroidal anti-inflammatory* drugs are reserved for more severe pain:
  - Indomethacin. The dosage is 50 to 150 mg/24 hr in divided doses;
  - Naproxen. The dosage is 250 mg bid with food.

    The analgesic, anti-inflammatory and antipyretic effects are related to inhibition of prostaglandin synthetase in subcutaneous fat tissue.

    NSAIDs provide rapid relief of local inflammation; they are prescribed for an average of 10 days.
- *Potassium iodide* (100 mg capsules or as SSKI) at a dose of 300 mg/day for one to two weeks is effective but there is a risk of hyperthyroidism associated with prolonged use.
- *Systemic corticosteroids* are only justified in severe cases, at doses of 0.5 to 1 mg/kg/day, after ruling out active infection and neoplastic disease.

Specific Treatment

Specific treatment of various causes is useful, including antibiotics for streptococcal and *Yersinia* infections and ATT for TB.

Despite a thorough workup, the cause of erythema nodosum cannot be determined in 15 to 40% of cases. Treatment in these cases is symptomatic and includes analgesics, NSAIDs, colchicine, hydroxychloroquine or potassium iodide.

OTHER PANNICULITIS

Lipodermatosclerosis

Typically seen in middle-aged to older individuals with chronic venous disorders (CVD).

Acute

- Painful, warm, red-purple, poorly defined plaques with variable induration.
- Favors the lower extremities, usually initially involves the skin above the medial malleolus (Figs 15.2 and 15.5).
- Sometimes involves lower abdominal pannus.

Chronic

Induration and hyperpigmentation of the lower legs with an 'inverted champagne bottle' appearance[Q] (Fig. 15.6).

Erythema Induratum

Most common cause is TB,[Q] though other systemic infections and disorders may also cause this presentation.

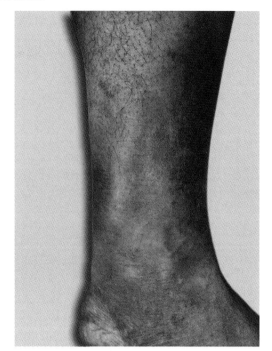

Fig. 15.5: Linear subcutaneous swelling of acute lipodermatosclerosis over the medial malleolus

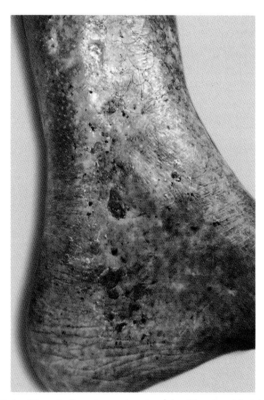

Fig. 15.6: Chronic lipodermatosclerosis with atrophie blanche

Seen more in females >> males; young to middle-aged.

Clinical features: Tender, inflamed nodules or plaques on posterior lower legs. They classically ulcerate and heal with a scar[Q] (Figs 15.2 and 15.7).

Histopathology: Neutrophilic vasculitis.

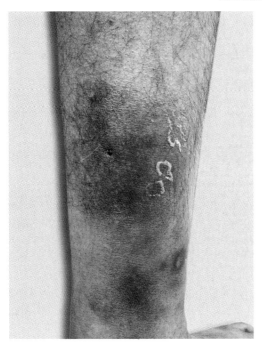

Fig. 15.7: Subcutaneous nodules which ulcerate and are seen in the posterior lower limbs (erythema induratum)

Chest X-ray and tuberculin skin test or IGRA can help to diagnose.

Metabolic Panniculitis

Lesions typically above the knees or even on the trunk. Oily liquid may drain spontaneously or on biopsy.

Pancreatic panniculitis: This occasionally may be the initial presentation of pancreatic disease (pancreatitis > cancer) or develop during its course.

Site: Usually favors lower legs but also arms, chest, and abdomen.

May become fluctuant, ulcerate, and drain an oily substance. Eosinophilia and polyarthritis are associated findings.

α_1-**antitrypsin deficiency panniculitis:** The clinical presentation is of painful red or purpuric nodules or plaques favoring the lower trunk or proximal extremities. May spontaneously ulcerate and drain an oily material.

Histopathology—liquefactive necrosis of dermis and SC septa.

Connective Tissue Panniculitis

Lupus profundus is the most classical form. It is also seen with dermatomyositis, systemic sclerosis, and rheumatoid arthritis.

Clinical Features

- Painful SC nodules or plaques in a characteristic pattern-on the face, shoulders, upper arms, breasts, hips, and buttocks (Figs 15.2 and 15.8). Notably spares the lower extremities.
- Overlying skin may be normal, depressed, bound down, or have changes of DLE ('lupus profundus')
- Can be associated with discoid LE (DLE) in at least one-third of cases.

Traumatic Panniculitis

Both physical trauma and cold may damage fat causing inflammation (Fig. 15.2).

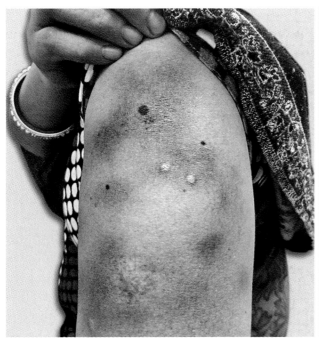

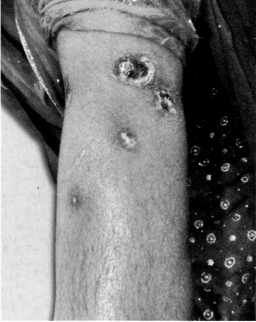

Fig. 15.8: Lupus panniculitis on the upper limb

15

- *Cold panniculitis* is often seen on hips and medial thigh of female equestrians due to riding in cold temperature with an added cause of tight clothes in that area. Also seen in cheeks of infants and children due to popsicles or ice cubes.
- *Artefactual panniculitis*: Fat is a favorite site for injection of foreign substances (urine, feces), illicit drugs, and other foreign substances.

Newborn

Subcutaneous Fat Necrosis[Q]

- Seen in full-term, usually healthy neonates
- Onset during the first 2–3 weeks of life
- Mobile, firm SC nodules or plaques, favoring the cheeks, shoulders, back, buttocks, and thighs
- Needle-shaped clefts on histopathology.

Sclerema Neonatorum

- Seen in premature, extremely ill neonates
- Onset during the first week of life
- Diffusely cold, rigid, board-like skin
- Needle-shaped clefts on histopathology.

Post-steroid Panniculitis

Onset usually within 10 days after the rapid withdrawal of systemic steroids. Firm red plaques on the cheeks, arms, and trunk. Needle-shaped clefts on histopathology.

15

CHAPTER 16

Adverse Drug Reactions

Chapter Outline

INTRODUCTION

It is often said that the phrase 'First do no harm' (Latin: Primum non nocere) is a part of the Hippocratic oath. Though the phrase does not appear in the oath its a good take on drug eruptions, which are never intentional and are difficult to predict for the first time in most patients. Drug eruptions can appear similar to many inflammatory skin diseases. Some cardinal features of a drug eruption are:

- Symmetric rash
- Sudden onset
- Itchy
- Self-limiting, if drug is discontinued.

CLASSIFICATION

Drug reactions can be classified in many ways. One useful approach is to separate predictable reactions occurring in normal patients from unpredictable reactions occurring in susceptible patients.

Predictable Adverse Reactions

- Overdosage (wrong dosage or defect in drug meta-bolism).
- Side effects (sleepiness from antihistamines).
- Indirect effects (antibiotics change normal flora).
- Drug interactions (alter metabolism of drugs; most commonly the cytochrome P-450 system).

Unpredictable Adverse Reactions

- Intolerance (normal side effect occurs at low dose).
- Allergic reaction (drug allergy or hypersensitivity; immunologic reaction to drug; requires previous exposure or cross-reaction).
- Pseudoallergic reaction (nonimmunologic activation of mast cells).
- Idiosyncratic reaction (unexplained reaction, not related to mechanism of action, without known or suspected immunologic mechanism).

PATHOGENESIS

In some instances, a drug reaction can be clearly assigned to an immunologic reaction type, although more often the mechanisms are not understood.

Pseudoallergic reactions (analgesics, contrast media, local anesthetics) are also common.

Type I: Urticaria, angioedema, anaphylaxis.

Type II: Thrombocytopenic purpura.

Type III: Leukocytoclastic vasculitis, serum sickness.

Type IV: Allergic contact dermatitis, some exanthems, photoallergic reactions.

The majority^Q of allergic drug reactions are caused by **type IV** cell-mediated immune reactions, which can present in a number of forms, most commonly a maculopapular eruption or morbilliform erythema. **Helper CD4+ T cells** occur more frequently in the more common morbilliform eruptions, while cytotoxic **CD8+ T** cells predominate in blistering eruptions (TEN, Stevens-Johnson syndrome) and fixed drug eruptions. *CD4—Morbilliform; CD8—Blistering, FDE.*

16

TYPES

The most common types of drug reactions are macular[Q] and maculopapular exanthems (40%), followed by urticaria and angioedema (37%).[Q] Fixed drug eruption (6%) and erythema multiforme/toxic epidermal necrolysis (5%) are the other frequently seen patterns. In *India* though *fixed drug eruption* is the commonest rash.[Q]

Most common causative drugs are:[Q]

1. *Antibiotics*:
   - β-lactam antibiotics—penicillins, cephalosporins
   - Sulfonamides—trimethoprim-sulfamethoxazole (be aware of cross-reactivity with sulfonamide derivatives, especially with the following drug classes: *diuretics*, *hypoglycemic*, and *anti-inflammatories*)
2. *Diuretics*:
   - Furosemide (contains a sulfonamide)
   - Hydrochlorothiazide (contains a sulfonamide)
3. *Nonsteroidal anti-inflammatory drugs* (NSAIDs)
4. *Antiepileptics*

CLINICAL FEATURES

Almost every drug can cause almost every type of reaction. Clinically, one must learn which reactions are most likely to produce certain findings. The various drug reactions are covered below in detail.

HISTORY

There are many methods of diagnosis of drug reactions including allergy testing and withdrawal of drugs but the most important step remains a proper history.

- The history is the most essential tool in diagnosing a drug reaction. Any exanthem in a hospitalized adult should be suspected of being a drug reaction. For patients coming in the OPD, ask about over-the-counter medications (laxatives, sleeping pills, herbal medications, ayurvedic medications, dyes, preserved foods).
- Determine the correct time course. If a patient is exposed to a medication for the first time, an allergic reaction cannot occur within the first 4–8 days. Reexposure, cross-reactions, or pseudoallergic reactions all occur more rapidly, sometimes almost instantaneously (anaphylaxis).

> In case of a drug-induced morbilliform eruption, skin rash can be delayed for as long as 1 week, but seldom longer.

- Does the patient have a known contact allergy to paracompounds? This could explain a reaction to sulfonamides, oral hypoglycemic agents, thiazide diuretics, local anesthetics of the ester-caine type.

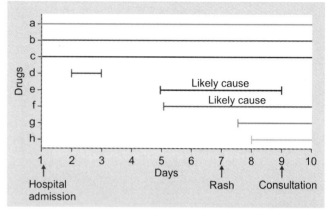

Fig. 16.1: A depiction of probable drug causes in relation to the *rash*

Similarly, ethylene diamine sensitivity can explain sensitivity to theophylline and related products.

- How was the drug administered? The likelihood of sensitization is topical >oral >intramuscular >intravenous. The best example is previous use of topical antihistamines sensitizing patient to oral agents.
- Does the patient have concurrent illnesses? HIV/AIDS predisposes to sulfamethoxazole/trimethoprim reactions, while infectious mononucleosis is associated with a high incidence of reactions to ampicillin.[Q]

A frequent problem encountered is when a patient is on multiple drugs. Two principles are useful to determine the likely cause:

1. New (started within 1 week of the rash)
2. Frequent offenders

In the example in Fig. 16.1, the *first step* is to list out the various drugs the patient has been given. The *second step* is to note the onset of each drug

- Here the drug 'a', 'b', and 'c' are unlikely to be the cause as the patient had been receiving these agents for months.
- Drug 'd' was stopped 4 days before the rash began, thus making it a less likely cause.
- Drug 'g' was started 6 hours after the rash appeared, and drug 'h' was started the following day.
- Drugs 'e' and 'f' were started 2 days before the rash and, therefore, have the best temporal relationship.

Drug 'e' is ampicillin, a well-known cause of rash, and drug 'f' is cetirizine, a rare cause of morbilliform eruptions. Therefore, drug 'e' is the likely cause of the rash.

COMMON REACTION PATTERNS

A simple classification is to divide the reactions into three types:

- Severe skin reactions

- Classic drug reactions
- Unique drug reactions

This is as it is important to differentiate a mild reaction from a severe one at the outset.

Severe Skin Reactions

Stevens-Johnson Syndrome and Toxic Epidermal Necrolysis

In most instances of severe skin reaction (SSR), skin findings are a clue to severe systemic ADR. But in rare instances, the cutaneous drug reaction is itself life-threatening.

Pathogenesis: Altered drug metabolism is the most likely explanation; a small number of drugs cause most SSRs. The reactions are probably type II or type IV immune reactions to the medication or its metabolites. It is very likely that the underlying diseases modify the metabolism of the drugs or alter the immune reaction to foreign substances.

The various causes are given in Table 16.1.

Clinical features: SSRs usually start with an erythema multiforme (EM)-like reaction, but then show increasing skin and mucosal involvement. A classification is given in Fig. 16.2.

Stevens-Johnson syndrome (SJS) refers to patients with prominent mucosal involvement, while toxic epidermal necrolysis (TEN) describes those with widespread loss of skin resembling a burn patient. An overview of the clinical features of EM, SJS, TEN is given in Table 16.2 and representative images are given in Figs 16.3 and 16.4A.

Of special importance for diagnosis is:

1. The target lesions in EM-like drug reactions are usually atypical, without classic rings, and favor the trunk.

Reaction	Trigger	Clinical features	% of skin surface affected	Mortality
Erythema multiforme	Herpes simplex	Classic, acral	<1%	0%
Erythema multiforme-like	Medications	Atypical, trunk, mucosa	<10%	1%
Stevens-Johnson syndrome	Medications (occasionally *Mycoplasma*)	Atypical, trunk, mucosa	<10%	6%
SJS/TEN	Medications	Atypical, trunk, mucosa	10–30%	25%
TEN	Medications	Atypical, trunk, mucosa	>30%	40%

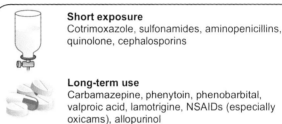

Short exposure
Cotrimoxazole, sulfonamides, aminopenicillins, quinolone, cephalosporins

Long-term use
Carbamazepine, phenytoin, phenobarbital, valproic acid, lamotrigine, NSAIDs (especially oxicams), allopurinol

Fig. 16.2: An overview of EM, SJS and TEN and the drugs causing SJS-TEN

2. Almost 90% of patients with SSR have mucosal involvement—oral, ocular, or genital.
3. The difference between SJS and TEN depends on the area of involvement with SJS (<10% of body area involved), SJS-TEN overlap (10–30% involvement) and TEN (>30% involvement)[Q] (Fig. 16.4B to D).

Differential diagnosis: Although drugs are implicated as cause in the majority of patients (80–85% cases),

Table 16.1	Causes of Stevens-Johnson syndrome and toxic epidermal necrolysis
Drugs Most common cause: The drugs causing it have been initiated <1 month and not more than 2 months after initiation.	• Antibiotics (**P**enicillins, **C**ephalosporins, **Q**uinolones, **S**ulfonamides) **PCQS**[Q] • Anticonvulsants (**P**henobarbital, **C**arbamazepine, **L**amotrigine) **PCL**[Q] • Allopurinol (most common cause in Europe and Israel) • Nonsteroidal anti-inflammatory drugs (NSAIDs, especially **oxicam**[Q] derivatives), nevirapine, abacavir, chlormezanone • Acetaminophen in children
Infections (Less common and generally believed to be more common in children)	• Bacterial:[Q] *Mycoplasma pneumoniae* (most common); less common: Yersinia, tuberculosis, syphilis, chlamydia, streptococci, Salmonella, Enterobacter, Pneumococcus • Fungal: Coccidiomycosis, histoplasmosis • Viral: Enterovirus, adenovirus, measles, mumps, influenza
Rare	• Immunizations: Smallpox, measles, diphtheria-pertussis-tetanus (DPT), Bacillus Calmette-Guérin (BCG), measles-mumps-rubella (MMR) • Acute LE, graft versus host disease, chemical or fumigant exposure (exposure to chlorotetraethylene), radiation therapy, inflammatory bowel disease

Table 16.2 A comparison of the features of EM, SJS, TEN

	EM	Stevens-Johnson syndrome	Toxic epidermal necrolysis
Etiology	HSV infection	Drugs Uncommon: *M. penumoniae*, viruses, immunization	
Systemic features	Usually none	• Fever, malaise, rash • Aphthous ulcers	• Same as SJS • Pulmonary symtoms
Morphology	*Targetoid (3 zones):* • Raised • Symmetric • Acral extremities	*Atypical targets (2 zones):* • Flat • Starts on trunk and palms and soles	• Papules, plaques, bulla • Desquamation >30% BSA • Painful • Positive Nikolsky sign[Q]
Mucosa	Few or none	• Oral • Conjunctivitis • Hemorrhagic crusts	Always Multiple mucosae Conjunctival edema

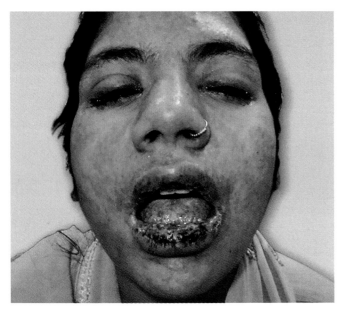

Fig. 16.3: Morbilliform rash with oral mucosa, eye and lip involvement in a visibly distressed patient—SJS

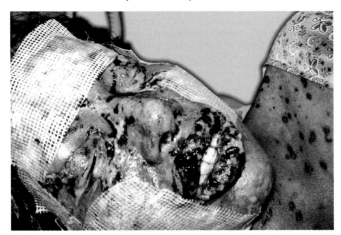

Fig. 16.4A: Extensive erosions, atypical target lesions, crusting of lip, SJS progressing to TEN

rarely other causes may elicit a similar clinical picture. Staphylococcal scalded skin syndrome (SSSS) is similar, but there is only loss of stratum corneum.

In transplantation patients, graft versus host disease and radiation dermatitis, or their combination, are impossible to separate.

Therapy: Problems include temperature control, fluid loss, and susceptibility to infection.

While IVIG has been tried in the west cyclosporine in the dose of 3–5 mg/kg/day for 7–10 days is also very useful in inducing reepithelization.

Systemic steroids in moderate to high doses (prednisolone equivalent in 1–2 mg/kg/d dose) for a period of 7–10 days, if instituted within first 72 hours is also effective.

DRESS

Various terms have been used for this reaction including, drug reaction with eosinophilia and systemic symptoms; drug rash with eosinophilia and systemic symptoms; drug-induced hypersensitivity syndrome; and drug-induced delayed onset multi-organ hypersensitivity syndrome (DIDMOHS).

When to suspect DRESS: The diagnosis of DRESS is suspected in a patient who received a new drug treatment in the previous two to six weeks and presents with the signs and symptoms given in Box 16.1.

The laboratory abnormalities include:
• Peripheral *eosinophilia* >700/μL or >10%
• *Lymphocytosis* (absolute lymphocyte count >4500/μL) and/or the finding of atypical lymphocytes
• Hepatitis
• If possible, test for Epstein-Barr virus (EBV), cytomegalovirus, human herpesvirus (HHV)-6, or HHV-7, as viral reactivation is suspected to be a marker of prolonged course and increased risk of complications.

Causative drugs are listed in Box 16.2.

As clinically DRESS may mimic SJS, it is important to differentiate the two and this is given in Table 16.3 and a representative image is given in Fig. 16.5.

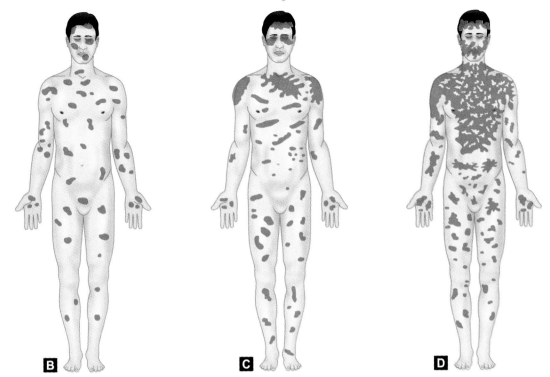

Fig. 16.4B to D: A depiction of SJS and TEN. The involvement of the area of skin determines the diagnosis: (B) <10% BSA SJS; (C) 10–30% BSA: Overlap of SJS/TEN; (D) >30% BSA: TEN

Box 16.1	Cardinal clinical features of DRESS

- Skin eruption (morbilliform or diffuse, confluent, and infiltrated) (2–6 weeks after drug)^Q
- Fever (38° to 40°C [100.4 to 104°F])
- Facial edema
- Enlarged lymph nodes^Q
- Internal organ involvement (hepatitis, pneumonitis, nephritis and hematological abnormalities).^{Q}

Box 16.2	Common agents implicated in causing DRESS

- Allopurinol
- Carbamazepine
- Dapsone
- Lamotrigine
- Minocycline
- Phenytoin^Q
- Sulfamethoxazole
- Sulfasalazine
- Vancomycin

Classic Drug Reactions

Maculopapular Exanthem

Most common reaction.^{Q} Classic 'rash' with erythematous macules, papules, and pruritus (Fig. 16.6). Biopsy often shows eosinophils.

Causative agents: Box 16.3.

Fixed Drug Eruption

A fixed drug eruption is a distinctive recurring reaction characterized acutely by erythematous and edematous plaques with a grayish center or frank bullae, and chronically by a dark postinflammatory pigmentation^Q (Figs 16.6 and 16.7).

Site: The glans penis seems to be a favoured site.^{Q} Other sites are the mouth^Q (lips and tongue), genitalia, face, and acral areas.

Table 16.3	Salient differences between DRESS and SJS	
	SJS/TEN	*DRESS*
Onset after drug use	SJS/TEN usually starts **4 to 28 days** after drug exposure	**2–6 weeks** after drug exposure
Mucosal involvement	At least **two** sites occur in over 90%	Mucosal affection is **mild**, limited to crusting of lips
Laboratory	**Leukopenia** is frequent and **lymphopenia**	**Eosinophilia** and atypical **lymphocytosis**
Liver	Mild elevation of liver enzymes Definite hepatitis <10%	**50%** have **hepatitis**
Kidney	Prerenal azotemia	Tubulointerstitial nephritis
Lung lesions	Necrosis of epithelial cells	Interstitial and alveolar infiltration

16

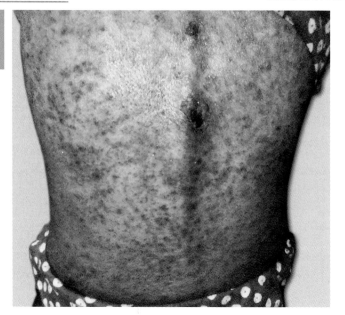
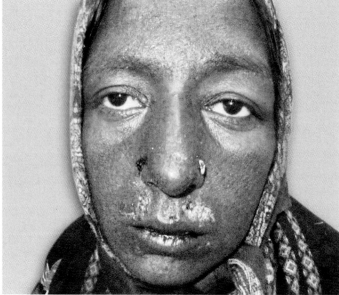

Fig. 16.5: Morbilliform rash on the trunk, facial edema with perioral swelling and crusting: DRESS

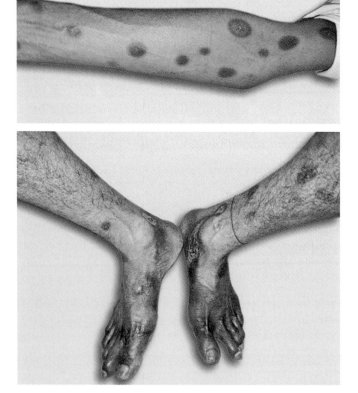

Fig. 16.6: Fixed drug eruption, note the marked post-inflammatory pigmentation

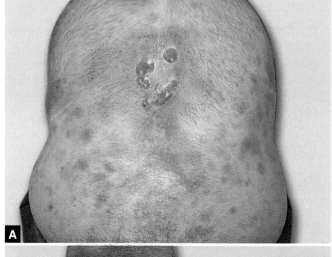

A

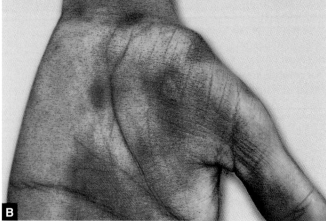

B

Fig. 16.7A and B: Bullous fixed drug eruption; (A) generalized on the trunk; and (B) localized on the palms

Box 16.3	Common causes of FDE
• Penicillin	• Benzodiazepines
• Ampicillin	• Carbamazepine
• Amoxicillin	• Cotrimaxazole
• Allopurinol	• Phenytoin
• Barbiturates	• Piroxicam

Patients with generalized bullous fixed drug eruption (GBFDE) (Fig. 16.7) can be misdiagnosed as having SJS/TEN, but in GBFDE, mucosal involvement is usually

Box 16.4 | **Common causes of drug-induced urticaria**

- Ampicillin
- Aspirin
- Barbiturates
- Dapsone
- Metronidazole
- NSAIDs
- ACE inhibitors
- Oral contraceptives
- Phenolphthalein
- Phenytoin
- Quinine
- Sulfonamides
- Tetracyclines

absent or mild and the clinical course is favorable with rapid resolution in 7 to 14 days after drug discontinuation. In India, quinolones-imidazoles have been noted to cause FDE most frequently.

Causative agents: Box 16.4.

Urticaria and Angioedema

Many drugs may cause this but salicylates[Q] are the most common, followed by angiotensin-converting enzyme (ACE) inhibitors. There are two main mechanisms of its causation:[Q]

- IgE-mediated (type I hypersensitivity) drug reaction, in which antibiotics (especially penicillins, cephalosporins, and sulfonamides) are implicated.

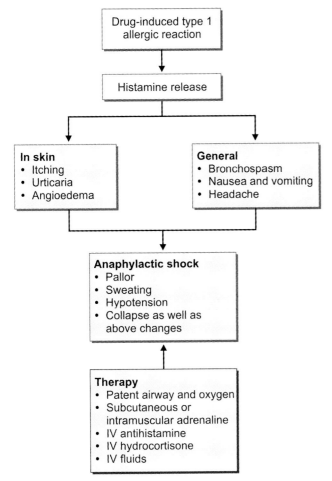

Fig. 16.8: Approach to management of anaphylaxis

- Non-IgE-mediated mechanism. Non-steroidal anti-inflammatory drugs (NSAIDs) and opiates which often work non-immunologically as histamine releasers.[Q]

Causative agents: Penicillin and related antibiotics, sulfonamides, aspirin, captopril, NSAIDs, insulin, contrast media. Angiotensin-converting enzyme (ACE) inhibitors are a common cause of angioedema;[Q] some tyrosine kinase inhibitors are also implicated.

Urticaria may be part of a severe and generalized reaction (anaphylaxis) which includes bronchospasm and collapse and in such cases adrenaline is the ideal treatment for anaphylaxis (Fig. 16.8).[Q]

Unique Drug Reactions

Acneiform and Rosacea-like Lesions

Follicular papulopustular eruption different from acne because of sudden onset (Fig. 16.9A and B).

Causative agents: ATT,[Q] oral contraceptives, androgens, corticosteroids,[Q] oral contraceptives (especially progesterone dominant),[Q] ciclosporin halogens (lithium, iodides,[Q] bromides). Epidermal growth factor inhibitors cause rosacea-like eruption.

Acute Generalized Exanthematous Pustulosis (AGEP)

Small nonfollicular pustules on an erythematous background appear within 24 hours, sometimes with fever and neutrophilia (Fig. 16.10).

Causative agents: Penicillin and macrolide antibiotics, terbinafine, hydroxychloroquine and diltiazem.

Allergic Contact Dermatitis

Patients are sensitized to a drug topically and then react severely when exposed systemically. Called baboon syndrome when severe and prominent in the genital region.

Causative agents: Antihistamines, benzocaine, neomycin, penicillin, and sulfonamides.

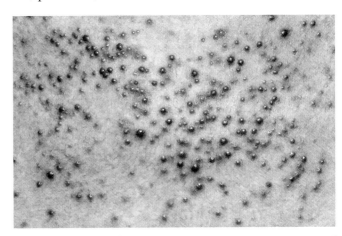

Fig. 16.9A: Acneiform eruption in a patient on androgens and whey protein

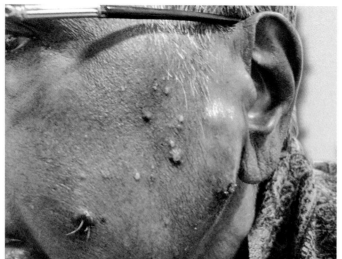
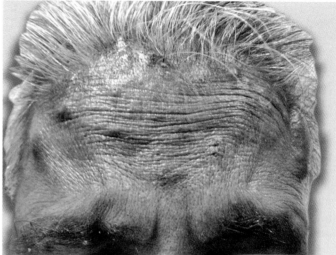

Fig. 16.9B: Gefitinib-induced acneiform eruption

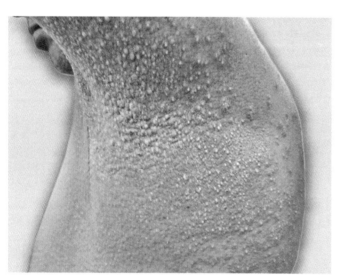

Fig. 16.10: Multiple pustules on an erythematous background in a case of AGEP

Acral Chemotherapy Reactions

Acral erythema (also called hand-foot syndrome[Q] or palmar-plantar erythrodysesthesia) occurs most often in patients with cancer treated with cytosine arabinoside, doxorubicin, capecitabine[Q] (an oral 5-fluorouracil derivative), or docetaxel.

The small molecule tyrosine kinase inhibitors sunitinib and sorafenib and others that target angiogenesis are also associated with a high incidence of hand-foot skin reaction,[Q] but the clinical and histologic patterns differ from the classic acral erythema caused by conventional cytotoxic agents.

In both types of acral reactions, dysesthesia of the involved areas (e.g. paresthesia, tingling, burning, painful sensation) precedes the development of the skin lesions.

- *Acral erythema* is most often characterized by a symmetric edema and erythema of the palms and soles, which may progress to blistering and necrosis
- *Hand-foot skin reaction* is characterized by well demarcated, bean to coin sized, hyperkeratotic, painful plaques with underlying erythema localized to the pressure areas of the soles.

Bullous Reactions

Rarely, drugs may trigger autoimmune bullous diseases. Vancomycin (IgA pemphigus) and penicillamine (bullous pemphigoid, pemphigus foliaceus and vulgaris) are the commonest drugs implicated. Bullae may also develop at pressure sites in drug-induced.

- *Linear IgA bullous disease*: Vancomycin,[Q] lithium, diclofenac, captopril, furosemide and amiodarone
- *Pemphigus*: The drugs most often implicated are penicillamine and other thiol (SH) compounds, including captopril[Q] or drugs such as piroxicam that are metabolized to thiols; penicillin and its derivatives, but not cephalosporins, also have been implicated.
- *Bullous pemphigoid*: Penicillamine and furosemide are most frequently implicated,[Q] although cases associated with captopril, penicillin and its derivatives, sulfasalazine, sulfapyridine, phenacetin, nalidixic acid, and topical fluorouracil.

Granulocyte-macrophage colony-stimulating factor can induce an eosinophilia and unmask a dormant bullous pemphigoid or *epidermolysis bullosa acquisita*.

- Like porphyria cutanea tarda, *pseudoporphyria*[Q] makes photoexposed skin fragile, prone to blisters and causes scarring, but porphyrin studies are normal. Suspect NSAIDs,[Q] furosemide,[Q] retinoids or tetracyclines.

Erythema Nodosum

Drugs can uncommonly cause erythema nodosum.

Causative agents: Oral contraceptives, antibiotics, amiodarone, hypoglycemic agents, NSAIDs, and sulfonamides.

Erythroderma

Drugs cause erythroderma after first producing a maculopapular exanthem or SSR.

Possible causative agents: Barbiturates, captopril, carbamazepine, cimetidine, NSAIDs, furosemide, sulfonamides, and thiazides.

Hyperpigmentation

Causative agents: ACTH, amiodarone,[Q] antimalarials[Q] (Fig. 16.11), arsenic, chlorpromazine, estrogens, minocyline,[Q] phenytoin, phenothiazine, psoralens (with UVA), and chemotherapy agents (busulfan,[Q] 5-fluorouracil,[Q] cyclophosphamide[Q]).

The common causes in India are to clofazamine[Q] (Fig. 16.12) and psoralens.

Hypertrichosis

Causative agents: Androgens,[Q] ciclosporin,[Q] minoxidil, phenytoin[Q] are most common; others include diazoxide, streptomycin, corticosteroids, penicillamine, and psoralens.

Minoxidil specially the 5% strength can lead to marked hypertrichosis on the face in females (Fig. 16.13).

Lichen Planus-like Eruptions

In this, the eruption mimics LP, but this mucosa is spared and scaling and eczematous elements may be seen (Fig. 16.14).

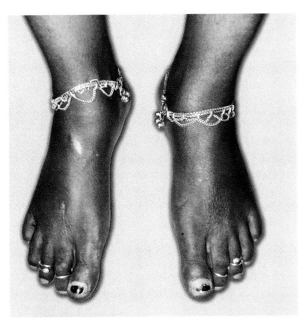

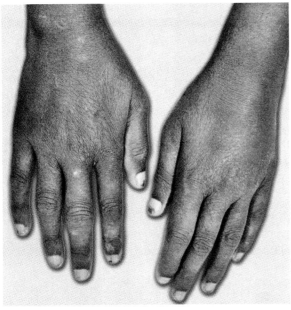

Fig. 16.11: HCQS-induced pigmentation on the exposed site

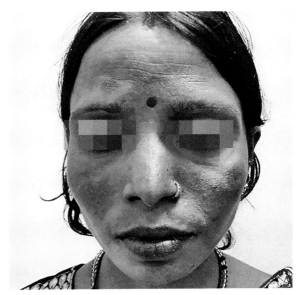

Fig. 16.12: Clofazimine-induced pigmentation over face in a patient on multidrug therapy for leprosy. Note the reddish brown color of lesions (*Courtesy*: Dr Pooja Arora)

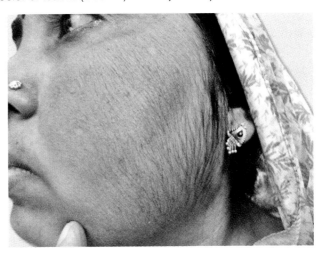

Fig. 16.13: Hypertrichosis on the face due to minoxidil 5% used on the scalp

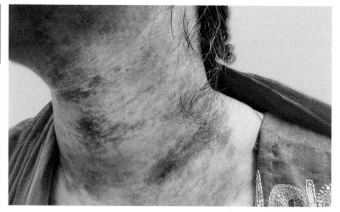

Fig. 16.14: Lichenoid drug rash due to an ayurvedic medication

Causative agents: Antimalarials, NSAIDs, gold, phenothiazines and PAS, beta-blockers, gold salts, and developing solutions for color film.

Lupus Erythematosus

Causative agents: Hydralazine,[Q] procainamide[Q] and terbinaline[Q] are most common; other causes include isoniazid, minocycline and biologicals. It is associated with antihistone antibodies.[Q]

SHIP—Sulfonamide, hydralazine, INH, procainamide.

Photoallergic and Phototoxic Reactions

Phototoxic eruptions are by far the most common drug-induced photo eruptions. They are caused by absorption of ultraviolet light by the causative drug, which releases energy and damages cells. Ultraviolet A (UVA) light is the most common wavelength implicated;[Q] ultraviolet B (UVB) light and visible light can elicit reactions with some drugs.

Photoallergic reactions[Q]: Benzodiazepines, griseofulvin, nalidixic acid, NSAIDs, phenothiazine, sulfonamides, sulfonylurea and thiazides. Most photoallergic reactions are caused by topical agents including biocides added to soaps (halogenated phenolic compounds) and fragrances such as musk ambrette and 6-methyl coumarin.

Phototoxic reactions[Q]: Amiodarone, furosemide, nalidixic acid, NSAIDs (especially piroxicam, diclofenac), psoralens, phenothiazine, and tetracyclines (especially doxycycline).[Q]

Psoriasiform Reaction[Q]

Agents worsening psoriasis include ACE antagonists, β-blockers, antimalarials, gold, interferons, lithium, and some oral contraceptives.[Q]

LIBAS—Liferium, Interferon, β-blockers, anti-malarials, ACE antagonist, Salicylates

Purpura

Drug-induced antibodies cross-react with and damage platelets.

Causative agents: Heparin, co-trimaxazole, gold salts, quinidine, quinine, and sulfonamides. Heparin-induced thrombocytopenia (HIT) occurs in around 5% of those receiving heparin.

Serum Sickness

This is a type III hypersensitivity[Q] response to foreign proteins with deposition of circulating immune complexes leading to fever, urticaria, edema, and arthralgias.

Causative agents: Penicillin,[Q] hydralazine, NSAIDs, para-aminosalicylic acid, sulfonamides, thiazides, and biologicals.

Vasculitis

Cutaneous small vessel vasculitis (CSVV) is caused by circulating immune complexes of drug and antibody (type III reaction).

CSVV typically presents with palpable purpura[Q] and/or petechiae; additional clinical findings include fever, urticaria, arthralgias, lymphadenopathy, low serum complement levels, and an elevated erythrocyte sedimentation rate.

Onset: In most patients, the clinical manifestations begin 7 to 10 days after exposure to the offending drug. However, the latent period may be as short as two to seven days with a secondary exposure or longer than two weeks with a long-acting drug such as penicillin G benzathine.

Drugs are overrated as cause but culprits include: Hydralazine, minocycline, propylthiouracil, and levamisole-adulterated cocaine.

Others are, ACE inhibitors, amiodarone, ampicillin, cimetidine, furosemide, NSAIDs, phenytoin, sulfonamides, and thiouracil.

Symmetrical Drug-related Intertriginous and Flexural Exanthema (SDRIFE)

As its name suggests, the rash presents as a sharply demarcated V-shaped erythema in the gluteal/perianal or inguinal/perigenital areas, often with involvement of at least one other flexural or intertriginous fold, in the absence of systemic symptoms (Fig. 16.15).

This newer acronym has superseded the previously used 'baboon syndrome'. It occurs hours to 2 days following drug exposure, is not associated with systemic symptoms and laboratory investigations are normal.

Causative agents: Amoxicillin, ceftriaxone, penicillin, clindamycin, and erythromycin are thought to be implied in about 50% of cases.

Xerosis

The skin can become rough and scaly in patients receiving oral retinoids,[Q] statins nicotinic acid[Q] or lithium.

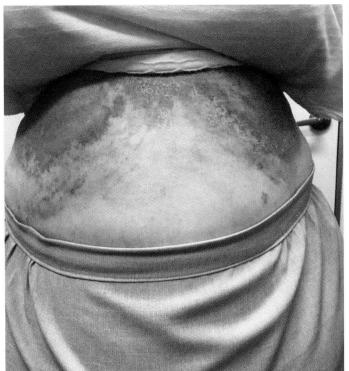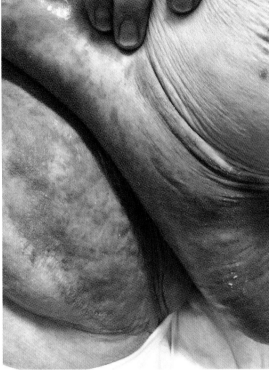

Fig. 16.15: Involvement of the flexures in a case of intertriginous drug eruption (*Courtesy*: Dr Shikha Chugh)

COMMON DRUGS/CLASSES AND THEIR REACTIONS

Antibiotics

Penicillins and sulfonamides are among the drugs most commonly causing allergic reactions. These are often morbilliform, but urticaria, erythema multiforme and fixed eruptions are common too. Viral infections are often associated with exanthems, and many rashes are incorrectly blamed on an antibiotic when, in fact, the virus was responsible. Most patients with infectious mononucleosis develop a morbilliform rash, if ampicillin is administered.[Q] Penicillin is a common cause of severe anaphylactic reactions, which can be life-threatening.

Minocycline can accumulate in the tissues and produce a brown or gray color[Q] in the mucosa, sun-exposed areas or at sites of inflammation, (lesions of acne[Q]). Minocycline can rarely cause the hypersensitivity syndrome reaction, hepatitis, worsen lupus erythematosus or elicit a transient lupus-like syndrome.

Anticonvulsants

Skin reactions to phenytoin, carbamazepine, lamotrigine and phenobarbitol are common and include erythematous, morbilliform, urticarial and purpuric rashes. TEN, erythema multiforme, exfoliative dermatitis, DRESS and a lupus erythematosus-like syndrome are fortunately rarer.

About 1% of patients taking lamotrigine develop Stevens-Johnson syndrome or TEN. A phenytoin-induced pseudolymphoma syndrome[Q] has also been described in which fever and arthralgia are accompanied by generalized lymphadenopathy[Q] and hepato-splenomegaly and, sometimes, some of the above skin signs. Long-term treatment with phenytoin may cause gingival hyperplasia[Q] and coarsening of the features as a result of fibroblast proliferation.

Highly Active Antiretroviral Drugs

Long-term highly active antiretroviral treatment (HAART) has commonly been associated with nail and skin hyperpigmentation,[Q] lipodystrophy,[Q] producing a gaunt facies with sunken cheeks. Interactions between highly active antiretroviral drugs and antituberculous drugs are common.

Steroids

Cutaneous side effects from systemic steroids include a ruddy face, cutaneous atrophy, striae, hirsutism, an acneiform eruption and a susceptibility to cutaneous infections, which may be atypical.

Penicillamine

Penicillamine can cause morbilliform eruptions or urticaria, but the drug has also been incriminated as a cause of hemorrhagic bullae at sites of trauma, of the extrusion of elastic tissue[Q] through the skin, and of pemphigus.

16

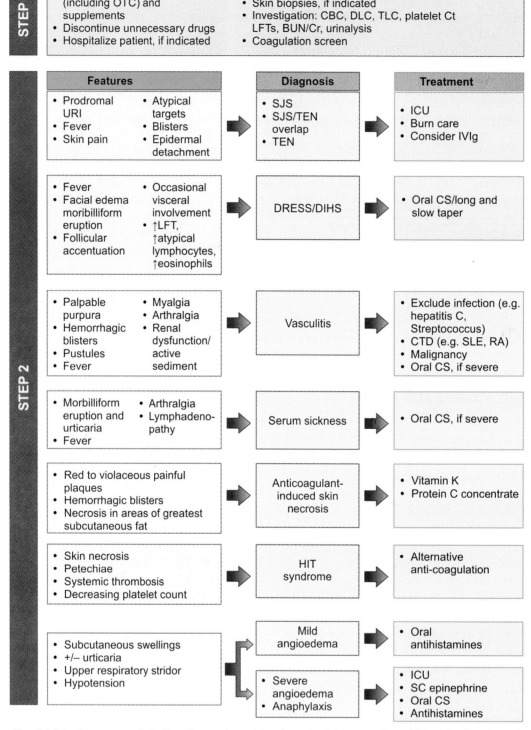

STEP 1
- Discontinue suspect drugs (including OTC) and supplements
- Discontinue unnecessary drugs
- Hospitalize patient, if indicated
- Consider alternative diagnoses
- Skin biopsies, if indicated
- Investigation: CBC, DLC, TLC, platelet Ct LFTs, BUN/Cr, urinalysis
- Coagulation screen

STEP 2

Features	Diagnosis	Treatment
• Prodromal URI • Fever • Skin pain	• Atypical targets • Blisters • Epidermal detachment	• SJS • SJS/TEN overlap • TEN	• ICU • Burn care • Consider IVIg
• Fever • Facial edema moribilliform eruption • Follicular accentuation	• Occasional visceral involvement • ↑LFT, ↑atypical lymphocytes, ↑eosinophils	DRESS/DIHS	• Oral CS/long and slow taper
• Palpable purpura • Hemorrhagic blisters • Pustules • Fever	• Myalgia • Arthralgia • Renal dysfunction/ active sediment	Vasculitis	• Exclude infection (e.g. hepatitis C, Streptococcus) • CTD (e.g. SLE, RA) • Malignancy • Oral CS, if severe
• Morbilliform eruption and urticaria • Fever	• Arthralgia • Lymphadeno-pathy	Serum sickness	• Oral CS, if severe
• Red to violaceous painful plaques • Hemorrhagic blisters • Necrosis in areas of greatest subcutaneous fat		Anticoagulant-induced skin necrosis	• Vitamin K • Protein C concentrate
• Skin necrosis • Petechiae • Systemic thrombosis • Decreasing platelet count		HIT syndrome	• Alternative anti-coagulation
• Subcutaneous swellings • +/− urticaria • Upper respiratory stridor • Hypotension		Mild angioedema	• Oral antihistamines
		• Severe angioedema • Anaphylaxis	• ICU • SC epinephrine • Oral CS • Antihistamines

Fig. 16.16: An approach to the diagnosis and treatment of drug eruptions (CS = Corticosteroid)

Oral Contraceptives

Reactions to these are less common now that their hormonal content is small. They may cause hair fall that may follow stopping the drug (telogen effluvium). Melasma,^Q hirsutism, erythema nodosum, acne and photosensitivity may also occur.

Biological Agents

The antitumour necrosis factor α therapies (etanercept, infliximab and adalimumab) are used extensively in the treatment of severe psoriasis and have all been associated with a lupus erythematosus-like cutaneous reaction. This may be associated with positive autoantibodies but rarely presents with systemic involvement. It usually settles on withdrawal of the drug.

Cetuximab and erlotinib are monoclonal antibodies to epidermal growth factor receptors (EGFR) used to treat bowel and lung cancers. These antineoplastic antibodies and their cousins commonly cause a distinctive widespread eruption with follicular pustules that resembles acne.[Q] This is because sweat and hair follicle cells express EGFR and the drug causes changes in these structures leading to follicular eruptions. Other side effects are xerosis, fissures of the palms and soles, altered hair growth and paronychia. These are dose-related and not allergic as they may be able to reinstitute the drug at lower dosage, after 1–2 weeks, without recurrence.

DIFFERENTIAL DIAGNOSIS

A possibility of drug-induced rash should always be kept in mind in a patient who develops a itchy symmetrical rash while on a drug. The clinical picture can mimic almost any inflammatory dermatoses. The most difficult situation is to distinguish between drug induced maculopapular rash and infective exanthem. The differential diagnosis of such rash includes:

- *A viral exanthem* and a drug eruption can be indistinguishable clinically specially the morbilliform rash. The difference is that a *drug eruption* is much more *pruritic*. Systemic features favor a viral exanthem.
- *Toxic erythemas* include scarlet fever, staphylococcal scalded skin syndrome eruptions, and Kawasaki syndrome (mucocutaneous lymph node syndrome). These three rashes have certain common features, including a sandpaper-like texture, mucous membrane involvement (scarlet fever and Kawasaki syndrome), the presence of fever, and a focus of infection or the presence of lymphadenopathy.

TREATMENT

Drug eruptions clear slowly with time after discontinuation of the responsible agent.

The time required for total clearing is usually 1 to 2 weeks.

For several days after the offending drug has been stopped, the eruption may actually worsen. This is particularly seen with drugs that have longer half life and where the drug metabolites may be responsible for the reaction like in antiepileptics induced rash. The decision whether the drug be stopped immediately will depend on the nature of rash and primary condition for which the drug(s) is being used and if a safer substitute is available. In serious reactions the suspected drug(s) needs to be stopped immediately along with institution of prompt supportive and specific therapy while in a non-serious rash a "carry through approach" continuing the drug, if it is essential may be undertaken. A close observation, however, to look for the progression of rash is essential as sometimes an initially benign looking rash may progress to more sinister rash later on.

Topical: Emollients

Systemic: Antihistamines (hydroxyzine (Atarax) 10–25 mg qid).

Systemic steroids: Usually required for serious reactions. In SJS/TEN a moderate to high doses for a short period (7–10 days) are generally helpful. In DRESS, a moderate dose (0.5–1.0 mg/kg/d) prednisolone equivalent, tapered gradually is employed for a fairly long period of time ranging from 3–6 months, to avoid internal organ damage and prevent long-term complications like autoimmunity. Steroids may also be sometimes required in drug-induced vasculitis, AGEP and acute urticaria/angioedema. Adrenaline is the drug of choice in the management of anaphylaxis.

The important aspect concerning ADR is recognizing severe drug reaction for which intensive care and systemic steroids are needed. Though this requires specialized texts, an approach to the diagnosis of these important drug eruption is detailed in Fig. 16.16.

Vesiculobullous Disorders

Introduction

Vesicles and bullae are accumulations of fluid within or under the epidermis. They can have varied causes, but in most cases, clinical diagnosis is based on some salient clinical features, which have to be confirmed by investigations. A brief approach to the diagnosis will be given below, which will be followed by a discussion on the various common entities that constitute the disorders under this heading.

Clinical Features

Symptoms: Burning and pain are almost invariable sensations of blisters; *pruritus* is particularly associated with pemphigoid diseases and dermatitis herpetiformis.[Q]

Morphology: The appearance of a blister is determined by the level at which it forms (Fig. 17.1). *Tense bullae*[Q] are characteristic of blistering diseases with *subepidermal split* level such as pemphigoid, whereas *flaccid bullae*[Q] that break easily are seen in bullous diseases with *intraepidermal split*, such as pemphigus.

If the blister does not have an underlying erythema, it is called monomorphic such as in monomorphic pemphigoid, and pseudoporphyria. Milia (horny pearls in the upper dermis) and scarring appear when the basement membrane is interrupted, such as in epidermolysis bullosa acquisita.[Q]

The **distribution** pattern of the lesions may be solitary (solitary bullous mastocytosis), grouped/ herpetiform (herpes simplex), circinate (linear IgA bullous disease), linear (phytophotodermatitis), or randomly (bullous pemphigoid).

The mucous[Q] membranes of body openings (eyes, nose, mouth, genitals) might be involved specially in pemphigus vulgaris.

Histology: Subepidermal blisters occur between the dermis and the epidermis. Their roofs are relatively thick and so they tend to be tense and intact. They may contain blood. Intraepidermal blisters appear within the prickle cell layer of the epidermis, and so have thin roofs and rupture easily to leave an oozing denuded surface. This tendency is even more marked with subcorneal blisters, which form just beneath the stratum corneum at the outermost edge of the viable epidermis, and therefore, have even thinner roofs.

The biopsy of a bulla can be interpreted based on its subparts and these subparts have antigens that determine various disorders (Fig. 17.2A). Broadly they are:

1. Epidermal keratinocytes
2. Intercellular binding substance—desmosome
3. Basement membrane zone—3 parts: Lamina lucida, lamina densa and sublamina densa
4. Dermis

The various antigens within these zones determine the various diseases seen.

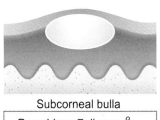

Subcorneal bulla	Intraepidermal bulla	Subepidermal bulla	
• Pemphigus Foliaceus[Q] • Bullous Impetigo • Miliaria Crystallina • Staphylococcal scalded skin syndrome • Sub-Corneal pustular dermatoses	• Pemphigus vulgaris[Q] • Acute eczema • Viral disoders • Miliaria rubra • Incontinentia pigmenti	• Bullous pemphigoid • Bullous erythema multiforme • Bullous lichen planus • Bullous lupus erythematosus • Epidermolysis bullosa • Dermatitis herpetiformis • Cicatricial pemphigoid • Pemphigoid gestationis • Linear IgA disease	• Porphyria cutanea tarda • Toxic epidermal necrolysis • Cold or thermal injury *BEDC: Mnemonic

*FCI: Mnemonic
F : Foliaceus
C : Crystallina, etc.
I : Impetigo

Fig. 17.1: Level of bulla in bullous disorders

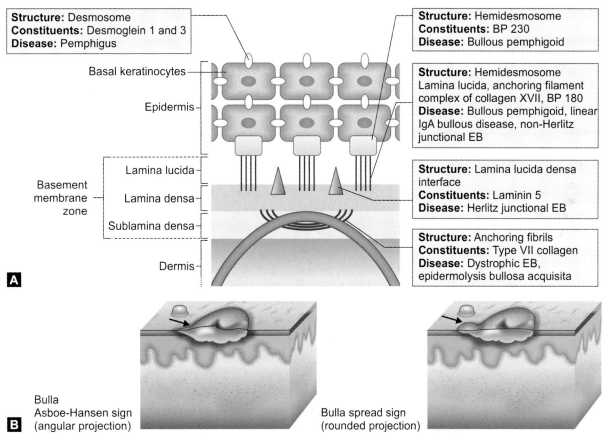

Fig. 17.2: (A) Main components of the skin and their clinical disorders; (B) A depiction of bulla spread sign

Signs

The dermatologist may evoke signs to disclose epidermal dislodgement with the (hand gloved!) fingers.

• *Nikolsky's sign*[Q]: Ability to split the epidermis on skin areas distant from the lesions of *normal*-appearing skin by a lateral pressure with a finger.

The Nikolsky's sign[Q] is positive in epidermal acantholysis such as in the pemphigus vulgaris, vegetans, foliaceus, erythematosus, and fogoselvagem subtypes of pemphigus and in staphylococcal scaled skin syndrome (SSSS).

• *Pseudo-Nikolsky's sign* (*epidermal peeling*): Ability to peel off the entire epidermis by a lateral pressure (rubbing) only on the *erythematous* skin areas. Positive in, SJS, TEN and burns.[Q]

• *Asboe-Hansen or Lutz sign* (*bulla spread sign*): Ability to enlarge a blister by applying mechanical pressure on the roof of intact blister (Fig. 17.2B).

INVESTIGATION

1. **Tzanck smear[Q]:** This is a simple procedure where the roof of the bulla is removed and the base is scraped and smeared on a glass slide, fixed and stained with Giemsa stain.[Q] The acatholytic cell is called a Tzanck cell and is a modified keratinocyte[Q] seen in pemphigus. In situations where DIF is not available, this proves to be a fast and economical method to confirm acatholysis.

2. **Biopsy:** The biopsy should include two-thirds blister cavity and one-third peribullous skin. One may draw a line that touches the blister (tangent) for orientation before giving local anesthesia and biopsy perpendicular to the tangent (Fig. 17.3). If the edematous papule or vesicle is small enough, it can be removed in its entirety for routine histology.

3. **DIF:** For direct immunofluorescence microscopy, which is a diagnostic test as it determines the antibody in the skin, a perilesional biopsy which can be taken from the *erythematous skin* 1–2 cm adjacent to a vesicle or bulla (lesional peribullous biopsy). They can be transported in Michel's solution. An overview of the technique, including IIF (see below) is depicted in Fig. 17.4.

   • In bullous pemphigoid (BP) and pemphigus vulgaris, a perilesional biopsy is done for direct immunofluorescence (DIF).
   • In dermatitis herpetiformis (DH), nearby normal skin is preferred for DIF.[Q]

   The various patterns of DIF are depicted in Fig. 17.5.

   Pemphigus: In this, the pattern is called fish net[Q] and is characterized by intercellular deposition of immunoglobulins and complement in a smooth or granular pattern (Fig. 17.6).[Q]

   Pemphigoid: Pemphigoid is characterized by a linear[Q] deposition of immunoreactants along the basement membrane (Fig. 17.7).

   Dermatitis herpetiformis is characterized by a granular deposition of IgA[Q] along the dermal–epidermal junction.

   Porphyria cutanea tarda and pseudoporphyria: A homogeneous deposition of particularly IgG along the dermal–epidermal junction and in vessel walls is typical in porphyria.

4. **Indirect immunofluorescence** microscopy is used to detect circulating antibodies in patient's serum.

   A **salt split test[Q]** is used to distinguish between EB acquisita and BP (Fig. 17.8).

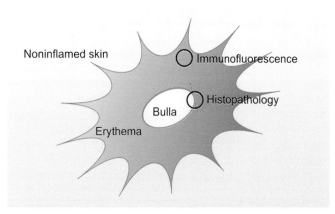

Fig. 17.3: A depiction of a bulla and the surrounding skin and the site for biopsy and IF

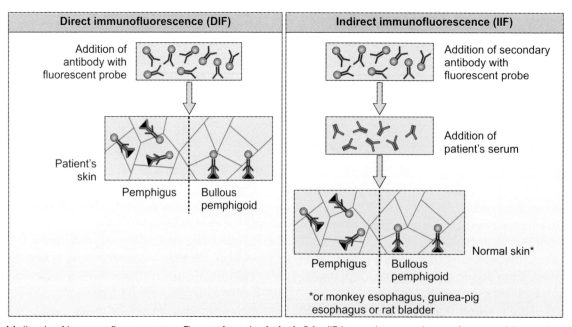

Fig. 17.4: Methods of immunofluorescence. The preferred **substrate[Q]** for IIF is monkey esophagus for pemphigus vulgaris, guinea-pig esophagus for pemphigus foliaceus, and human skin for the pemphigoid group and LABD

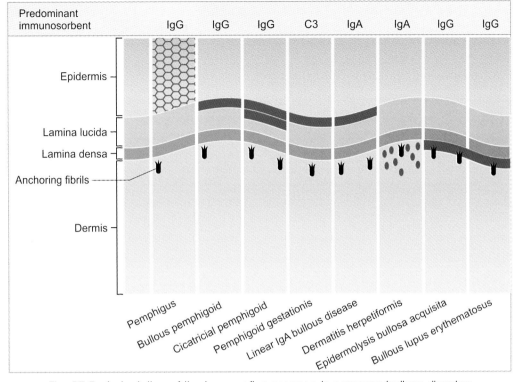

Fig. 17.5: A depiction of the immunofluorescence in common bullous disorders

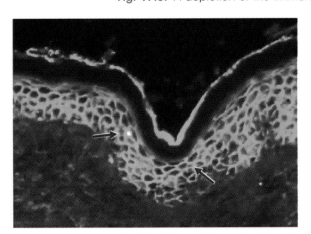

Fig. 17.6: Fish net pattern⁰ of deposition of antibodies in pemphigus vulgaris

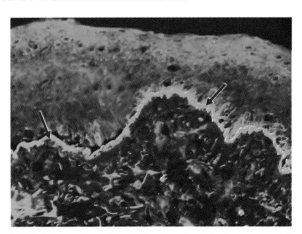

Fig. 17.7: Linear deposition⁰ of antibodies in bullous pemphigoid

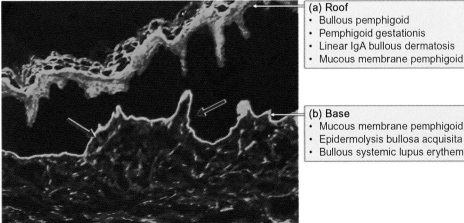

(a) Roof
- Bullous pemphigoid
- Pemphigoid gestationis
- Linear IgA bullous dermatosis
- Mucous membrane pemphigoid

(b) Base
- Mucous membrane pemphigoid
- Epidermolysis bullosa acquisita
- Bullous systemic lupus erythematosus

Fig. 17.8: Salt split test wherein the split is in the level of lamina lucida⁰

Table 17.1 An overview of the common autoimmune bullous disorders

Disease	Clinical features	Etiology	Histology/DIF
Bullous pemphigoid	Tense blisters on an urticated base[Q]	IgG autoantibodies to basement membrane antigen **BP180** or **BP230**	Subepidermal blisters Linear IgG
Dermatitis herpetiformis	Itchy small blisters and vesicles	IgA autoantibodies to gluten tissue transglutaminase in the gut and epidermis	Subepidermal blisters, papillary tips abscesses **Granular IgA** in dermal papillary tips[Q]
Pemphigus vulgaris	Fragile blisters and erosions Mucosa +[Q]	Desmogleins 1 and 3 Antibodies[Q]	Suprabasal bulla **Intercellular IgG**
Pemphigus foliaceus	Superficial scaly erosions Mucosa (–)	Desmoglein 1[Q]	Subcorneal bulla DIF-like pemphigus
Paraneoplastic pemphigus	Skin erosions Mucosa (+)	Desmogleins 1 and 3, desmoplakin	Suprabasal acantholysis

5. **ELISA** is a quantitative assay for monitoring disease activity and is specially useful in pemphigus. Pemphigus foliaceus has antibodies to desmoglein 1 but not to desmoglein 3, while mucosal dominant pemphigus vulgaris has IgG to desmoglein 3 only and mucocutaneous pemphigus vulgaris to both desmogleins 1 and 3.

A depiction of the basement membrane zone is given in Fig. 17.2 that helps to understand the site of damage in various bullous disorders. An overview of the common conditions is given in Table 17.1 and details follow.

The list of conditions that will be covered includes primarily the autoimmune bullous diseases a classification of which is given in Table 17.2 and the genetic disorder epidermolysis bullosa.

Table 17.2 List of autoimmune bullous disorders

Loss of intraepidermal adhesion	
Pemphigus vulgaris	• Classic pemphigus vulgaris • Pemphigus vegetans
Pemphigus foliaceus	• Fogo selvagem (endemic variant) • Pemphigus erythematosus (Senear-Usher) • Drug-induced pemphigus
Others	• Paraneoplastic pemphigus • IgA pemphigus
Loss of subepidermal adhesion	
Pemphigoid	• Bullous pemphigoid • Pemphigoid gestationis • Cicatricial pemphigoid • Other variants
Linear IgA disease	• Chronic bullous disease of childhood • Adult form
Others	• Epidermolysis bullosa acquisita • Dermatitis herpetiformis

SUBCORNEAL AND INTRAEPIDERMAL DISORDERS

Pemphigus Group

Pemphigus refers to a group of disorders with loss of intraepidermal adhesion because of autoantibodies directed against proteins of the desmosomal complex that hold keratinocytes together. The desmosome is a complex structure, with many of its components targets for autoantibodies. In pemphigus, desmogleins 1 and 3 are important and they have a variable distribution in the epidermis.

> The **1** (Dsg 1) is more at the **top** (stratum granulosum), while the **3** (Dsg 3) is more at the **bottom** (S. basale).[Q]

Desmoglein 3 is crucial for cell adhesion and is found in the oral mucosa and the lower layers of the epidermis, while desmoglein 1 is almost only present in the skin and most expressed in the upper layers. Thus pemphigus foliaceus never involves the mucosa and has superficial erosions, while pemphigus vulgaris often presents with oral disease and may have full-thickness acantholysis (*see* Fig. 17.9).

3OL: Desmoglein 3, Oral mucosa, Lower epidermis.

> Antibodies against Dsg 1 cause pemphigus foliaceus while those against Dsg 3 cause pemphigus vulgaris.

The cause is an immune response dominated by T cells that are desmoglein-specific and produce IL-4. These cells then induce B cells which produce antibodies against the desmogleins.

1. Pemphigus Vulgaris (PV)

Definition

Severe, potentially fatal disease with intraepidermal blister formation on skin and mucosa caused by autoantibodies against desmogleins.

Pemphigus vulgaris is particularly common in Ashkenazi Jews[Q] and people of Mediterranean or Indian origin. There is linkage between the disease and certain human leukocyte antigen (HLA) class II alleles.

Pathogenesis

Patients develop antibodies against desmoglein 3 (Dsg 3) and later desmoglein 1 (Dsg 1) (Fig. 17.9). The bound antibodies activate proteases that damage the desmosome, leading to acantholysis.

Occasionally, drugs can cause pemphigus vulgaris and pemphigus foliaceus. Agents containing sulfhydryl groups (penicillamine, captopril, piroxicam)[Q] are more likely to cause pemphigus foliaceus;[Q] those without sulfhydryl groups tend to cause pemphigus vulgaris. The latter group includes beta-blockers, **p**enicillin, and **r**ifampicin **(PCR)**.[Q]

Clinical Features

Sites: Oral mucosa, scalp, face, mechanically stressed areas, nail fold, intertriginous areas (can present as intertrigo).

The flaccid blisters are not stable, as the epidermis falls apart; therefore, erosions and crusts common (Figs 17.10 and 17.11).

Nikolsky sign and bulla spread sign are positive in this group.

- *Oral involvement*: In 70%[Q] of patients, PV starts in the mouth with painful erosions (Fig. 17.10). Other

mucosal surfaces can also be involved. Caused by anti-Dsg 3 antibodies, with Dsg 3 being the main desmoglein in the mucosa. Additional localized disease, often on the scalp.

- Generalized disease because of development of antibodies against Dsg 1 which is present in skin along with Dsg 3. Painful, poorly healing crusted erosions and ulcers; blisters hard to find (Fig. 17.11).

Course

The course of all forms of pemphigus is prolonged, even with treatment, and the mortality rate of pemphigus vulgaris is still at least 15%.[Q] Most patients have a terrible time with weight gain and other side effects from systemic corticosteroids and from the lesions, which resist healing.

Investigation

1. *Histology*: When a fresh lesion is biopsied (small excision, not punch biopsy), acantholysis is seen (free-floating, rounded keratinocytes)[Q] with retention of basal layer keratinocytes (**'row of tombstone'** effect—suprabasal blisters[Q]). Earliest change is eosinophilic spongiosis (Fig. 17.12).

2. *Direct immunofluorescence*: Perilesional skin shows deposition of IgG (100%), C3 (80%) or IgA (20%), as well C1q in early lesions. Antibodies surround the individual keratinocytes (Fig. 17.6). This is known as the 'fish net pattern'.[Q]

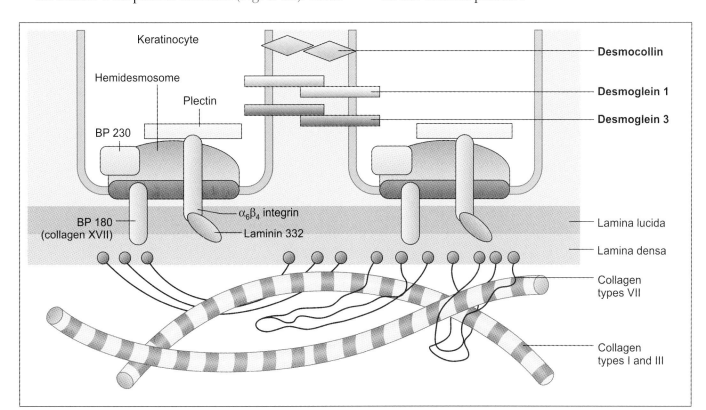

Fig. 17.9: A color depiction of the components of the intercellular adhesion molecule (desmosome) involved in pemphigus

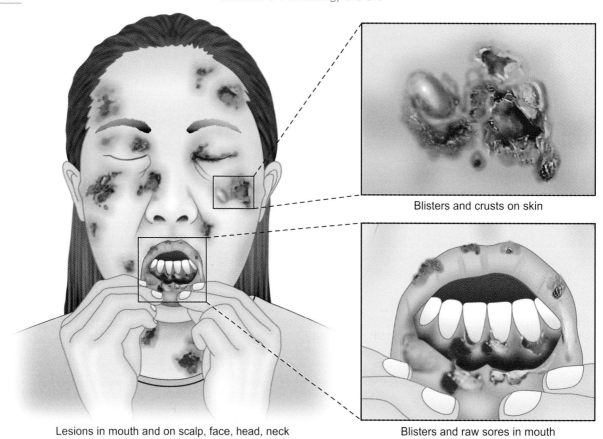

Blisters and crusts on skin

Lesions in mouth and on scalp, face, head, neck

Blisters and raw sores in mouth

Fig. 17.10: A depiction of the flaccid bulla, erosions and marked mucosal involvement in pemphigus vulgaris

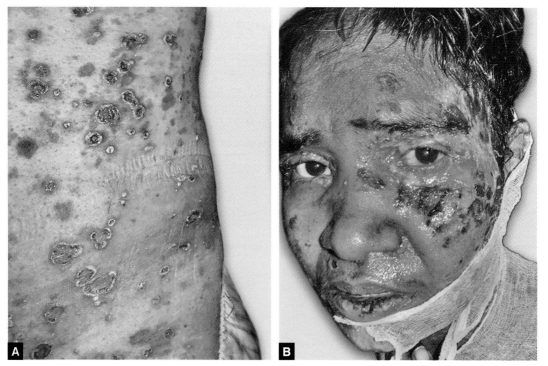

Fig. 17.11A and B: Pemphigus vulgaris: (A) Multiple flaccid bulla and erosions; (B) Erosions on the face with oral and lip involvement

3. *Indirect immunofluorescence*:[Q] Using monkey esophagus, 90% of sera show positive reaction; titer can be used to monitor disease course.

4. *ELISA*: Can be used to identify anti-Dsg 3 with mucosal disease or anti-Dsg 1 or anti-Dsg 3 with widespread disease, also help in monitoring disease course.

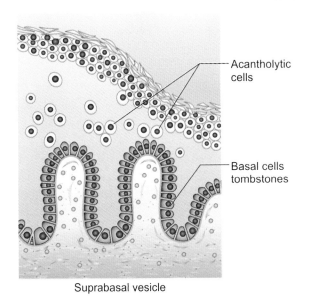

Fig. 17.12: The three components of pemphigus vulgaris—suprabasal bulla, acantholytic cells and the basal cells that are intact but lose their intercellular connection, resembling a **row of tombstones**

Check for associated diseases, especially *thymoma*[Q] and myasthenia gravis.[Q]

Differential Diagnosis

Because the blister is superficial, other eroding diseases must be considered.

Staph-scalded skin: Patients have sheets of exfoliating skin related to a staph-producing toxin. Mucosa spared.

TEN: Clinically ill patients with significant crusting of the lips, nose, and eyes.

Other: Herpetic eruptions, impetigo, IgA pemphigus, and vasculitis.

Therapy

1. Systemic corticosteroids[Q] are necessary for long periods of time. The main cause of morbidity and mortality today in patients with pemphigus vulgaris is corticosteroid side effects. For this reason, corticosteroids are *always* combined with steroid-sparing agents. Patients should be screened for osteoporosis and latent tuberculosis before embarking on long-term corticosteroid therapy. Osteoporosis prophylaxis may be warranted.
2. *Combination pulse therapy:* Treatment of choice. Every 3–4 weeks, pulse of prednisolone 1.0 g daily plus single dose of cyclophosphamide 7.5–15.0 mg/kg; in interval cyclophosphamide 1–2 mg/kg daily. Prednisolone-azathioprine therapy:
   • Start with prednisolone 1.5–2.0 mg/kg and azathioprine 2.5 mg/kg. Goal is to suppress blister formation within 1 week; if this is not achieved; double the prednisolone dose.

• Once blister formation is suppressed, logarithmic tapering to maintenance dose of prednisolone 8 mg daily and azathioprine 1.5 mg/kg daily.
3. *Alternative immunosuppressive agents:* Chlorambucil 0.1–0.2 mg/kg daily; cyclosporine 5.0–7.5 mg/kg daily; mycophenolate mofetil 2.0 g daily, cyclophosphamide.
4. *Therapy-resistant course:* Drastic measures include high-dose intravenous immunoglobulins or column immune absorption of autoantibodies. The immunosuppressive therapy must be continued or a rebound invariably occurs. Rituximab[Q] is a humanized murine monoclonal antibody to CD20 that may knock out B cells, pre-B cells and antibody production and though expensive is a highly effective agent for pemphigus. The consensus dosage of rituximab in pemphigus is a cycle of 2 × 1000 mg with a 2-week interval. The cycle is repeated after 6 and 12 months.

2. Pemphigus Vegetans

Definition

Rarest variety of pemphigus[Q] with hyperkeratotic verruciform reaction (vegetans).[Q]

Clinical Features

Pemphigus vegetans is a subtype of PV in which lesions accumulate in body folds (axillae, submammary and groin) and around orifices (lips, anus). The lesions consist of pustules (Hallopeau type)[Q] or papillomas (Neumann type) or a combination of both.

Variants

a. *Pemphigus vegetans—Neumann type:* Originally typical PV, then development of white macerated plaques in involved areas.
b. *Pemphigus vegetans—Hallopeau type:* Also known as pyodermite végétante, limited to intertriginous areas, starts as pustules that evolve into vegetating lesions.

Histology: Can be tricky; pseudoepitheliomatous hyperplasia and numerous eosinophils; acantholysis can be hard to find.

3. Pemphigus Foliaceus

Definition

Form of pemphigus with superficial blisters caused by autoantibodies against Dsg 1.[Q]

All age groups affected; not infrequently children.

A rare variant is the endemic pemphigus also known as fogo selvagem[Q] which is presumed to be infectious in origin.

Pathogenesis

Autoantibodies against Dsg 1[Q], the main desmoglein in the upper epidermis.

More often drug-induced[Q] than PV. Usual agents have sulfhydryl groups such as captopril, penicillamine, and piroxicam.

Clinical Features

Sites of predilection include scalp, face, chest, and back (seborrheic areas; Fig. 17.13)[Q] with diffuse scale and erosions. Can progress to involve large areas (exfoliative erythroderma).[Q] Facial rash is sometimes in a butterfly pattern. Oral mucosa usually spared[Q] (Dsg 1 is not expressed in oral epithelia). Individual lesions are slowly developing slack blisters that rupture easily, forming erosions and red-brown crusts (Fig. 17.14A and B).

Sometimes these patients are misdiagnosed and can proceed to erythroderma (Fig. 17.14C).

Intact blisters are very short lived (in comparison to pemphigoid).

Investigation

1. *Histology*: Subcorneal blister forms in stratum corneum or stratum granulosum; acantholysis rarely seen; usually just a denuded epithelium and sparse dermal perivascular inflammation. Not always useful.
2. Direct and indirect immunofluorescences show *superficial* deposition of IgG in fishnet pattern.
3. ELISA reveals IgG antibodies against Dsg 1.

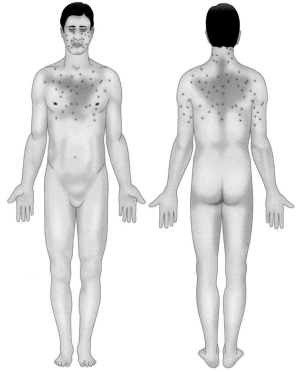

Fig. 17.13: Distribution of lesions in pemphigus foliaceus

Differential Diagnosis

Frequently misdiagnosed, as blisters are so uncommon. Depending on clinical variant, possibilities include drug reaction, photodermatosis, seborrheic dermatitis, and lupus erythematosus.

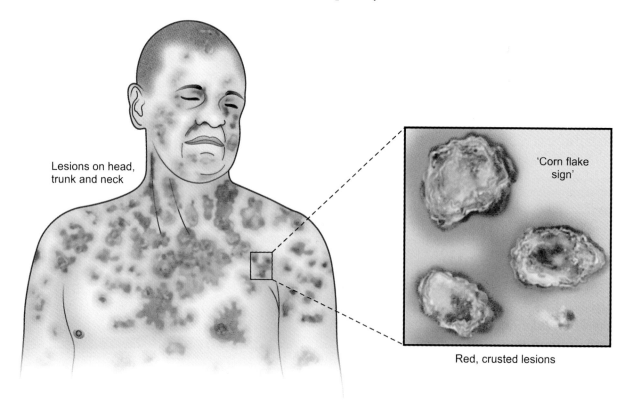

Lesions on head, trunk and neck

'Corn flake sign'

Red, crusted lesions

Fig. 17.14A: Morphology of pemphigus foliaceus lesions

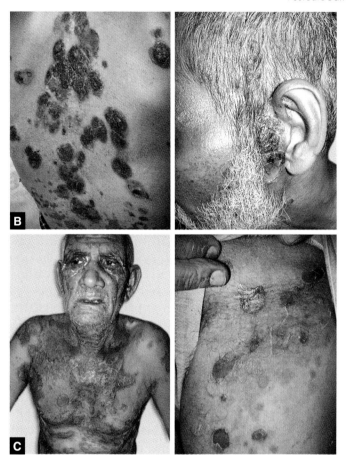

Fig. 17.14B and C: (B) Crusted plaques with underlying erosions in the seborrheic areas seen in pemphigus foliaceus; (C) A case of pemphigus foliaceus in erythroderma. The image on the right shows Nikolsky's sign

Therapy

Same approach as PV but usually **more responsive to therapy**. Dapsone may be helpful.

4. Rare Variants of Pemphigus

There are numerous other variants of pemphigus, some that are rare and others that are frequently misdiagnosed and are being described in Table 17.3; details of which are beyond the scope of this book (Table 17.3).

Hailey-Hailey Disease

Hailey-Hailey disease (familial benign chronic pemphigus)^Q is an autosomal dominant non-immune blistering condition resulting from mutations in the ATP2C1 gene located on chromosome 3.^{Q}

Pathogenesis^Q

The gene encodes a calcium–manganese pump^Q essential for desmosomal adhesion and keratinization Mutations result in suprabasal keratinocyte acantholysis^Q and dyskeratosis.^{Q}

Sweating, heat and maceration tend to aggravate this disorder.

Clinical Features

Clinically, this manifests as flaccid vesicopustules and superficial erosions coalescing to form larger scaly circinate plaques. These have a predilection for sites of skin friction, typically the neck, submammary and

Table 17.3	Uncommon variants of pemphigus		
Disorder	*Clinical features*	*Histology and DIF*	*Treatment*
Pemphigus erythematosus (Senear-Usher syndrome)^Q	Erythema and crusting in butterfly distribution and seborrheic areas. Overlap of P. foliaceus and SLE^Q	Superficial acantholysis and blister DIF: IgG: Intraepidermal and C3: DEJ ANA: (+)	Prednsiolone Dapsone Sunscreen
IgA pemphigus	**Subcorneal pustular variant:** Lesions are broad annular erythematous patches with peripheral flaccid pustules and central crusting (Fig. 17.15A). Often serpiginous or arciform borders. Favor flexures and trunk; never mouth (Fig. 17.15B), pruritic. **Intraepidermal neutrophilic dermatosis** (sunflower lesions^Q are considered typical—multiple pustules arranged like a flower)	Usually just a pustule is seen DIF: IgA	Dapsone Steroids
Paraneoplastic pemphigus*	Most often associated with non-Hodgkin lymphoma,^{Q} leukemia, Castleman tumor, or thymoma.^{Q} Severe, persistent painful stomatitis Polymorphic skin findings	IgG antibodies against plakins and desmogleins confirm the diagnosis	Prednisolone Rituximab Tumor resection chemotherapy

*If a patient is sick and has lesions resembling erythema multiforme, lichen planus, and a blistering disease, be highly suspicious of paraneoplastic pemphigus.

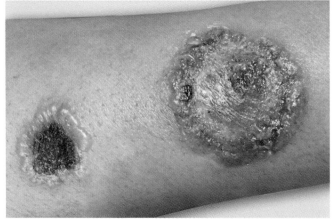

Fig. 17.15A: Peripheral vesicles and bulla surrounding central crusted lesion: IgA pemphigus

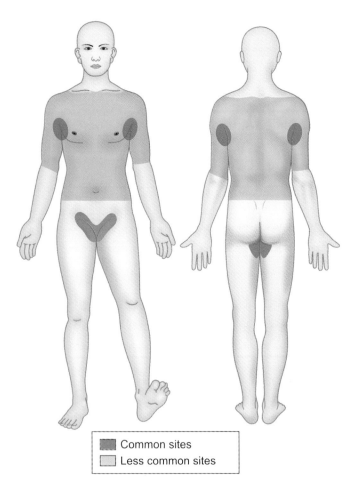

Common sites
Less common sites

Fig. 17.15B: Distribution of lesions in IgA pemphigus

intertriginous areas.^Q Secondary infection, both fungal and bacterial, is common. The histology is said to have a characteristic appearance called 'dilapidated brick wall' appearance.^Q DIF is negative.^Q

Therapy

There is no universally effective treatment. Mild cases can usually be managed with topical corticosteroids,

antibiotics, antifungals or vitamin D analogues. More severe cases may require systemic therapy with ciclosporin, methotrexate, dapsone or retinoids. There are case reports of successful outcomes with various surgical and ablative laser procedures.

Miscellaneous Subcorneal and Intraepidermal Disorders

Bullous impetigo: This is a pyoderma and a common cause of blistering in children wherein purulent flaccid bulla are seen containing pus and are frequently grouped or located in body folds. It is caused by *Staphylococcus aureus* and is amenable to oral and topical antibiotics.

Staphylococcal scalded skin syndrome: This disorder is a close differential of TEN wherein a toxin (exfoliatin) secreted by some strains of *S. aureus* makes the skin painful and red which later on peels like a scald. The infective foci (*Staphylococcus*) is usually hidden (e.g. conjunctiva, throat, wound, furuncle) and the toxin causes dyshesion of desmoglein 1,^Q which is also the target antigen in pemphigus foliaceus.

Miliaria crystallina: This is a sweat gland disorder where sweat accumulates under the stratum corneum leading to the formation of vesicles without underlying redness.^Q This can follow fever or heavy exertion. The vesicles look like droplets of water lying on the surface, but the skin is dry to the touch. The disorder is self-limiting and needs no treatment.

Subcorneal pustular dermatosis: The lesions are small groups of pustules rather than vesicles and the pustules begin as vesicles. Oral dapsone is the treatment of choice. Many patients have IgA antibodies to intercellular epithelial antigens.

SUBEPIDERMAL IMMUNOBULLOUS DISORDERS

The pemphigoid group includes mainly three diseases all characterized by autoantibody-mediated inflammation at the dermal–epidermal junction (DEJ): Bullous pemphigoid (BP), cicatricial pemphigoid (CP), and epidermolysis bullosa acquisita (EBA).

Pathogenesis

The usual cause is immunoglobulin (Ig)G antibodies against:
• Molecules in the *hemidesmosome*, which anchor keratinocytes to the basement membrane (*non-scarring*).
• Molecules that anchor the basement membrane to the dermis (then often *scarring*).

The various antigens and the disorders that develop as a consequence towards the antigens are seen in Fig. 17.16.

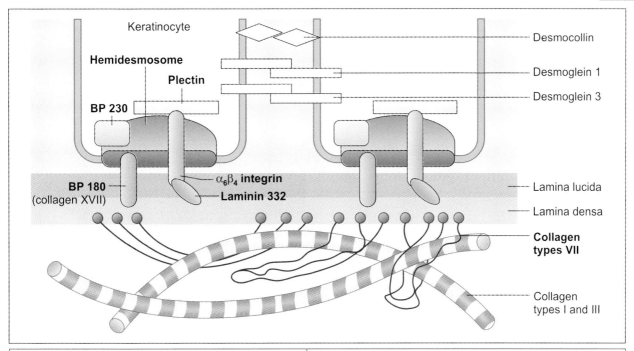

BP: Antibodies—type XVII collagen (BP180) and secondarily against-intracellular plakin (BP230).
(Both molecules anchor keratinocytes to the basement membrane)
Linear IgA disease: Antibodies recognize an N-terminal of BP180.

CP: Antibodies are against laminin 332, α$_6$β$_4$-integrin (ocular form) or C-terminal components of BP180.
(All involved in the basement membrane and its connections to the dermis)
EBA: Antibodies type VII collagen (anchoring fibrils) in the papillary dermis.

Fig. 17.16: The pemphigoid disorders—various antigens are depicted in color in the diagram

Bullous Pemphigoid (BP)

Subepidermal blistering disease caused by autoantibodies to components of the hemidesmosomes in the basement membrane zone (BMZ). BP is the most common auto-immune bullous disease mainly affecting elderly[Q] and affects men more than females.

Pathogenesis

Figure 17.16 depicts the components of the basement membrane zone including the hemidesmosome and extracellular proteins, which anchor the epidermis to the dermis. Autoantibodies are directed against two hemidesmosomal proteins:

• BP 230 or BP antigen 1 (BPAG1),[Q] a 230 kD[Q] component of the inner plaque of the hemidesmosome.
• BP 180 or BP antigen 2 (BPAG2),[Q] a 180 kD[Q] transmembrane glycoprotein also known as type XVII collagen. BP 180 is more likely to be more involved in the initial immune response, since it is transmembrane.

Antibody binding alone does not cause the problem. Antibody-initiated inflammation mediated by mast cells and complement is the key factor. The blood and tissue eosinophilia[Q] often lead to intense pruritus,[Q] which may precede the other disease manifestations by weeks.

Drugs: They can rarely lead to BP (benzodiazepine, furosemide, penicillin, sulfasalazine),[Q] also sunlight, and ionizing radiation.

Clinical Features

In some patients, before blisters develop, pruritus,[Q] dermatitis, and urticarial lesions may be seen. Tense bullae on an erythematous base are characteristic.[Q] In pigmented skin, the background redness may not be seen (Figs 17.17 and 17.18). As the epidermis is the blister roof, the blisters are very stable and hence are tense.[Q]

• Bullae are **stable**, often become quite **large**, contain enough fluid to show a fluid level and almost never involve mucosal surfaces.
• **Hemorrhagic bullae** due to their proximity with the vessels of the dermal papillae are classical.

Mucosa is involved in 20% of the cases. Nikolsky's sign is negative.[Q]

Predilection sites are the trunk, abdomen, and **flexural**[Q] aspects of the extremities.

Neurological diseases may predate the onset of the disease; including cerebrovascular disease, Parkinson's disease, epilepsy and multiple sclerosis, and are risk factors for bullous pemphigoid.

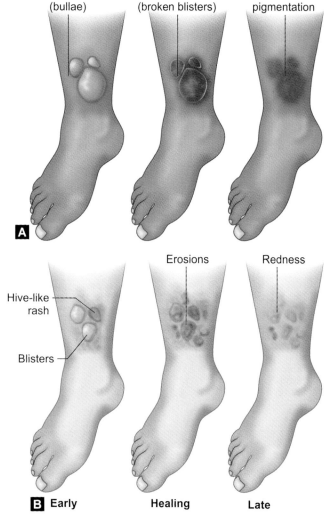

Fig. 17.17A and B: A depiction of the stages of bullous pemphigoid (above—pigmented skin, below—Caucasian skin types)

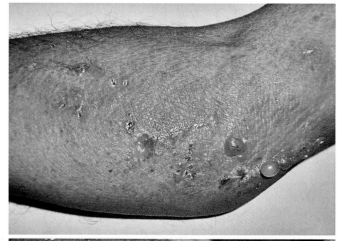

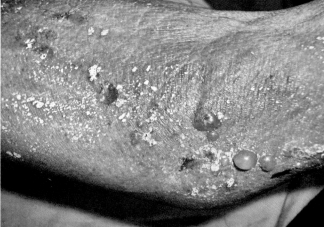

Fig. 17.18: Tense bulla on erythematous, usually *urticated* skin classical of bullous pemphigoid

Histology

- In the prebullous lesions, the presence of unexpected eosinophilia is a good clue. Later subepidermal blister formation.
- Two forms: A cell-rich form that contains many eosinophils and neutrophils and a cell-poor form with a sparse infiltrate.

Investigation

- Elevated sed rate, eosinophilia, increased IgE in 60%.
- Direct immunofluorescence: Best taken from erythematous area at periphery, not blister itself; linear band of IgG and C3 along BMZ.[Q]
- Indirect immunofluorescence: Using NaCl split skin, the autoantibodies usually attach to just the roof of the blister,[Q] but can appear on the dermal side or in both locations. They are seen in 70% of patients.
- ELISA identifies antibodies against both BP 230 and BP 180 in 60–80% of patients. Those directed speci- fically against the NC16 epitope of BP 180 correlate best with disease course.

Differential Diagnosis

Epidermolysis bullosa acquisita, linear IgA disease, generalized bullous fixed drug reaction, other bullous drug reactions, erythema multiforme, bullous systemic lupus erythematosus. DIF is the most reliable method of differentiating BP from other subepidermal disorders.

Treatment

- Mainstay is systemic corticosteroids:
  - Prednisolone 1 mg/kg daily.
  - As soon as control is reached, tapering to maintenance dose of 8 mg daily.
  - Try to taper to alternate-day dosage for adrenal-sparing effect.
- Most widely used steroid-sparing agent is azathioprine; mycophenolate mofetil also appears promising. Methotrexate 15–20 mg weekly is also effective; it can be combined with high potency topical corticosteroids during the 4–6 weeks of induction.

- Some patients do well on high-potency topical corticosteroids; worth a try with localized disease or systemic problems (especially diabetes mellitus).

Pemphigoid Gestationis

Synonym: Herpes gestationis.

This is pemphigoid occurring in pregnancy, or in the presence of a hydatidiform mole or a choriocarcinoma.[Q]

Pathogenesis

Due to an HLA mismatch between the mothers (HLA-B8, -DR3, or -DR4) and fathers (HLA-DR2), the child is sensitized against placental antigens, BP 180[Q] and less often BP 230.

Clinical Features

Sites: Protuberant abdomen and extremities; mucosal involvement 20%.

Grouped, periumbilical, tense blisters with pruritus develop in second or third trimester and persist until delivery.[Q] Rarely appear postpartum. Resolve within 3 months. Occasionally recur with menses or ingestion of oral contraceptives. Tends to be worse in next pregnancy.[Q]

Investigation

- Histology: Subepidermal blister, usually with cell-rich pattern.
- Direct immunofluorescence: Band of C3[Q] along BMZ; occasionally IgG; all the others uncommon.
- Indirect immunofluorescence: The IgG antibodies cannot always be demonstrated directly, but their strong complement-fixing properties allow identification (herpes gestationis factor). On NaCl split skin, the IgG attaches to the blister roof.

Therapy

Topical corticosteroids first; then systemic prednisolone 20–40 mg daily, which should be continued through delivery.

Mucous Membrane Pemphigoid
(Cicatricial Pemphigoid)

Mucous membrane pemphigoid is an autoimmune skin disease showing IgG and C3 deposition at the basement membrane zone. Chronic subepidermal blistering disease favoring mucous membranes, especially mouth and eyes.

Pathogenesis

Poorly understood; several different target antigens—BP 180, BP 230, laminin 5, $\alpha_6\beta_4$-integrin, laminin 332 and type VII collagen (in anchoring filaments). The finding of anti-laminin 332 antibodies indicates a potential for occult malignancy.[Q]

Clinical Features

The condition differs from bullous pemphigoid as:
- One that its blisters and ulcers occur mainly on mucous membranes such as the conjunctivae, the mouth and genital tract and the lesions heal with scarring[Q] (Fig. 17.19).
- Bullae on the skin itself are less common (25–30% of cases).
- Localized form is known as Brunsting-Perry disease with persistent plaques on which recurrent blisters develop. These patients have lesions of the head and neck without mucosal disease, caused by antibodies against laminin 332.

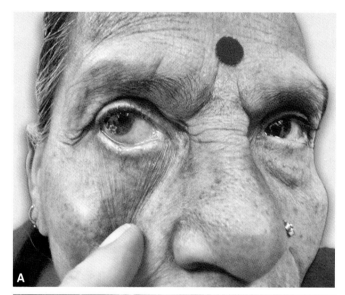

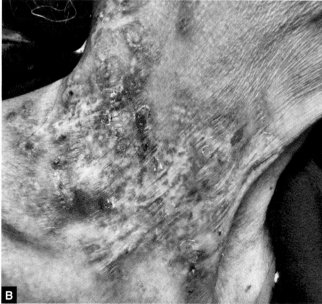

Fig. 17.19A and B: Cicatricial pemphigoid: (A) Ocular involvement with scarring and; (B) localized lesions of the neck

Treatment

The condition tends to persist and treatment is relatively ineffective, although very potent local steroids, dapsone, systemic steroids and immunosuppressive agents are usually tried. Good eye hygiene and the removal of in growing eyelashes are important.

Epidermolysis Bullosa Acquisita (EBA)

This is a rare subepidermal blistering disease with predilection for areas subject to mechanical forces. It is seen in adults in 4th–5th decades; not to be confused with epidermolysis bullosa.

Pathogenesis

Autoantibodies directed against type VII collagen,[Q] a component of the lamina densa.[Q]

Clinical Features

Acral mechanobullous form closely resembles porphyria cutanea tarda; fragile skin and blisters on backs of hands healing with milia and scarring; nail dystrophy.

It can be differentiated from BP by two important features—blisters arise in response to trauma on otherwise normal skin and milia[Q] are seen after the lesions heal. While the entire pemphigoid group can heal with milia, they are most common in EBA. No preceding urticaria and pruritus.

Inflammatory form is very similar to BP with stable blisters; less often resembles cicatricial pemphigoid or dermatitis herpetiformis; heals with scarring; sometime scarring alopecia. About 50% of patients have mucosal involvement.

Investigation

- *Direct immunofluorescence*: Deposition of IgG (rarely IgA) in BMZ.
- *Indirect immunofluorescence*: IgG with ability to bind complement found in 50%. The antigen lies on the dermal side of the lamina densa, in contrast to the bullous pemphigoid antigens, which lie on the epidermal side—a difference that can be demons-trated by immunofluorescence after the basement membrane is split at the lamina densa by incubating skin in a saline solution (the 'salt-split' technique).[Q]
- ELISA identifies antibodies against type VII collagen.

Differential Diagnosis

Before the ability to identify antibodies to type VII collagen, EBA was diagnosed as BP with negative immunofluorescence or as porphyria cutanea tarda with negative urine studies. Bullous lupus erythemato-sus also has antibodies to type VII collagen but is clinically quite different.

Therapy

The first-line therapy for EBA is a combination of low-dose corticosteroids, colchicine, or dapsone.

Colchicine is often used as a first-line drug in a dose of 0.5–1 mg/day. Dapsone is prescribed at a dose of 25 mg/day that is gradually increased to 100 mg/day.

Corticosteroids are only effective for the inflammatory form, but not as effective as in pemphigoid. With localized disease, try topical corticosteroids first. Prednisolone 60–80 mg daily, combined with azathio-prine 1–2 mg/kg daily, cyclosporine 3–5 mg/kg daily or cyclophosphamide 50 mg daily; steroid component tapered as soon as improvement seen.

Plasmapheresis can help to spare systemic medica-tions. Intravenous immunoglobulin (IVIG) and rituximab have both been tried.

Linear IgA Disease of Adults (LAD)

Children: Chronic bullous disease of childhood.

This is a subepidermal blistering disease caused by deposits of IgA along BMZ. It is seen more commonly in females (female: male ratio 2:1).

Pathogenesis

Multiple target antigens have been identified and there are two types of antigens—those that stain lamina lucida and those that attach to type VII collagen in sublamina densa-type. The major target antigens is the 120 kDa LAD-1 antigen and the 97 kDa LAD antigen 1.

Several drugs[Q] cause LAD; most common is vanco-mycin but also penicillin, sulfamethoxazole/trimetho-prim, vigabatrin.

Clinical Features

LAD may be identical to dermatitis herpetiformis but without gastrointestinal involvement, or resemble BP or even cicatricial pemphigoid with ocular involvement. Over 50% have mucosal involvement; sometimes limited to these tissues. The classic arrangement of lesions is called the **'string of pearls or crown of jewels'** appearance (Fig. 17.20).[Q]

Children: Most common subepidermal blistering disorder in childhood.[Q] It occurs before 5 years of age and resolves spontaneously.

The lesions are distributed periorifacially (abdomen, groin, axillae, and face) in a rosette fashion. Mucosal disease very common (as high as 90%).

Investigation

1. IgA antibodies in a linear pattern[Q] best seen with direct immunofluorescence.

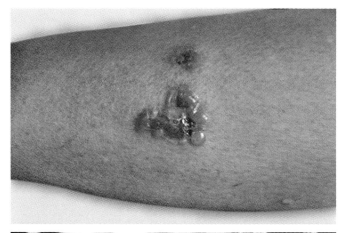

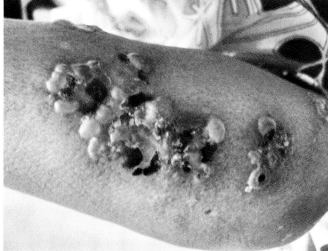

Fig. 17.20: Tense blisters clustered together in the so-called 'string of pearls' appearance.^{Q} Linea IgA bullous disorders

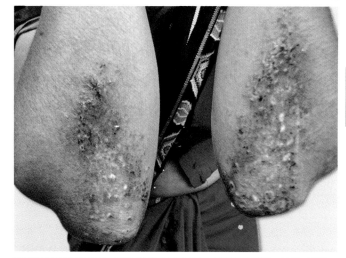

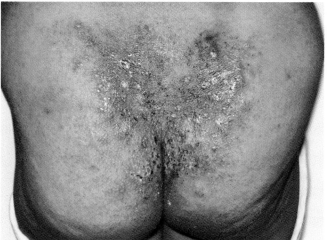

Fig. 17.21: Dermatitis herpetiformis^Q: Intensely itch, papules, vesicles and are seen on the extensor aspects and are excoriated

2. Additional tests should include eye examination and jejunal biopsy to exclude celiac disease.

Treatment

Dapsone (0.5–2.0 mg/kg) is usually effective,^{Q} but more for the sub-lamina densa type. Corticosteroids work best for lamina lucida type.

Dermatitis Herpetiformis (DH)

Pruritic vesicular disease caused by IgA autoantibodies directed against epidermal transglutaminase^Q and presenting with granular pattern in papillary dermis.

Clinical Features

The classic clinical presentation of DH is a very itchy^Q polymorphous skin eruption comprising of erythema, urticarial plaques, papules, vesicles, excoriations, and purpura sometimes in **herpetiform configuration**.

The lesions are distributed typically on the extensor surfaces of the body,^{Q} such as the knees, elbows (Fig. 17.21), and shoulders, in the so-called **vertical distribution**. Large blisters are rarely seen.

Hallmark is intensely pruritic or burning tiny vesicles, which are usually scratched^Q away by the time the patient presents. The disease has a fluctuating course driven mostly but not always by gluten ingestion and improves under UV light (seasonal flare-ups).

Patients often are not able to tolerate iodine^Q and flare with exposures, such as when eating seafood. Gluten-sensitive enteropathy^Q (sprue, adult coeliac disease),^{Q} demonstrable by small bowel biopsy, is always present,^{Q} but most patients do not have diarrhea, constipation or malnutrition as the enteropathy is mild, patchy and involves only the proximal small intestine. Palmoplantar purpura and enamel defects of the secondary teeth are less commonly noted.

Occasional association with other autoimmune diseases such as diabetes mellitus, pernicious anemia, thyroid disease, and vitiligo.

Pathogenesis

There is a strong genetic predisposition for DH. In patients with HLA-DQ2, HLA-B8, HLA-DQ8^Q

17

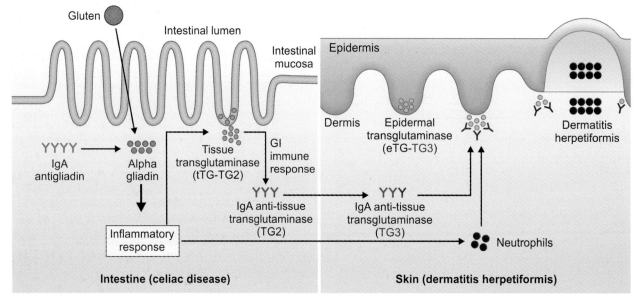

Fig. 17.22: Pathogenesis of dermatitis herpetiformis

phenotype, an autoimmune reaction develops after the ingestion of gluten (Fig. 17.22).

- First, tTG (tissue transglutaminase) modifies gliadin, the alcohol-soluble fraction of gluten to an antigen, which binds to the HLA-DQ2/HLA-DQ8 molecule to evoke cellular and humoral (anti-gliadin antibodies) immune reactions.

- The humoral and cellular immune reactions lead to inflammation and damage of the gut mucosa, resembling changes seen in celiac disease. The subclinical gluten sensitivity is obligate to develop DH.

- These antibodies cross react with epidermal transglutaminase (eTG) leading to neutrophilic abscess, and are localized to the dermal papilla.

Rare patients with enteropathy have skin involvement; a few patients with skin findings have symptomatic bowel disease, but most (90%) have an abnormal bowel biopsy.

Complications of gluten-sensitive enteropathy include diarrhea, abdominal pain, anemia and, rarely, malabsorption. Small bowel lymphomas have been reported.

Investigation

- Pathology: Neutrophilic papillary tip microabscess[Q] are the hallmark. Often associated with eosinophils.[Q] Edema leads to subepidermal blister formation (Fig. 17.23).

- Direct immunofluorescence: Granular deposits of IgA[Q] in dermal papillae; along BMZ.

- Indirect immunofluorescence: IgA antibodies against smooth muscle endomysium (source of tissue transglutaminase) present in 80%.

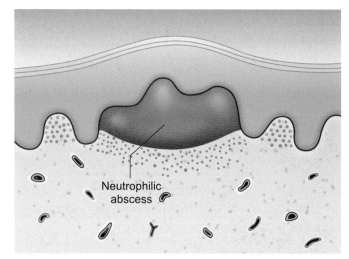

Fig. 17.23: Histology of dermatitis herpetiformis

- Serum antibody tests for antiendomysial antibodies or tissue transglutaminase[Q] can help diagnose the enteropathy.

Differential Diagnosis

Dermatitis herpetiformis is probably one of the most incorrectly thought of diagnosis in any case of pruritus where there is no obvious cause.

Scabies, BP before the development of blisters, prurigo simplex, excoriated eczema and insect bites are the common differentials.

Treatment

Gluten-free diet (GFD) is the first choice of treatment.[Q] Every patient with DH should be informed about this; however, consistent adherence on GFD is difficult (Table 17.4). Unfortunately, the effect of GFD takes time.

Table 17.4	Gluten-free diet
Avoid	*Allowed*
Grains and starches **B**arley, **R**ye, **O**ats, **W**heat*	Rice, corn, millet, coconut-flour, Buckwheat, amaranth quinoa, potato, soyabean, tapioca
Grain products: Cream of wheat, wheat-germ, oatmeals, and others	Gluten-free bread and cookies, rice cakes
Commercial breads, cakes, cookies, crackers, pasta	
Malt, coffee substitutes, beer	
Caution with sausage, processed meats or fish, spices, cheeses (gluten binders), cheese substitutes, soups, sauces, puddings	

*BROW—mnemonic

The skin rash disappears in months after the cessation of gluten, and gluten rechallenge causes flare-up of the disease within days. A patient with symptoms of celiac disease should be referred to a gastroenterologist.

Dapsone[Q] is amazingly effective; hours to days after the first dose, the pruritus disappears. Usually a low dose of 25–50 mg suffices.

Epidermolysis Bullosa
(Mechanobullous Disorders)

This is a group of disorders with mechanical defects leading to easy blistering, caused by defective structural proteins. Though there are numerous types and the details of which is beyond the scope of this book, it is important to note that this disorder is the first bullous disorder where genetic mapping has been done[Q] and is thus amenable to *in utero* diagnosis. An overview of the disorder is given in Fig. 17.24.

The full classification is beyond the scope of this chapter but an working classification of the common conditions is given in Table 17.5. The site of genetic defect is depicted in Fig. 17.24. The milder variants have an intraepidermal involvement while the deeper the defect more severe the clinical course.

Diagnostic Approach

Clinical examination and family history can only point to possible diagnosis. The gold standard method for the diagnosis of epidermolysis bullosa was transmission electron microscopy;[Q] however, limited expertise and availability of this technique has seen it surpassed by immunofluorescence microscopy (IFM)[Q] with standardized antibodies against the various structural proteins. Final diagnosis based on antigen mapping of skin biopsy and identification of genetic defect.

Clinical Features

- Clinically, all forms of EB look similar, with fragile skin so that slight trauma produces blisters or erosions.[Q]
- The skin may heal with pigmentary changes, milia, or scarring.

EB simplex: Least disturbing form of EB; patients tend to easily develop blisters from minor mechanical

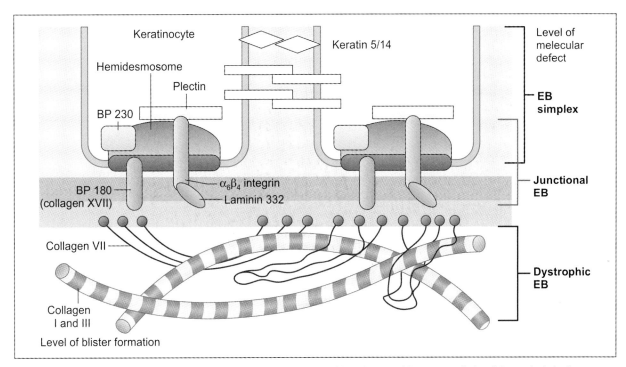

Fig. 17.24: A color depiction of the antigens and site of involvement in congenital epidermolysis bullosa

Table 17.5	Classification of EB	
Disorder	*Site of bulla*	*Genetic defect*
Epidermolysis bullosa simplex (usually autosomal dominant)	Intraepidermal	Keratins 5 and 14^Q
Junctional epidermolysis bullosa (autosomal recessive)	Lamina lucida	Components of the hemidesmosome-anchoring filaments (e.g. laminins, integrins and bullous pemphigoid 180 molecule)
Dystrophic epidermolysis bullosa (autosomal dominant/ recessive)	Beneath lamina densa	Type VII collagen

trauma such as crawling on knees and elbows or (later in life) walking.

Defect: The most common mutations is in keratins 5 and 14,^Q which are paired and expressed low in the epidermis, either in the basal layer or just above (Fig. 17.25). All have autosomal dominant inheritance except the form associated with muscular dystrophy.

The common types include:
- Epidermolysis bullosa simplex—localized (formerly Weber-Cockayne type), presenting in childhood with blistering at sites of trauma (hands, elbows and feet).
- Generalized variant (Koebner type).
- Dowling-Meara type, featuring herpetiform blisters on the trunk.
- Keratin 5 (and perhaps 14) is also involved in transfer of melanin to keratinocytes, so some forms of EBS have mottled pigmentation. Hyperhidrosis and palmoplantar keratoderma can be associated.

- Generalized EBS with scarring, as well as muscular dystrophy or pyloric stenosis: Patients have a defect in plectin. A protein that binds keratin filaments to hemidesmosomes.

Clinical features: Blisters form within or just above the basal cell layers of the epidermis and so tend to heal *without* appreciable *scarring* (Fig. 17.26).

Nails and mucosae are not involved.

The blistering tends to be worse after sweating and wearing and ill-fitting shoes.

Treatment: Blistering can be minimized by avoiding trauma, wearing soft well-fitting shoes and using foot powder. Large blisters should be pricked with a sterile needle and dressed. Their roofs should not be removed. Local antibiotics may be needed. In most instances, patients learn how to avoid and treat blisters and thus are able to cope well with life.

EB junctional type: Mutations involve proteins involved in the formation of the dermoepidermal junction; all have autosomal-recessive inheritance and tend to scar.

Defect: The separation occurs in the lamina lucida of the basement membrane, usually following mutations in the genes responsible laminin-332^Q formation (Fig. 17.25).

Defects can also be seen in the components of the hemidesmosme (Fig. 17.25) like collagen XVII (bullous pemphigoid antigen 2), laminin 5 or $\alpha_6\beta_4$ integrin.

Clinical features
- *Most severe type: JEB Herlitz*: Patients have defects in laminin and tend to develop widespread, poorly healing erosions, with fluid loss and infections, often leading to death in the first two years of life. The perioral and perianal skin is usually involved, as are the nails and oral mucous membrane.
- *JEB non-Herlitz* (also known as generalized atrophic bullous epidermolysis bullosa [GA-BEB]) is caused

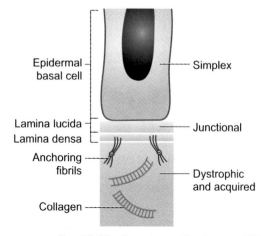

Simplex	:	Keratin 5, 14
Junctional	:	Hemidesmosome (BPAg2, $\alpha_6\beta_4$ integrin)
		Lamina lucida (laminin 1, laminin 5)
		Lamina densa (type IV collagen)
		Anchoring filments (laminin 332)
Dystrophic	:	Anchoring fibrils (type VII collagen)

Epidermal basal cell — Simplex

Lamina lucida — Junctional
Lamina densa
Anchoring fibrils — Dystrophic and acquired
Collagen

Fig. 17.25: Overview of the types of EB and site and antigen involved

17

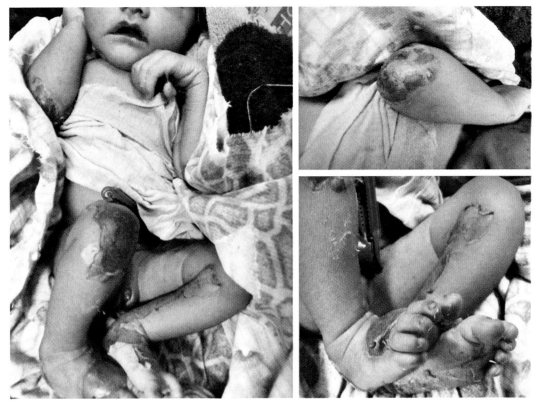

Fig. 17.26: EB simplex: Multiple erosions localized to the trauma-prone areas

by mutations in BP180 (now known as collagen XVII) and is characterized by widespread blisters, alopecia, and nail and dental problems but a less severe course (Fig. 17.27).

- *JEB and pyloric atresia* usually have mutations in α6β4 integrin.

Dystrophic EB: Most severe form; mutations in type VII collagen,[Q] the main component of the anchoring fibrils in the papillary dermis (Fig. 17.28); invariable scarring, often mutilating.[Q]

Dominant dystrophic epidermolysis bullosa (Cockayne-Touraine-Pasini).

In the autosomal dominant type, blisters appear in late infancy and are localized to the friction sites (e.g. the knees, elbows and fingers), healing with scarring and milia formation. The nails may be deformed or even lost but the mouth is not affected. The only treatment is to avoid trauma and to dress the blistered areas.

Recessive dystrophic epidermolysis bullosa (Hallopeau-Siemens).

Patients have two abnormal collagen VII molecules and very fragile skin.

Recessive dystrophic epidermolysis bullosa (generalized severe subtype) is a fatal form of epidermolysis bullosa wherein extensive, sometimes hemorrhagic, subepidermal blisters start in infancy, and heal with scarring; the condition can be so severe that the nails are lost and webs form between the digits. The hands

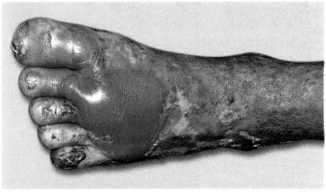

Fig. 17.27: A case of junctional EB with involvement of the nail and skin with areas of pigmentary loss and scarring

and feet may become useless balls, having lost all fingers and toes (mitten hands).[Q]

The teeth, mouth and upper part of the esophagus are all affected; esophageal strictures may form. Squamous cell carcinomas of the skin (20× risk) and renal failure are late complications.

Treatment: Being a genetic disorder, effective therapies for any of the subtypes have not been established.[Q] The mainstays of treatment are avoidance of skin trauma, meticulous wound care, adequate pain relief and monitoring for secondary complications. Treatment of recessive dystrophic epidermolysis bullosa with phenytoin, and systemic steroids are disappointing.

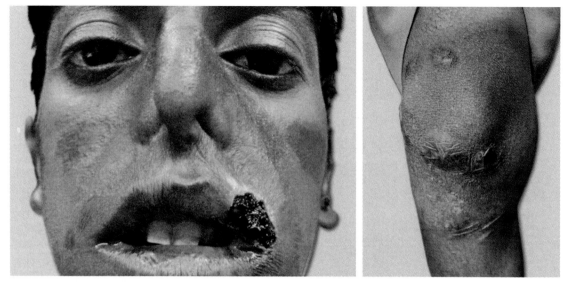

Fig. 17.28: A case of dystrophic EB post-erosive stage. Note the marked scarring and remnant activity of disease

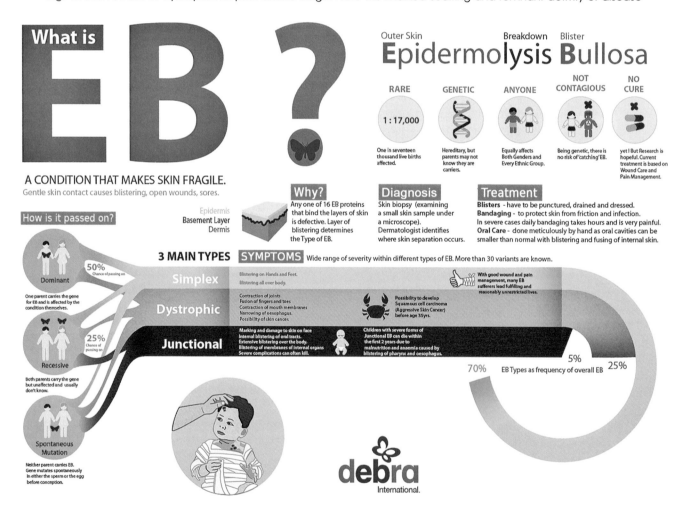

Fig. 17.29: Infographic on epidermolysis bullosa

Gene therapy^Q to replace the mutated DNA may be possible, if a safe vector can be found to insert the 'corrected' sequence. Silencing autosomal dominant inherited mutations with small interfering RNA (siRNA) also shows promise. Cell therapies with keratinocyte, dermal fibroblast, bone marrow-derived stem cell or patient-specific induced pluripotent stem cell injections may be useful.

A summary of this important disorder is given in Fig. 17.29 as a quick overview and reference.

Pigmentary Disorders and Tumors

Disorders of Skin Pigmentation

Melanin is formed from the essential amino acid phenylalanine[Q] through a series of enzymatic steps in the liver and skin. Tyrosine is formed in the liver by the hydroxylation of the essential amino acid phenylalanine under the influence of phenylalanine hydroxylase (Fig. 18.1).

The melanin is made within the melanosomes (Fig. 18.2), which are of a size of 0.1 × 0.7 μm and are of two types—eumelanosomes (containing eumelanin), or pheomelanosomes (containing pheomelanin). These melanosomes pass into the dendritic processes of the melanocyte to be further transferred into neighboring keratinocytes (Fig. 18.2). The melanosomes are then engulfed into lysosomal packages (melanosome complexes) and distributed throughout the cytoplasm. The ratio of melanocytes to keratinocytes is about 1:36, that is one melanocyte supplies melanin to about 36 keratinocytes.[Q]

What determine a person's skin color is the activity of those melanocytes and their interactions with their keratinocyte neighbors.[Q] Darker skin individuals have melanocytes that produce more and larger melanosomes. Also these melanosomes are efficiently transferred to keratinocytes and more slowly degraded in the melanosome complexes.[Q]

Control of Melanogenesis

Melanogenesis can be increased by several stimuli, the most important of which is UVR. Tanning represents a protective mechanism by our skin against future UV damage and is of two types involves two distinct reactions.

1. *Immediate pigment darkening (IPD)*, also called the Meirowsky phenomenon, follows exposure to long wave ultraviolet (UVA 320–400 nm).[Q] This pigment darkening occurs over minutes to days, dependent on UV dose and constitutive skin color,

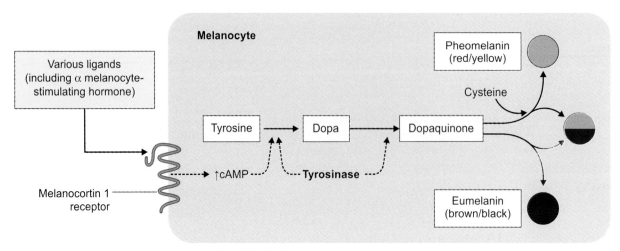

Fig. 18.1: Pathway of melanogenesis

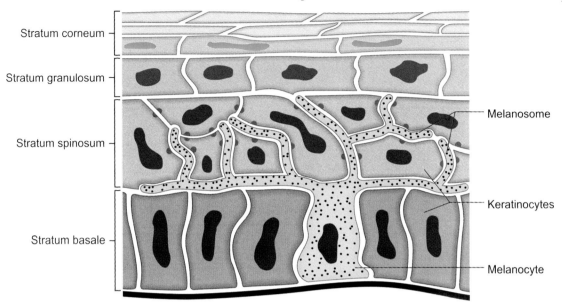

Fig. 18.2: Melanocyte and its interaction with keratinocytes. The melanosomes are transferred from the melanocyte to the keratinocyte

and is responsible for the well-known phenomenon of a 'false tan'. It is not caused by melanin synthesis but oxidation of preformed melanin and redistribution of melanin from perinuclear melanosomes to peripheral dendrites.

2. *Delayed tanning* (*DT*), the production of new pigment occurs some 3–4 days after exposure to medium-wave ultraviolet (UVB: 290–320 nm)[Q] and UVA and is maximal at 7 days.
   - UVR results in DNA damage, which leads to the activation of p53.
   - This in turn induces both keratinocytes and melanocytes in the skin to secrete pro-opiomelanocortin.
   - Alpha melanocyte-stimulating hormone (α-MSH), a cleavage product of pro-opiomelanocortin, then binds the melanocortin 1 receptor on melanocytes and signals for the upregulation of microphthalmia transcription factor (MITF).
   - MITF has a central role in melanogenesis by inducing the proliferation of melanocytes, increasing tyrosinase activity and melanosome production, and increasing the transfer of new melanosomes to their surrounding keratinocytes.

Estrogens and progestogens (and possibly testosterone too) may, in some circumstances, stimulate melanogenesis, either directly (by acting on estrogen and progestogen receptors in the melanocyte) or by increasing the release of MSH peptides from the pituitary.

Classification

A simple method of classification is based on the onset of the disorder (congenital and acquired), the type of

pigmentation and the etiology of the same, which depends on either melanin or melanocyte variations.
- *Hyperpigmentation*:
  - Excess melanin or other pigments (iron, silver, tattoos). If other pigments, then endogenous vs. exogenous.
  - Increased melanin production and transfer (café au lait macule) *vs.* increased number of melanocytes (lentigines, melanocytic nevi, malignant melanoma).
- *Hypopigmentation*: Loss of melanin (albinism) *vs.* loss of melanocytes (vitiligo).

HYPOPIGMENTATION DISORDERS

There are various causes of a pigmentary loss of the skin depending on various steps of melanogenesis. A simple overview is given in Fig. 18.3 based on disorders that damage the melanocytes and those that affect tyrosinase.

A more elaborate classification is based on the distribution of the disorders (Fig. 18.4 and Table 18.1).

Albinism

This is a family of disorders with disturbances in either melanin production or formation and transfer of melanosomes and typically affect skin and eyes.

In oculocutaneous albinism (OCA, autosomal recessive), melanin is missing in the skin, hair, and eyes. In ocular albinism, the defects are primarily in the eye.

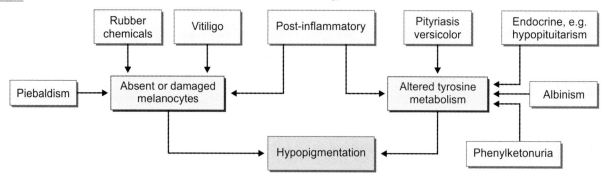

Fig. 18.3: Overview of hypopigmentation disorders based on the main pathogenetic steps

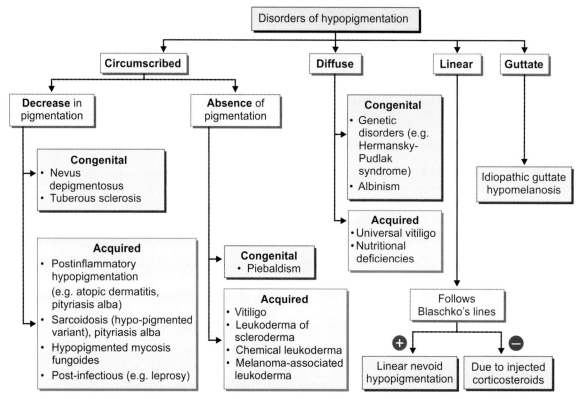

Fig. 18.4: Approach to diagnosis of hypopigmented disorders based on distribution

Table 18.1	Disorders of hypopigmentation	
Generalized involvement (whole body)	Congenital	Albinism, Chédiak-Higashi syndrome, Hermansky-Pudlak syndrome, phenylketonuria
	Acquired	Panhypopituitarism
Localized involvement	Congenital	Piebaldism Waardenburg syndrome, hypomelanosis of Ito, nevus depigmentosus, tuberous sclerosis
	Acquired	Vitiligo, postinflammatory hypopigmentation, pityriasis alba, idiopathic-guttate-hypomelanosis, chemical leukoderma

Tyrosinase-negative albinism

Pathogenesis: Mutation in tyrosinase gene; melanosomes contain no melanin.[Q]

Clinical features: Most severe form of albinism:[Q]

- Skin: White hair, white to pale pink skin, no pigmented nevi, risk for UV-induced tumors (actinic keratoses, squamous cell carcinomas).
- Eyes: Gray translucent iris, red reflex, photophobia, nystagmus, loss of vision.

Diagnostic approach: Hair bulb negative for tyrosine, ophthalmologic examination.

Tyrosinase-positive albinism

Pathogenesis: Most common form of albinism;[Q] tyrosinase is present; melanin formed and melanosomes start to form but rarely mature completely.

Mutation in protein P blocks formation of eumelanin, but other forms are still produced.

Clinical features:
- Skin: White skin and hair at birth; later slight pigmentation, often yellow-red hair; may have a few freckles.
- Eyes: Some pigment presence; defects less severe than above.

Diagnostic approach: Hair bulb positive for tyrosinase, ophthalmologic examination.

There are other types of albinism and are uncommon and can have associated systemic and immunological defects. These include:

- *Hermansky-Pudlak syndrome*: Tyrosinase-positive albinism plus platelet defects.
- *Chédiak-Higashi syndrome and Griscelli syndrome*: Pigmentary dilution[Q] with a gray sheen, macrophage defects with severe infections.

Treatment

Avoidance of sun exposure, and protection with opaque clothing, wide-brimmed hats and sunscreen creams, are essential and allow albinos in temperate climates to live a relatively normal life. Early diagnosis and treatment of skin tumors is critical.

Piebaldism

Uncommon genodermatosis with circumscribed hypomelanosis; autosomal dominant[Q] inheritance.

Mutation in KIT gene on chromosome 4q12 that causes altered migration of melanocytes from the neural crest to the skin during embryogenesis.

Clinical Features

These patients often have a white forelock of hair[Q] and patches of depigmentation lying symmetrically on the limbs, trunk and central part of the face, especially the chin[Q] (Fig. 18.5). Typically, patients have pigmented islands within white patches.[Q]

Associated syndromes: *Waardenburg syndrome*:[Q] Piebaldism (with a white forelock in 20% of cases), dystopia canthorum (lateral displacement of the inner canthus of each eye), a prominent inner third of the eyebrows, irides of different[Q] color and deafness.

Nevus Depigmentosus

Localized area of depigmentation, usually following Blaschko lines, caused by aberrant transfer of melanosomes.

Clinical Features

Sharply demarcated permanent area of depigmentation present at birth, which grows with child; usually respects the midline[Q] (Fig. 18.6).

Differential Diagnosis

Nevus anemicus is a pharmacologic nevus,[Q] which is pale because of vasoconstriction. Hence nevus depigmentosus becomes red with rubbing; nevus anemicus does not. Diascopy can also be used to differentiate between the two.

Therapy

Camouflage with cosmetics as for vitiligo.

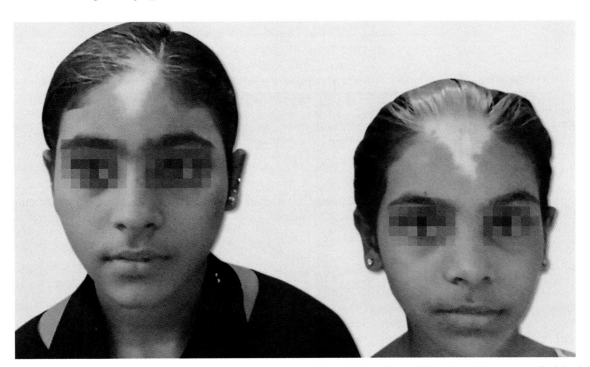

Fig. 18.5: White forelock and characteristic, triangular amelanotic patch on the mid-forehead in a case of piebaldism

18

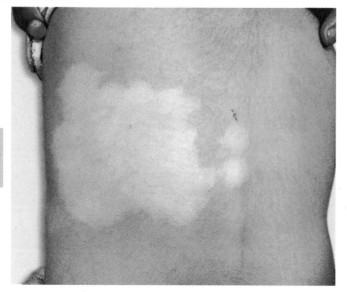

Fig. 18.6: Nevus depigmentosus. Hypomelanotic patch with a decrease but not absence of pigmentation. The segmental nature can be confused with hypomelanosis of Ito

Hypomelanosis of Ito

This is not a single disease, but is best described as a manifestation of genomic mosaicism, and thus associated with wide variety of underlying defects, including mental retardation and severe neurological defects.

Clinical Features

Widespread areas of hypopigmentation following Blaschko lines (Fig. 18.7); individual lesions identical to nevus depigmentosus.

Diagnostic Approach

History, extensive physical examination, cytogenetic testing.

Vitiligo

Acquired localized depigmentation of skin, hair, and occasionally mucosa, of unknown etiology, characterized by complete loss of melanocytes.[Q]

Pathogenesis

Etiology not well understood. Theories include:
- Autoimmune destruction of melanocytes.
- Neural pathways,[Q] because of relation to stress.
- Metabolic abnormalities: Accumulation of toxic metabolites.
- 'Self-destruct' action because of aberrant tetrahydrobiopterin and catecholamine synthesis.

Clinical Features

The most common presentation of vitiligo is totally amelanotic (i.e. milk- or chalk-white)[Q] macules or patches surrounded by normal skin. The borders are usually 'scalloping' convex, as if the depigmenting process were 'invading' the surrounding normally pigmented skin.

Lesions enlarge centrifugally overtime, though the rate may be slow or rapid.

Trichrome vitiligo[Q] features a hypopigmented zone between normal and totally depigmented skin (Fig. 18.8). The intermediate zone does not have a gradation of color from white to normal, but rather a fairly uniform hue. The number of melanocytes is also intermediate in this zone, suggesting slower centrifugal progression than in typical vitiligo.

In **quadrichrome vitiligo**[Q], a fourth darker color is present at sites of perifollicular repigmentation (Fig. 18.9).

Pentachrome vitiligo[Q] with five shades of color black, dark brown, medium brown (unaffected skin), tan and white has also been described.

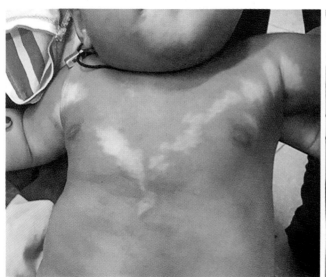
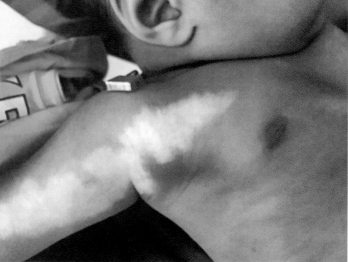

Fig. 18.7: Hypomelanosis of Ito: 'S' shaped whorled pattern of hypopigmented macules along lines of Blaschko in an infant

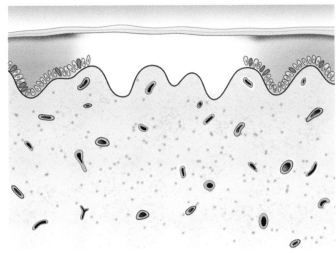

Fig. 18.8: Vitiligo: Epidermis—complete *absence* of pigment and melanocytes. Dermis—normal

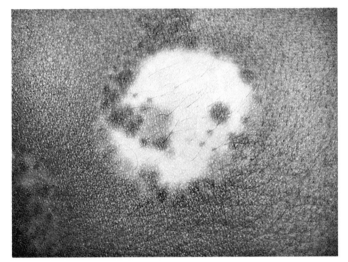

Fig. 18.9: A case of quadrichrome vitiligo. Apart from the three zones at the periphery (trichrome), there is perifollicular pigmentation. Note the presence of pigmented hair which is a good prognostic sign

One of the manifestations of vitiligo is the isomorphic Koebner phenomenon (IKP), characterized by the development of vitiligo at the sites of trauma (e.g. a laceration, burn or abrasion).[Q]

Classification

Degree of involvement highly variable, ranging from a few macules to almost complete depigmentation (Fig. 18.10) and some representative images are depicted in Fig. 18.11:

1. **Localized:**
   - *Focal*: One or more patches in the same area.
   - *Segmental*: Limited to a dermatome or Blaschko lines.
   - *Mucosal*: Only affected mucous membranes (rare).

2. **Generalized:**
   - *Acrofacial*: Distal extremities and facial, especially periorificial.
   - *Vulgaris* (*common*): Disseminated lesions without region predilection.
   - *Universal*: Complete or almost complete depigmentation.

Prognosis

Course highly variable and unpredictable. Spontaneous repigmentation that is cosmetically satisfactory for the patient occurs only rarely. Speckled repigmentation in a patch indicates that melanocytes from the outer root sheath of the hair follicle are producing melanin. Important to establish, if the vitiligo is stable or progressive, as this influences choice of therapy.

Laboratory evaluation: Thyroid function tests including autoantibodies, anti-parietal cell antibodies, total IgE, ANA, glucose.

Treatment

The cosmetic disfigurement from vitiligo can be devastating to affected patients specially in India. Treatment is often unsatisfactory for those with extensive and long-standing disease. In the white patches, pigment cells are only present deep in the hair follicles and treatments mostly try to get melanocytes to divide and migrate into affected skin. The established therapy of vitiligo can be described as varially effective but an overview is given in Table 18.2.

Table 18.2	Treatment of vitiligo		
Age	*Type*	*lst choice*	*2nd choice*
<5 years	Focal (<5%)	Topical steroids	UVB (311 nm), topical PUVA
	Segmental	Topical steroids +UVA	
	Widespread (>5%)		
>5 years	Focal (<5%)	Topical corticosteroids (+UVA)	UVB (311 nm), topical
	Segmental	Minigrafts	PUVA, oral PUVA (>12 years), minigrafts (if stable)
	Widespread (>5%)	UVB (311 nm)	
Adults	Eyelids, lips, nipples, penis	Minigrafts	Oral PUVA (>12 years), topical corticosteroids (+UVA)
	Resistant, involving >80%	Total depigmentation	

18

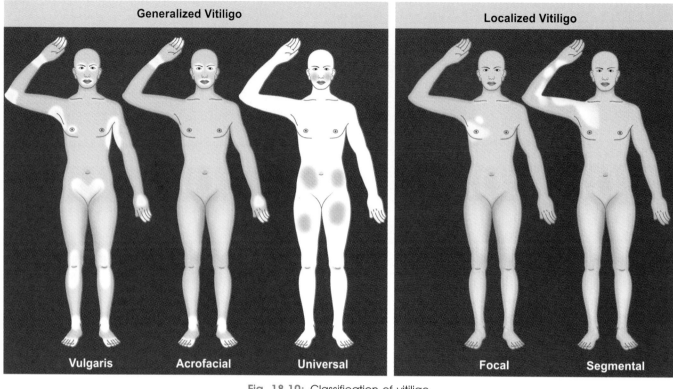

Fig. 18.10: Classification of vitiligo

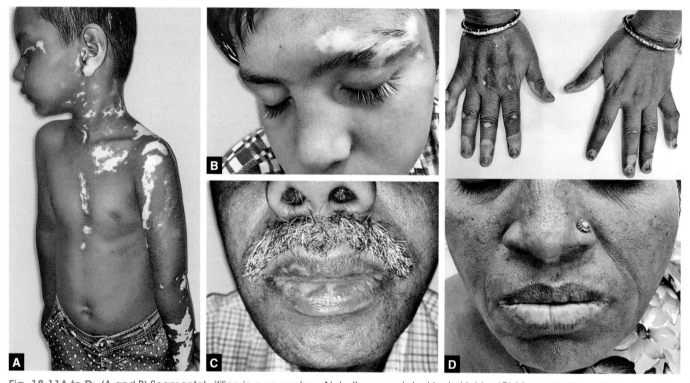

Fig. 18.11A to D: (A and B) Segmental vitiligo in a young boy. Note the associated leukotrichia; (C) Mucosal vitiligo; (D) Lip tip vitiligo

The *aims* of vitiligo *treatment* are repigmentation and stabilization of the depigmentation process. The choice of therapy depends on the extent, location, and activity of disease as well as the patient's age, skin type and motivation to undergo treatment. In general, a period of at least 2–3 months is required to determine whether a particular treatment is effective. The areas of the body that typically have the best response to medical therapy are the face, neck, mid-extremities and trunk, while the distal extremities and lips are the most resistant to treatment.

Medical therapy

1. *Corticosteroids*: This is administered in vitiligo affecting < 20% of the body surface area and can achieve >75% repigmentation with either class 1 (superpotent) or class 2–3 (high-potency) topical corticosteroids.

   Oral steroids has been used in a pulse form, but should be used *only* for cases with documented *instability* of disease. Though a common practice is to give betamethasone (betnesol 1 mg) twice a week, a safer alternative is to administer a short-acting steroid to avoid side effects. An option that we follow is to administer deflazaort (0.25–1 mg/kg) in an alternate day dosage.

2. *Topical drugs* like tacrolimus 0.1%, topical calcipotriol have been used and are useful, if given alternating with topical steroids to avoid side effects. Good results are obtained when these agents are used for facial lesions and/or combined with sun exposure.

3. *Topical PUVA* is an option but unless supervised tend to cause side effects. Topical 8 methoxyposralen can be administered but requires careful sunlight exposure after 20 minutes beginning with 1 minute alternate day, gradually increasing to 5 minutes over months.

4. *Oral PUVA*: This form of therapy was first used by the Egyptians and ancient Indians. In India, PUVA solution is still the most cost-effective option for treating vitiligo, which uses sunlight as the source of UV light.

Psoralen photochemotherapy involves the use of psoralens combined with UVA. The psoralen most commonly utilized is 8-methoxypsoralen (8-MOP, methoxsalen), though if sunlight is the source (PUVAsol) 4,5′, 8-trimethylpsoralen (TMP, trioxsalen) should be administered.

Oral PUVA treatments using 8-MOP (0.4–0.6 mg/kg) are typically administered two times weekly. For patients with vitiligo, the initial dose of UVA is usually 0.5–1.0 J/cm², which is gradually increased until minimal asymptomatic erythema of the involved skin occurs. A cheaper protocol, if sunlight is used, is to give TMP (Neosoralen Forte) 0.6 mg/kg/d and after 2 hours expose to sunlight (11 AM–3 PM) for 5–10 minutes on alternate days.

The response rate of PUVA is variable; although the majority of patients obtain cosmetically acceptable improvement, complete repigmentation is achieved in only a few patients. The total number of PUVA treatments required is generally between 50 and 300.

Phototherapy: NB-UVB (311 nm)^Q has become the gold standard of therapy for vitiligo. The mean repigmentation achieved is 41–68% with 3 to 6 months of therapy. It has consistently been shown to be effective, although is not curative.

Surgical modalities: Where pigment is absent in hair follicles or in skin without hair follicles, autologous skin grafts can be performed. The two most common procedures transplant either minigraft implants of 1 mm cylinders or epidermal roofs of suction-raised blisters from unaffected skin. Melanocyte and stem cell transplants, in which single cell suspensions are made from unaffected skin and applied to dermabraded vitiliginous skin, are also useful but are still being investigated.

Postinflammatory Hypopigmentation

This is a common disorder consequent to eczema, pityriasis versicolor, psoriasis, sarcoidosis and lupus erythematosus (Fig. 18.12). It may also result from cryotherapy or a burn. In general, the more severe the inflammation, the more likely pigment is to decrease rather than increase. These problems are most significant in darker-skinned individuals.

Pityriasis Alba

This disease mainly affects children between the age of 3 and 16 years and is clinically obvious in dark-skinned individuals.

Pathogenesis

The exact cause is unknown, though it is formally recognized as postinflammatory hypomelanosis.

The following factors have been incriminated in its pathogenesis:
- Excessive and unprotected sun exposure.
- Frequent bathing with hot water, frequent washing of face with soap-based cleansers.
- Cutaneous signs of atopy which are associated with pityriasis alba.

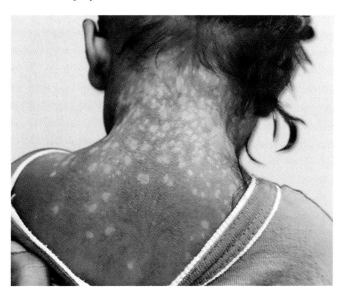

Fig. 18.12: Macular postinflammatory hypopigmentation consequent to pityriasis versicolor

Clinical Features

Pityriasis alba is characterized by multiple ill-defined hypopigmented macules and patches surmounted by fine,^{Q} 'bran-like' (pityron, Greek for bran) scales^Q (Fig. 18.13) and may persist for months or years before solving spontaneously. The early lesion is a mildly erythematous, slightly scaling patch with an indistinct elevated margin. In children, the face is the most common area of involvement, although it can occur at any location and may have one to several lesions. The lesion/patch appears to get worse and flakier in winters, when the skin is dry. However, it is more noticeable in the summer when the pale skin stands out against a tan.

Differential Diagnosis

Diagnosis is based on the clinical examination. A biopsy is rarely needed. In children, face is involved in one-third of cases of tinea versicolor. Thus, in doubtful cases, KOH skin scrapping can be performed. The white spots in vitiligo are distinguished by sharp demarcation, complete depigmentation and lack of scales.

Treatment

Treatment is not often necessary as spontaneous resolution occurs. Emollients can be used for the dry scaling, and 1% hydrocortisone cream is used for the inflammatory reaction.

Chemical Depigmentation

It usually occurs as an occupational leukoderma^Q in workers exposed to phenols.

P-tertiary-butylphenol^Q is the most important agent, especially in 'Bindi-induced' depigmentation. Other phenols that can cause this condition are monobenzy-lether of hydroquinone (used in treatment of

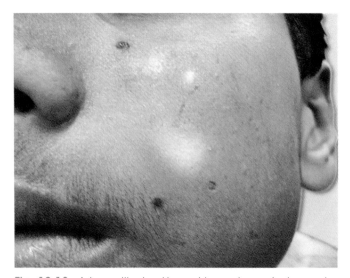

Fig. 18.13: A boy with dry skin and hypopigmented macules (pityriasis alba)

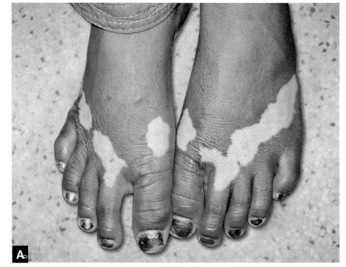

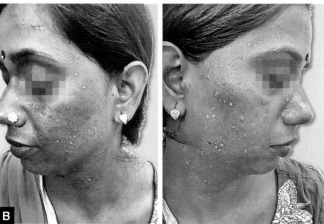

Fig. 18.14A and B: (A) Chemical leukoderma due to rubber chappals; (B) A patient with hydroquinone-induced depigmentation

hyperpigmentation) and 4-tertiarybutyl catechol. These cause a lethal effect on melanocytes.

The dorsa of hands and feet (Fig. 18.14A and B) are commonly affected though it can occur on sites that are not exposed to the chemical.

Idiopathic Guttate Hypomelanosis

Idiopathic guttate hypomelanosis (IGH—white spots on the arms and legs) is characterized by 2 to 5 mm porcelain white spots with sharply demarcated borders. They are located on the exposed areas of hands, forearms, and lower legs of middle-aged and older people (Fig. 18.15). The pathogenesis of IGH is not clearly known.

It could be a part of the normal ageing process. Chronic exposure to UV radiation can be areas another factor as lesions occur on sun-exposed sites.

DISORDERS OF HYPERPIGMENTATION

These disorders can be consequent to either an increase in melanocytes or overactive melanocytes (Fig. 18.16). These disorders can be classified clinically according

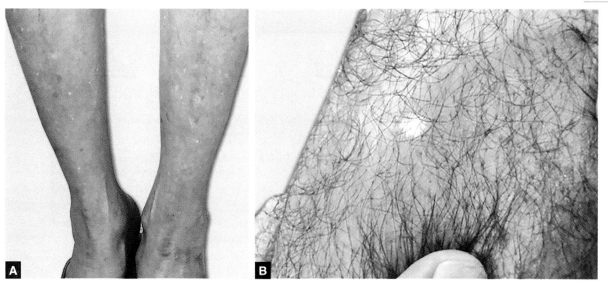

Fig. 18.15A and B: (A) Idiopathic guttate hypomelanosis sharply demarcated depigmented macules; (B) Idiopathic guttate hypomelanosis (IGH)

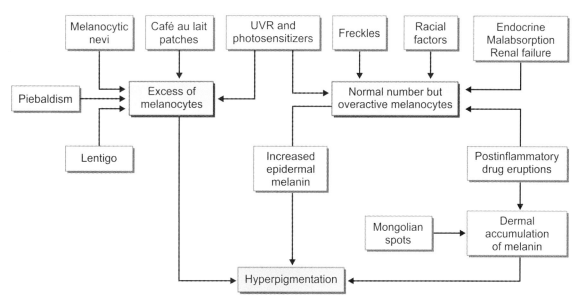

Fig. 18.16: Overview of hyperpigmentation disorders based on the main pathogenetic steps

to the distribution of the lesions and the onset (Fig. 18.17). A simpler method is to classify them on the basis of the color, that is brown color denotes epidermal disorders and bluish color is imparted by dermal disorders (Table 18.3).

Brown Hyperpigmentation

Café au lait Macule (CALM)

Circumscribed tan macule, usually present at birth (Fig. 18.18A and B).

Clinical features: Irregular tan macules and patches varying in size from 1 to many cm. More than five café au lait[Q] macules >1.5 cm suggest neurofibromatosis 1, but the macules can be sporadic or associated with a variety of syndromes.

Histology: Increased pigment in basal layer, normal number of melanocytes, giant melanosomes.

Freckles

Localized hyperpigmentation caused by sun exposure; waxes and wanes with seasons.

Clinical features: Much more common in skin types I and II; especially among redheads. Usually appear in childhood, flaring each summer; irregular brown macules of varying shades of tan and brown.

Histology: Increased melanin,[Q] normal melanocytes (Fig. 18.19A to C).

Differential diagnosis:

• Lentigo and junctional nevus can look like a freckle.

18

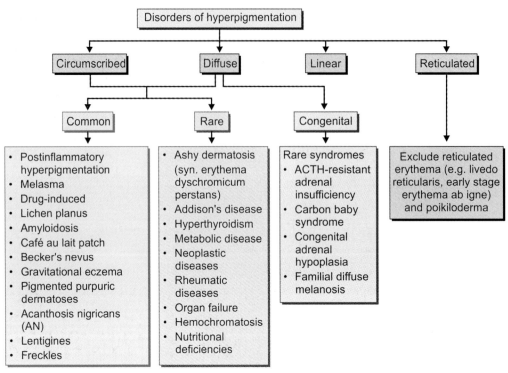

Fig. 18.17: A clinical classification of disorders of hyperpigmentation

Table 18.3	Classification based on predominant color	
Brown hyperpigmentation	Diffuse	**Metabolic:** Hemochromatosis, Wilson disease,[Q] porphyria, hepatic failure, renal failure, Addison disease, tumors producing MSH or ACTH, ACTH therapy.
		Drugs or chemicals: Antimalarials, arsenic, chlorpromazine, estrogens, minocycline,[Q] phenytoin, phenothiazine, psoralens (with UV); chemotherapy agents (busulfan, 5-fluorouracil, cyclophosphamide).
		Disease-related: Systemic sclerosis, Whipple disease, mycosis fungoides, Sézary syndrome
	Localized	• Tumors and nevi: Freckle, lentigo, syndromes with lentigines, café au lait macule, seborrheic keratosis, melanocytic nevus, Becker nevus
		• Melasma
		• Phototoxic dermatitis: Berloque dermatitis[Q]
		• Medications: Bleomycin (flagellate streaks[Q]), 5-fluorouracil (over veins)
		• Burns, ionizing radiation, trauma
		• Postinflammatory hyperpigmentation following dermatoses or trauma
Gray or blue hyperpigmentation	Diffuse	Hemochromatosis, metastatic melanoma with circulating melanin, bismuth, silver, gold, systemic ochronosis
	Localized	Nevus of Ota,[Q] nevus of Ito,[Q] Mongolian spot,[Q] blue nevus, incontinentia pigmenti, macular amyloidosis, fixed drug reaction, erythema dyschromicum perstans, exogenous ochronosis

- *Actinic lentigo*: This does not darken with sun exposure and is acquired later in life. In contrast, freckles darken after sun exposure and are present from early childhood.
- *Lentigo simplex*: This is acquired in childhood, but the lentigines are not confined to sun-exposed skin.
- *Junctional nevi*: Darker pigmentation and lack of change after sunlight exposure favor a diagnosis of junctional nevus.

Therapy: Sunscreens, light avoidance, as freckles are marker for increased risk of skin cancers.

Others believe that freckles should be accepted as normal. Prevention by sunlight avoidance is effective but not practical.

Lentigo

They are light or dark brown macules, ranging from 1 mm to 1 cm across. Although usually discrete, they

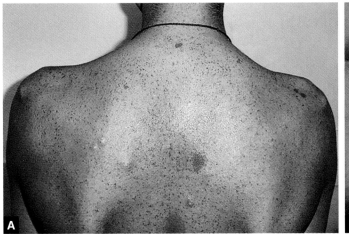
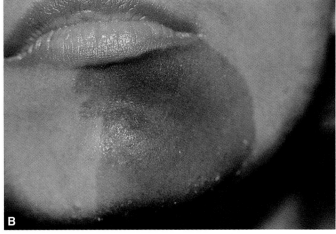

Fig. 18.18A and B: (A) A case of neurofibromatosis with a multiple brown CALM and multiple lentigines; (B) A single CALM on the face in a patient

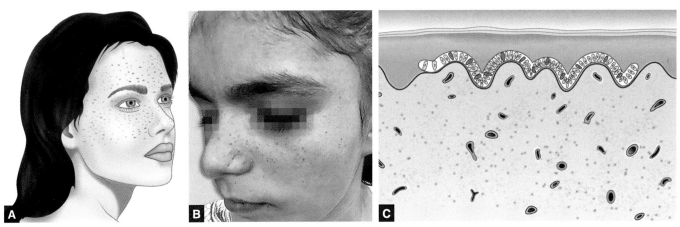

Fig. 18.19A to C: (A and B) Ephelides, also known as freckles, are most frequently encountered in fair-skinned individuals on sun-exposed skin. Sun exposure causes accentuation; (C) Histology of a freckle with increased melanin in the normal melanocytes

may have an irregular outline. Lentigo simplex presents with a dark brown small macule with increased melanocytes[Q] in the basal layer (Fig. 18.20A).

Simple lentigines arise most often in childhood as a few scattered lesions, often on areas not exposed to sun, including the mucous membranes (Fig. 18.20B).

Senile or *solar lentigines* are common after middle age on the backs of the hands (age spots or liver spots) and on the face.

Sometimes they are associated with systemic findings and a few important syndromes are:

- *Peutz-Jeghers syndrome*[Q]: Profuse lentigines on and around the lips, buccal mucosa, gums, hard palate, hands and feet. The syndrome is associated with polyposis of the small intestine, which may lead to recurrent intussusception and, rarely, to malignant transformation of the polyps. 10% of affected women have ovarian tumors.

- *Cronkhite-Canada syndrome*: This consists of multiple lentigines on the backs of the hands and a more diffuse pigmentation of the palms and

volar aspects of the fingers. Other findings include, gastrointestinal polyposis, alopecia and nail abnormalities.

- *Leopard syndrome*:[Q] This is an acronym for generalized lentiginosis associated with cardiac abnormalities demonstrated by ECG, ocular hypertelorism, pulmonary stenosis, abnormal genitalia, retardation of growth and deafness.

Differential diagnosis: In contrast to freckles, lentigines have increased *numbers* of *melanocytes* (Fig. 18.20A). They should be distinguished from freckles, from junctional melanocytic nevi and from a lentigo maligna. Lentigo maligna appears as an irregularly colored (varying shades of brown and black), irregularly bordered macule on sun-exposed regions of the body.

Treatment: Treatment is usually unnecessary and prevention, by sun avoidance and the use of sunscreens, is the best approach. Melanin-specific high energy lasers (e.g. Q-switched ruby laser, 694 nm; Q-switched alexandrite laser,[Q] 755 nm; Nd:YAG laser,[Q] 1064 nm) can be used.

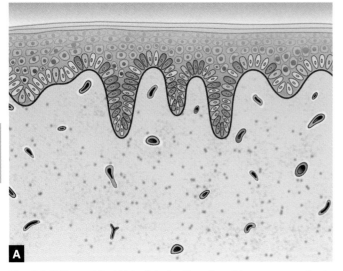
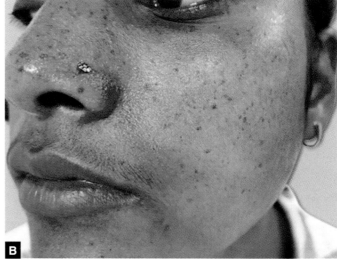

Fig. 18.20A and B: (A) Actinic lentigo. Small brown macules in sun-exposed skin of a middle-aged person. Epidermis—increased basal layer pigmentation resulting from increase in melanocytes and melanin; rete ridges are elongated; (B) Multiple lentigines in a female

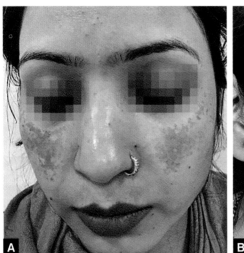
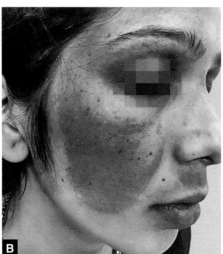
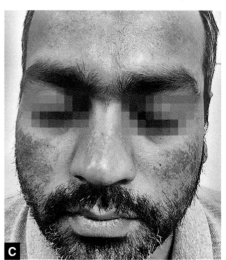

Fig. 18.21A to C: (A) A young female with melasma involving the malar area. The lesions started in pregnancy; (B) A 35-year-old female with malar and mandibular melasma. Also note the presence of freckles of cheeks; (C) Malar melasma in a 35-year-old male. Melasma is rare in men. Unlike females, hormones play little role in pathogenesis. UV light and mustard oil are implicated as causative factors in male melasma

Topical therapies are also effective for lightening lentigines such as daily application of 0.1% tretinoin cream, 2–4% hydroquinone or a combination of these with or without a retinoid, alpha-hydroxy acid, or topical corticosteroid.

Melasma

Synonyms: Chloasma, mask of pregnancy.[Q]

This is a common disorder with combined epidermal and dermal hyperpigmentation of forehead, cheeks, and perioral area[Q] (Fig. 18.21A to C).

Pathogenesis: Risk factors include:
- Sun exposure
- Pregnancy[Q]
- Use of oral contraceptives[Q] (or tumors secreting estrogens)
- Rarely caused by phenytoin

The exact cause of melasma is unknown. The theory is that the melanocytes in the affected skin produce greater amounts of melanin than they do in the uninvolved skin. This hyperfunctioning of the melanocytes is thought to be triggered by UV exposure,[Q] hormonal or other systemic conditions such as thyroid disease. These stimuli can cause increased levels of nitric oxide, which stimulates tyrosinase activity, causing increased localized melanin production.

Clinical features: Irregular brown hyperpigmentation, sometimes with blue tones, often speckled.

Sometimes mask-like pattern. Typically worsens with sun exposure.

Three patterns of hypermelanosis are observed and are described as centrofacial, malar, and mandibular. The central facial pattern is the most common[Q], affecting the forehead, cheeks, nose, upper lip, and chin. The malar and mandibular patterns exclusively affect the cheeks, nose, and the mandible.

The melanocytes in the areas of involvement are increased in number as well as in activity, producing a greater number of melanosomes.

Therapy: It is difficult to treat melasma as the melanin is present at varying depths in the dermis and epidermis. Also minor sun exposure can reactivate the process which is an issue in India. Any treatment regimen must include strict sun avoidance, including broad-spectrum sunscreen and hats.

> • Despite advanced and expensive therapies, melasma is often recalcitrant and recurrent.
> • Caution should be used as over treatment or aggressive therapies that cause inflammation, may in turn cause more hyperpigmentation, specially in Indian skin.

1. *Topical agents*: HQ (hydroquinone[Q]) is useful and the optimal effect is achieved with preparations containing 2–5% hydroquinone applied for 6–10 weeks. After this, maintenance treatment should be with preparations containing no more than 2% hydroquinone. Commonly the hydroquinone may be combined with a topical steroid and a retinoid for short-term use. Caution should be observed as prolonged unsupervised application of HQ can cause exogenous ochronosis.

   Fluocinolone 0.01% plus hydroquinone 4% plus tretinoin 0.05% solution is a commonly used preparartion (modified Kligman regimen[Q]).

   Other topical lightening agents include tyrosinase inhibitors such as kojic acid and azelaic acid.

2. *Superficial chemical peels[Q]* help to remove epidermal melanin and are thus a useful adjunct to topical treatment. Glycolic acid peels are the most efficacious of the peeling agents but require expertise for proper application and in Indian skin salicylic acid peels are better.

3. Lasers have a variable effect (Q-switched ruby, Q-switched alexandrite, CO_2 and Er:YAG,) and in Indian skin can worsen melasma and result in dyspigmentation. New fractionated lasers show promising results but not in Indian skin.

Laser treatment has not been consistently effective, and the side effects may be greater than the benefits.

Becker's Nevus

Becker's nevus is a relatively common anomaly affecting 0.5% of young men and women.

Clinical features

Site: Usually occurs in the scapular region.[Q] It can occur on other sites of the body like face, neck, and distal extremities.

It usually develops in adolescence as an irregular asymmetrical area of hyperpigmentation which may later thicken and develop coarse dark hairs[Q] (Fig. 18.22). The prominence in adolescence with increased hair growth (hypertrichosis) shows that it is androgen dependent.

Treatment: It can be treated with[Q] switched Nd:YAG or alexandrite laser.

Blue and Gray Hyperpigmentation

Erythema Dyschromicum Perstans/Ashy Dermatosis

This is a poorly understood dermatosis with inflammatory phase and late postinflammatory dermal melanosis. It is often confused with lichen planus pigmentosus, which some authors believe to be the same entity.

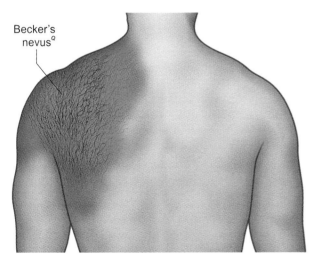

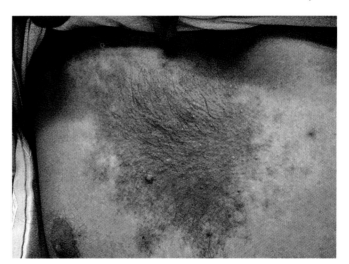

Fig. 18.22: Very large, light brown to black patch (Becker's nevus) with increased amount of darker hair growth

18

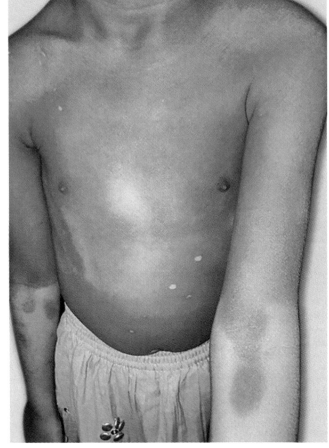

Fig. 18.23: Bluish macule on the trunk in a child with EDP

Clinical features: Early lesions are erythematous macules favoring the trunk; they slowly evolve into blue-gray (ashy) macules with indistinct borders, often coalesce (Fig. 18.23). Totally asymptomatic.

Therapy: Nothing well established; both chloroquine and PUVA have proponents.

Deposition of Metallic Salts/Drugs

A number of heavy metals can be deposited in the skin, usually imparting various shades of blue and gray. The most common agents are shown in Table 18.4. Hyperpigmentation caused by medications is also listed in Table 18.5.

Exogenous Ochronosis (EO)

EO is a cutaneous disorder that occurs due to use of chemical substances on the face. It is synonymous with endogenous ochronosis.

Clinical findings: EO is characterized by the presence of asymptomatic bilaterally symmetrical speckled blue black to gray brown macules (Fig. 18.24) on the face mainly the malar areas, lower cheeks, temples and neck. In early stages, it resembles melasma.

EO most commonly occurs due to use of topical hydroquinone (used as a skin lightening agent) but

Table 18.4	Hyperpigmentation caused by heavy metals[Q]	
Silver	Nose drops, silver nitrate sticks	Argyria
Gold	Arthritis medication	Chrysiasis
Iron	Multiple blood transfusions, excessive ingestion	Siderosis
Arsenic	Fowler solution, skin tonics, old insecticides	Arsenical melanosis
Lead	Paints with lead	Plumbism with gingival[Q] hyperpigmentation

Table 18.5	Pigmentation due to drugs[Q]
Amiodarone	Diffuse blue-gray hyperpigmentation in sun-exposed areas[Q]
Minocycline	• Dark blue to black macules in acne scars or over cysts • Hyperpigmented patches in light-exposed areas (slowly reversible)[Q] • Hyperpigmentation of mucosal surfaces, especially mouth
Antimalarials	Gray hyperpigmentation, especially facial and pretibial, as well as on gingiva and palate.
Chemotherapy agents	• Generalized hyperpigmentation: 5-fluorouracil • Localized hyperpigmentation: Bleomycin, cyclophosphamide • Linear hyperpigmentation: 5-Fluorouracil (over veins), bleomycin (flagellate, presumably following scratching)

has also been described with use of phenol, resorcinol, quinine, mercury, picric acid and oral antimalarials.

The cause is competitive inhibition of the enzyme homogentisic oxidase by hydroquinone leading to accumulation of homogentisic acid and its metabolic products that polymerise to form the ochronotic pigment in the papillary dermis.

Treatment: Ideal therapy is with a laser.

Dermal Melanocytosis

Blue-gray usually congenital lesions contain dermal melanocytes. The deeper location of the melanin is responsible for the blue-gray-black tones.

Nevus of Ota[Q]: It is a dermal melanocytic[Q] hamartoma that presents as bluish-brown patchy hyperpigmentation on the face along the first or second branches of the trigeminal nerve (Fig. 18.25).

Clinical features: Lesions are usually present at birth or occur during the first year of life. It can also appear around puberty.

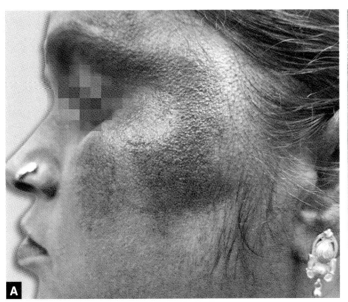
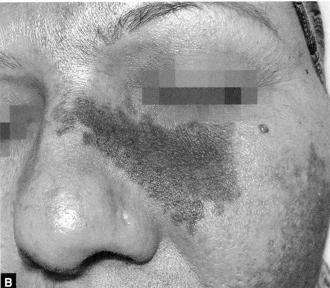

Fig. 18.24A and B: Blue-gray pigmentation: (A) Ochronosis due to use of fairness creams; (B) A case of localized ochronosis due to use of HQ 4%

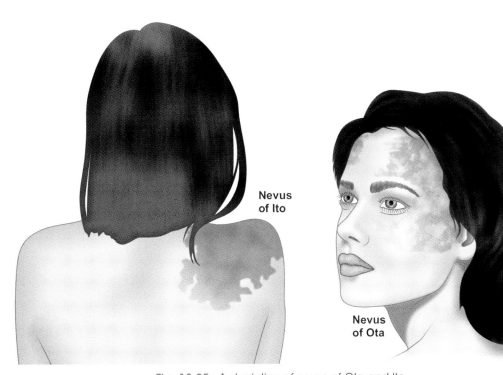

Nevus of Ito

Nevus of Ota

Fig. 18.25: A depiction of nevus of Ota and Ito

The condition is characterized by unilateral, irregular, patchy bluish gray to brown hyperpigmentation in the periorbital region, temple, malar prominence, nose and forehead (Fig. 18.26).

Ocular involvement occurs in 60% of cases in the form of scleral and conjunctival pigmentation. Rarely, bilateral lesions can occur.

Treatment: Q-switched lasers[Q] are the mainstay of treatment but results depend on the age of the patient and the depth of pigmentation.

Mongolian spot: A blue-gray patch over the sacrum,[Q] which is present in 90% of Asian, but uncommon in white babies; it tends to regress.

Nevus of Ito: Unilateral blue-gray patch on the shoulder and scapular region; also occurs most frequently in Asians.

MELANOCYTIC NEVI AND THEIR VARIANTS

A nevus (mole) is a benign neoplasm of pigment-forming cells, the nevus cell. In this section, nevus is used to mean melanocytic nevus. They may be

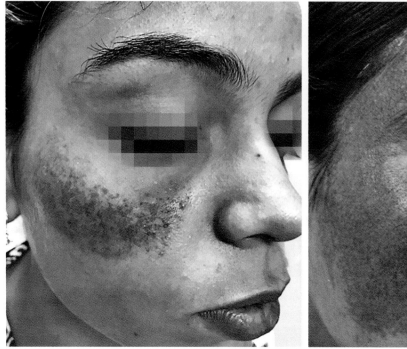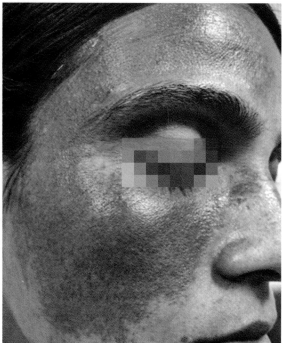

Fig. 18.26: Female patients with nevus of Ota

congenital or acquired. Most appear at puberty or in young adulthood. They may flare during pregnancy. Nevus cells are derived from the neural crest.^{Q} Morphologically, one can recognize the nevus cell because it has no dendritic processes and groups together in nests within the epidermis and dermis (Fig. 18.27).

An average individual has 10–50 nevi, some of which regress. These nevi are symmetrical and regular, tan, brown or black macules or papules, usually less than 5 mm in diameter.

Nevi are traditionally classified on their histological pattern:
- Junctional nevi—melanocytes at the dermal–epidermal junction (DEJ)
- Dermal nevus—melanocytes in the dermis
- Compound nevus—melanocytes in both sites.

There are numerous other clinical variants which are described as special type of nevi.

Clinical Features of Benign Nevi

The junctional nevus is a light to dark brown macule. (Fig. 18.28A).

Compound and intradermal nevi are flesh-colored or brown, smooth- or rough-surfaced papules that occur in older children and adults (Fig. 18.28B and C).

Nevi can occur anywhere on the body, but are increased on areas of sun exposure. The lesions have a continued progression thus they begin as junctional nevi, and in adolescence and adulthood, some (not all) of the nevus cells migrate downward into the dermis

forming the compound nevi and then finally in adulthood, these nevi may continue to migrate so that all of the nevus cells relocated in the dermis (to form the intradermal nevi).

> The clinical appearance of benign nevi changes with aging and they involute or fade around the sixth or seventh decade.

Special Types of Nevi

1. Spitz
2. Blue
3. Dysplastic/atypical
4. Congenital
5. Halo nevi

Spitz: The Spitz nevus (benign juvenile melanoma) is composed of spindle and epithelioid nevus cells. It is a smooth, round, slightly scaling, pink nodule that occurs most frequently in children (Fig. 18.29). The most important aspect of dealing with this lesion is to recognize that it is a nevus and not a melanoma, and to avoid extensive surgical intervention.

Blue nevi are small, steel-blue macules, papules, and nodules that usually begin early in life. Their importance in diagnosis is their similar appearance to nodular melanoma. If any doubt exists, a biopsy should be performed.

Congenital nevi (Fig. 18.30) are present at birth or shortly thereafter; they are usually elevated and have uniform, dark brown pigmentation with discrete borders.^{Q} Of newborns, 1% have congenital nevi. Often they contain hairs (Fig. 18.31).

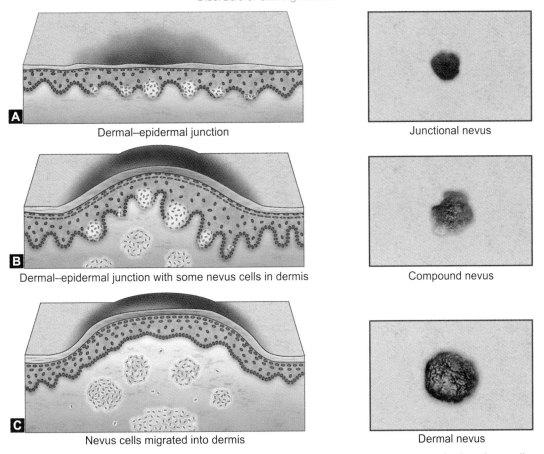

Fig. 18.27A to C: A depiction of the clinic histological appearance of common acquired melanocytic nevi

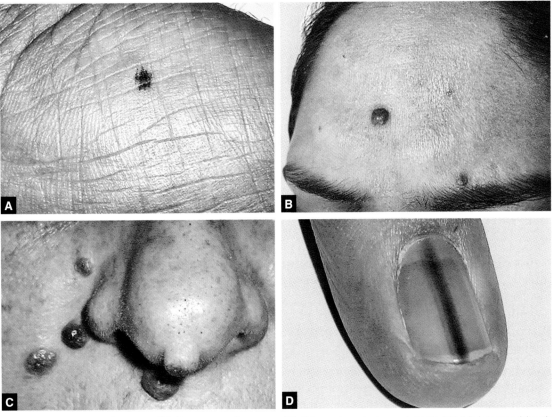

Fig. 18.28A to D: (A) Junctional nevus; (B) Compound nevus; (C) Skin-colored dermal nevi; (D) Melanonychia striata due to junctional nevus

18

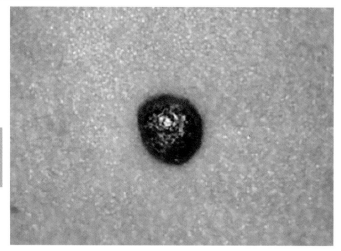

Fig. 18.29: Spitz nevus presenting as a solitary dome-shaped, hyperpigmented nodule

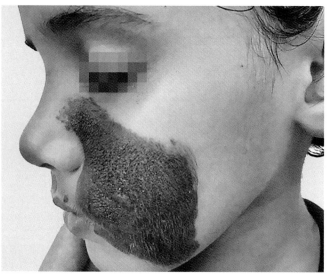

Fig. 18.30: An intermediate-sized congenital melanocytic nevus in a 6-year-old girl. Note the hair growth on the lesion

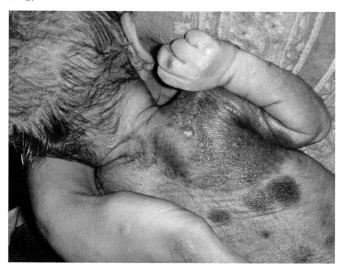

Fig. 18.31: Congenital nevus with thickening of skin and hypertrichosis

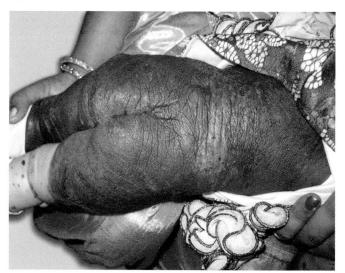

Fig. 18.32: Bathing trunk nevus^Q

They have been divided into three types—small (<1.5 cm in diameter}, medium (1.5–20 cm), and large (>20 cm). Congenital nevi are melanoma precursors.^Q The risk is very small for small lesions (<1%) but large congenital nevi (>20 cm across or covering 5% of body area) have a 6 to 12% chance of developing into a malignant melanoma.^Q

Giant lesions covering a large portion of the body (bathing trunk nevus) including the dorsal midline are at risk for neurocutaneous melanosis (Fig. 18.32).

Small congenital nevi have little to no increased risk of transformation into melanoma and, therefore, do not need to be removed prophylactically.

Dysplastic nevi: Occasionally, patients have multiple large atypical nevi that continue to develop throughout life. Clinically, the *atypical mole* is more than 5 mm, is variegated in color with a pink background, and has an irregular, indistinct border.

Atypical moles were initially recognized as markers for increased risk of melanoma in family members with inherited malignant melanoma, the familial atypical mole and melanoma syndrome or dysplastic nevus syndrome. In these families, virtually all members with atypical moles developed a melanoma in their lifetime, whereas family members without atypical moles did not.

Subsequently, investigators discovered that approximately 5% of the healthy Caucasian population in the United States has atypical moles. The risk of developing a melanoma in these individuals, is unclear, and in majority of them, melanoma never develops.

The clinical^Q **ABCDE** rule is helpful for separating unequivocally benign nevi from dysplastic or atypical nevi and melanomas. It is not helpful for separating the latter two groups. The rule is as follows (Fig. 18.33):

• **A**symmetry
• **B**order (irregular, leakage of pigment)

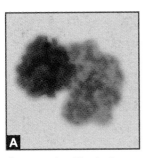

Asymmetry: The lesion lacks a mirror image on any plane

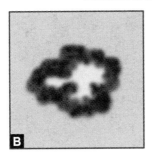

Border: The margins of the lesion are irregular

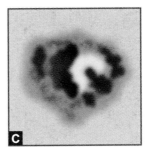

Color: Multiple colors are present in the lesion

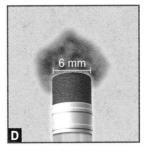

Diameter: Lesions larger than 6 mm are suspect

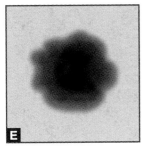

Evolving: The lesion is changing over time

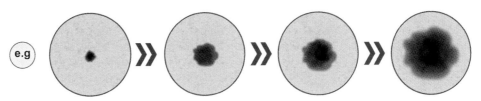

Fig. 18.33A to E: A depiction of the ABCDE rule for diagnosing cases of melanoma

- **C**olor (multiple colors)
- **D**iameter (>5 mm).

Some experts add the 'E' to this rule.

> Another method of identifying a atypical nevi is the so-called 'ugly duckling sign'[Q], that is identifying a mole that is different from the others.

Halo nevus[Q]: Also known as Sutton nevus, this lesion is surrounded by a halo of depigmentation (Fig. 18.34). The nevus may become pale or even disappear. Adults with multiple halo nevi should be checked for a melanoma, which may trigger an antimelanocyte immune response.

Treatment

In Indian skin, the risk of melanoma is negligible. There is no indication to remove common melanocytic nevi (moles) unless they are irritated. But in most clinical set ups, removal of moles is possibly the commonest cosmetic procedure and most patients who ask for removal do it for no medical reason. We have analysed our data and found that for small moles possibly lasers (ablative) may be useful but for a larger lesion, RF is a good option. In ideal situations, the excised lesion should be analysed histologically for melanoma.

For congenital nevi, a staged excision is advisable. For dysplastic nevi, a histological evaluation in necessary.

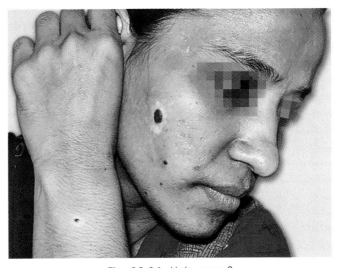

Fig. 18.34: Halo nevus[Q]

MALIGNANT MELANOMA

Malignant melanoma is a cancerous neoplasm of pigment-forming cells, melanocytes, and nevus cells.

Epidemiology

Its incidence is 15–20:100 000 in Northern Europe and USA; this is a lifetime risk of developing melanoma of 2%. The risk is inversely related to skin color.

The peak age is around 60 years but this varies with the type of melanoma; superficial spreading melanoma appears much sooner than lentigo maligna melanoma. Acrolentiginous melanoma is equally common in all races, and thus the most common melanoma of darker individuals.[Q]

Over half of all melanomas are <0.75 mm thick, so that >95% of patients never develop metastases.

Pathogenesis

A brief overview is given here (Fig. 18.35A), though in pigmented skin, the incidence is less. Thus most of these factors apply largely to Caucasian skin.

- *Both UVB and UVA* increase the risk of melanoma. Intermittent excessive exposure—such as bad sunburns during childhood—correlates better with superficial spreading and nodular melanoma, while chronic long-term exposure fits with lentigo maligna melanoma.
- *Genetic contributions* are usually complex. For example, pale-skinned individuals with mutations in the MCR1 gene have a 17-fold increased risk of developing a melanoma with BRAF mutation.

> Familial atypical mole and melanoma syndrome should be suspected:
> 1. Personal or family history of melanoma and
> 2. Numerous (>50) atypical nevi

- *Melanoma genes*: A series of gene mutations have been associated with melanoma. Mutations involve either signal transduction of a tyrosine kinase receptor (c-Kit, EGFR. FGFR, ErbB-2) (Fig. 18.35B).

Genetic testing may be considered when three family members have melanoma; an individual has three melanomas, or three cancer events (melanoma or pancreatic cancer) occur in a family.

> Rule of 3s for familial melanoma genetic testing:
> - 3 melanomas in a family,
> - 3 melanomas in an individual,
> - 3 cancers (melanoma or pancreatic) in a family.

Clinical Features

The various types are depicted in Table 18.6 and Fig. 18.36.

SSM (Fig. 18.36A): The most common type of melanoma is the superficial spreading melanoma.[Q] This lesion is irregular in color (red, white, black, dark brown, and blue), surface (macule, papule, or nodule), and border (notched), and may occur anywhere on the body. It is found most frequently on the upper back in males, and on the upper back and lower legs in females.

Nodular melanoma (Fig. 18.36B and D) is a rapidly growing, blue-black, smooth or eroded nodule. It occurs anywhere on the body. It begins in the vertical growth phase, so is less likely to be diagnosed in a premetastatic stage.

Lentigo maligna melanoma (Fig. 18.36C) occurs on sun-exposed skin, especially the head and neck. It is

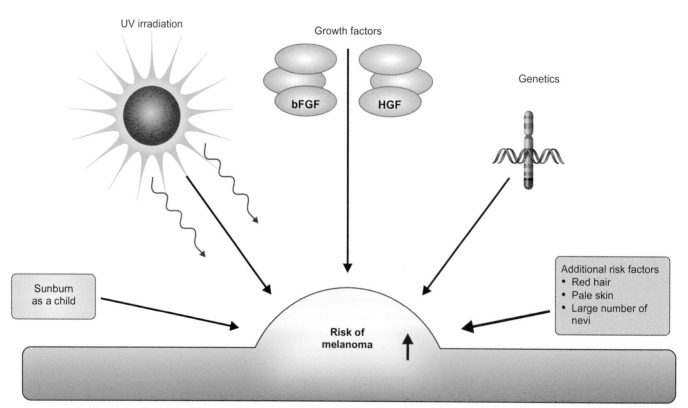

Fig. 18.35A: Overview of the factors that cause melanoma

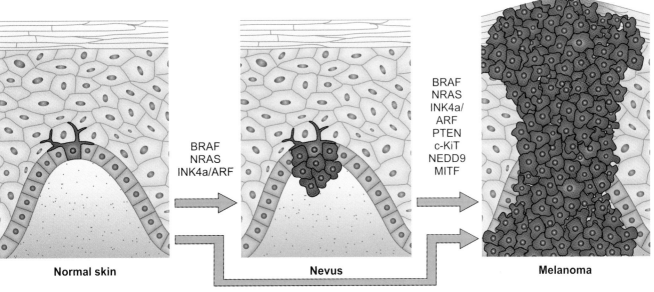

Fig. 18.35B: Gene mutation that predict melanoma

Table 18.6 Clinical features of melanoma

Type	Location	Median age (years)	Premetastatic	Frequency (%)[a]	Ethnicity
Lentigo maligna	Sun-exposed surfaces (head, neck)	70	5–15 years	10	Caucasian
Superficial spreading	All surfaces (back, legs)	47	1–7 years	27	Caucasian
Nodular	All surfaces	50	Months to 2 years	9	Caucasian
Acral lentiginous	Palms, soles, nail beds	61	Months to 8 years	1	Blacks, Asian

[a]53% of melanomas are unclassified.

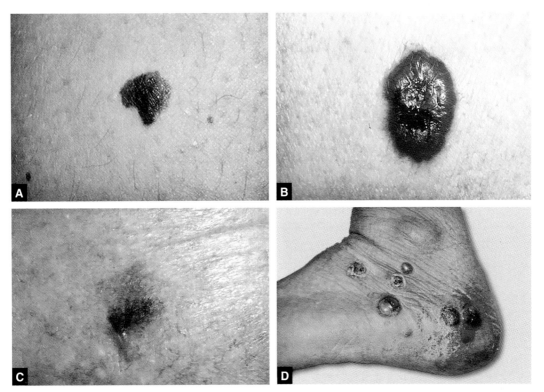

Fig. 18.36A to D: (A) Superficial spreading melanoma *in situ*; (B) Nodular malignant melanoma; (C) Lentigo maligna presenting as a hyperpigmented lesion with irregular borders located on the forehead; (D) Acral variant

multicolored, with dark brown, black, red, white, and blue hues, and it is elevated in areas. It is preceded by lentigo maligna (*in situ* melanoma[Q]), which extends peripherally and is an unevenly pigmented, dark brown and black macule. Lentigo maligna often reaches a diameter of 5 to 7 cm before showing signs of invasion.

Acral lentiginous melanoma (Fig. 18.36E) occurs on the palms, soles, and distal portion of the toes or fingers. It is an irregular, enlarging, black growth similar to a lentigo maligna melanoma. The vertical growth phase in this type of melanoma can be deceptive, showing only a small degree of papular elevation associated with a deep component. In contrast to the other melanomas, acral lentiginous melanoma is most frequent in the Black and Asian populations.[Q]

Diagnosis

Biopsy: All suspicious pigmented lesions must undergo biopsy, by excision with narrow 2 to 3 mm margins of normal skin or by deep shave biopsy. Definitive treatment by wide surgical excision should not be undertaken until confirmation of malignant melanoma has been made histologically.[Q]

Clark and Breslow[Q] correlated survival with tumor thickness. Breslow, using an ocular micrometer, measured tumor thickness from the stratum granulosum to the depth of invasion.[Q] These measurements are reproducible and are the preferred method of calculating tumor thickness and, thus, of predicting 5-year survival (Fig. 18.37).

Investigative approach: This varies with the type of melanoma. The usual approach is to excise a suspicious lesion, get a histological diagnosis and then plan the definitive surgery.[Q]

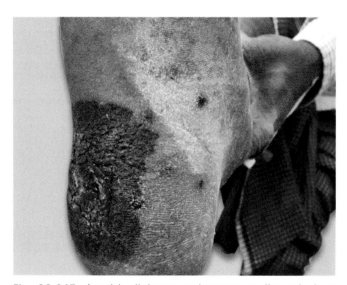

Fig. 18.36E: Acral lentiginous melanoma on the sole in a 45-year-old male

Breslow's[Q] thickness (mm)
5-year survival (%)
Granular layer
Epidermis
Papillary dermis
Reticular dermis
Subcutaneous fat
1.0
2.25
3.0
99
75
44
22

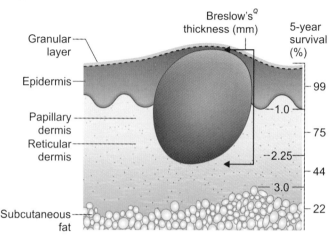

Fig. 18.37: Survival is related to depth of invasion (thickness measured in millimeters)

Box 18.1	Prognostic factors in melanoma[Q]

- Tumor depth (TD) in mm
- Ulceration
- Mitoses in thin melanomas
- Invasion of lymphatics or blood vessels by tumor cells
- Positive sentinel lymph node biopsy

An investigative approach is detailed in Fig. 18.38.

The various prognostic factors based on the investigations are listed in Box 18.1.

Therapy

The survival of patients with malignant melanoma depends on early diagnosis, when surgical excision is often curative. An overview of the therapy is given in Fig. 18.39. Radiolymphatic sentinel node mapping and biopsy have been used for melanomas larger than 1 mm in thickness in patients with clinically negative lymph nodes.

Surgical Excision

The margin of normal skin excised around the melanoma increases with the depth of invasion, or thickness: *in situ*,

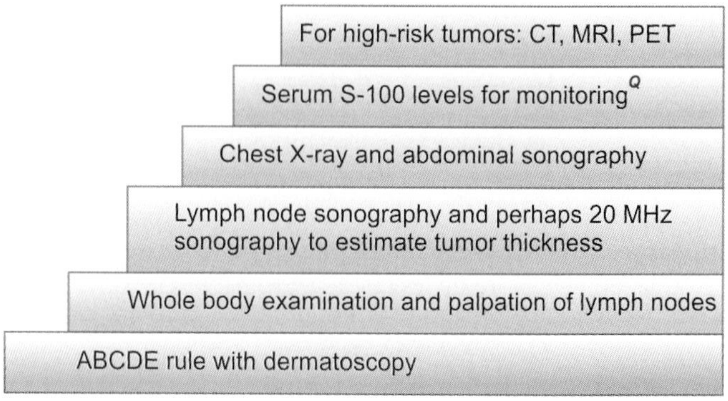

For high-risk tumors: CT, MRI, PET
Serum S-100 levels for monitoring[Q]
Chest X-ray and abdominal sonography
Lymph node sonography and perhaps 20 MHz sonography to estimate tumor thickness
Whole body examination and palpation of lymph nodes
ABCDE rule with dermatoscopy

Fig. 18.38: An investigative approach in melanoma

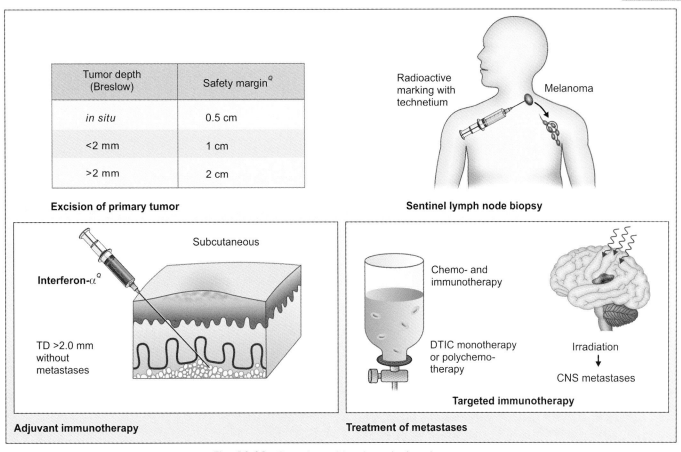

Tumor depth (Breslow)	Safety margin^Q
in situ	0.5 cm
<2 mm	1 cm
>2 mm	2 cm

Excision of primary tumor

Radioactive marking with technetium

Melanoma

Sentinel lymph node biopsy

Interferon-α^Q

Subcutaneous

TD >2.0 mm without metastases

Adjuvant immunotherapy

Chemo- and immunotherapy

DTIC monotherapy or polychemo-therapy

Irradiation

↓

CNS metastases

Targeted immunotherapy

Treatment of metastases

Fig. 18.39: Overview of treatment of melanoma

Box 18.2 | **Oncotherapy for metastasis**

- Immunotherapy—interferon α-2b, interleukin, ipilimumab, nivolumab, pembrolizumab
- Kinase inhibitors—vemurafenib, dabrafenib, trametinib, cobimetinib
- Oncolytic virus—talimogene laherparepvec

0.5 cm margin; thickness less than 2 mm, 1 cm margin; thickness more than 2 mm, 2 cm margin.

Oncological Therapy

Numerous medical agents have been tried largely for a malignant melanoma that has metastasized, and is best managed by a medical oncologist familiar with these agents—chemotherapy, radiation, immuno-therapy, kinase inhibitors, and oncolytic virus (Box 18.2).

Radiation therapy is used for palliation of bone and brain metastasis, and when lentigo maligna is so large that surgical removal is technically difficult.

Benign and Malignant Tumors

SKIN TUMORS

Skin tumors, represent a diverse group of varied disorders, which have been classified in various ways, but a simple method is by dividing the entities into the source of origin, epidermal, dermal and the potential for malignancy (Table 19.1).

Table 19.1	Classification of skin tumors	
	Epidermis and appendages	**Dermis**
Benign	• Seborrheic keratosis • Skin tag • Beckers nevus • Linear epidermal nevus • Melanocytic nevus • Sebaceous nevus • Syringoma • Epidermal/pilar cyst • Milium • Chondrodermatitis Nodularis helicis	• Hemangioma • Lymphangioma • Glomus tumor • Pyogenic granuloma • Dermatofibroma • Neurofibroma • Neuroma • Keloid • Lipoma • Mastocytosis
Premalignant	• Actinic keratosis • Bowen's disease	Large plaque parapsoriasis
Malignant	• Basal cell carcinoma • Squamous cell carcinoma • Malignant melanoma • Paget's disease of the nipple	• Mycosis fungoides • B cell Lymphoma • Kaposi's sarcoma • Dermatofibro-sarcoma protuberans • Merkel cell carcinoma • Metastases

The term **nevus** refers to a skin lesion that has a localized excess of one or more types of cell in a normal cell site. Nevi may be composed mostly of keratinocytes (e.g. in epidermal nevi), melanocytes (e.g. in congenital melanocytic nevi), connective tissue elements (e.g. in connective tissue nevi) and a mixture of epithelial and connective tissue elements (e.g. in sebaceous nevi). In this context, such nevi are known as hamartomas or malformations.

TUMORS OF THE EPIDERMIS

Benign Disorders of the Epidermis

Seborrheic Keratosis
(Basal Cell Papilloma, Seborrheic Wart)

This is a common benign epidermal tumor, and is seen commonly in elderly patients or those exposed to sunlight.

The exact cause is unknown but include, an autosomal dominant inheritance, following an inflammatory dermatosis or uncommonly a sudden eruption of hundreds of itchy lesions is associated with an internal neoplasm (Leser-Trelat sign),[Q] usually in adenocarcinoma of the gastrointestinal tract.

Clinical features: Seborrheic keratoses usually arise after the age of 50 years, but flat lesions may be visible earlier. They are seen commonly on the face and trunk.

A distinctive 'stuck-on' appearance is classic and the lesions may be flat, raised, filiform or pedunculated; the surface may be smooth or verrucous. The surface may have greasy scaling and scattered keratin plugs ('currant bun' appearance). They are largely benign in nature (Fig. 19.1).

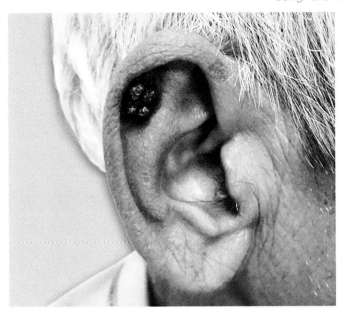

Fig. 19.1: Hyperpigmented verrucous papules on the pinna in an elderly male. Note the **'stuck on'** appearance seborrheic keratosis

Dermatosis papulosa nigra: It is a common variant of seborrheic keratoses affecting black adults. Multiple pigmented papules, just raised or filiform, appear on the face and neck but may extend to the trunk (Fig. 19.2). The condition may be inherited as an autosomal dominant trait.

Stucco keratosis: This variant of seborrheic keratoses is seen most often around the ankles after the age of 50. They have a similar 'stuck on' appearance to seborrheic

warts and are small (1–2 mm) white keratotic papules that are easily lifted off the skin with a finger nail, without bleeding.

Investigation: Biopsy is needed only in rare cases.

Treatment: Seborrheic keratoses can be left untreated, but those that are ugly or easily traumatized ones can be removed with a curette or by destructive means including cryotherapy and electrodessication.

Skin Tags (Acrochordon)

These common benign outgrowths of skin affect mainly the middle-aged and elderly. There is no known cause but sometimes it is familial. Skin tags are most commonly seen in obese individuals,[Q] acanthosis nigricans or in diabetic patients.[Q]

Clinical features: Skin tags are soft skin-colored or pigmented pedunculated papules commonly found around the neck and within the major flexures (Fig. 19.3).

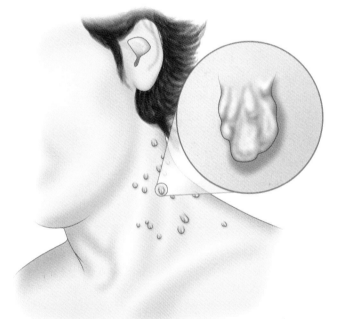

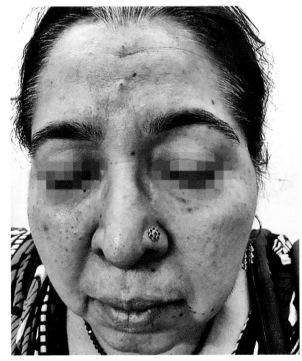

Fig. 19.2: Dermatosis papulosa nigra: Multiple hyperpigmented papules over the face in a 50-year-old female. This is a clinical variant of seborrheic keratoses

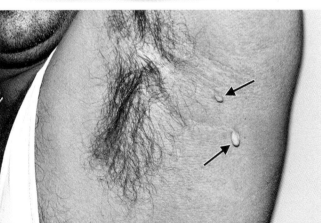

Fig. 19.3: Skin tags are benign outgrowth of skin seen commonly on the flexures in obese individuals

Treatment: Small lesions can be snipped off with fine scissors, frozen with liquid nitrogen or destroyed by electrocautery. There is no way of preventing new ones from developing.

Melanocytic Nevi

Melanocytic nevi (moles) are localized benign tumors of melanocytes. These have been discussed in detail in Chapter 18.

Epidermal Nevus

This lesion is an example of cutaneous mosaicism and so tends to follow Blaschko's lines[Q] (Fig. 19.4). Epidermal nevi are the prototype of cutaneous mosaicism (Fig. 19.5). A mutation in early embryonic life leads to a localized area of abnormal skin. The umbrella term 'epidermal nevus' is accepted although many skin components can be involved.

There are many different methods of classifying epidermal nevi but the two common ones are:

a. True epidermal nevi with only epidermal changes versus organoid nevi which also have dermal or adnexal involvement.

b. Hard or verrucous nevi versus soft or papillomatous nevi.

Clinical features and variants

• *Linear epidermal nevus*: An epidermal nevus is always present at birth, but sometimes not recognized as it may be flat, perhaps slightly pigmented, and only later become hyperkeratotic and raised (Fig. 19.6A). Soft and hard epidermal nevi can be distinguished; the former is papillomatous, similar to a skin tag or fleshy melanocytic nevus, while the latter is warty.

• *Nevus sebaceous* (Fig. 19.6B): These nevi usually occur on the scalp, with a bald patch at birth that becomes thicker and keratotic in puberty.[Q] Secondary benign neoplasms (trichoblastoma, syringocystadenoma papilliferum) can arise over time within a nevus sebaceous. Rarely, malignant transformation into a basal cell carcinoma can occur in adult life.

• *Becker nevus*[Q] (Fig. 19.6C): In this, there is a slightly hyperpigmented area, typically on the shoulder; at puberty it becomes hairy; patients may have proliferation of the arrector pili muscles (smooth muscle nevus) with frequent goose bumps.

• *Nevus comedonicus*: Many plugged follicular structures, resembling comedones of acne.

• *ILVEN*: ILVEN is an acronym for inflammatory linear verrucous epidermal nevus. ILVEN is exceptional in that it appears later in life.[Q] It is characterized by linear psoriasiform or dermatitis streaks, usually on extremities (Fig. 19.6D).

• *Epidermolytic nevus*: Verrucous nevus that is not clinically distinct but histopathology reveals epider-

molytic hyperkeratosis. Patients with cutaneous and gonadal mosaicism can then have a child with congenital bullous ichthyosiform erythroderma.[Q]

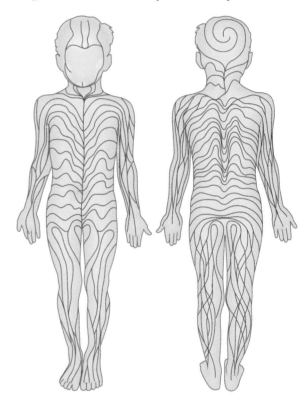

Fig. 19.4: Lines of Blaschko. Epidermal nevi often follow these embryological lines

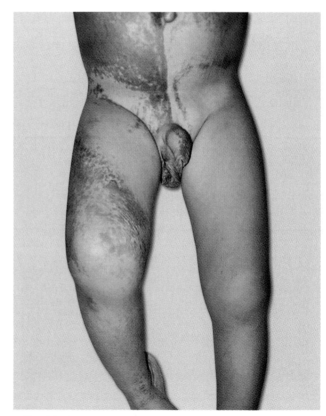

Fig. 19.5: Epidermal nevus along the lines of Blaschko

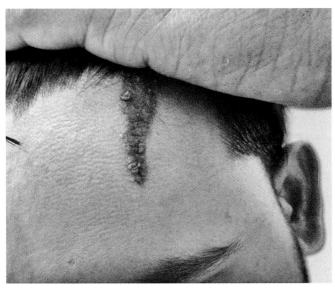

Fig. 19.6A: Epidermal nevi with both a soft component and raised rough verrucous component

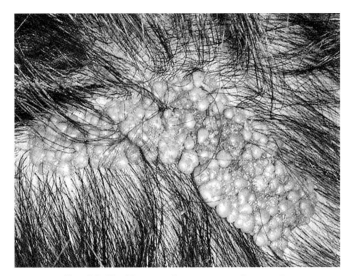

Fig. 19.6B: Nevus sebaceous on the scalp

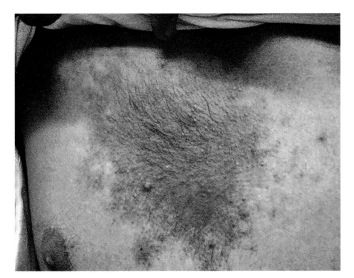

Fig. 19.6C: Raised hyperpigmented plaque with increased hair and localized acne—Becker's nevus

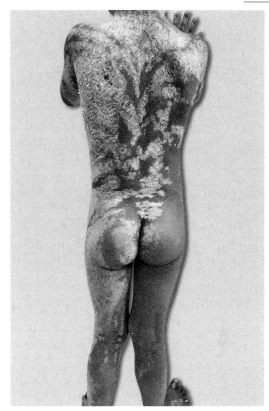

Fig. 19.6D: Scaly, bilateral, epidermal nevi along the lines of Blaschko

- *CHILD* (congenital hemidysplasia with ichthyosiform nevus and limb defects)[Q] characterized by psoriasiform persistent patches that strikingly respect the midline and often favor the flexures (ptychotropism); there are also skeletal defects.
- *Proteus syndrome*: Soft epidermal nevi in Blaschko lines, cerebriform connective-tissue nevi of the feet, macrodactyly.

Epidermoid and Pilar Cysts

Epidermoid cyst: Most arise from the **infundibulum**, the upper part of the hair follicle above the site of entry of the sebaceous duct. Some are true inclusion cysts following trauma, usually to palms or soles, where a

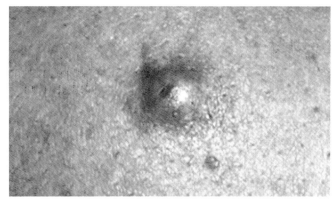

Fig. 19.7A: Epidermoid cyst with a central punctum

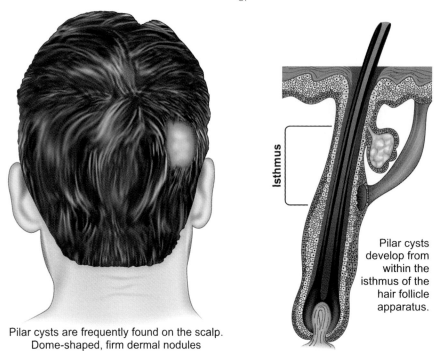

Pilar cysts are frequently found on the scalp.
Dome-shaped, firm dermal nodules

Isthmus

Pilar cysts
develop from
within the
isthmus of the
hair follicle
apparatus.

Fig. 19.7B: Pilar cysts are frequently found on the scalp. Dome-shaped, firm dermal nodules

fragment of epidermis is embedded in dermis; others follow severe acne. Often incorrectly called sebaceous cysts, these are common and can occur on the scalp, face, behind the ears and on the trunk. They often have a **central punctum**; when they rupture, or are squeezed, foul-smelling cheesy material comes out (Fig. 19.7A).

Pilar cyst: Most lesions are on scalp (90%); rest on face, neck, and upper trunk (Fig. 19.7B). They are firmer than epidermoid cyst, *no central pore*; contents compact keratin with cheesy nature and smell.

Treatment is by excision, or by incision followed by expression of the contents and removal of the cyst wall. Failure to remove the entire cyst wall may result in recurrence.

Milia

Milia are small subepidermal keratin cysts. They are common on the face in all age groups and appear as tiny white millet seed-like papules of 0.5–2 mm in diameter and occasionally can be larger (Fig. 19.8). They

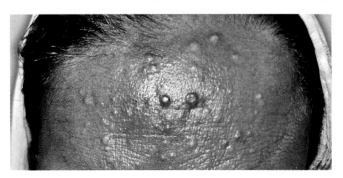

Fig. 19.8: Multiple milia on the forehead of a female patient

are seen also following subepidermal blistering (e.g. in epidermolysis bullosa). The contents of milia can be picked out with a sterile needle or pointed scalpal blade (No. 11) without local anesthesia.

Premalignant Disorders

Actinic Keratosis

This is a UVB-induced precancerous condition as melanin protects against its development, actinic keratosis is not seen in black skin. Conversely, albinos are especially prone to develop them.

Clinical features: They affect the middle-aged and elderly in temperate climates and younger people in the tropics. The pink or gray rough scaling macules or papules seldom exceed 1 cm in diameter and the rough surface is better felt than seen. AK occurs in the areas of heaviest sun exposure—the forehead, bald scalp, cheeks, nose, tips of the ears, and lower lip, as well as the backs of the hands and forearms (Fig. 19.9).

About 1% of actinic keratoses are expected to change into invasive squamous cell carcinoma.[Q]

A flat pale seborrheic keratosis is identical clinically; hyperkeratotic lesions may be confused with warts.

Therapy: There are many treatment options including, freezing with liquid nitrogen, curettage with electro-desiccation or cautery and excision.

Medical therapy includes, topical 5-fluorouracil cream, topical imiquimod 3 times weekly for 6 weeks and photodynamic therapy.

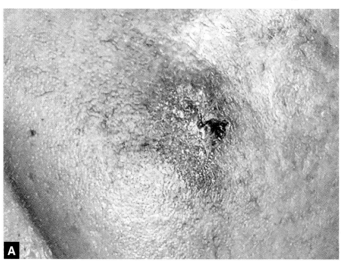
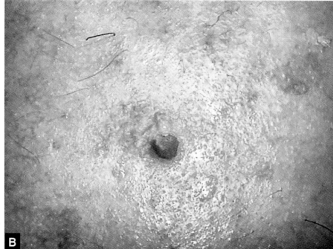

19

Fig. 19.9: Actinic keratoses on the face (A) and on the scalp (B)

Bowen Disease

This is essentially a squamous cell carcinoma *in situ*.[Q] This is an SCC *in situ* but not on sun-exposed skin.

Pathogenesis: Formerly most common triggers were radiation and arsenic; nowadays human papilloma virus (HPV) seems to a common cause[Q] in Bowenoid papulosis.

Clinical features: It is a 1–3 cm slightly raised patch, tan to red-brown with variable scale[Q] (Fig. 19.10A and B). Over years, Bowen disease tends to evolve into an invasive squamous cell carcinoma. It is often mistaken for a patch of dermatitis.[Q]

Other possibilities include tinea, psoriasis, warts, actinic keratosis, superficial basal cell carcinoma, extramammary Paget disease.

> Always biopsy therapy resistant patches of dermatitis or psoriasis to exclude Bowen's disease, superficial BCC or lymphoma.

Therapy: Excision, curettage and electrodesiccation, laser ablation, or cryosurgery.

Erythroplasia of Queyrat (Fig. 19.11)

This is an SCC *in situ* on the transitional epithelium of the penis, female genitalia, or mouth. It presents as a harmless-looking red 'velvety patch' with a sharp border.[Q]

Arsenical Keratoses

Exposure to inorganic arsenic[Q] (iatrogenic, industrial exposure, ground water) causes a variety of changes. Similar lesions may develop with chronic exposure to pitch and tar, as well as ionizing radiation. Standard therapy suffices.

This problem is endemic in some parts of the world and in India is localized to the Eastern part of the country including West Bengal along the riverine belt.[Q]

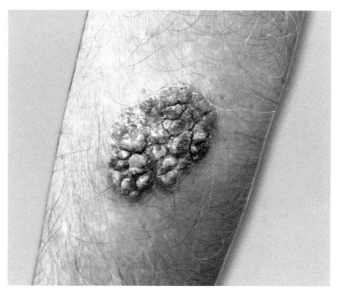

Fig. 19.10A: A case of Bowen's disease on the hands of an elderly male (Dr Aastha Gupta, RML Hospital)

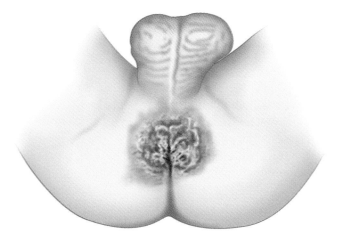

Fig. 19.10B: Perianal Bowen's disease can have an insidious onset and be misdiagnosed as tinea or dermatitis. Biopsy of any dermatitis not responding to therapy should be a consideration for the treating clinician

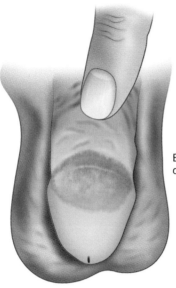

Erythroplasia
of Queyrat

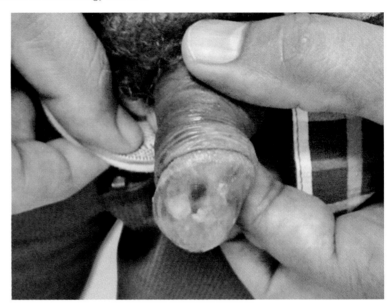

Fig. 19.11: A depiction of an erythematous persistent plaque on the genitalia: Erythroplasia of Queyrat

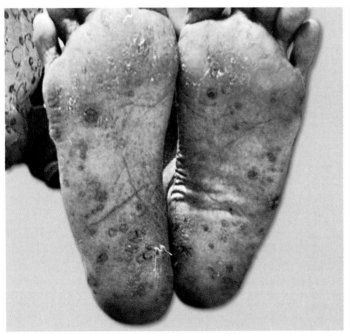

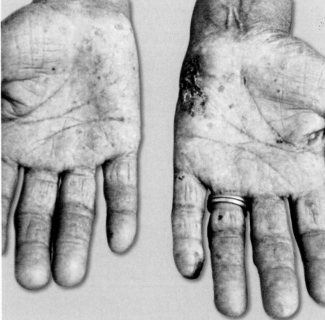

Fig. 19.12: Multiple punctate hyperkeratotic papules on the palms and soles in a case of arsenical keratosis

The clinical features are characterized by hypo- and hyperpigmentation, described as 'rain drops on a dusty road'.^{Q} In addition, SCC *in situ* develops in arsenical keratoses on the palms and soles (Fig. 19.12), as well as more typical Bowen disease elsewhere.^{Q} Superficial BCC also occur.

Cutaneous Horn

This clinical diagnosis describes a protuberant mass of compacted keratin (horn). The clue is at the base of the horn, where on histological examination one may find a wart, seborrheic keratosis, or SCC (*in situ* or invasive) (Fig. 19.13).

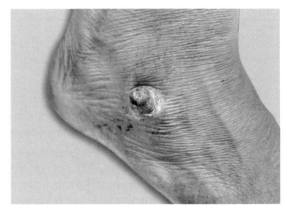

Fig. 19.13: A cutaneous horn

Leukoplakia

Leukoplakia is the generic name for white plaques on the mucosa. SCC *in situ* of the lower lip is seen in actinic cheilitis. It is usually scaly or crusted but sometimes white.

In the mouth, **danger areas**[Q] are the "side of the tongue and the gutter between the labial and gingival mucosa". Oral speckled leukoplakia (leukoplakia plus erythroplakia) is almost always SCC *in situ*. Risk factors include tobacco, heat and HPY.

Malignant Epidermal Tumors

Basal Cell Carcinoma (Rodent Ulcer)

BCC is the **most common form** of skin cancer[Q] and is seen on the face of the middle-aged or elderly males. It is locally invasive, does not metastasize[Q] and is also known as the **rodent ulcer**.[Q] It grows slowly and may eventually become locally destructive, but almost never metastasizes.

Etiology: Prolonged sun exposure, fair-skinned individuals, farmers, scars (caused by radiation exposure, vaccination or trauma) and tar and oils that can act as cocarcinogens with ultraviolet radiation. Previous treatment with arsenic can predispose to multiple basal cell carcinomas. Multiple basal cell carcinomas are found in the nevoid and genetic conditions such as xeroderma pigmentosum, albinism and Bazex syndrome.

The key factor appears to be altered regulation of the *sonic hedgehog pathway*.[Q] A summary of the pathogenetic factors are listed in Fig. 19.14.

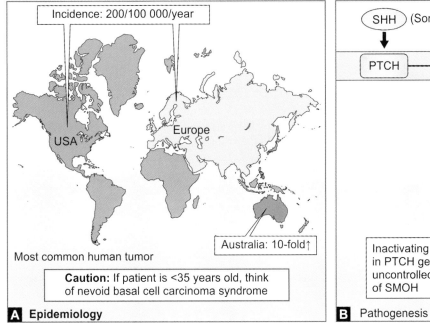

A Epidemiology

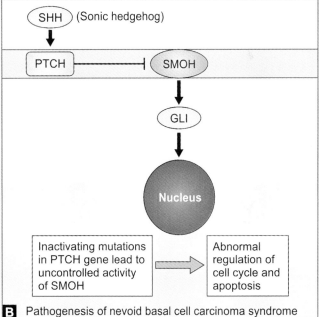

B Pathogenesis of nevoid basal cell carcinoma syndrome

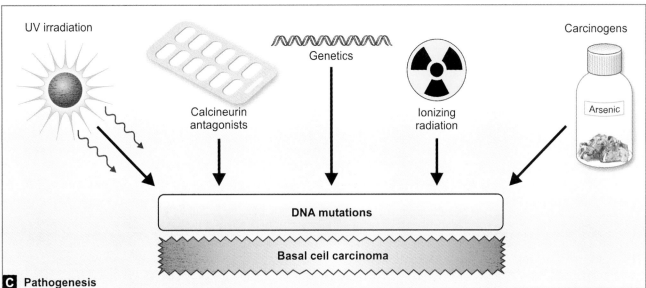

C Pathogenesis

Fig. 19.14A to C: A summary of the factors that cause BCC

Clinical features

a. *Nodular type*: This is the most common type.[Q] It begins as a small glistening translucent, sometimes umbilicated, skin-colored papule leads to central necrosis which forms an ulcer with an adherent crust and a rolled pearly edge[Q] (Fig. 19.15A and B). Classically telangiectatic vessels are seen on the tumor's surface.

b. *Superficial (multicentric)*: This is seen on the trunk. The lesion is classically described as a red, pink or brown scaly thin plaque with a fine edge (Fig. 19.15C). Such lesions can grow to more than 10 cm in diameter. This is the most common type of BCC in arsenic toxicity and immunosuppression.[Q]

c. *Cystic*: The lesion has a tense, translucent, look with marked telangiectasia.

d. *Morphoeic (cicatricial, sclerosing, infiltrative)*: This is a slowly expanding yellow or white waxy plaques with an ill-defined edge, which might show ulceration and crusting.

e. *Pigmented*: Pigment may be present in all types of basal cell carcinoma, causing all or part of the tumor to be brown or have specks of brown or black within[Q] it (Fig. 19.15D and E). It is more commonly seen in pigmented skins.

f. *Fibroepithelioma (Pinkus tumor)*:[Q] This is a fleshy nodule usually on the flank with a unique histological

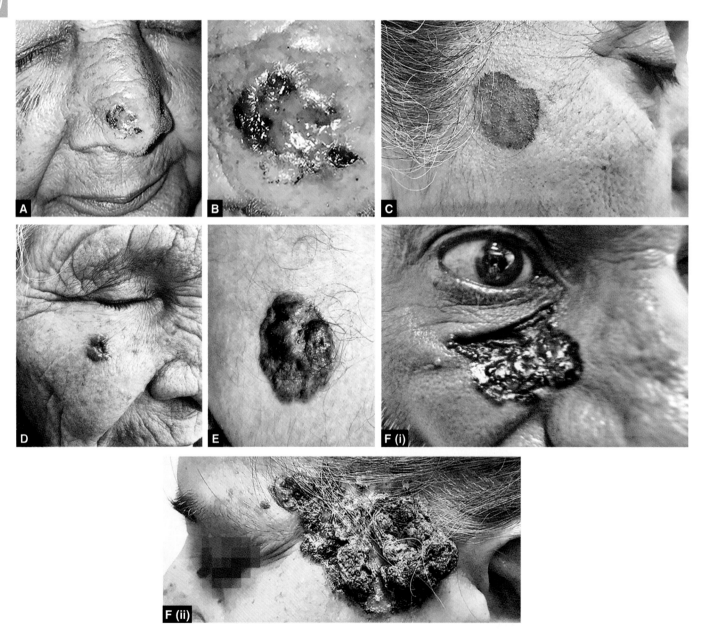

Fig. 19.15A to F: Basal cell carcinoma: (A and B) Shiny translucent papule with smooth surface and telangiectasias. Note the rolled out border; (C) Superficial BCC; (D) Pigmented basal cell carcinoma: Hyperpigmented papule with rolled out border present over the cheeks in an elderly female; (E) Pigmented basal cell carcinoma; (F) Ulcerative basal cell carcinoma, also called **rodent ulcer**. The characteristic border can be appreciated

appearance; lacy interconnecting basaloid tumor strands are dominated by mesenchymal proliferation.

g. *Ulcerated BCC*: When BCCs are ignored they can reach considerable size, as they are usually painless and simply ignored. There is marked, central ulceration with hemorrhage and crusting occurs (Fig. 19.15F).

Differential diagnosis

1. Nodular basal cell carcinoma: Intradermal melanocytic nevus, giant molluscum contagiosum or a keratoacanthoma.
2. Pigmented BCC: Seborrheic warts and malignant melanomas.
3. Cicatricial BCC: Morphea or a scar.
4. Superficial BCC: Psoriasis or with nummular eczema.

Histology (Fig. 19.16)**:** Small, darkly blue staining basal cells grow in well-defined aggregates which invade the dermis.

The outer layer of cells is arranged in a **palisade**.[Q]

Treatment: There is no single treatment of choice for all basal cell carcinomas. Treatment should be tailored to the type of tumor, its site and the age and general health of the patient. The 5-year cure rate for all types of basal cell carcinoma is over 95% but regular follow-up is advisable to detect local recurrences.

1. Surgical excision with histologic control and cosmetic closure is the treatment of choice (MOHS surgery)[Q]. This is specially useful for **recurrent, sclerosing, or otherwise difficult** BCC.

    For discrete nodular or cystic lesions, excision with 4 mm of surrounding normal skin, is the treatment of choice.
2. Alternatives, all of which have somewhat higher recurrence rates. They include:
    • *Cryosurgery*: Suitable for superficial BCC. Two freeze-thaw cycles should be used.
    • *Radiation therapy*: Best for elderly patients with numerous lesions or in difficult locations.

• *Photodynamic therapy*: Useful for superficial and small lesions; new procedure, so long-term recurrence rates not well-established.
• *Curettage and electrodesiccation or cautery*: Formerly widely used for superficial or small lesions; scarring and high recurrence rate limit its use today to exceptional situations.
• Topical imiquimod or 5-fluorouracil can be used over a long period of time, usually 3× weekly for 6 weeks, for superficial BCC.
• Hedgehog pathway inhibitors like vismodegib and sonidegib.

An overview of the therapeutic modalities is depicted in Fig. 19.17.

Squamous Cell Carcinoma (SCC)

SCC is the **second most common** malignant skin tumor (most common in black individuals and in organ transplant patients)[Q] and most common mucosal malignancy.[Q] It is a destructive growth with a *risk of lymphatic and hematogenous spread*[Q] for tumors thicker than 5 mm.

Pathogenesis (Fig. 19.18)**:** The main factor implicated is UVB exposure (ultraviolet-induced mutations in the p53 tumor suppressor gene), but there are many other factors including HPV (types 16 and 18; 31, 33, and 38),[Q] radiation therapy, arsenic exposure, chemical carcinogens (tar, pitch), heat-induced (kangri cancer) and immunosuppression and chronic inflammation and scars.[Q]

Clinical features: SCC develops out of actinic keratoses, so they have the same distribution—sun-exposed skin of the face, forearms, and backs of the hands (Figs 19.19 and 19.20). Lesions that are larger, thicker, crusted, ulcerated, or resistant to therapy may be SCC. Rapidly enlarging anaplastic lesions may start as ulcers with a granulating base and an indurated edge.

The growth rate and risk of metastasis is highly variable and the prognosis is best for lesions on skin arising from actinic keratoses; worst for lip, penis, and vulva SCC (Fig. 19.21A to D).

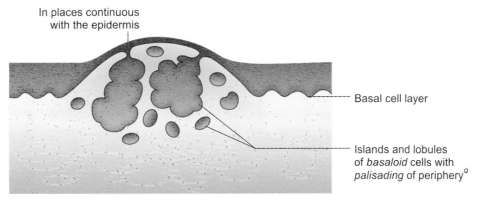

Fig. 19.16: A depiction of the histology of BCC

19

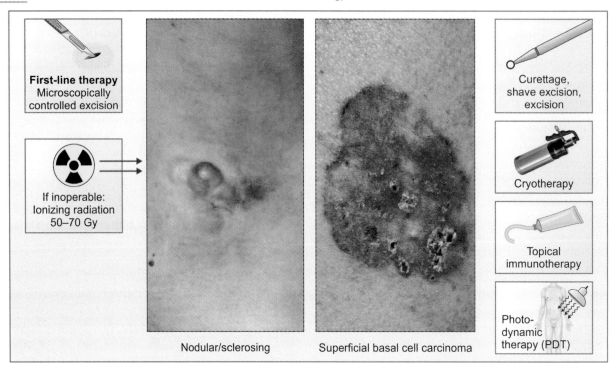

First-line therapy
Microscopically
controlled excision

If inoperable:
Ionizing radiation
50–70 Gy

Curettage,
shave excision,
excision

Cryotherapy

Topical
immunotherapy

Photo-
dynamic
therapy (PDT)

Nodular/sclerosing   Superficial basal cell carcinoma

Fig. 19.17: Treatment modalities for BCC

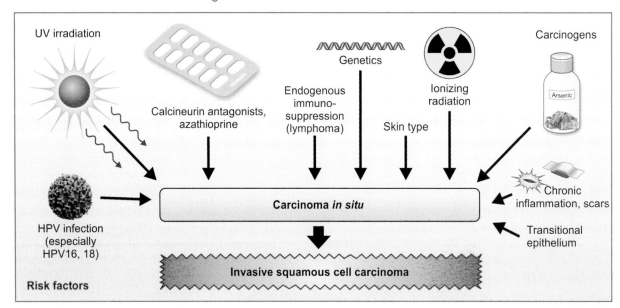

UV irradiation

Calcineurin antagonists,
azathioprine

Genetics

Endogenous
immuno-
suppression
(lymphoma)

Skin type

Ionizing
radiation

Carcinogens

Arsenic

Carcinoma *in situ*

HPV infection
(especially
HPV16, 18)

Risk factors

Chronic
inflammation, scars

Transitional
epithelium

Invasive squamous cell carcinoma

Fig. 19.18: Overview of the factors that predispose to the formation of SCC

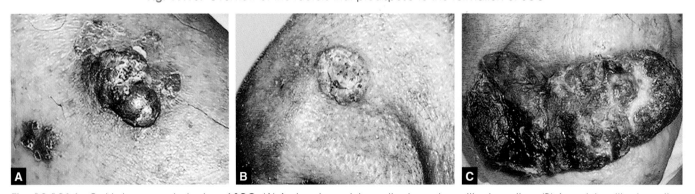

Fig. 19.19A to C: Various morphologies of SCC: (A) A chronic nodule on the lower leg with ulceration; (B) A nodule with ulceration of the nose; (C) An exophytic tumor of the lower lip

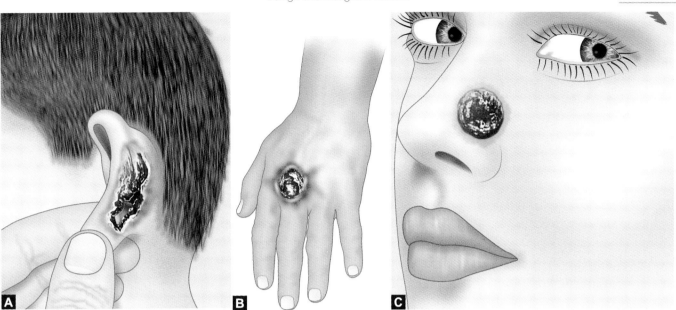

Fig. 19.20A to C: (A) Large ulcerative tumor destroying the ear. Squamous cell carcinomas arising on the ear have a higher rate of metastasis; (B) Large nodule on the dorsal hand; (C) Large crateriform squamous cell carcinoma: These tumors can be locally invasive and destructive. On occasion, they can also metastasize

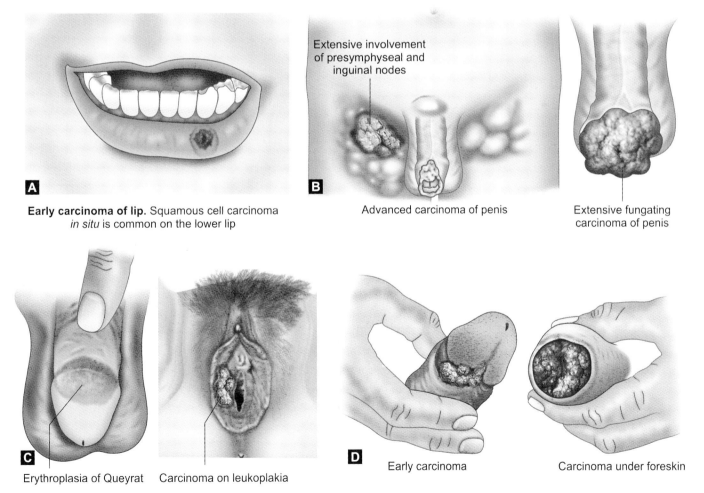

Early carcinoma of lip. Squamous cell carcinoma *in situ* is common on the lower lip

Extensive involvement of presymphyseal and inguinal nodes

Advanced carcinoma of penis

Extensive fungating carcinoma of penis

Erythroplasia of Queyrat   Carcinoma on leukoplakia

Early carcinoma

Carcinoma under foreskin

Fig. 19.21A to D: (A) Lower lip—most common site on face; arises from actinic cheilitis or tobacco overuse; (B) SCC seen usually on the glans; main factors are HPV infection and smegma; (C) SCC on the genitalia—often related to HPV16 and 18; rarely associated with lichen sclerosus et atrophicus or even lichen planus; (D) SCC on glans penis, similar in etiology to vulval SCC

- Lower lip—most common site on face; arises from actinic cheilitis or tobacco[Q] (Fig. 19.21A).
- Border and tip of the tongue—mostly in pipe smokers; high risk of metastases.
- Penis—usually on the glans; main factors are HPV infection and smegma, as SCC is much less common in circumcised men[Q] (Fig. 19.21B).
- Vulva—often related to HPV16 and 18; rarely associated with lichen sclerosus et atrophicus or even lichen planus (Fig. 19.21C).

Other factors that predict metastasis are given in Table 19.2.

Histology: Keratinocytes are in disarray, with marked variation in cell size and nuclear features. Individual cell keratinization. Degree of keratinization reflects degree of differentiation and is used in staging schemes (Fig. 19.22).

Well-differentiated tumors have swirls of keratinization (squamous eddies).[Q] The most important prognostic parameters are tumor depth and fibrotic stromal reaction (desmoplastic SCC).[Q]

Diagnostic approach: Clinical examination and biopsy.

Table 19.2	Factors that determine propensity of metastasis of SCC[Q]
Site	Tongue, penis, and vulvar carcinomas
Type	Sclerosing SCC
Chronic inflammation	Chronic draining sinuses, chronic ulcers, areas of previous X-radiation or thermal injury
Size	>2 cm in diameter
Depth	>2 mm in depth or invading to the subcutaneous tissue*
Other factors	Poorly differentiated tumors; perineural involvement; SCC in the immunosuppressed cases, and those with lymphoproliferative disorders.

*Those of 2–6 mm, around 4% metastasize; and of those >6 mm, 20% metastasize.

Therapy

1. Excision with histologic control of margins[Q] (Mohs surgery)
2. All other approaches are less than ideal; they include radiation therapy, photodynamic therapy, laser ablation, and cryosurgery.
3. Inoperable or metastatic SCC are usually treated with palliative protocols with drugs like methotrexate or cisplatin combined with doxorubicin or 5-fluorouracil. The outlook depends primarily on tumor thickness.

An overview of medical and surgical therapy is given in Fig. 19.23.

Paget's Disease (Apocrine Ductal Carcinoma)[Q]

Intraductal carcinoma[Q] of the breast extending to involve nipple with invasion of epidermis by malignant cells. 0.5 –1 % of breast carcinomas.

Clinical features: It presents as a well-defined red scaly plaque which spreads slowly over and around the nipple.[Q]

The condition is sharply marginated and **unilateral**, (Fig. 19.24) whereas eczemas are usually poorly marginated and affect both nipples.[Q] Nipple adenoma is a benign breast tumor which typically has a crusted surface.

Extramammary Paget's disease affects other sites bearing apocrine glands and is caused by an underlying ductal carcinoma. The perineum[Q] is the next most common site after breast. The classic morphology is of erythematous eroded scaly patch in the axillae or anogenital region (Fig. 19.24).

Therapy: Surgery and follow-up management following guidelines for carcinoma of the breast.

TUMORS OF THE DERMIS

Vascular Malformations and Tumors

These disorders are either present at birth (port wine stains) or appear soon after (hemangioma). They can

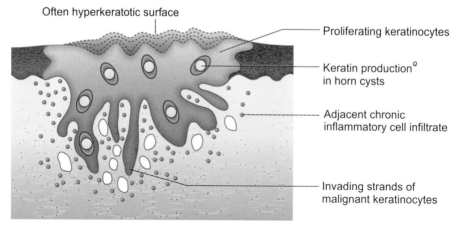

Often hyperkeratotic surface

Proliferating keratinocytes

Keratin production[Q] in horn cysts

Adjacent chronic inflammatory cell infiltrate

Invading strands of malignant keratinocytes

Fig. 19.22: Histology of SCC

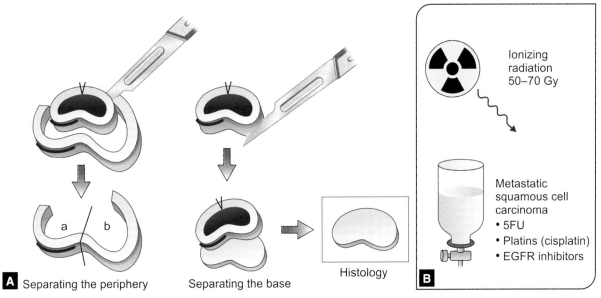

Fig. 19.23A and B: (A) Steps of Mohs surgery; (B) Medical therapy

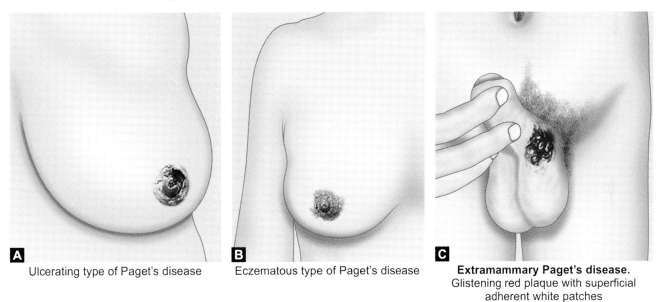

Ulcerating type of Paget's disease

Eczematous type of Paget's disease

Extramammary Paget's disease.
Glistening red plaque with superficial adherent white patches

Fig. 19.24A to C: A depiction of Paget's disease

be classified clinically into two types—vascular malformations and hemangiomas (Table 19.3).

We will focus on the common disorders as the uncommon conditions including the arteriovenous malformations are beyond the scope of this book.

Nevus Flammeus (Port-Wine Stain)

Congenital localized vascular malformation consisting of dilated capillaries.

Classification:

- *Medial form*: Usually nape or forehead (stork bite[Q] nevus) (Fig. 19.25).

  Also known as Salmon patches: The forehead and the upper eyelids are also called stork bites.[Q] Nuchal lesions may remain unchanged,[Q] but patches in other areas usually disappear within a year.

Table 19.3	Vascular malformations and tumors
Malformations	*Hemangiomas*
• Present at **birth**[Q] • Do not involve (*Port-wine stain: **Persists**)[Q] ('salmon' patch is exception)	• Usually appear **after birth**[Q] • Involute by 9 years
1. **Capillary** ('salmon' patch and 'port-wine' stain) 2. **Arterial** 3. **Venous** 4. **Combined**	1. **Superficial (capillary)** 2. **Deep (cavernous)** 3. **Mixed**

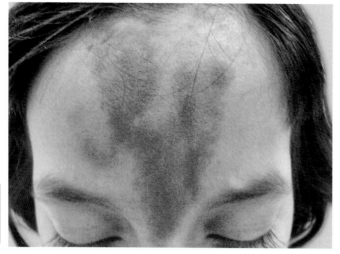

Fig. 19.25: Port-wine stain on the forehead, also called 'stork bite'

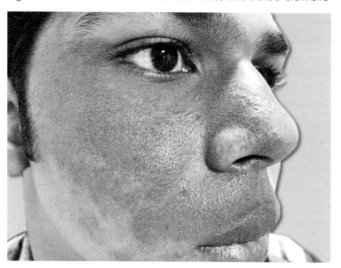

Fig. 19.26: PWS on the lateral aspect of face which tends to persist

- *Lateral form*: Follows peripheral or cranial nerve (Fig. 19.26).

Clinical features: Circumscribed, flat pink or deeper red area; present at birth—grows with child. In adult life, tendency to thicken, develop papules (Fig. 19.27). Median lesions may regress during infancy; lateral ones do not. Median lesions are not associated with other abnormalities; lateral ones may be.

Syndromes

a. *Sturge-Weber syndrome:*[Q] Unilateral nevus flammeus in distribution of 1st or 2nd branch of trigeminal nerve with ipsilateral vascular abnormalities of meninges or cortex.
(*STURGE: Sporadic, Tram track calcification, U/L port-wine stain, Retardation, Glaucoma, Epilepsy*)

b. *Klippel-Trénaunay-Weber syndrome:*[Q] Nevus flammeus involving a limb, with hypertrophy of underlying bones and muscles. There may be underlying venous (Klippel-Trénaunay) or arteriovenous fistulae (Parkes-Weber).

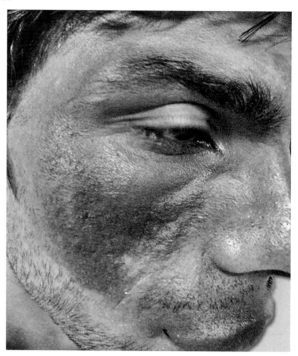

Fig. 19.27: Thickening and hypertrophy of skin with associated PWS

Investigation: Children with lateral lesions should be followed for vascular, neurologic, or orthopedic problems.

Therapy: Camouflage; capillaries can be destroyed with pulsed dye (PDL)[Q] or copper vapor laser; later papules destroyed with Nd:YAG laser.

Treatment sessions can begin in babies and anesthesia is not always necessary. Early intervention before 1 year of age may result in better clearance.

Venous Malformation (Cavernous Hemangioma)

Venous malformations are deeper, softer and unlikely to regress spontaneously. They are readily compressible (Fig. 19.28). Because of their slow flow, venous malformations are subject to thromboses and thus can be painful.

Lymphangiomas

Group of lymphatic malformations and proliferations involving skin and soft tissue.

Clinical features

- *Lymphangiectases*: Small dilated primarily clear vesicles. Appear secondary to lymphatic obstruction or chronic lymphedema (Fig. 19.29).
- *Lymphangioma circumscriptum*: Congenital lesion that may first become apparent in childhood; multiple grouped vesicles, clear to red-blue, usually described as resembling frogs pawn.
- *Cystic hygroma*[Q]: Congenital deep unilocular lymphatic malformation;[Q] typically involves soft tissue of face, neck; less often axilla or groin.

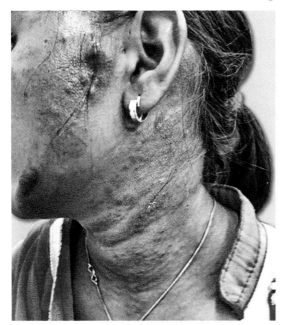

Fig. 19.28: Compressible blue swelling on the neck in a case of segmental venous malformation

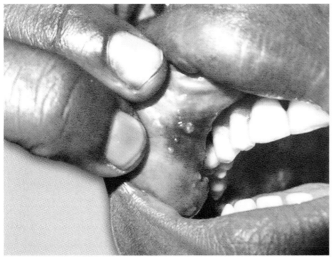

Fig. 19.29: Translucent vesicles in a case of lymphangioma

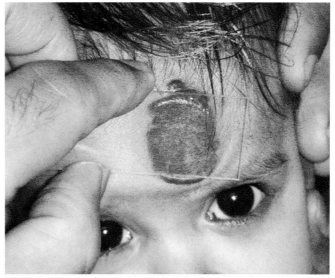

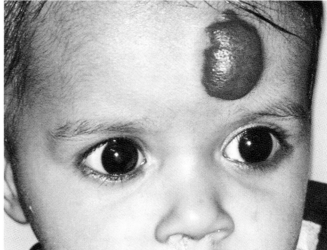

Fig. 19.30: Compressible red nodules in hemangioma

Regression is complete by the age of **5 years** in **50%** of children and in **90%** by the age of **9 years**, leaving only an area of slight atrophy.[Q]

To differentiate hemangiomas from malformation (port-wine stain), the following questions are useful:

Question	Hemangioma	Malformation
Present at birth?	Usually no; appears in first weeks of life	Yes
Growing?	Yes	No
Regressing?	Yes	No

Variants include:

Congenital: Congenital hemangiomas typically are large nodules with a rim of dilated vessels. No sex predilection. Fully developed at birth[Q]; lack Glut-1; divided into RICH (rapidly involuting congenital hemangioma) and NICH (noninvoluting).

Multiple—if there are more than **five** hemangiomas, look for liver involvement.

Hemangioma (*Capillary Hemangioma*)

This is the most common vascular lesion,[Q] which typically appears at birth or just thereafter and almost always resolve spontaneously.[Q]

They are more common in girls, preterm infants with low birth weight, in infants from multiple gestations and from mothers of advanced maternal age.

They are composed of Glut-1 + endothelial cells similar to the placental microvasculature.[Q]

Clinical features: Raised red to purple soft nodules that can become very large. About 30% can be seen at birth, but most appear later and all continue to grow. Tumors can be compressed, but do not disappear with diascopy (Fig. 19.30). During the first months of life, hemangiomas can continue to grow.

19

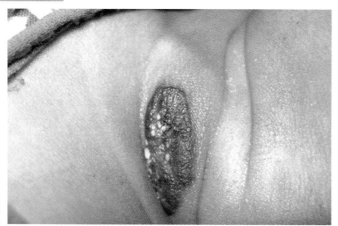

Fig. 19.31: Ulcerated hemangioma on the vulva

Syndromal: PHACE syndrome[Q] (**p**osterior fossa Dandy-Walker malformation, segmental **h**emangioma (mainly facial), **a**rterial anomalies, **c**ardiac anomalies (coarctation), **e**ye anomalies F:M:: 9:1).

Complications include:
- Obstruction of vital structures: Eyes, nose, mouth.
- Bleeding: Serious events surprisingly rare but ulceration is common (Fig. 19.31).
- Rarely, Kasabach-Merritt syndrome[Q] develops with consumptive coagulopathy and risk of bleeding

Therapy: Most hemangiomas do not need treatments.

Small lesions can be treated with intense pulsed light source, pulsed dye[Q] or Nd:YAG laser (also intralesional); treatment should be started early, not awaiting till growth phase.

Aggressive periorificial lesions:
- Intralesional or systemic corticosteroids (prednisolone 20–30 mg daily for 2–3 weeks).
- In 2008, beta-blockers were noted serendipitously to dramatically improve proliferating hemangiomas, and propranolol [Q] at a dose of 2–3 mg/kg/day in 2–3 divided doses and this is now the mainstay of treatment for complicated hemangiomas. Careful monitoring of blood sugar and blood pressure is necessary during the 2–10 months course of treatment.

Pyogenic Granuloma

This is a misnomer as no infective foci has been linked to this disorder. It is a rapidly growing capillary hemangioma which usually developing after trauma.[Q]

Clinical features: Typically eroded, often weeping or friable tumor that reaches several cm in size over week (Fig. 19.32). It is usually preceded by a definite history of trauma.

Many different clinical patterns:
- Common on digits, especially nail folds.

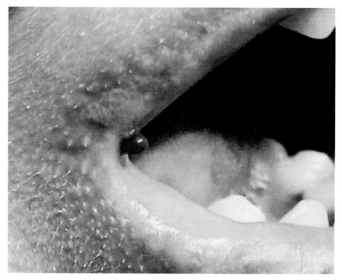

Fig. 19.32: Pyogenic granuloma

- Next most likely site is interdental gingiva, common during pregnancy (epulis of pregnancy).
- Satellite lesions are common, as are satellite recurrences (central lesion removed; many small peripheral lesions recur).

Treatment: Lesions should be removed by curettage under local anesthetic with cautery to the base. Rarely, this is followed by recurrence or an eruption of satellite lesions around the original site.

Miscellaneous Benign Dermal Tumors

Dermatofibroma

This is an extremely common reactive fibrous proliferation and is most commonly consequent to arthropod assault and folliculitis.

Clinical features: These lesions are usually seen on the legs and on compression a dermatofibroma becomes *depressed*, rather than protruding as would a melanocytic nevus (dimple sign or Fitzpatrick sign[Q]) (Fig. 19.33).

Histologically, the proliferating fibroblasts merge into the sparsely cellular dermis at the margins.

A simple lesion may be left alone but, if there is any diagnostic doubt, it should be excised.

Neuroma

This rare benign tumor is usually solitary and is consequent to a nerve injury at the site of trauma or a surgical wound.

The morphology is non-specific but the tumor is frequently painful, even with gentle pressure.

ENGLAND is a useful acronym for painful tumors (Eccrine spiradenoma, Neuroma, Glomus tumor, Leiomyoma, Angiolipoma, Neurofibroma (rarely) and Dermatofibroma (rarely).

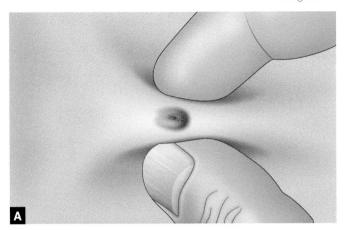

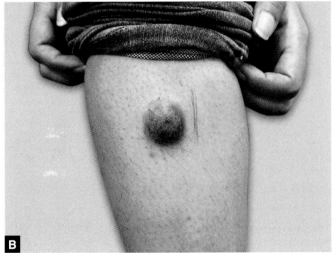

Fig. 19.33A and B: Dermatofibroma: (A) Dermonstrating the dimple sign; (B) Pigmented firm nodule classic of dermatofbroma

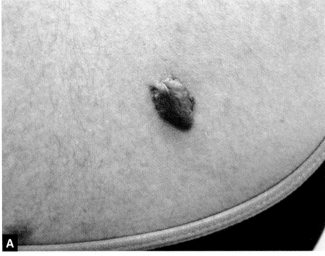

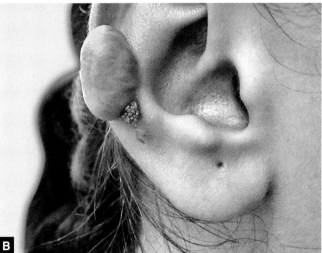

Fig. 19.34A and B: (A) An early keloid on the trunk; (B) A keloid on the ear lobe a common site due to ear piercing by 'jewellers'. Note the verruca adjoining the keloid

Hypertrophic Scars and Keloids

This is consequent to excessive connective tissue proliferation following an injury; a hypertrophic scar remains confined to the boundaries of the original insult, while a keloid proliferates beyond these limits.[Q]

Etiopathogenesis: Predisposing factors are:
1. *Ethnic factors*: Far more common in blacks.
2. *Location*: Sternum,[Q] shoulders, neck (after thyroid operation), ear lobes (piercing), ankles, shins, over clavicle, edge of chin, and other sites where skin tension is generally increased.
3. *Type of injury*: Burns and infections more often form keloids, leading to contractures and impaired function, as well as considerable cosmetic defects.

Clinical features: Firm skin-colored to red nodules and plaques (Fig. 19.34A and B). Keloids have irregular 'fingers' growing at the periphery.[Q] Both may be tender, painful, or pruritic.

Treatment: Silicone sheeting and intralesional steroid injections are helpful but treatment should be given early. Silicon gel sheeting for at least 12 hours daily is useful but though early studies were promising recent ones are not as promising.

Lipomas

Lipomas are the most common benign tumors[Q] and are composed of mature fat cells in the subcutaneous tissue. They are usually solitary but may be multiple. They are most commonly situated on the proximal parts of the limbs but can occur at any site. Clinically *'slip sign'* can be appreciated.

They need to be removed, only if there is doubt about the diagnosis, or if they are painful, unsightly or interfere with activities such as sitting back against a chair.

Mastocytosis (Urticaria Pigmentosa)

This term describes the various conditions in which the skin, and occasionally other tissues, contains an excess of mast cells. All types are characterized by a tendency for the skin to wheal after being rubbed (Darier's sign).[Q]

Malignant Tumors

Kaposi Sarcoma

This is an uncommonly seen (In India) virally induced, usually multifocal tumor with many clinical forms. It is caused by human herpesvirus 8 (HHV 8).[Q]

Clinical features

a. *Classic Kaposi sarcoma*: Usually affects elderly men of Jewish or Mediterranean background; slowly growing red-brown patches and plagues on feet or legs; when advanced, nodules, ulceration and rarely systemic involvement (Fig. 19.35A and B). Excellent prognosis. Patients tend to die with, rather than from, classic Kaposi sarcoma. These tumors are very sensitive to radiotherapy, which is the treatment of choice during the early stages.

b. *Endemic African Kaposi's sarcoma* is seen primarily in men who are HIV seronegative in Africa. Clinical presentation is similar to the classic form, but endemic Kaposi's sarcoma is more likely to involve the lymph nodes.

c. *Iatrogenic Kaposi sarcoma*: Associated with immuno-suppression; resolves if immune status can be restored. Usually diffuse subtle lesions, but can resemble HIV-associated Kaposi sarcoma.

d. *HIV-associated Kaposi sarcoma*: Disseminated Kaposi sarcoma, usually in homosexual men, often with oral involvement or facial involvement, but can occur anywhere. Early lesions are oval macules and papules that follow skin tension lines. The advent of highly active antiretroviral therapy (HAART) is useful to treat this condition and even multiple

lesions of HIV-associated Kaposi's sarcoma usually resolve with this treatment.

Treatment: Therapy must be adjusted to the clinical situation. In HIV/AIDS, highly active antiretroviral therapy (HAART) is most important. In elderly asymptomatic individuals, no treatment, cryotherapy, or local radiation therapy (20–30 Gy) is best. In advanced KS, systemic IFN-α (3×10^6 thrice weekly) or liposomal anthracydines are preferred.

Lymphomas and Leukemias

A simple classification is detailed below which suffices for students though a more comprehensive classification exists. It is convenient to group them into two broad categories:

1. Disorders that arise in the *skin* or preferentially involve:
   - Cutaneous T cell lymphoma (mycosis fungoides) and its variants.
   - Sézary syndrome
   - Lymphoma associated with HIV infection.
2. Those arising *extracutaneously*, but which sometimes involve the skin:
   - Hodgkin's disease
   - B cell lymphoma
   - Leukemia.

Mycosis fungoides (MF): This is a slowly evolving epidermotropic cutaneous T cell lymphoma[Q] characterized by a proliferation of small- to medium-sized CD4 T cells with cerebriform nuclei.[Q]

Clinical features: In most cases, the disorder undergoes a transition from a patch to the tumor stage (Fig. 19.36)

a. *Patch stage*: Macules and patches, slightly erythematous and scaly, often with cigarette paper surface (wrinkled appearance, also called pseudoatrophy); sites of predilection include buttocks, trunk, upper thighs, upper arms (Fig. 19.37). Less often there is involvement of flexures, scalp, and palms. The initial cases resemble psoriasiform dermatitis. The bizarre shapes of the patches and their asymmetrical distribution are suggestive of MF. Another feature is the varying shades of color of the patches.

b. *Plaque stage*: Gradual thickening of patches with increased scale.

c. *Tumor stage*: Usually after many years, abrupt development of thick, often ulcerated tumors arising from the plaques.

The patch stage of CTCL may be difficult to diagnose clinically, but the plaque and tumor stages are usually characteristic.

The first two phases of the disease may last for 20 years or more, but the tumor stage is often short, with spread and death usually within 3 years.

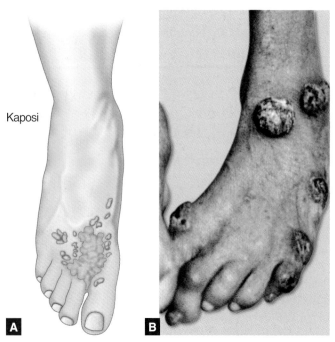

Kaposi

A   **B**

Fig. 19.35A and B: Purple ulcerated nodules of Kaposi sarcoma

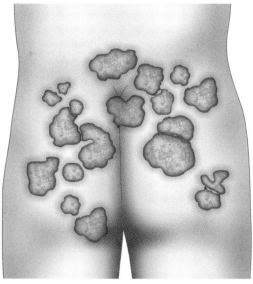
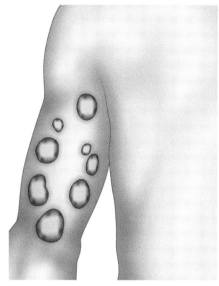

Patch stage of mycosis fungoides on the buttocks. Atrophic poikilodermatous patches are frequently encountered on the buttocks

Annular plaques

Fig. 19.36: A depiction of the morphology of the patch stage

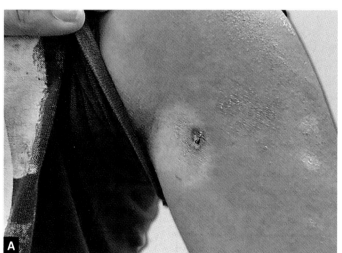
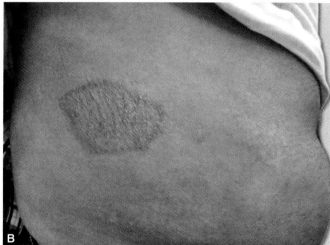

Fig. 19.37A and B: Patch stage of MF: (A) Scaly macules and plaques; (B) Atrophic hypopigmented plaques

Variants:

- *Subcutaneous panniculitis-like T cell lymphomas:* This resembles an ulcerating panniculitis, especially lupus panniculitis profundus. Subcutaneous nodules on the trunk and extremities are accompanied by general malaise, fever, chills, and weight loss.
- *Anaplastic large cell CD30+ lymphomas:* This presents as rapidly growing tumors that sometimes regress spontaneously. About 10% have regional lymph node involvement.
- *Granulomatous slack skin:* This affects young patients. Indurated plaques become atrophic and the skin then becomes pendulous in the affected areas.
- *Pagetoid reticulosis:* This is seen most often on the acral parts and again affects the young. It appears as a slow-growing psoriasiform or verrucous plaque.

- *Folliculotrophic mycosis fungoides:* This usually appears as itchy pink scaly plaques with follicular prominence, most commonly on the head and neck. This is followed by alopecia although this may be subtle.
- *Sézary syndrome*^{Q}: *Triad* of erythroderma is associated with pruritus and lymphadenopathy. Abnormal T lymphocytes with large convoluted nuclei are found circulating in the blood (Sézary cells).

Histology: The histological characteristics:

1. Intraepidermal lymphocytic microabscesses (Pautrier microabscesses)^Q
2. A band of lymphoid cells in the upper dermis, infiltrating the epidermis
3. Atypical lymphocytes.

Immunophenotyping and T cell receptor gene rearrangement studies may sometimes, but not always, be helpful in reaching a definitive diagnosis. Many biopsies, over several years, may be needed to prove that a suspicious rash is indeed an early stage of CTCL.

Treatment: An overview of the therapy is given here as details of intervention depend on the staging of the disease.

- *Patch stage*: Moderately potent or potent local steroids with UVB treatment, is useful in the patch stage. As they frequently have a dry skin, they should be encouraged to moisturize their skin.
- *Plaque stage*: PUVA, oral retinoids and α-interferon, are helpful. If lesions become more indurated, electron beam therapy[Q] may be used. Topical nitrogen mustard paint may also be used.
- *Tumor stage*: Individual tumors respond well to low-dose radiotherapy.
- *Sézary syndrome*: Treatment with extracorporeal photopheresis (irradiation of psoralenized blood with UVA in a machine) or with a targeting monoclonal antibody carrying diphtheria toxin may help destroy circulating malignant cells.

Extracutaneous lymphomas

Hodgkin's disease: Though an extremely uncommon presentation, sometimes it may present as severe generalized pruritus. Thus such patients should be examined for lymphadenopathy and hepatospleno-megaly. Rarely Hodgkin's disease may affect the skin directly, as small nodules and ulcers.

Leukemia: Skin involvement is an uncommon finding and it presents as plum-colored plaques or nodules or, less often, a thickening and rugosity of the scalp (cutis verticis gyrata). Commonly the rash associated with leukemia are non-specific red papules (leukemids). Other non-specific manifestations include pruritus, herpes zoster, acquired ichthyosis and purpura.

B cell lymphomas: B lymphocytic lymphomas presenting with skin lesions are rare. They appear as scattered plum-colored nodules.

CUTANEOUS METASTASES

Tumors that commonly metastasize to the skin can be recalled with the acronym **BLOCK** (**b**reast, **l**ung, **o**vary, **c**olon, **k**idney) (Fig. 19.38).

Breast carcinoma accounts for 70% of all cutaneous metastases in women,[Q] followed by the lungs, kidney, and ovaries.

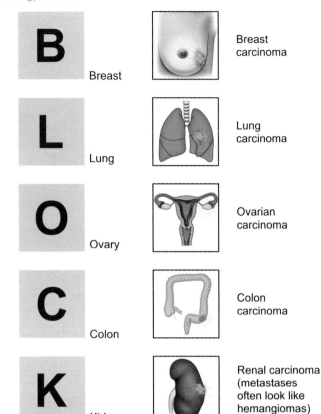

Fig. 19.38: Mnemonic for the common sources of skin metastases

In men, lung carcinoma[Q] is the commonest followed by colorectal and renal cancers.

Melanoma is responsible for 20–30% of all cutaneous metastases.[Q]

Clinical Features

Suddenly appearing red-brown papules and nodules, usually multiple but occasionally solitary, are typical. Sometimes there are dues to the possible underlying tumor, although a final answer depends on the pathology of the primary and metastatic lesions.

Carcinoma en cuirasse[Q] is metastatic breast carcinoma which is both erythematous, resembling erysipelas, and sclerotic. Metastases that block lymphatic drainage create obstruction and a 'peau d'orange' effect. Breast carcinoma also commonly goes to the eyelids and scalp. Metastases can appear 10–15 years after the primary tumor.

Renal cell carcinoma metastases are often very vascular and mistaken for a hemangioma; this is common on the scalp.

Gastric and ovarian carcinomas may metastasize to the umbilicus[Q] (Sister Mary Joseph nodule).[Q]

Disorders of Vascular System

Disorders of Blood Vessels and Lymphatics

Acrocyanosis

This type of 'poor circulation' is often familial and is seen common in females. The hands, feet, nose, ears and cheeks become blue-red and cold while the palms are often cold and clammy (Fig. 20.1). The condition is caused by arteriolar constriction and dilatation of the subpapillary venous plexus, and to cold-induced increases in blood viscosity. Patients have normal peripheral pulses, in contrast to those with peripheral arterial occlusive disease. The management is warm clothes and avoidance of cold.

Erythrocyanosis

This occurs in fat, often in young women.

Purple-red mottled discoloration is seen over the fatty areas such as the buttocks, thighs and lower legs. It is aggravated by cold and causes an unpleasant burning sensation. It is self-limiting but other disorders may occur at this site (e.g. perniosis, erythema induratum, lupus erythematosus, sarcoidosis, cutaneous tuberculosis and leprosy). Weight reduction is often recommended.

Pernio

Synonym: Chilblain.

This is a localized erythema caused by exposure to damp cold.[Q]

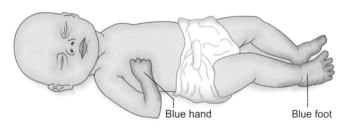

Blue hand   Blue foot

Fig. 20.1: A depiction of acrocyanosis

Pathogenesis: It is triggered by modest cold (freezing temperatures not required) coupled with moisture and involves the toes. The cause is a combination of arteriolar and venular constriction, the latter predominating on rewarming with exudation of fluid into the tissues.

Clinical features: Blue-purple papules and nodules (Fig. 20.2) which have a slow onset, are seen on the toes and can also involve shins, thighs, fingers; more common in women who are overweight and not physically active. They are painful, and itchy or may be associated with burning on rewarming. Occasionally, they may ulcerate.

Differential diagnosis: Lupus erythematosus (chilblain lupus), sarcoidosis (lupus pernio). In both instances, permanent and not cold-related.

Therapy: Protection from cold; if severe and chronic, topical calcium channel blockers (usually nifedipine) may help. The blood pressure should be monitored at the start of treatment and at return visits. The vasodilator nicotinamide (500 mg three times daily) may be helpful alone or in addition to calcium channel blockers. The condition usually resolves in 2–3 weeks.

Erythromelalgia

This is a rare paroxysmal condition in which the extremities (most commonly the feet) become red, hot, swollen and painful (Fig. 20.3) when exposed to heat, and relieved by cooling. The condition may be sporadic or familial.

Secondary erythromelalgia is associated with a myeloproliferative disease (e.g. polycythemia rubra vera or thrombocythemia), lupus erythematosus, rheumatoid arthritis, diabetes, degenerative peripheral vascular disease or hypertension.

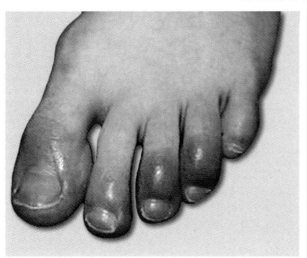
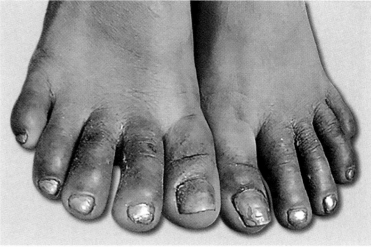

Fig. 20.2: Perniosis on the toes

20

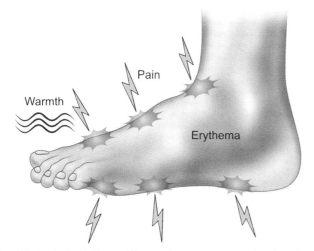

Fig. 20.3: A depiction of the various components of erythromelalgia

Treatment

Elevation and cooling of the extremities can be helpful. Small doses of aspirin give symptomatic relief. Topical therapies include capsaicin cream and lidocaine patch. Alternatives include non-steroidal anti-inflammatory drugs (NSAIDs), gabapentin, beta-blockers, pentoxifylline and the serotonin re-uptake inhibitor venlafaxine.

Telangiectases

Irreversible dilation of cutaneous capillaries and postcapillary venules. They appear as linear, punctate or stellate crimson-purple markings.

Classification

Primary telangiectasias (congenital or without obvious cause):
- Generalized essential telangiectasia
- Unilateral nevoid telangiectasia syndrome
- Poikiloderma syndromes
- Ataxia-telangiectasia

- Hereditary benign telangiectasia
- Hereditary hemorrhagic telangiectasia
- Telangiectasia macularis eruptiva perstans (combination of telangiectasia and mast cell disease).

Secondary telangiectases:
- Mycosis fungoides (poikiloderma vascular atrophicans variant)
- Rosacea
- Dermatomyositis
- Systemic sclerosis, especially CREST syndrome
- Lupus erythematosus
- Xeroderma pigmentosum
- Sun-damaged skin
- Erythema ab igne
- Portal hypertension
- Carcinoid syndrome

Nevus Araneus

Synonym: Spider nevus.

Definition: Acquired vascular lesion consisting of central dilated arteriole and radiating capillaries.

Clinical features: 2–4 mm red papule from which extend fine telangiectasia (thus spider nevus) seen on the face and neck (Fig. 20.4). Associated with pregnancy, liver disease,[Q] and CREST syndrome.

Therapy: Destruction of central vessel with laser or intense pulsed light source (IPL).

Livedo

It is defined as a net-like blue-red erythema.

Pathogenesis

Livedo results from reduced arteriolar flow and accumulation of deoxygenated blood in venules. This cyanosis of the skin is net-like (reticulated) or marbled

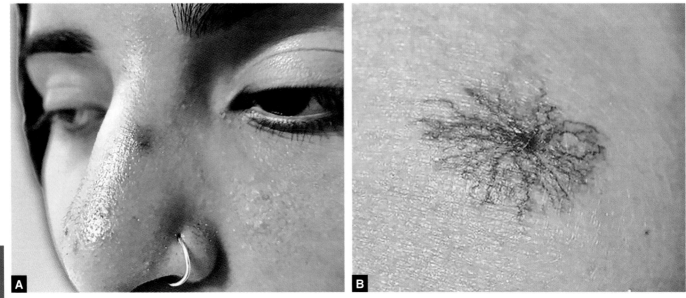

Fig. 20.4A and B: (A) Spider nevi. (B) A close up with radiating capillaries around a central arteriole

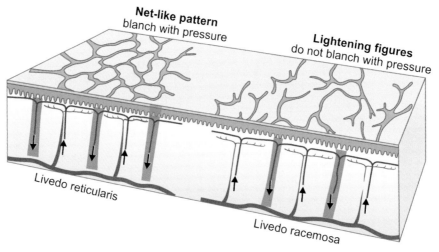

Fig. 20.5: Anatomical basis of livedo reticularis and racemosa

and is caused by stasis in the capillaries furthest from their arterial supply: at the periphery of the inverted cone supplied by a dermal arteriole (Fig. 20.5). There are two forms:

a. *Livedo reticularis*: Functional or physiologic, transient; result of vasoconstriction.[Q]

b. *Livedo racemosa*: Pathologic, permanent; result of vascular occlusion or malformation.[Q]

Clinical Features

Livedo reticularis more common on legs; if arms or trunk involved, think of livedo racemosa.

Transient: Results from exposure to cold or other triggers; also known as cutis marmorata.[Q]

Livedo racemosa is persistent, progressive; associated with variety of underlying diseases; always requires investigation (Table 20.1). The biopsy shows fibrin in

vessel wall, thrombi in small vessels and extravasation of erythrocytes.

Table 20.1	Diseases associated with livedo racemosa	
Inflow impaired (arterial)	*Outflow impaired (venous)*	*Hyperviscosity*
Arteriosclerosis	Leukocytoclastic vasculitis	Cryoglobulinemia
Cholosterol emboli	Thrombi	Thrombocytosis
Sneddon syndrome	Emboli	Macroglobulinemia
Arteritis: polyarteritis nodosa, connective tissue disease, thrombo-angiitis obliterans		Cold agglutinin disease
		Anti-phospholipid syndrome

Therapy

Livedo reticularis: None required, or warming. Livedo racemosa: Treat associated disease.

Antiphospholipid syndrome: Some patients with an apparently idiopathic livedo reticularis develop progressive disease in their peripheral, cerebral, coronary and renal arteries. Others, usually women, have multiple arterial or venous thromboembolic episodes accompanying livedo reticularis. Recurrent spontaneous abortions and intrauterine fetal growth retardation are also features. Prolongation of the activated partial thromboplastin time (APTT) and the presence of antiphospholipid antibodies (either anticardiolipin antibody or lupus anticoagulant, or both) help to identify this syndrome. Systemic lupus erythematosus should be excluded.

Erythema Ab Igne

This appearance is also determined by the underlying vascular network. Its brownish pigmented, reticulated erythema, with variable scaling, is caused by damage from long-term exposure to local heat[Q] or infrared source—usually from an open fire, hot water bottle, heating pad (Fig. 20.6) or, in recent years, *laptops*.[Q]

Flushing

This transient vasodilatation of the face may spread to the neck, upper chest and, more rarely, other parts of the body. There is no sharp distinction between flushing and blushing though the latter is provoked by emotional stimuli. The various causes are listed in Table 20.2.

1. *Paroxysmal flushing* (hot flushes), common at the menopause, is associated with the pulsatile release of luteinizing hormone from the pituitary, as a consequence of low circulating estrogens and failure of normal negative feedback.

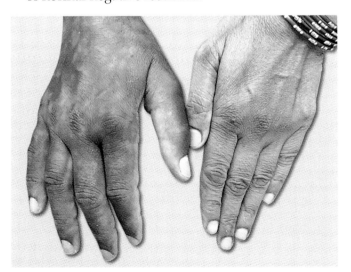

Fig. 20.6: Use of a heating pad on the right hand causing erythema ab igne

Table 20.2	Causes of flushing
Physiological	• Emotional (blushing) • Menopausal (hot flushes) • Exercise
Foods	• Hot drinks • Spicy foods • Additives (monosodium glutamate) • Alcohol (especially in Oriental people)
Drugs	• Vasodilators including nicotinic acid,[Q] hydralazine • Nitrates and sildenafil • Calcium channel blockers including nifedipine • Disulfiram or chlorpropamide + alcohol • Cholinergic agents
Pathological	• Mastocytosis • Carcinoid tumors • Pheochromocytoma • Dumping syndrome • Migraine headaches
Rosacea	—

2. *Alcohol-induced flushing* is caused by the vasodilatory effects of alcohol and accumulation of acetaldehyde.
3. *Drug-induced fumaric acid therapy* for psoriasis; rarely others (mast cell degranulators, hormones, chemotherapy agents, nicotinic acid, IL-2).
4. *Mastocytosis*: Red-brown macules and papules, sometimes with telangiectases; occasionally flushing.
5. *Pheochromocytoma*: Increased blood pressure, tachycardia; attacks for flushing.
6. *Rosacea*[Q]: Some patients present with flushing with no other signs; later papules, telangiectases and small pustules, almost exclusively on face; triggered by alcohol, nicotine, spices, heat.

ARTERIAL DISEASE

Raynaud Syndrome/Phenomenon

Vascular spasms of digital arteries with distinct clinical patterns; often associated with autoimmune diseases (Fig. 20.7).

Epidemiology: Female:male ratio 4:1.

Classification

Raynaud phenomenon is the classical clinical **triad**[Q] of ischemia (white), cyanosis (blue), and reactive hyperemia (red) occurring sequentially in a digit.

 (*PCR— pallor,*[Q] *cyanosis, redness*)

 Primary Raynaud syndrome (**Raynaud disease**)[Q] is the presence of Raynaud phenomenon for more than 2 years without evidence of an underlying disease.

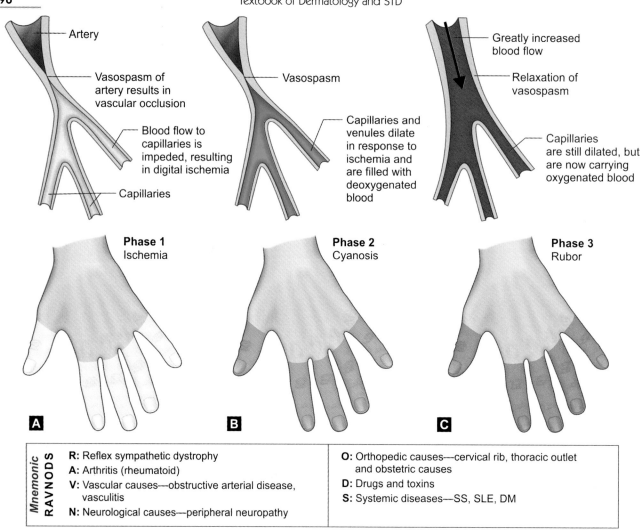

Fig. 20.7: Depiction of the three phases of Raynaud's phenomenon and the common causes

Secondary Raynaud syndrome: Same clinical findings, but associated with a variety of disorders:

- Collagen-vascular disorders[Q] (especially systemic sclerosis or mixed collagen-vascular disorder, but any of the others is possible).
- Exogenous factors: Vibration (jackhammer operator), repeated hammering (hypothenar hammer syndrome); injuries, postoperative; cold exposure; reflex sympathetic dystrophy (Sudeck atrophy).
- Gammopathy with hyperviscosity syndrome; polycythemia vera, Waldenström macroglobulinemia.
- Combination of vasculitis and hyperviscosity: Paroxysmal nocturnal hemoglobinuria, cold agglutinin disease, cryoglobulinemia, hot-cold hemolysin.
- Obstructive arterial disease: Arteriosclerosis, thromboangiitis obliterans (Buerger disease), thrombosis, thoracic outlet syndrome.
- Neurological diseases with peripheral manifestations.

- *Medications*: Amphetamines, beta-blockers, clonidine, oral contraceptives, ergot derivatives[Q]—both in medications and in biological products, cytostatic agents (bleomycin, vinca alkaloids); heavy metals, vinyl chloride.
- Others: Paraneoplastic, hypothyroidism.

Clinical Features

Triad (*PCR*) explained by pathophysiology:

- *Pallor* (*white*): Sudden vasospasm; cold numb fingers (cadaver digit).
- *Cyanosis* (*blue*): Venous constriction persists even in face of arterial relaxation; cyanosis.
- *Rubor* (*red*): Restored blood flow, pain, throbbing.

  Features usually include:
  – Bilateral
  – Start in only one digit
  – Develop persistent finger swelling
  – Cuticle thickens, proximal nail fold is thinned with telangiectases.
  – Occasional involvement of toes, nose, or ears.

Diagnostic Approach

Careful history, confirming presence of white-blue-red triad and searching for triggering factors (as below):

1. Occupation: Working outdoors, fishing industry, using vibrating tools, exposure to chemicals such as vinyl chloride.
2. Examination of peripheral and central vascular system for proximal vascular occlusion.
3. Drug history: Such as beta-blockers, oral contraceptives, bleomycin, migraine therapy
4. Symptoms of other autoimmune rheumatic disorders:
   - Arthralgia or arthritis
   - Cerebral symptoms
   - Mouth ulcers
   - Alopecia
   - Photosensitivity
   - Muscle weakness
   - Skin rashes
   - Dry eyes or mouth
   - Respiratory or cardiac problems

Clinical and laboratory evaluation to rule out the causes of secondary Raynaud syndrome, including, ANA, anti-DNA antibodies, anticardiolipin antibodies, cold agglutinins, cryoglobulins, serum protein electrophoresis, blood viscosity test.

Some patients with isolated Raynaud's phenomenon have positive antinuclear antibodies and abnormal nailfold capillaroscopy. These cases are at increased risk of developing a defined connective tissue disease, with up to 50% of such cases progressing within 10 years. This forms an important group of cases that may facilitate very early diagnosis of SSc (VEDOSS).[Q]

Therapy

If an underlying disease is found, it should be treated. The Raynaud phenomenon is managed in the same way regardless of cause.

1. Avoidance of cold: Warm gloves, hand warmers.
2. Calcium channel blockers are treatment of choice[Q]; nifedipine 5 mg tid (start initially at 5 mg a day) if orthostatic hypotension is problem, try diltiazem 60–120 mg daily or verapamil 240–360 mg daily, though the latter are less effective than nifedipine.
3. Other vasodilators such as prazosin also useful, start with 1 mg daily; may increase slowly to as high as 6 mg daily.
4. Calcitonin 100 IU IV daily for 10–14 days, or calcitonin nasal spray 100 IU 1–3 × weekly.
5. Prostaglandins or prostacyclins: All very expensive; given IV either continuously in hospital or daily for 6–8 hours over 5 days:
   - Alprostadil (PGI2).
   - Epoprostenol (prostacyclin).
   - Iloprost trometamol.
6. Topical nitroglycerine paste: May help to avoid fingertip necrosis.
7. Supplemental measures: Physical therapy, infrared light, windmilling (swinging hands like windmill to force blood to periphery).

Pressure Ulcer

This is due to a sustained or repeated pressure on the skin over bony prominences that lead to ischemia and consequently to pressure sores. These are common in patients over 70 years old who are confined to hospital, especially those with a fractured neck of femur. The morbidity and mortality of those with deep ulcers is high.

Etiology

The skin and underlying tissues need to be continually nourished with oxygen and nutrients. Pressure blocks the blood flow, and, if prolonged, can lead to tissue death. Healthy people get neurological signals that cause them to shift position. The main factors responsible for pressure sores are:

1. Prolonged immobility and recumbency (e.g. caused by paraplegia, arthritis or senility).
2. Vascular disease (e.g. atherosclerosis).
3. Neurological disease causing diminished sensation (e.g. in paraplegia).
4. Malnutrition, severe systemic disease and general debility.

Clinical Features

The sore begins as an area of erythema which progresses to a superficial blister or erosion. If pressure continues, deeper damage occurs with the development of a black eschar which, when removed or shed, reveals a deep ulcer, often colonized by *Pseudomonas aeruginosa*. The skin overlying bony prominences, such as the sacrum, greater trochanter, ischial tuberosity, the heel and the lateral malleolus, is especially at risk (Fig. 20.8).

Category/stage I: Nonblanchable erythema: Intact skin with non-blanchable redness of a localized area usually over a bony prominence (Fig. 20.9A). Darkly pigmented skin may not have visible blanching; its color may differ from the surrounding area (Fig. 20.9B).

The area may be painful, firm, soft, warmer or cooler as compared to adjacent tissue. Category/Stage I may be difficult to detect in individuals with dark skin tones.

Category/stage II: Partial thickness skin loss: Partial thickness loss of dermis presenting as a shallow open ulcer with a red pink wound bed, without slough or bruising (Fig. 20.9C). May also present as an intact or open/ruptured serum-filled blister. Presents as a shiny or dry shallow ulcer without slough or bruising. Bruising indicates suspected deep tissue injury.

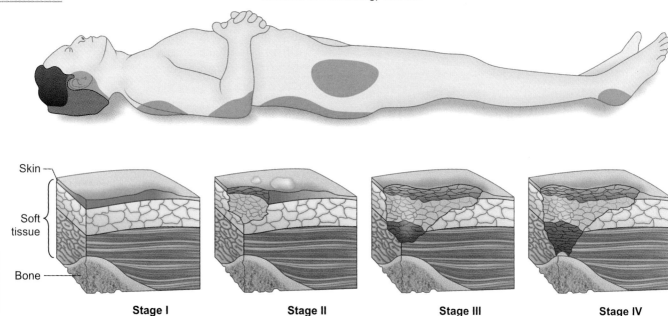

Skin

Soft tissue

Bone

| Stage I | Stage II | Stage III | Stage IV |

Fig. 20.8: Common sites (above) and stages (below) of a pressure ulcer

Category/stage III: Full thickness skin loss: Full thickness tissue loss. Subcutaneous fat may be visible but bone, tendon and muscle are not exposed (Fig. 20.9D). Slough may be present but does not obscure the depth of tissue loss. May include undermining and tunneling.

The depth of a Category/Stage III pressure ulcer varies by anatomical location. The bridge of the nose, ear, occiput and malleolus does not have subcutaneous tissue and Category/Stage III ulcers can be shallow.

Category/stage IV: Full thickness tissue loss: Full thickness tissue loss with exposed bone, tendon or muscle (Fig. 20.9E). Slough or eschar may be present on some parts of the wound bed.

Unstageable: Depth unknown: Full thickness tissue loss in which the base of the ulcer is covered by slough (yellow, tan, gray, green or brown) and/or eschar (tan, brown or black) in the wound bed (Fig. 20.9F).

Stable (dry, adherent, intact without erythema or fluctuance) eschar on the heels serves as 'the body's natural (biological) cover' and should not be removed.

Suspected deep tissue injury: Depth unknown: Purple or maroon localized area of discolored intact skin or blood-filled blister due to damage of underlying soft tissue from pressure and/or shear (Fig. 20.9G). The area may be preceded by tissue that is painful, firm, mushy, boggy, warmer or cooler as compared to adjacent tissue.

Deep tissue injury may be difficult to detect in individuals with dark skin tones. Evolution may include a thin blister over a dark wound bed. The wound may further evolve and become covered by thin eschar. Evolution may be rapid exposing additional layers of tissue even with optimal treatment.

Management

Stage I Ulcer

1. Prevention: By turning recumbent patients regularly and using antipressure mattresses and positioning devices such as foam wedges.

   Whether lying in bed or sitting in the chair, frequent repositioning, definitely no less than at least every 2 hours, is essential.

2. For stage I, petrolatum is an effective moisturizer

3. Treatment of malnutrition and the general condition.

Advanced stage: The initial management of stages II, III, and IV is the same as that for stage I, in relation to off loading the pressure with surfaces and repositioning.

Management decisions should be based on ulcer presentation. For example, a wound with cellulitis, bad odor, or frank pus may require a local or systemic anti-infective treatment.

• Debridement: Regular cleansing with normal saline or 0.5% aqueous silver nitrate. Antibacterial preparations locally and absorbent dressings. Appropriate systemic antibiotic, if an infection is spreading.

• Selection of dressings is based on the goal of care, and not on wound etiology. Stages III and stage IV ulcers may require packing to fill the void or 'dead space' left from tissue destruction. Packing deep wounds is important to prevent infection and abscess formation.

• Presence of frank pus and odorous exudate demand microbiologic analysis.

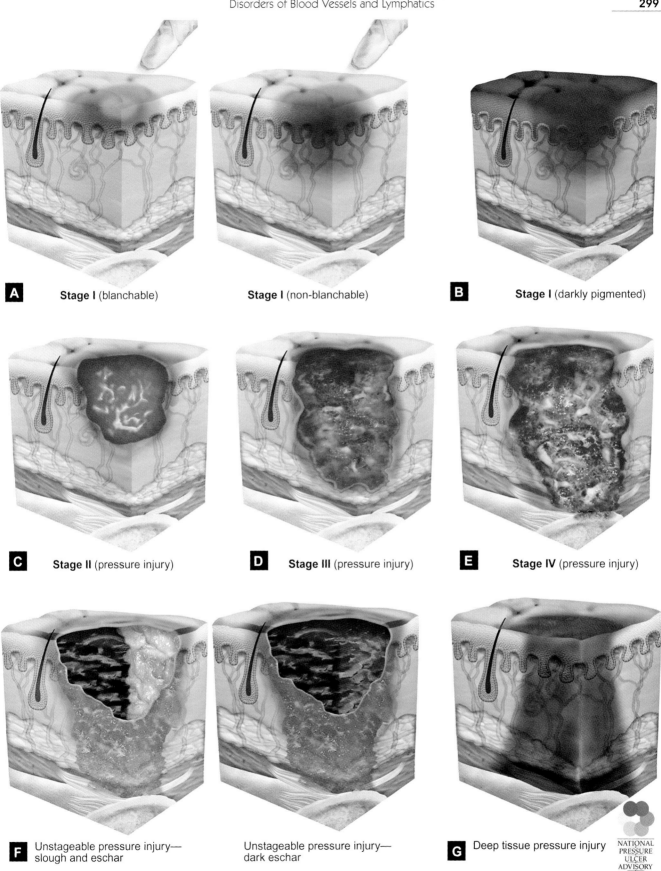

A   **Stage I** (blanchable)   **Stage I** (non-blanchable)   **B**   **Stage I** (darkly pigmented)

C   **Stage II** (pressure injury)   **D**   **Stage III** (pressure injury)   **E**   **Stage IV** (pressure injury)

F   Unstageable pressure injury—slough and eschar   Unstageable pressure injury—dark eschar   **G**   Deep tissue pressure injury

NATIONAL
PRESSURE
ULCER
ADVISORY
PANEL

Fig. 20.9A to G: (A) Stage I: Pressure injury—blanchable vs non-blanchable; (B) Stage I: Pressure injury—darkly pigmented; (C) Stage II pressure injury; (D) Stage III pressure injury; (E) Stage IV pressure injury; (F) Unstageable pressure injury—slough and eschar; unstageable pressure injury—dark eschar; (G) Deep tissue pressure Injury

VENOUS DISEASE

Deep Vein Thrombosis

Pathogenesis

Risk factors include trauma, lack of physical activity (especially absolute bed rest), aberrant coagulability (following surgery, miscarriage, or pregnancy), use of oral contraceptives, underlying malignancy, smoking, long airplane flights, and excessive physical activity in poorly trained individuals (Sunday mountain climbers).

A list of causes is given in Table 20.3 (*VBC: Venous defects, blood flow defects and clotting defects*).

Clinical Features

The onset may be 'silent' or heralded by pain in the calf, often about 10 days after immobilization following surgery or a long haul aeroplane flight, parturition or an infection.

The leg becomes **swollen and cyanotic** distal to the thrombus, often accompanied by fever, chills, and tachycardia. The calf may hurt when handled or if the foot is dorsiflexed **(Homan's sign)**.[Q] Sometimes a pulmonary embolus is the first sign of a silent deep vein thrombosis (DVT).

> - If a patient has unexplained calf pain, leg edema, tense muscles or tenderness, always think of DVT.
> - In bedridden patients, the signs and symptoms are often less dramatic.

Investigation

Clinical diagnosis extremely difficult and unreliable; must always be confirmed.

a. *D-dimer test*[Q]:
  - Fibrin split products, which always appear when clotting occurs

b. *Compression sonography*: Method of choice.[Q]

Treatment

Immediate anticoagulation is the most important step; low-molecular-weight heparin given subcutaneously and oral coumarin should be started. The platelet count (risk of heparin-induced thrombocytopenia) and prothrombin time or international normalized ratio (INR) should be monitored. When an INR of 2–3 has been reached for 3 days, heparin therapy can be stopped. The oral anticoagulants should be continued for 3–6 months. Compression therapy should also be instituted immediately.

DVT after a surgical operation is less frequent now, with early postoperative mobilization, regular leg exercises, the use of elastic stockings over the operative period and prophylaxis with low dose heparin. There is no evidence that aspirin taken before a long flight reduces the incidence of DVTs, but elastic stockings and leg exercises during the flight are sensible precautions.

Superficial Thrombophlebitis

The term thrombophlebitis (inflammation of vein) refers to a less serious issue as compared to phlebo-thrombosis (primary thrombosis, far more serious).

Pathogenesis

The elements of the Virchow triad[Q] (vessel wall damage, increased coagulability, delayed blood flow) remain the crucial factors for thrombosis.

Table 20.3	Causes of deep vein thrombosis
Vein wall defects	• Trauma (surgery and injuries) • Chemicals (intravenous infusions) • Neighboring infection (e.g. in leg ulcer) • Tumor (local invasion)
Blood flow defects	• Stasis (immobility, operations, long aircraft flights, pressure, pregnancy, myocardial infarction, heart failure, incompetent valves) • Impaired venous return
Clotting defects	• Platelets increased or sticky (thrombocythemia, polycythemia vera, leukemia, trauma, splenectomy) • Decreased fibrinolysis (postoperative) • Deficiency of clotting factors (e.g. antithrombin, proteins C and S, factor V Leiden) • Alteration in clotting factors (oral contraceptive, infection, leukemia, pregnancy, shock and hemorrhage) • Antiphospholipid antibody • Prothrombin gene mutation
Others	• Malignancy (thrombophlebitis migrans) • Smoking • Behçet's syndrome • Inflammatory bowel disease

Clinical Features

This is inflammation in a thrombosed vein characterized by pain, erythema and tenderness at the sites of inflammation. If the affected vein is varicose or superficial, it will be red and feel like a tender cord. The leg may be diffusely inflamed, making a distinction from cellulitis difficult. There may be fever, leukocytosis and a high ESR.

One-third of patients with thrombophlebitis have deep vein thrombosis at the same time. Duplex sonography should be performed to rule out deep thrombosis or an ascending phlebitis in a varicosity, which can also cause a pulmonary embolus, if it reaches the junction of the great saphenous vein and femoral vein.

Therapy

- Compression therapy with class II stockings or relatively firm elastic wraps.
- Often, low-molecular-weight heparin in either prophylactic or a weight-adjusted dosages is used.
- No bedrest. NSAIDs.
- If the junction is involved, emergency surgery.

Leg Ulcers

Leg ulcers are a common disorder which most often seen by dermatologist, as the diagnosis is initially based on visual recognition. Specialist in ulcers and surgeons invariably manage them! The common causes are listed in **Fig. 20.10**.

Venous Leg Ulcer

The cause of this symptom complex is believed to be related to venous hypertension consequent to a defect in the venous drainage of the leg. This requires three sets of veins: Deep veins surrounded by muscles; superficial veins; and the veins connecting these together—the perforating or communicating veins. When the leg muscles contract, blood in the deep veins is squeezed back, against gravity, to the heart (the **calf muscle pump**) and reflux is prevented by valves. When the muscles relax with the help of gravity, blood from the superficial veins passes into the deep veins via the communicating vessels.

If the valves in the deep and communicating veins are incompetent, the calf muscle pump now pushes blood into the superficial veins leading to capillary bed, leading to (Fig. 20.11):

- Extravasation of erythrocytes, and
- Accumulation of leukocytes and inflammatory cytokines including transforming growth factor-β1(TGF-β1). This prompts a cascade of events, including the release of oxygen-free radicals and matrix metalloproteinases, which causes local tissue destruction, fibrosis and ulceration. The constellation of clinical findings is known as **lipodermatosclerosis[Q]**.

Clinical Features

Symptoms: The patients complain of pain, burning, aching, heaviness, itching, cramping, swelling and restless legs. These symptoms generally worsen after prolonged standing and at the end of the day.

Signs:

Site: Typically, venous ulcers occur over or proximal to the medial malleolus,[Q] but they may occur anywhere below the knee. Ulceration is most common found in the gaiter area,[Q] from the mid-calf to the medial malleolus.[Q]

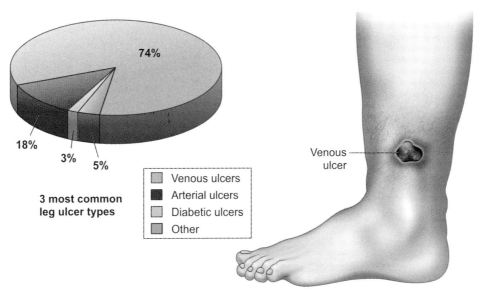

Fig. 20.10: A depiction of the causes of common leg ulcers and the site of venous ulcer

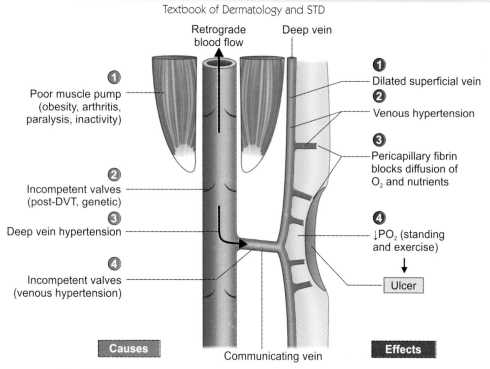

Poor muscle pump
(obesity, arthritis,
paralysis, inactivity) — ①

Incompetent valves
(post-DVT, genetic) — ②

Deep vein hypertension — ③

Incompetent valves
(venous hypertension) — ④

Retrograde blood flow

Deep vein

① Dilated superficial vein

② Venous hypertension

③ Pericapillary fibrin blocks diffusion of O_2 and nutrients

④ ↓PO_2 (standing and exercise)

↓

Ulcer

Causes

Communicating vein

Effects

Fig. 20.11: An overview of the factors that predispose to venous ulcers

The other features include:
- Red or bluish discoloration (corona phlebectasia)
- Edema
- Loss of hair
- Brown pigmentation (mainly hemosiderin from the breakdown of extravasated red blood cells) and scattered petechiae.
- Prominent varicose veins and incompetent perforating branches (blowouts) between the superficial and deep veins, which are best felt with the patient standing.
- Atrophie blanche (ivory white scarring with dilated capillary loops).
- Induration, caused by fibrosis and edema of the dermis and subcutis—sometimes called lipodermatosclerosis. This, if untreated, can lead to a indurated hyperpigmented bound—down skin around the mid-calf resembling an inverted champagne bottle.[Q]

A depiction of a venous ulcer is seen in Fig. 20.12.

Complications

1. Bacterial superinfection is common, but needs systemic antibiotics only if there is pyrexia, a purulent discharge, rapid extension or an increase in pain, cellulitis, lymphangitis or septicemia.
2. Eczema is common around venous ulcers.
3. Allergic contact dermatitis is a common complication and should be suspected, if the rash worsens, itches or fails to improve with local treatment. Lanolin, parabens (a preservative) and neomycin are the most common culprits.

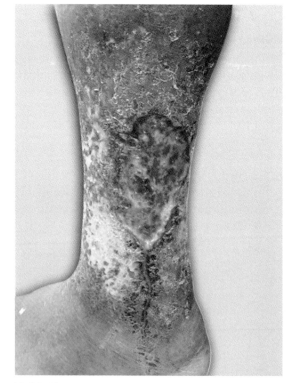

Fig. 20.12: The associated physical signs of chronic venous insufficiency, such as hyperpigmentation, chronic scarring, and skin contraction in the ankle region, are readily identified. Note the classic characteristics of venous disease: (1) irregular edges, (2) shallow ulcer, (3) evidence of hyperpigmentation (hemosiderosis), and (4) location above the medial malleolus.

4. Malignant change can occur. If an ulcer has a hyperplastic base or a rolled edge, biopsy may be needed to rule out a squamous cell carcinoma.

Differential Diagnosis of Leg Ulcers

The most common cause of leg ulcers remains venous ulcers[Q] (Fig. 20.10). The other causes that are important include arterial and neuropathic causes as depicted in Fig. 20.13.

The differentiation between venous ulcers and other common causes of leg ulcer is given below.

1. **Arterial ulcer**

   Risk factors: Peripheral arterial disease, cigarette smoking, diabetes, and hyperlipidemia.

   Symptoms: Intermittent claudication.[Q] The patient experiences pain around the calf muscles during exercise early in the disease and at rest in late disease. The pain tends to be relieved when the patient places the leg in a dependent position.

   Site: Toes, dorsum of foot, heel, calf and shin, and are unrelated to perforating veins.

   Morphology: Arterial ulcers present in distal locations, often over bony prominences such as the toes. They tend to have a round, punched-out[Q] appearance with sharp edges. The base of the ulcer is often dry and may be covered with necrotic debris, presenting as an eschar. These ulcers are sometimes so deep that bone or tendon might be visible. Perhaps the most important clinical feature in making a diagnosis of an arterial ulcer is the absence of pedal pulses (Fig. 20.14).

2. **Trophic ulcer:** Ulcer over pressure points of plantar foot, surrounded by callus, foot deformities.

3. **Vasculitic ulcers:** These ulcers start as painful palpable purpuric lesions, turning into small punched-out ulcers (Fig. 20.15). The involvement of larger vessels is heralded by livedo and painful nodules that may ulcerate.

4. **Thrombotic ulcers:** Skin infarction, leading to ulceration, may be caused by embolism or by the increased coagulability of polycythemia or cryoglobulinemia.

5. **Infective ulcers:** Uncommonly ulcers can be caused by tuberculosis, leprosy, atypical mycobacteria, diphtheria and deep fungal infections, such as sporotrichosis or chromoblastomycosis.

6. **Panniculitic ulcers:** These may appear at odd sites, such as the thighs, buttocks or backs of the calves. The most common types of panniculitis that ulcerate are lupus panniculitis, panniculitic T cell lymphoma, pancreatic panniculitis and erythema induratum.

7. **Malignant ulcers:** Those caused by a squamous cell carcinoma are the most common, but both malignant melanomas and basal cell carcinomas can also present as ulcers. Ulcers can form over CD30 anaplastic large cell lymphomas, panniculitic T cell lymphomas and tumor stage mycosis fungoides.

8. **Pyoderma gangrenosum:** These large and rapidly spreading ulcers may be circular or polycyclic, and have a blue, indurated, undermined or pustular margin.[Q]

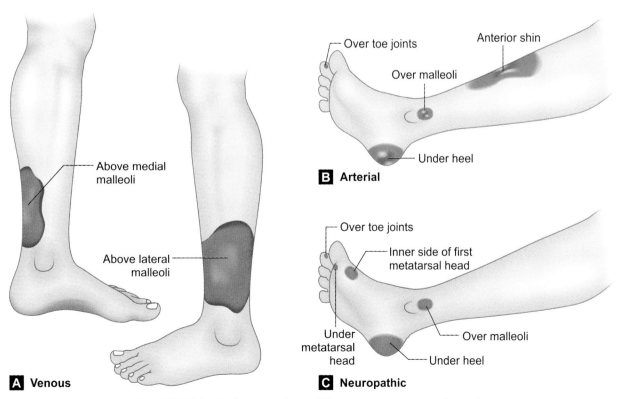

Fig. 20.13A to C: A comparison of the common causes of leg ulcer

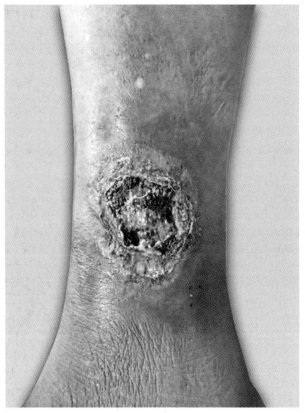

Fig. 20.14: A depiction of an arterial ulcer. Note the lack of edema, dry skin, loss of hair and regular margins. There are also signs of a venous component, though this is a minor sign

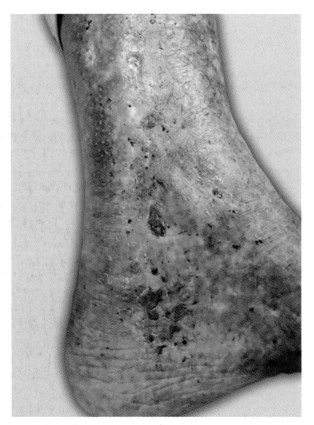

Fig. 20.15: Stellate ulcers which are painful in a case of small vessel vasculitis

Investigation

Most chronic leg ulcers are venous in origin, but the other common causes are arterial insufficiency and neuropathic diseases. In patients with venous ulcers, a search for factors that can lead to leg edema and poor wound healing is useful, including, obesity, peripheral artery disease, immunosuppression, malnutrition, diabetes, cardiac failure or arthritis.

a. Blood glucose
b. Full blood count to detect anemia, which will delay healing
c. Culture for pathogens
d. Color flow duplex ultrasound^Q is the gold standard in the diagnosis of venous incompetence. Doppler ultrasound may help to assess arterial circulation when atherosclerosis is likely. It seldom helps, if the dorsalis pedis or posterior tibial pulses can easily be felt. If the maximal systolic ankle pressure divided by the systolic brachial pressure (ankle brachial pressure index) is greater than 0.8, the ulcer is unlikely to be caused by arterial disease.
e. Cardiac evaluation for congestive failure.

Treatment

The treatment of leg ulcers requires a specialized team but an overview is given below, based on certain basic principles.

1. Venous ulcers will not heal, if the leg remains swollen and the patient chair-bound. Pressure bandages, leg elevation, weight reduction and walking exercise are more important except when atherosclerotic ulcers is to be treated as it has a compromised arterial supply.
2. Topical measures specially antibiotics are rarely of great help as isolating bacteria on culture is all to common without being necessarily pathogenic. Most ulcers, despite positive bacteriology, are not much helped by systemic antibiotics.
3. Admission to hospital for elevation and intensive treatment may be needed, but the results are not encouraging as patients may stay in the ward for many months only to have their apparently well-healed ulcers breakdown rapidly when they go home as a result of non-compliance with therapy.
4. Never put topical steroids on ulcers.
5. Watch out for contact allergy to local applications.

A. Compression and mobilization: The compression should be graduated so that it is greatest at the ankle and least at the top of the bandage and this helps to reduce edema and aids venous return. The bandages are applied over the ulcer dressing, from the forefoot to just below the knee. Bandages can be kept for 2–7 days at a time and are left on at night.

The combined layers give a 40–50 mmHg compression at the ankle. Once an ulcer has healed, a graduated compression stocking from toes to knee (or preferably thigh), should be prescribed, providing pressures of 25–35 mmHg at the ankle.

- The compression hoses sold at many retail stores are not to be used for therapeutic compression—as they have 0 to less than 20 mmHg compression.
- 'Diabetic socks' are not compression hoses, which is a common misconception.

B. Elevation of the affected limb: This helps in venous drainage, decreases edema and raises oxygen tension in the limb.

Patients should rest with their bodies horizontal and their legs up for at least 2 hours every afternoon. The foot of the bed should be raised by at least 15 cm, it is not enough just to put a pillow under the feet.

C. Walking: Walking, in moderation, is beneficial, but prolonged standing or sitting with dependent legs is not.

D. Topical therapy

1. *Cleansing*: Daily washing in tub or shower; moist compresses with physiologic saline (0.9%). Compresses with 5.0% saline are more effective but may be irritating or painful. Olive oil is useful for removing crusts and residual creams or ointments.

2. *Superinfection with exudation*: Antiseptic solutions with moist compresses. For resistant infections, Culture and sensitivity; then consider fusidic acid ointment or mupirocin ointment. In most instances, systemic antibiotics are preferable.

3. *Dermatitis therapy*: Always exclude allergic contact dermatitis caused by topical agent or preservative. Common allergens include balsam of Peru, wool wax alcohols, cetylsterol alcohol, emulgators, preservatives (parabens), antibiotics (especially neomycin, gentamicin, chloramphenicol). Use of any of these agents should be considered carefully.

E. Dressing

1. *Clean ulcers*: Low-adherent dressings are useful in patients with fragile skin. They reduce adherence at the wound bed and allow passage of exudate to an overlying dressing. They are usually made of paraffin tulle, either plain or impregnated with various agents (e.g. chlorhexidine, xeroform, povidone iodine) and need be changed only once or twice a week. The area should be cleaned gently with saline before the next dressing is applied.

Semipermeable films (Tegaderm) are porous to air and water vapor, but not fluids or bacteria, and are suitable for shallow ulcers with low to medium exudate, in which they encourage a moist wound healing.

2. *Infected ulcer*: Useful preparations include 0.5% silver nitrate, 0.25% sodium hypochlorite, 0.25% acetic acid, potassium permanganate (1 in 10 000 dilution) and 5% hydrogen peroxide, all made up in aqueous solution, and applied as compresses with or without occlusion. Helpful creams and lotions include 1.5% hydrogen peroxide, 20% benzoyl peroxide, 1% silver sulfadiazine, 10% povidone-iodine.

F. Systemic therapy

1. Antibiotics are not always helpful as, just because bacteria can be isolated from an ulcer does not mean that antibiotics should be prescribed. Ulcers need not be 'sterilized' by local or systemic antibiotics. Indications are, spreading infections characterized by an enlarging ulcer, increased redness around the ulcer and lymphangitis. Antibiotics should cover streptococcal or staphylococcal infection, metronidazole (*Bacteroides* infection) and ciprofloxacin (*Pseudomonas aeruginosa* infection).

2. If there is an arterial component, consider low-dose aspirin, low-dose heparin, pentoxifylline; prostacyclin infusions possible but value not proven.

G. Surgical intervention: This is of two types one for the incompetent vein and for the non-healing ulcer.

PURPURA

This disorder is characterized by spontaneous small areas of bleeding into the skin. The lesions of purpura consist of petechiae, tiny pinpoint areas of bleeding, as well as ecchymoses, which are larger. The various important types include:

- *Petechiae*: Flat lesions, macules ≤4 mm, typically initially bright red and then fade to a rust color.
- *Ecchymosis*: Flat lesions, macules and/or patches, >5 mm,[Q] typically initially red or purple, but may fade to yellow, brown, or green.
- *Palpable purpura*: Elevated, round or oval, red or purple papules and/or plaques sometimes barely palpable.
- *Retiform purpura*: Stellate or branching lesions, with angular or geometric borders. These are often palpable plaques, but can present as nonpalpable patches as well.

This entity is conventionally divided into two variants, namely *inflammatory* and *non-inflammatory*, the latter is because of blocking of the vessels. The inflammatory variant is usually seen in autoimmune disorders.

Table 20.4 A classification of purpura based on the clinical presentation

Petechiae	Platelet function disorder	• Congenital (vWD: usually AD) • Acquired (drug-induced, liver disease, uremia, dysproteinemia, acquired vWD)
	Thrombocytosis	Myelofibrosis may be primary or secondary to other malignancy
	No platelet abnormality	• Pigmented purpuric eruptions, capillaritis • Hypergammaglobulinemic purpura of Waldenstrom • Intravascular, local pressure, or trauma
Ecchymosis	Procoagulant defects	• Anticoagulant therapy • Liver disease • Vitamin K deficiency • DIC (Fig. 20.16) • Platelet disorders
	Decreased dermal support of vessels and minor trauma	• Solar or senile purpura[Q] (Fig. 20.17) • Corticosteroid therapy • Scurvy (vitamin C deficiency) • Systemic amyloidosis[Q] • Genetic disease (Ehlers-Danlos syndrome, PXE)
Palpable purpura, inflammatory[Q]	Leukocytoclastic vasculitis[Q]	• Henoch-Schönlein purpura • Urticarial vasculitis • Mixed cryoglobulinemia • Rheumatic vasculitis
	Anti-neutrophilic cytoplasmic antibody (ANCA)	• Wegener's granulomatosis • Churg-Strauss syndrome • Microscopic polyangiitis
Retiform purpura with inflammation		• Rheumatic vasculitis (e.g. RA and SLE) (Fig. 20.18) • Polyarteritis nodosa • ANCA vasculitides
Retiform purpura, non-inflammatory	Platelet occlusion	• Heparin necrosis (Fig. 20.19) • Thrombocytosis • Paroxysmal nocturnal hemoglobinuria (PNH) • TTP • Cold-related gelling or agglutination • Occlusion secondary to organism invading vessel (Fig. 20.20)
	Systemic coagulopathies	• Inherited hypercoagulable states • Warfarin necrosis[Q] • Purpura fulminans • Antiphospholipid antibody or lupus anticoagulant
	Emboli	• Cholesterol • Endocarditis • Oxalate
	Reticulocytes	• Sickle cell disease • Calciphylaxis

There are numerous causes of purpura and a clinical presentation based classification is given in Table 20.4 and etiological classification is detailed in Table 20.5.

Investigation

Though the most common cause of purpura is trauma,[Q] especially to the thin sun-damaged skin of elderly forearms (senile purpura Fig. 20.17), there are numerous other causes as can be seen in Table 20.6 which required detailed investigations. A brief guideline for investigations is given in Table 20.3. For clinician, an approach is given in Flowchart 20.1 which is based on clinical presentation of purpura and presence of palpable lesions which is seen in vasculitis.

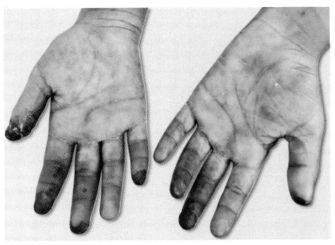

Fig. 20.16: DIC leading to peripheral symmetrical gangrene

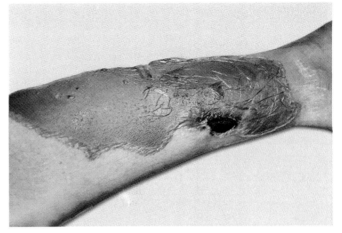

Fig. 20.19: Retiform purpura, non-inflammatory, (platelet occlusion—heparin necrosis)

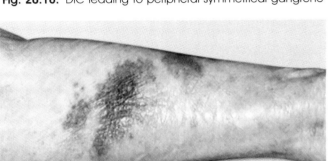

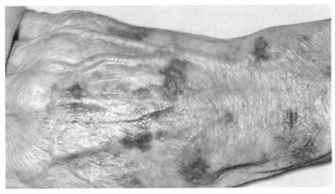

Fig. 20.17: Senile pupura most commonly seen on the limbs

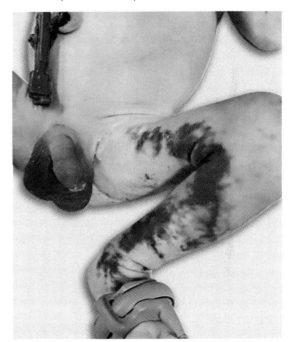

Fig. 20.20A: Occlusion secondary to infective pathology and sepsis involving the vessel

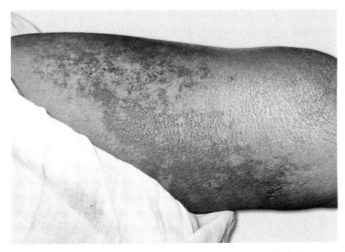

Fig. 20.18: Inflammatory retiform purpura in SLE

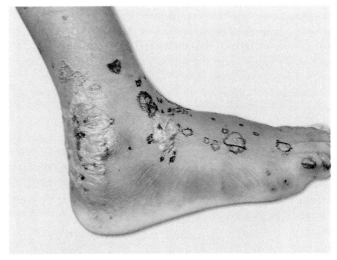

Fig. 20.20B: Purpura and ecchymosis in meningococcemia

Table 20.5 An etiological classification of pupura

Platelet defects	• Thrombocytopenia • Idiopathic • Connective tissue disorders • Disseminated intravascular coagulation • Hemolytic anemia • Hypersplenism • Giant hemangiomas • Bone marrow damage • Drugs
Coagulation defects	• Inherited defects (e.g. hemophilia, Christmas disease) • Connective tissue disorders • Disseminated intravascular coagulation • Paraproteinemias • Acquired defects (e.g. liver disease, anticoagulant therapy, vitamin K deficiency, drugs)
Vascular defect	• Raised intravascular pressure (coughing, vomiting, venous hypertension, gravitational) • Vasculitis (including Henoch-Schönlein purpura) • Infections (e.g. meningococcal septicemia, Rocky mountain spotted fever) • Drugs (carbromal, aspirin, sulfonamides, quinine, phenylbutazone and gold salts) • Painful bruising syndrome
Others	• Senile purpura • Topical or systemic corticosteroid therapy • Scurvy (perifollicular purpura) • Lichen sclerosus et atrophicus • Systemic amyloidosis

Pigmented Purpuric Dermatoses (PPD)

Pathogenesis: Increased hydrostatic presence, often coupled with mild venous insufficiency, is the main factor. Drugs are an overrated cause.

Clinical features: Primary lesions are 2–3 mm red-brown macules on the feet or shins.

Variants include (Fig. 20.21):
• Schamberg purpura[Q]—most common form, multiple red-brown macules.
• Lichen aureus—solitary yellow-brown patch usually over an incompetent vein other forms that may be annular, lichenoid, or eczematoid; sometimes the lesions coalesce.

Histopathology: Perivascular lymphocytic infiltrates (lymphocytic vasculitis).

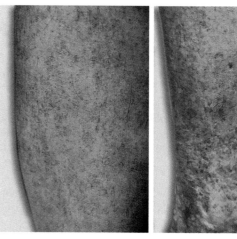

Fig. 20.21: Pigmented purpuric macules and papules on the lower leg: PPD

Table 20.6 Investigations to arrive at the cause of purpura

Petechiae	• CBC with differential and peripheral smear • If **anemic**, check reticulocyte count, LDH, haptoglobin, and bilirubin • If **hemolysis** is present, check PTT, PT/INR, fibrinogen, D-dimer, Coombs, ANA • If inconclusive, consider bone marrow biopsy • ANA, anti-Ro, anti-La
Ecchymosis	↑PT/INR, ±↑PTT
Palpable purpura and retiform inflammatory purpura	• Skin biopsy, BUN/Cr, urinalysis • ↓Complement (e.g. CH50, C4, C3, C1q) may relate to a variety of systemic processes, e.g. SLE, malignancy, and infection • ANA and ↓complement (SLE) • RF, anti-CCP (RA) • ANA, RF, anti-Ro or La (Sjögren's) • ANCA (90%), c-ANCA: Wegener's granulomatosis • ANCA (50%), p-ANCA (anti-MPO), or c-ANCA: Churg-Strauss • ANCA (70%), p-ANCA: Microscopic polyangiitis
Retiform purpura noninflammatory	• CBC • Platelet count, skin biopsy, PT/INR, PTT • Protein C and S, D-dimer, fibrin degradation products • Hyperphosphatemia, elevated calcium phosphate product (>70 mg/dL)

Flowchart 20.1: Approach to diagnosis of purpura

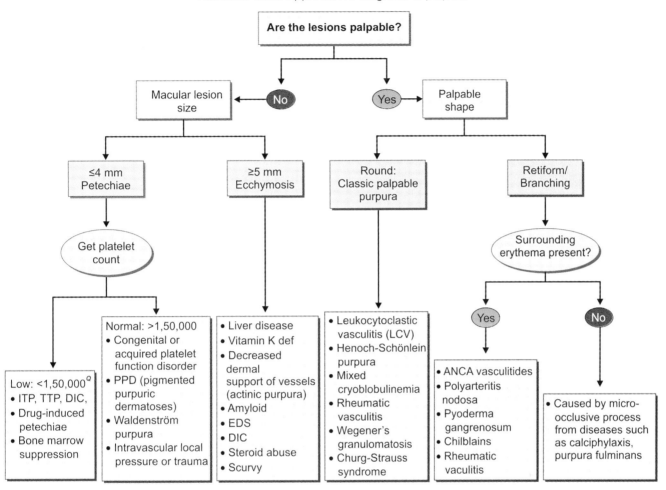

Flowchart 20.2: An overview of variants of primary lymphedema

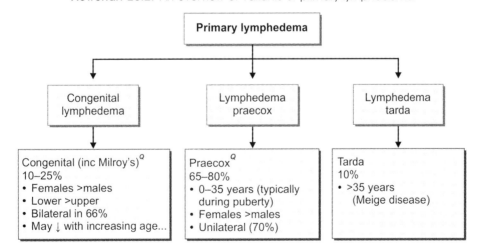

Therapy: Topical corticosteroids are used for pruritus. Support hose may slow progression.

DISORDERS OF THE LYMPHATICS

Lymphedema

The skin overlying chronic lymphedema is firm and pits poorly. Long-standing lymphedema may lead to gross, almost furry, hyperkeratosis, as in the so-called 'mossyfoot'.

Cause

Lymphedema may be primary or secondary. The primary forms are developmental defects, although signs may only appear in early puberty or even in

Table 20.7	Cause of secondary lymphedema
Lymphatic obstruction	• Filariasis • Granuloma inguinale • Tuberculosis • Tumor
Lymphatic destruction	• Surgery • Radiation therapy • Tumor
Recurrent lymphangitis	• Erysipelas • Infected pompholyx
Uncertain etiology	• Rosacea • Melkersson-Rosenthal syndrome[Q] (facial nerve palsy, fissuring of tongue and lymphedema of lip) • Yellow nail[Q] discoloration, pleural effusion, lower limb lymphedema

adulthood. An overview of the primary types is given in Flowchart 20.2.

Sometimes lymphedema involves only one leg. Secondary causes are listed in Table 20.7.

Treatment

Therapy that helps to reduce the swelling is the ideal method of therapy. For this, the treatment methods include:
• Multilayer compression bandaging,
• Manual lymphatic drainage by an experienced physiotherapist
• Exercise and skin care.

Prevention of infection is essential to prevent continued lymphatic damage and antibiotics should be given at the first sign of lymphangitis or erysipelas. If erysipelas recurs, long-term penicillin should be given.

Vasculitis and Neutrophilic Disorders

Introduction

The term vasculitis exemplifies disorders that show inflammation within the vessel wall, with endothelial cell swelling, necrosis or fibrinoid change.

The clinical manifestations depend upon the size of the blood vessel affected. The classical triad is 'Painful, Palpable, Purpura'[Q]—which describe the lesions seen.

Classification

The size of diseased vessels has been the major criterion for classifying these disorders in most schemes, as size is a major determinant of their clinical symptoms. Large size signifies the aorta and its branches; medium size signifies vessels that, while smaller than the major branches of the aorta, contain an internal elastic membrane as well as muscular media and adventitia. Small size denotes capillaries, and postcapillary venules and arterioles. This classification has stood the test of time and is displayed in Fig. 21.1 and Table 21.1.

Also vasculitis may be primary or associated with underlying disorder (autoimmune disease, drug reaction, infection, malignancy, serum sickness).

Though, in dermatology, the small vessel vasculitis is often seen, other vasculitis can also affect the small vessels and have skin manifestations.

Investigation

Investigation aims to establish and confirm the diagnosis, the extent and severity of organ involvement, and disease activity.

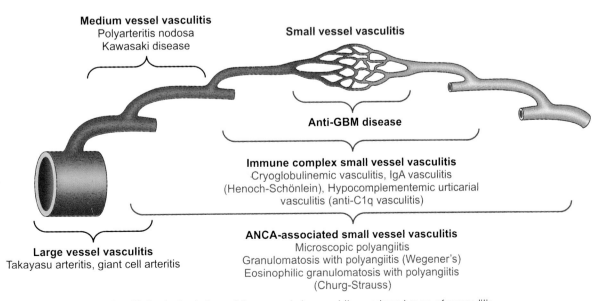

Fig. 21.1: A depiction of the vessel size and the various types of vasculitis

Table 21.1 Names for vasculitides adopted by the 2012 International Chapel Hill Consensus Conference on the Nomenclature of Vasculitides

	Primary	*Secondary*
Large vessel vasculitis (LVV)[Q]	• Takayasu's arteritis (TAK) • Giant cell arteritis (GCA)	• Syphilis • Tuberculosis
Medium vessel vasculitis (MVV)[Q]	• Polyarteritis nodosa (PAN) • Kawasaki's disease (KD)	HBV associated PAN
Small vessel vasculitis (SVV)[Q]	Antineutrophil cytoplasmic antibody (ANCA)-associated vasculitis (AAV) 1. Microscopic polyangiitis (MPA) 2. Granulomatosis with polyangiitis (Wegener's) (GPA) 3. Eosinophilic granulomatosis with polyangiitis (Churg-Strauss) (EGPA)	Drugs (propylthiouracil, hydralazine)*
	Immune complex SVV 1. Antiglomerular basement membrane (anti-GBM) disease 2. Cryoglobulinemic vasculitis (CV) 3. IgA vasculitis (Henoch-Schönlein) (IgAV) 4. Hypocomplementemic urticarial vasculitis (HUV) (anti-C1q vasculitis)	• Cryoglobulinemic vasculitis (HCV) • RA, SLE, Sjögren's syndrome • Serum sickness • Drug induced (sulfonamides, penicillins, thiazide diuretics and many others)
Single-organ vasculitis (SOV)	Cutaneous leukocytoclastic angiitis	
Variable	• Behçet's • Cogan's	

1. *Urine analysis*: This is the most important investigation because the severity of renal involvement is one of the key determinants of prognosis. Detection of proteinuria or hematuria in a patient with systemic illness needs further investigation.

2. *Blood tests*: Leukocytosis suggests a primary vasculitis or infection. Eosinophilia suggests eosinophilic granulomatosis with polyangiitis or a drug reaction.

3. *Liver function tests*: Abnormal results suggest viral infection (hepatitis A, B, C) or may be non-specific.

4. *Immunology*: Antineutrophil cytoplasmic antibodies are associated with the primary systemic necrotizing vasculitides.

   ANCA are found in about 75% of the three small vessel vasculitis.[Q] Cytoplasmic ANCA is highly specific for Wegener's granulomatosis.[Q] Perinuclear ANCA associated with myeloperoxidase antibodies occur in microscopic polyangiitis[Q] and eosinophilic granulomatosis with polyangiitis (Churg-Strauss).[Q]

   • 75% of patients with *WG* are *cANCA* positive
   • 40–75% of CSS patients are positive for either cANCA or pANCA
   • pANCA is found in about 50% of MPA
   • Either ANCA can be found in any of these three disorders, and are absent in 5–30%

   Rheumatoid factors and antinuclear antibodies may indicate vasculitis associated with connective tissue disease.

5. *Biopsy*: Tissue biopsy is important to confirm the diagnosis before treatment with potentially toxic immunosuppressive drugs. The choice of tissue to biopsy is crucial.

6. *Other investigations*:
   • Angiography can show aneurysms.
   • Blood cultures, viral serology and echocardiography are important to exclude infection and other conditions that may present as systemic multisystem disease.

An approach to the diagnosis of vasculitis based on major investigations is given in Flowchart 21.1.

Treatment

Though the details of therapy will be covered in the text that follows a general intervention based on the size of the vessels is given in Table 21.2. For skin involvement dapsone and colchicine are also effective.

SINGLE-ORGAN VASCULITIS

Leukocytoclastic Vasculitis

Synonyms: Hypersensitivity angiitis, CSSV, 'palpable purpura'.[Q]

It is defined as an inflammation of dermal venules with immune complex deposition and fibrinoid necrosis. This is the most common type of cutaneous vasculitis.[Q]

Flowchart 21.1: Investigative approach to diagnosis of vasculitis

Biopsy
(24–48 hours old)
- Lesions: Nodule, purpura, NOT from the ulcer
- Routine histology and direct immunofluorescence

Baseline Investigations
- CBC with differential platelet count, ESR, C reactive protein
- LFT, BUN and creatinine, urinalysis, stool, occult blood

Specific tests based on clinical diagnosis
- Antistreptolysin O and anti-DNAse B titers; hepatitis B/C and HIV serologies; throat, urine or blood culture as indicated
- Cryoglobulins
- CH50/C3/C4, if suspect urticarial vasculitis (also C1q if low C4)
- Rheumatoid factor, ANA, anti-ENA antibodies (e.g. anti-Ro), ANCA

Disease Specific Investigations

1. ANCA-associated vasculitis:
   - Chest X-ray, CT of chest and sinuses
   - Electromyogram/nerve conduction studies, echocardiogram/electrocardiogram, and biopsy of the respiratory tract (upper or lower), nerve, kidney or muscle
2. Classic (systemic) polyarteritis nodosa
   - Mesenteric/renal/celiac angiogram
   - Consider biopsy of muscle, nerve, kidney or testicles

Table 21.2	Relationship between vessel size and response to induction treatment			
Dominant vessel	Corticosteroid alone	Cylophosphamide and corticosteroids	Rituximab	Other treatment
Large arteries	+++	–	–	+
Medium arteries	+	++	–	++[a]
Small vessel (ANCA-associated)	+	+++	+++	+
Small vessel (Immune complex)	++	+/–	+	++[a]

[a]Includes plasmapheresis, anti-viral therapy for hepatitis B-associated PAN and HCV-associated cryoglobulinemia, and IVIg for Kawasaki disease.

Epidemiology: Favors children and young adults; in older patients, often drug reaction or reflection of systemic vasculitis.

Pathogenesis

Many possible triggers are shown in Table 21.3 and Fig. 21.2. Usually immune complexes are formed, then deposited in the venules, where they activate complement and establish an inflammatory reaction that damages the vessel wall (Fig. 21.3).

Clinical Features

The hallmark of leukocytoclastic vasculitis is purpura Fig. 21.4. More advanced lesions are often palpable. Other lesions may be urticarial, pustular, or necrotic.

The most common clinical findings are purpura (99%), papules (40%), ulcerations (30%), pustules (20%), urticaria (10%), subcutaneous nodules (10%), and livedo racemosa (5%).

Sites: Lower legs (100%), arms (15%), mucosa (15%), external ears (10%), and conjunctiva (5%).

Histology: Necrotic vessel wall with fibrin, nuclear dust (leukocytoclasia), and exocytosis of erythrocytes.

Differential Diagnosis

Septic vasculitis (gonorrhea, meningococcemia, candidiasis, many others); livedo vasculitis. Leukocytoclastic vasculitis is common in Wegener's granulomatosis and polyarteritis nodosa; a positive biopsy does not exclude systemic vasculitis.

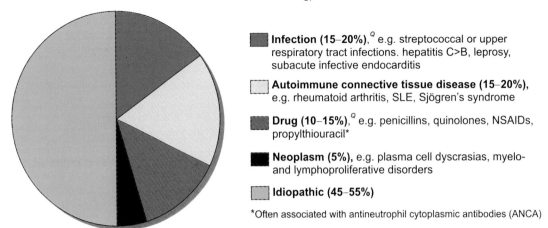

■ **Infection (15–20%),**[Q] e.g. streptococcal or upper respiratory tract infections. hepatitis C>B, leprosy, subacute infective endocarditis

□ **Autoimmune connective tissue disease (15–20%),** e.g. rheumatoid arthritis, SLE, Sjögren's syndrome

■ **Drug (10–15%),**[Q] e.g. penicillins, quinolones, NSAIDs, propylthiouracil*

■ **Neoplasm (5%),** e.g. plasma cell dyscrasias, myelo- and lymphoproliferative disorders

□ **Idiopathic (45–55%)**

*Often associated with antineutrophil cytoplasmic antibodies (ANCA)

Fig. 21.2: Etiology of cutaneous small vessel vasculitis

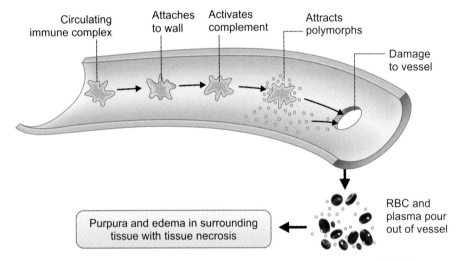

Fig. 21.3: A depiction of the steps involved in the causation of CSSV

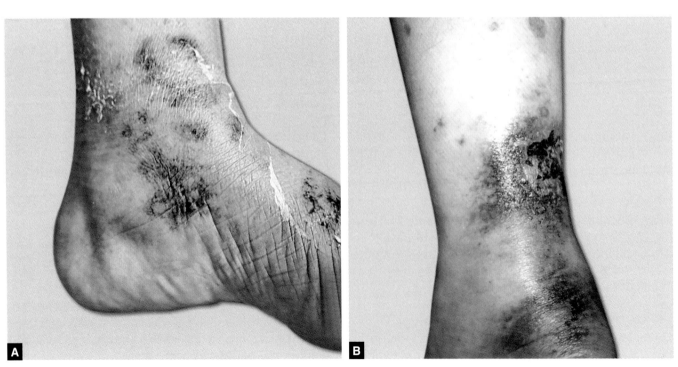

Fig. 21.4: (A) Stellate purpura; and (B) Ulcerative forms of cutaneous vasculitis

Table 21.3 Cause of CSSV and the possible investigations

Infections: streptococci, tuberculosis, hepatitis B and C	Throat culture, antistreptolysin, chest radiograph, hepatitis serology
Lupus erythematosus, Sjögren syndrome	Antinuclear antibodies, autoantibodies
Rheumatoid arthritis	Rheumatoid factor
Cryoglobulinemia	Cryoglobulins
Gammopathy	Serum protein electrophoresis
Complement defects	CH50, C3, C4
Serum sickness	History: Vaccines, antithymocyte globulin, streptokinase, immunoglobulins
Drugs	ACE inhibitors, NSAIDs, phenytoin, sulfonamides, thiouracil

Investigation

Investigations should be directed toward identifying the cause and detecting internal involvement (Table 21.3).

- History may indicate infections; myalgias, abdominal pain, claudication, mental confusion and mononeuritis may indicate systemic involvement.
- Chest X-ray, ESR and biochemical tests monitoring the function of various organs are indicated.
- The *most important test* is urine analysis, checking for proteinuria and hematuria, because vasculitis can affect the kidney subtly and so lead to renal insufficiency.
- Skin biopsy will confirm the diagnosis of small vessel vasculitis.
- Direct immunofluorescence can be used to identify immune complexes.

Therapy

If acute insult, treat the trigger.
- Often no therapy is needed; bed rest and compression stockings help.
- *Corticosteroids*: Prednisolone 60 mg for 3–5 days.
- If recurrent, *dapsone* 0.5–2.0 mg/kg daily or colchicine 0.5–1.0 mg daily.

> Development of systemic features such as arthralgia, abdominal pain, or hematuria should prompt assessment for systemic vasculitis and is indicative of a worse prognosis.

Erythema Elevatum et Diutinum

Chronic cutaneous vasculitis with formation of fibrotic plaques.

Clinical features: Symmetrical, slowly-developing red-brown papules and nodules favoring backs of hands, over the digital joints and knees and elbows.[Q]

Therapy: Limited disease; intralesional or high-potency topical corticosteroids. More widespread or resistant disease: Dapsone 0.5–2.0 mg/kg daily.

Granuloma Faciale

Chronic form of leukocytoclastic vasculitis causing red-brown facial plaques.[Q]

Clinical features: Usually solitary or limited number of red-brown plaques limited to face, typically cheeks, chin, forehead or ears. Occasionally, multiple or scattered lesions. Lesions are soft, poorly circumscribed, and asymptomatic, but a cosmetic problem.

Histology: Name is misnomer, as lesion is not a granuloma.[Q] Perivascular infiltrate of neutrophils and eosinophils; initially leukocytoclastic vasculitis. Characteristic Grenz zone[Q] between normal epidermis and infiltrate.

Therapy: Intralesional corticosteroids, laser destruction, cryotherapy. Dapsone 0.5–2.0 mg/kg daily sometimes induces prompt remission.

Cutaneous Polyarteritis Nodosa

Cutaneous polyarteritis nodosa is a chronic relapsing arteritis of subcutaneous and deep dermal small and medium-sized vessels. By definition, visceral organs are spared. Progression to systemic disease is rare.

Clinical features: The cutaneous lesions are painful nodules which may ulcerate and occur most frequently on the lower legs.

There may be marked livedo reticularis. There are no diagnostic markers and the diagnosis is made on the typical lesions and histology.

Therapy: Treatment usually requires glucocorticoids in moderate doses. Other agents that have been used include sulphapyridine, dapsone, and stanazolol.

SYSTEMIC VASCULITIS

Small Vessel Vasculitis

Microscopic Polyangiitis

Necrotizing vasculitis with a few immune deposits, always involving smallest blood vessels but capable of affecting medium-sized vessels and with tropism for kidneys and lungs[Q] (pulmonary-renal syndrome).[Q]

Clinical features:

General findings: Fever, weight loss.

Skin: Leukocytoclastic vasculitis (30–40%).

Kidneys: Pauci-immune necrotizing glomerulonephritis with casts (70%).

Lungs: Pulmonary vasculitis with alveolar hemorrhage and hemoptysis (10–15%).

Serology: 60% positive for pANCA.^{Q}

Therapy: Prednisone and cyclophosphamide, as in polyarteritis nodosa.

Wegener's Granulomatosis (Granulomatosis with Polyangiitis)

Definition: Systemic vasculitis with aseptic granulomatous inflammation, primarily involving upper and lower respiratory tracts, as well as kidneys.^{Q}

- Almost any organ system can be affected.
- The ACR in 1990 developed classification criteria, which are widely used in clinical trials (Box 21.1).

Clinical features (Fig. 21.5)

- *1st stage*: General signs and symptoms such as fever, and malaise. Symptoms in the ear, nose and throat (such as epistaxis, crusting and deafness) are associated with this condition.
- *2nd stage*: Lower airway problems: Cough, dyspnea, hemoptysis, pleurisy.
- *3rd stage*: Generalized involvement including skin.

Box 21.1 | ACR criteria for classification of Wegener's granulomatosis

1. *Nasal or oral inflammation*: Development of painful or painless oral ulcers or purulent or bloody nasal discharge.
2. *Abnormal chest radiograph*: Chest radiograph showing the presence of nodules, fixed infiltrates or cavities.
3. *Urinary sediment*: Microhematuria (>5 red cells per high power field) or red cell casts in urinary sediment.
4. *Granulomatous inflammation*: Histological changes showing granuloma on biopsy, inflammation within the wall of an artery or in the perivascular or extravascular area (artery or arteriole).

Note: For purpose of classification, a person shall be said to have Wegener's granulomatosis, if at least 2 of these 4 criteria are present. The presence of any 2 or more criteria yields a sensitivity of 88.2% and specificity of 92.0%.

Frequency of organ involvement: Lungs (95%), upper airway (90%), kidneys (85%), joints (70%), eyes (60%), ears (60%), skin (45%), nerves (20%), heart (10%).

Skin: Polymorphic picture including leukocytoclastic vasculitis, urticarial vasculitis, necrotizing pyodermas (mini-pyoderma gangrenosum), panniculitis.

Histology

Triad^Q of (1) necrotizing leukocytoclastic vasculitis, (2) necrosis, and (3) granuloma formation. The granulomas

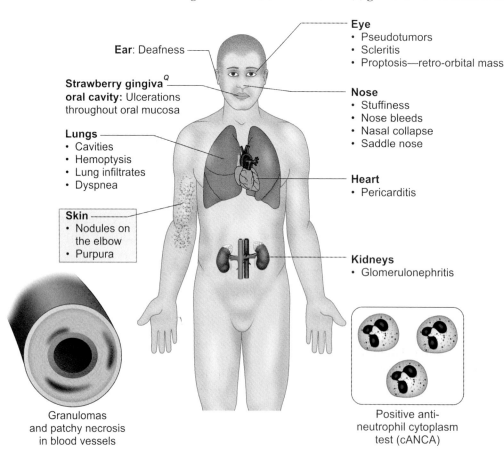

Fig. 21.5: Clinical features of Wegener's granulomatosis

can be in the vessel walls; they can be palisading (thus microscopically mistaken for granuloma annulare) or rich in giant cells.

Investigation

- Tissue diagnosis: *Usually* airway or renal biopsy; sometimes skin biopsy helps.
- Investigate upper airways, lungs, and kidneys.
- **cANCA positive** in 50% during early phases, 90% when generalized.

Differential diagnosis

- Pulmonary disease: Microscopic polyangiitis, infections.
- Kidneys: Other causes of glomerulonephritis.
- Destructive upper airway disease: NK/T cell lymphoma (nasal type), formerly known as lethal midline granuloma.

Therapy

Fauci regimen: Prednisone 1 mg/kg daily and cyclophosphamide 2 mg/kg daily. If not responsive, either agent can be increased. Once response occurs, taper prednisone with goal of stopping. Cyclophosphamide is continued for at least 1 year at the standard dose before being slowly tapered.

Many other immunosuppressive regimens are under investigation, such as cyclophosphamide induction followed by methotrexate. Recurrences or localized disease can often be treated with cotrimoxazole.

Churg-Strauss Syndrome

A rare systemic granulomatous vasculitis favoring small vessels with a **triad** of (1) asthma, (2) granulomatous vasculitis of lungs and skin, and (3) eosinophilia of tissues and blood.^{Q}

The ACR criteria are given in Box 21.2.

Clinical features

- *Asthma* is present in over 80% and often the presenting symptom, present for years before other features develop. Pulmonary infiltrates and vasculitis come later. Nasal and sinus disease is not destructive.
- Multiple other organs involved: Mononeuritis multiplex (60%), kidneys (50%), heart (40%), gastrointestinal tract (40%).
- Skin: Involved in 70%: Purpura, nodules, and urticarial vasculitis.

Investigation

Tissue diagnosis: Skin or lung biopsy.

Investigate lungs and other organs on the basis of signs and symptoms.

Laboratory: ESR, hypereosinophilia, elevated IgE, cryoglobulins, immune complexes.

Box 21.2 | **ACR criteria for classification of CSS**

1. *Asthma*: History of wheezing or diffuse high pitch rales on expiration.
2. *Eosinophilia*: >10% on white cell differential count.
3. Mononeuropathy or polyneuropathy: Development of mononeuropathy, multiple mononeuropathies, or polyneuropathy (i.e. glove/stocking distribution) attributable to systemic vasculitis.
4. *Pulmonary infiltrates, non-fixed*: Migratory or transient pulmonary radiographs (not including fixed infiltrates) attributable to a systemic vasculitis.
5. *Paranasal sinus abnormalitiy*: History of acute or chronic paranasal or tenderness or radiographic opacification of the paranasal sinuses.
6. *Extravascular eosinophils*: Biopsy including artery, arteriole, or venule showing accumulations of eosinophils in extravascular areas.

Note: For purposes of classification, a person shall be said to have Churg-Strauss syndrome, if at least 4 of these 6 criteria are present.

Both cANCA and p-ANCA^Q can be positive; estimated 20% for each.

Therapy

Very steroid responsive: Initially use prednisolone 1 mg/kg daily. Reserve immunosuppressive agents (cyclophosphamide, mycophenolate mofetil, cyclosporine) for treatment failures or life-threatening disease.

Henoch-Schönlein Purpura^Q

Appears primarily in children, purpura associated with gastrointestinal distress and arthralgias^Q; IgA immune complexes^Q in kidneys and skin (**Fig. 21.6A**).

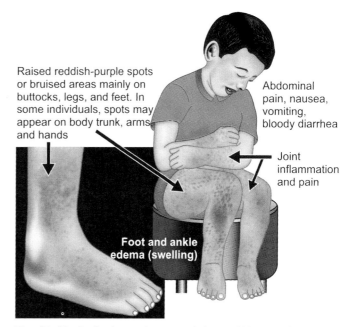

Raised reddish-purple spots or bruised areas mainly on buttocks, legs, and feet. In some individuals, spots may appear on body trunk, arms and hands

Abdominal pain, nausea, vomiting, bloody diarrhea

Joint inflammation and pain

Foot and ankle edema (swelling)

Fig. 21.6A: Typical symptoms and signs of Henoch-Schönlein purpura

Clinical features: The classic tetrad^Q is: (1) Purpura (universal), (2) Arthritis (82%), (3) Nephritis (40%); (4) Abdominal pain (63%), or gastrointestinal hemorrhage (33%). It typically presents following an upper respiratory tract infection (Fig. 21.6B to D).

The ACR criteria of diagnosis are given in Box 21.3.

Investigation: Assessment of organ involvement in all patients:

- Urinalysis (proteinuria, hematuria, red cell casts), should be performed urgently in all patients in whom HSP is suspected.
- Renal function (creatinine clearance, quantification of protein leak, if present, using either 24-h protein excretion or urine protein/creatinine ratio).
- Blood pressure.
- Serological investigations: ANA, ANCA, RF should all be negative. A positive ANA or ANCA suggests the presence of a connective tissue disease or other vasculitis.
- Complement levels are normal.
- Biopsy: A renal biopsy should be considered in both children and adults, if there is significant proteinuria or hematuria that persists (in children >1 year). IgA-dominant immune deposits are observed in the walls of small vessels and in the renal glomeruli.^{Q}

In the kidney, the earliest lesion is focal or diffuse proliferative glomerulonephritis.^{Q} The appearances may be indistinguishable from IgA nephropathy. Immunofluorescence reveals diffuse mesangial IgA deposition.

Differential diagnosis: The classical features of palpable purpura, arthritis, and gastrointestinal involvement makes the diagnosis relatively easy in children. In adults, other types of vasculitis should be considered, especially in those who are ANCA or ANA positive.

Box 21.3	**ACR classification criteria for Henoch–Schönlein purpura**

1. *Palpable purpura*: Slightly elevated purpuric rash over one or more areas of the skin not related to thrombocytopenia.
2. *Bowel angina*: Diffuse abdominal pain worse after meals, or bowel ischemia, usually bloody diarrhea.
3. *Age at onset <20 years*: Development of first symptoms at age 20 years or less.
4. *Wall granulocytes on biopsy*: Histological changes showing granulocytes in the walls of arteries or venules.

Note: For purpose of classification, a patient shall be said to have Henoch-Schönlein purpura, if at least 2 of these 4 criteria are present. The presence of any 2 or more criteria yields a sensitivity of 87.1% and specificity of 87.7.

Prognosis: Overall, prognosis is determined by the extent of renal involvement. In Henoch-Schönlein purpura, the presence of nephritis^Q predicts a worse long-term prognosis.

Most patients have a good prognosis and the illness is self-limiting,^{Q} resolving within 2–3 weeks. Up to 50% of children have recurrences typically purpura and abdominal pain. Hematuria and proteinuria may persist for up to 1 year in 50% of children.

Treatment: Most patients do not need specific therapy, as the condition is self-limiting. NSAIDs help arthralgia, but should be avoided in those with significant renal involvement. The role of corticosteroids is controversial.

Acute Hemorrhagic Edema

Target-like purpura in infant and small children.

Urticarial Vasculitis

This is a small vessel vasculitis characterized by burning urticaria-like lesions (rather than itching found in true urticaria), which last for longer than 24 hours,^{Q} sometimes leaving bruising and then pigmentation^Q (hemosiderin) at the site of previous lesions^Q (Fig. 21.7).

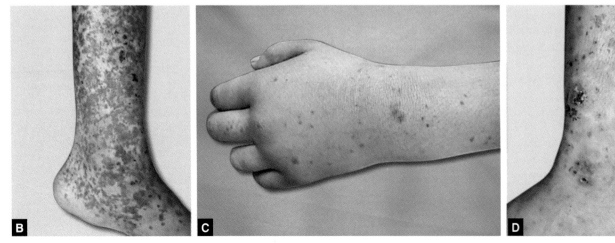

Fig. 21.6B to D: (B) Palpable purpura; (C) Joint swelling; (D) healing with pigmentation (Henoch-Schönlein purpura)

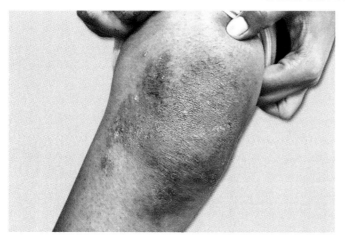

Fig. 21.7: Note the urticarial lesions with central pigmentation in a case of urticarial vasculitis

There may be foci of purpura in the wheals, low serum complement levels, elevated ESR and sometimes angioedema. General features include malaise and arthralgia.

Medium Vessel Vasculitis (MVV)

Polyarteritis Nodosa

Definition: A multisystem vasculitis characterized by formation of microaneurysms in medium-sized arteries[Q].

Rare; most commonly affects middle-aged men. Association with hepatitis B;[Q] also with HIV/AIDS.[Q]

Clinical features (Fig. 21.8): In the early stages, the symptoms can be non-specific and a high index of suspicion is required to achieve an early diagnosis.

- *General symptoms*: Fever, weight loss, arthralgias.
- *Skin*: Frequently involved; livedo racemosa, digital gangrene, subcutaneous nodules, ulcers, leukocytoclastic vasculitis.

Cutaneous polyarteritis nodosa: Disease limited to skin for long periods of time; nodules and ulcers, usually on legs.

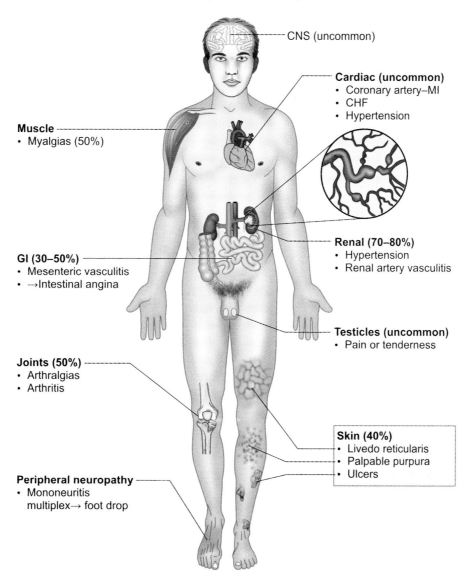

Fig. 21.8: Clinical findings in polyarteritis nodosa

21

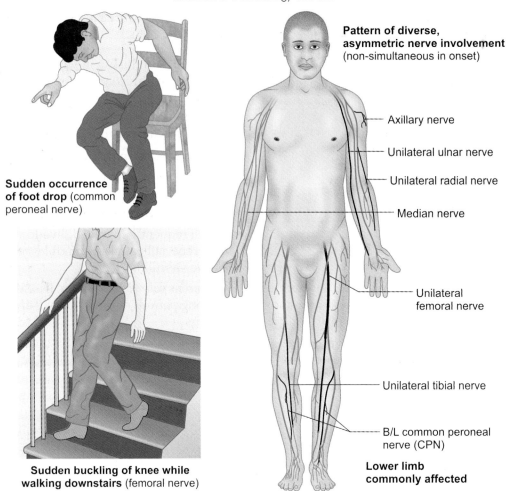

Sudden occurrence of foot drop (common peroneal nerve)

Sudden buckling of knee while walking downstairs (femoral nerve)

Pattern of diverse, asymmetric nerve involvement (non-simultaneous in onset)

— Axillary nerve

— Unilateral ulnar nerve

— Unilateral radial nerve

— Median nerve

— Unilateral femoral nerve

— Unilateral tibial nerve

— B/L common peroneal nerve (CPN)

Lower limb commonly affected

Fig. 21.9: Clinical presentation of neuropathy in polyarteritis nodosa (PAN)

- *Gastrointestinal tract*: 'Intestinal angina'—postprandial abdominal pain because of inadequate blood supply; drastic problems include ischemic bowel perforation and mesenteric artery thrombosis or rupture.
- *Peripheral neuropathy* (Fig. 21.9): Vasculitic neuropathy in up to 80%; involves larger peripheral nerves (mononeuritis multiplex) with sensory and in some instances motor problems.
- *Kidney*: Almost 100% involvement, but usually *subclinical* except for hypertension.
- *Heart*: Can lead to myocardial infarction or congestive heart failure.
- *CNS*: Risk of strokes, as well as hypertensive changes.

  The ACR criteria are given in Box 21.4.

Histology: Segmental involvement makes it hard to find lesions. Initial inflammatory infiltrate is neutrophilic, later replaced by mononuclear cells with intimal proliferation, finally granulomas and fibrosis.

Investigation

- *Histologic confirmation*: Usually skin or muscle biopsy from affected area.

- *Imaging*: Angiography can reveal microaneurysms in gastrointestinal or renal arteries.
- A few changes indicate severity of disease: Elevated sedimentation rate, anemia, thrombocytosis, microscopic hematuria.
- Check for HBsAg positivity.
- ANCA positive in 5%.

Differential diagnosis

- Microscopic polyangiitis (glomerulonephritis, alveolar hemorrhage, pANCA).
- Kawasaki (children, acute picture)
- Wegener (head and neck, lungs, cANCA)
- Leukocytoclastic vasculitis (little systemic involvement)
- Lupus erythematosus (other skin findings, ANA, autoantibodies).

Therapy: Systemic corticosteroids: Prednisolone 1 mg/kg daily; can start with pulse therapy 1.0 g daily for 3 days. If unresponsive or with major organ involvement, add cyclophosphamide (2 mg/kg daily) or other immunosuppressive agents. If patient is HBsAg positive, then start therapy with prednisone and plasma exchanges, followed by IFN and lamivudine—consult hepatology.

Box 21.4	ACR (1990) classification criteria for PAN

1. *Weight loss*: Loss of 4 kg or more of body weight since the illness began, not due to dieting of other factors.
2. *Livedo reticularis*: Mottled reticular pattern over the skin of portions of the extremities or torso.
3. *Testicular pain or tenderness*: Pain or tenderness of the testicles, not due to infection, trauma, or other causes.
4. *Myalgias, weakness, or leg tenderness*: Diffuse myalgias (excluding shoulder or hip girdle) or weakness of muscles or tenderness of leg muscles.
5. *Mononeuropathy or polyneuropathy*: Development of mononeuropathy, multiple mononeuropathies, or poly-neuropathy.
6. *Diastolic BP >90 mmHg*: Development of hypertension with diastolic BP >90 mmHg.
7. Elevated blood urea or creatinine: Elevated BUN >40 mg/dL or creatinine 1.5 mg/dL, not due to dehydration or obstruction.
8. *Hepatitis B virus*: Presence of hepatitis B surface antigen or antibody in serum.
9. *Arteriographic abnormality*: Arteriogram showing aneurysms or occlusion of the visceral arteries, not due to arteriosclerosis, fibromuscular dysplasia, or other non-inflammatory causes.
10. *Biopsy of small or medium vessel*: Histological changes showing the presence of sized artery containing PMN granulocytes or granulocytes and mononuclear leukocytes in the artery wall.

Note: For purposes of classfication, a patient shall be said to have PAN, if at least 3 of these 10 criteria are present. The presence of any 3 or more criteria yield a sensitivity of 82.2% and specificity of 86.6%.

Mucocutaneous Lymph Node Syndrome
(Kawasaki Disease)

Systemic vasculitis in children (usually <5 years) with acute onset and involvement of coronary arteries.

Diagnostic criteria: Criteria have been developed by the Japanese Kawasaki Research Committee (Box 21.5).

Clinical features (Fig 21.10): Six main findings present in 95% (except for cervical lymphadenopathy):

- Unexplained high **temperature**
- Bilateral **conjunctivitis**
- Oral involvement with pharyngeal erythema and strawberry tongue[Q]
- Maculopapular or urticarial **exanthem**
- **Acral edema**, palmoplantar erythema and then characteristic desquamation of fingertips after 10–14 days[Q]
- Cervical lymphadenopathy (50%)
- Coronary artery disease[Q]: The real problem is coronary artery inflammation with the formation of aneurysms, occurs in around 20% of untreated patients in week 2–3.

Diagnosis certain when **five of six** features present, or **four plus coronary artery disease**.

Box 21.5	Diagnostic criteria for Kawasaki disease

1. Fever persisting for 5 days
2. Bilateral conjunctival congestion
3. Oromucosal findings
   - Reddening of lips
   - Strawberry tongue[Q]
   - Diffuse injection of oral and pharyngeal mucosa
4. Polymorphous exanthem
5. Peripheral extremities
   - Initial stage:
     - Reddening of palms and soles
     - Indurative edema
   - Convalescent stage: Membranous desquamation from fingertips
6. Acute non-purulent cervical lymphadenopathy

Note: At least five items are required for a diagnosis of KD. If coronary aneurysms are noted on 2D echocardiography or coronary angiography then 4 items are sufficient.

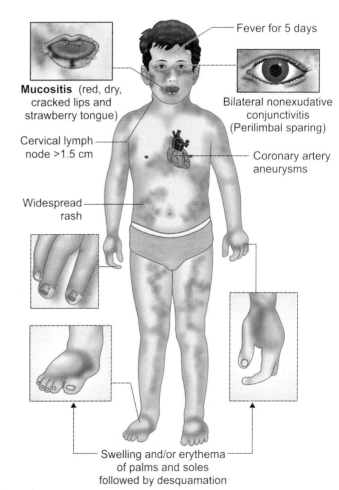

Fig. 21.10: A depiction of the various manifestation of Kawasaki disease

In older children, cardinal signs and symptoms are often missing so life-threatening cardiac disease may be overlooked (incomplete Kawasaki disease).

Therapy: High-dose intravenous immunoglobulins^Q (single dose 2 mg/kg over 8 hours) plus aspirin 30–40 mg/kg daily until defervescence, then 3–5 mg/kg daily for 2 months. If aneurysms are present, consult with cardiology regarding further anticoagulation and management.

Large Vessel Vasculitis
Takayasu's Arteritis (TA)

The Chapel Hill Consensus Conference defined TA as: Granulomatous inflammation of the aorta and its major branches. Usually occurs in patients younger than 50.

Clinical features: The occurrence of stroke in a young person^Q especially when associated with a high ESR or CRP should heighten suspicion of TA.

The criteria of diagnosis are given in Box 21.6.

Giant Cell Arteritis

Arteritis, often granulomatous, usually affecting the aorta and/or its major branches, with a predilection for the branches of the carotid artery. Often involves the temporal artery. Onset usually in patients >50 years and often associated with polymyalgia rheumatica.

Clinical features (Fig. 21.11): In the early stages, the symptoms can be non-specific and a high index of suspicion is required to achieve an early diagnosis.

Symptoms

- *Systemic*: Fever, weight loss, myalgia, arthralgia. Morning stiffness across the shoulder and hip girdles is suggestive of co-existent PMR (polymyalgia rheumatica).
- *Headache*: The characteristic feature is new onset or change in character from previous headache. The headache is located typically in the temples.
- *Visual disturbance*: This may occur suddenly without warning and may be bilateral.

Transient visual loss may be a warning of impeding acute visual loss, which may be profound.

Jaw claudication and limb claudication.

Signs

- *Vascular*: The temporal arteries may be tender, thickened, and non-pulsatile. Bruits may be audible over affected arteries, especially in the carotid and supraclavicular regions.
- *Eye*: Signs anterior ischemic optic neuropathy. Formal slit-lamp examination by an ophthalmologist may be required. The optic disc may be pale with profound loss of acuity to counting fingers or less.

Box 21.6 | ACR classification criteria for Takayasu arteritis

1. *Age <40 years old*: Development of symptoms or signs related to Takayasu arteritis at age <40 years.
2. *Claudication of extremities*: Development and worsening of fatigue and discomfort in muscles of one or more extremity while in use, especially the upper extremities.
3. *Decreased brachial arterial pulse*: Decreased pulsation of one or both brachial arteries.
4. *BP difference >10 mmHg*: Difference of >10 mmHg in systolic blood pressure between arms.
5. *Bruit over subclavian arteries or aorta*: Bruit audible on auscultation over one or both subclavian arteries or abdominal aorta.
6. *Arteriogram abnormality*: Arteriographic narrowing or occlusion of the entire aorta, its proximal branches, or large arteries in the proximal upper or lower extremities, not due to atherosclerosis, fibromuscular dysplasia, or similar causes; changes usually focal or segmental.

Note: For purposes of classification, a patient shall be said to have Takayasu's arteritis, if at least 3 of these 6 criteria are present. The presence of any 3 or more criteria yield a sensitivity of 90.5% and specificity of 97.8%.

Box 21.7 | ACR criteria for classification of GCA

1. *Age at onset >50 years*: Development of symptoms or findings beginning aged 50 years or older.
2. *New headache*: New onset or new type of localized pains in the head.
3. *Temporal artery abnormality*: Temporal artery tenderness to palpation or decreased pulsation, unrelated to atherosclerosis of cervical arteries.
4. *Increase in ESR*: ESR >50 mm/h by Westergren method.
5. *Abnormal artery biopsy*: Biopsy specimen with artery showing vasculitis characterized by a predominance of mononuclear infiltration or granulomatous inflammation.

Note: For purposes of classfication, a patient shall be said to have giant cell arteries, if at least 3 of these 5 criteria are present.

Diagnostic criteria: The ACR in 1990 developed classification criteria, which are widely used in clinical trials. They have a specific city of 91.2% and sensitivity of 93.5%. There are no validated diagnostic criteria, but the accepted criteria are given in Box 21.7.

Variable Vessel Vasculitis
Behçet Syndrome

Definition: Systemic vasculitis with recurrent aphthae, genital ulcerations,^{Q} and involvement of many other organs.

Pathogenesis: Complex; in Japan, strong association with HLA-B51;^{Q} heat shock proteins (especially HSP60) may be involved in stimulating γδ+ T cell response insusceptible individuals; infectious triggers (streptococci, herpes simplex) also long suspected.

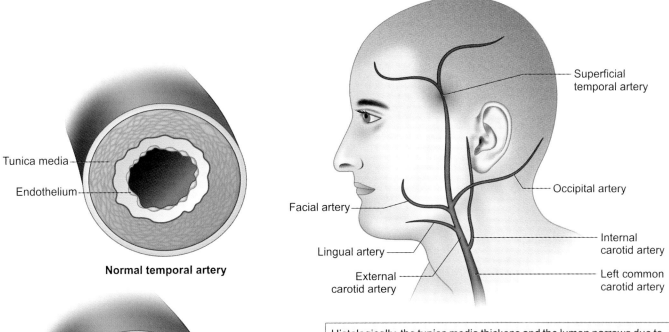

Histologically, the tunica media thickens and the lumen narrows due to tunica interna fibrosis. Inflammatory cells can be seen invading the tunica media, eosinophils. Giant cells can occasionally be seen populating areas around the internal elastic membrane.

- Giant cell arteritis (GCA) can alternatively be called *cranial arteritis* *or temporal arteritis*, reflecting the most commonly affected vessels.
- CGA is the inflammation of the lining of the arteries and is a relatively common vasculitis among older adults.
- Common symptoms of GCA include blurring or loss of vision, headaches, and jaw pain. Other areas, such as head and neck, can also be affected by GCA.

Fig. 21.11: Features of giant cells arteritis

Clinical features: *Main features* (**triad**) (Box 21.8):[Q]
- Recurrent oral aphthae, at least 3 in 12 months (100%).
- Indolent genital ulcers (90%).
- Chronic recurrent uveitis (50%).

Other features:
- Skin: Erythema nodosum (80%), recurrent thrombophlebitis, pathergy (pustular response at site of trauma).
- Large vessel vasculitis: Pulmonary artery aneurysms (arterial-bronchial fistula formation), aortic aneurysms.
- Arthritis and arthralgias: Favor hands, wrists, ankles, knees.
- Gastrointestinal ulcers, distal ileum and cecum.
- CNS: Stroke, aseptic meningitis.
- Kidney disease and peripheral neuropathy rare.

Diagnosis is based on the criteria as given in Box 21.8.

Pathergy test[Q]**:** Inject 0.1 mL of physiologic NaCl with fine needle on forearm; read after 24–48 hours. Pustule

Box 21.8	**International study group diagnostic criteria for Behçet's disease**

Recurrent oral ulceration (aphthous or herpetiform) observed by a physician or the patient at least three times over one 12-month period.

And two of the following:
- Recurrent genital ulceration.
- Eye lesions: Anterior uveitis, posterior uveitis, cells in the vitreous by slit lamp examination, or retinal vasculitis.
- Skin lesions: Erythema nodosum, pseudofolliculits, papulopustular lesions, or acneiform nodules in post-pubescent patients not on steroids.
- Positive pathergy test.

or papule suggests diagnosis; histology shows neutrophilic infiltrate or vasculitis.

Therapy

Oral and genital lesions: Topical or intralesional corticosteroids. Cyclosporine most effective for uveitis; azathioprine also effective.

Other systemic therapy:
- Colchicine 0.5–1.5 mg daily.
- Dapsone 0.5–2.0 mg/kg daily.
- Corticosteroids/immunosuppressive agents.

NEUTROPHILIC DERMATOSES

Sweet Syndrome

Acute neutrophilic illness with fever, leukocytosis, and erythematous succulent cutaneous plaques.

Epidemiology: Female: male ratio 3.5:1, more common in spring and fall.

Clinical features

1. Prodrome and arthralgias
2. Succulent plaques, with irregular border (rocky island pattern); sometimes illusion of vesiculation[Q]—look vesicular but are solid when pressed; plaques may be dotted with pustules
3. Oral lesions seen in 20%

Histology: Distinctive band of subepidermal edema with band-like infiltrate rich in neutrophils. Later nuclear dust and ingestion of neutrophils by macrophages (bean bag cells).

Therapy: Prednisolone[Q] 60 mg daily tapered over 2–3 weeks. If recurrent, consider methotrexate, clofazimine, or thalidomide.

Pyoderma Gangrenosum

(Neutrophilic, Pathergy, Cribriform Scarring)[Q]

Neutrophilic dermatosis, noninfectious, with rapid tissue destruction.

Mechanism still unknown; abnormal neutrophil trafficking and immunologic dysfunction are the best guesses. Association with inflammatory bowel disease, rheumatoid arthritis, and monoclonal gammopathy (usually IgA) is clear; less often associated with lymphomas and leukemias.

Clinical features: Ulcer with prominent undermined border[Q] and boggy necrotic base. Grows rapidly. May start as pustule. Can become extremely large and extend to fat, fascia, or even muscle. Heals with cribriform (sieve-like) scars. Displays **pathergy:** Skin trauma (needle stick, insect bite, biopsy) can trigger lesions.[Q]

Therapy: Treat associated disease.

Topical therapy usually inadequate; exception is intralesional corticosteroids in early lesions. Systemic corticosteroids are mainstay: Prednisolone 1–2 mg/kg daily tapered as healing occurs. Cyclosporine (and presumably also tacrolimus and pimecrolimus) is amazingly effective, suggesting that T cells play a role in the primary pathogenesis. Inhibitors of TNF-α are also dramatically effective, even though no role for this cytokine had been expected in pyoderma gangrenosum.

Disorders of
Skin Appendages

Acne Vulgaris

Acne vulgaris remains not only one of the commonest skin problems, but can have a deep psychological impact of adolescent age as it affects the face.

Because of the visible nature of the condition and the potential for permanent scarring, acne is frequently associated with psychological distress, depression, and decrease in self-esteem.

EPIDEMIOLOGY

Acne is primarily a disorder of adolescence although all age groups may be affected by its many variants. The onset of acne frequently correlates with puberty and presents between the ages of 10 and 13 years in both sexes. Males tend to develop acne somewhat later in adolescence, but develop disease of greater severity. Females tend to have a less severe, but a more chronic course. Also, post-adolescent acne, both persistent and late onset, is more common in women.

- Acne affects approximately 85% of young people between the ages of 12 and 24 years.
- Peak prevalence occurs between the ages of 15 and 20 years. The majority of teenage boys can expect clearing of lesions between 20 and 25 years of age.

Individuals at increased risk for acne include patients with endocrine disorders such as polycystic ovarian syndrome (PCOS)^Q, hyperandrogenism, Cushing syndrome, and precocious puberty.

ETIOPATHOGENESIS

The etiology of acne has four major features. It is now believed that subclinical inflammation is the initiating

event and that the inflammation continues throughout the entire process (Figs 22.1 and 22.2).

1. **Androgen-induced seborrhea^Q (excess grease):** The more sebum (grease) the greater degree of acne. Sebum is produced by the pilosebaceous glands, which are predominantly found on the face, back and chest. Evidence suggests that in most patients, the seborrhea is due to increased response of the sebaceous glands to normal levels of plasma androgens^Q as a result of enhanced end organ sensitivity. This is due to action of enzyme 5α reductase in sebaceous gland

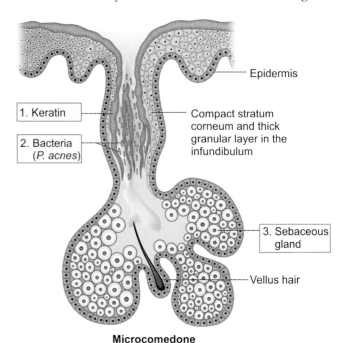

Fig. 22.1: A depiction of the main pathogenic factors of acne vulgaris

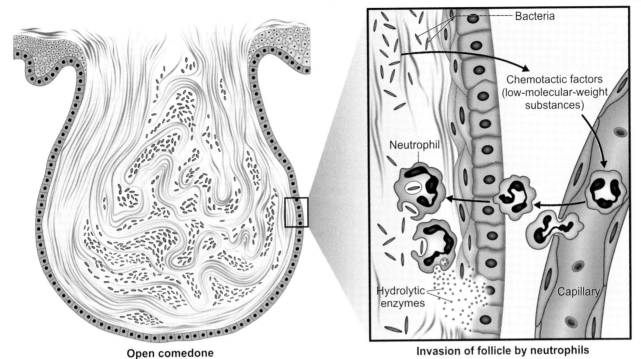

Open comedone   **Invasion of follicle by neutrophils**

Fig. 22.2: Role of inflammation in the causation of acne

which converts testosterone to the more potent dihydrotestosterone (DHT).

2. **Comedone formation (blackheads, whiteheads and microcomedones), also known as comedogenesis:** It is due to an abnormal proliferation and differentiation of ductal keratinocytes[Q] leading to occlusion of the pilosebaceous canal. It is controlled, in part, by androgens. In prepubertal subjects, comedones are seen early and they precede the development of inflammatory lesions.

3. **Colonization of the pilosebaceous duct with *Propionibacterium acnes*[Q] (*P. acnes* now called *Cutibacterium acnes*):** It is a later stage in the development of acne lesions (especially inflammatory lesions). The seborrhea and comedone formation alter the ductal microenvironment, which results in colonization of the duct. Cutibacterium also forms biofilms in the infundibulum of the pilosebaceous gland and this affect the responsiveness of *C. acnes* to antibiotics.

4. **Production of inflammation[Q]:** Pro-inflammatory agents released by *C. acnes* include lipases, which damage the follicular wall and trigger inflammation, as well as chemotactic factors, which firstly recruit CD4-lymphocytes, and later neutrophils and monocytes to the affected area (Fig. 22.2).

FACTORS WHICH MODIFY ACNE

- *Hormonal factors*: About 70% of females will notice an aggravation of the acne just before or in the first few days of the period. In adult and persistent acne in females (>25 years) polycystic ovarian syndrome

(PCOS) and other endocrinological disorders play a role.

- UV light can benefit acne, but in India, acne commonly worsens in summers specially in the humid months.
- *Stress*: This is a controversial issue—there is some evidence that stress makes acne worse but data to support this view is limited. Stress may manifest itself as acne excoriée, where patients, usually females, habitually scratch the spots the moment they appear.
- *Diet*: Although the evidence for a link between diet and acne is not strong, some people with acne have reported improvement in their skin when they follow a low-glycemic index diet:

- Increase the consumption of whole grains, fresh fruits and vegetables, fish, olive oil, garlic.
- Decrease the consumption of high-glycemic index[Q] foods such as sugar, biscuits, cakes, ice-creams, cheese and bottled drinks.

- *Cosmetics* (*acne venenata*): Excessive use of cosmetics specially foundations, night creams and sunscreen, without understanding the skin type can itself cause acne cosmetica. Most cosmetics are oil based and more suited for countries with cold, dry climate, their use in tropical climate like India may predispose to acne. If cosmetics are used, they should be water-based and used sparingly. A simple way of arriving at an ideal moisturizer is the so-called 'transparency rule'—more

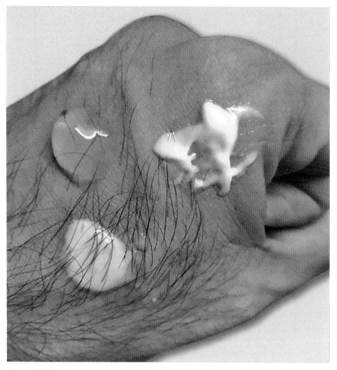

Fig. 22.3: The gel-based near transparent moisturizer^Q is the ideal moisturizer for an acne prone skin

transparent the moisturizers less is the acnegenicity (Fig. 22.3). If cosmetics are used, they should be water-based and used sparingly.

- *Drugs*^Q: The following drugs may cause or exacerbate acne:
  - Topical and oral corticosteroids
  - Anabolic steroids
  - Lithium
  - Ciclosporin
  - Progesterone
  - Testosterone
  - Antidepressants
  - Anticonvulsants—carbamazepine, phenytoin, phenobarbitone
  - Isoniazid
  - Anticancer drugs, specifically the epidermal growth factor receptor (EGFR) drugs
  - Anabolic steroids can also trigger or worsen typical acne (body builder's acne).
- *Picking*: Acne excoriee or Picker's acne, is a condition, usually seen in adolescent females, who habitually scratch the spots the moment they appear, resulting in post-inflammatory hyperpigmentation and scars (Fig. 22.4).
- *OTC products*: Most advertized over the counter products fail to clear acne. Worse, most of them have the wrong base and can be sticky, tacky and comedogenic. Also the active ingredients are less active than therapeutic acne medications.

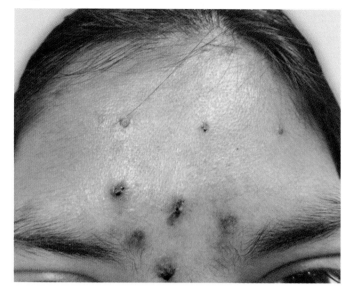

Fig. 22.4: Acne excoriée because of frequent picking of the lesion

CLASSIFICATION

There are several subtypes of acne. Some of them occur because of physiologic changes associated with normal development.

1. *Neonatal and infantile acne*: Comedones and papules in pustules in newborn because of adrenal activity and androgen transfer from the mother and are usually transient (Fig. 22.5).

   Infantile acne: True acne in infants; it starts at 3–6 months and is seen usually in boys, and persists. Parents often give a history of acne and children are at risk for severe acne later.

2. *Mid-childhood acne* is observed in children aged 18 months to 7 years. Acne in this age range is rare and implies more significant systemic problems such as Cushing syndrome, premature adrenarche, congenital adrenal

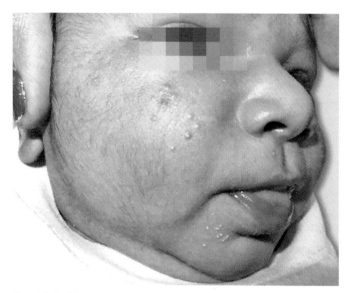

Fig. 22.5: Neonatal acne on the cheeks with milia on the chin

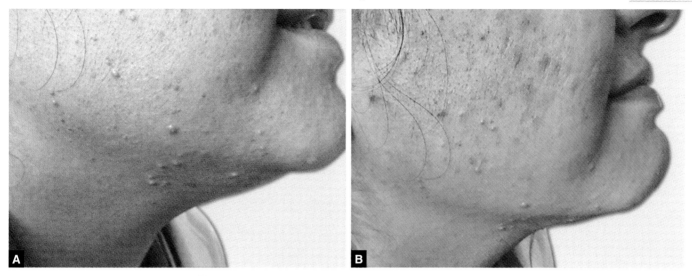

Fig. 22.6A and B: Persistent acne in females involving the jawline

hyperplasia, gonadal/adrenal tumors, or true precocious puberty.[Q] These patients require an extensive endocrinological evaluation.

3. *Preadolescent acne*: This is the fourth type of acne within the childhood spectrum and encompasses ages 8 to 12 years. Typically, comedones are evident on the face and neck, but are less common on the torso. This may be an indicator of emerging puberty.

4. *Adolescent acne* is a common occurrence, and about 70% of the time occurs at puberty and lasts, in general, approximately 5 years.

5. *Postadolescent acne*: This is acne seen or persisting >25 years and is seen most commonly in women. Tends to flare in the week prior to menstruation and up to one-third of these women have hyperandrogenism.

   Site: Papulonodules on the lower face, jawline, and neck (Fig. 22.6A and B).[Q]

6. *Acne conglobata*[Q] is the most severe form of acne and typically arises in adolescent males, although it does not exclude females. It presents with nodules, abscess formation, malodorous draining sinus tracts and both hypertrophic and atrophic scars (Fig. 22.7). Multiporous grouped comedones are typical of acne conglobata.

7. *Acne fulminans* occurs uncommonly but with an explosive onset in the teenage male population. In essence, the morphology is like acne conglobate with systemic features.[Q] Acne fulminans rarely is triggered when high-dose systemic retinoids are initiated. Associated systemic symptoms are common.

8. *Acne associated with a syndrome*: Examples include Apert, PAPA, PASH, and SAPHO.

   The other types are listed in Box 22.1 (Figs 22.8 and 22.9).

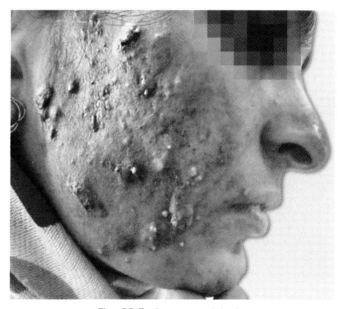

Fig. 22.7: Acne conglobata

Box 22.1	Acne variants
Acne excoriée	Habitual picking, usually by young women, in a vain attempt to eradicate them (Fig. 22.8)
Acne mechanica	Caused by friction from chin straps, sports padding, or equipment
Chloracne	Due to occupational exposure to toxins like chlorinated or halogenated chemicals Large comedones and pustules face, trunk, genitals, and extremities
Acne cosmetica	Adolescent females who wear a lot of makeup. Comedones, papules, pustules
Acne associated with endocrine abnormalities	Often accompanied by hirsutism, menstrual irregularities, and virilizing characteristics, pustules and cysts (Fig. 22.9)

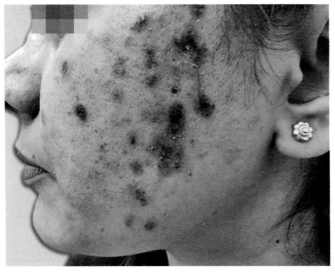

Fig. 22.8: Acne excoriée: The picking of the lesion leaves patchy pigmentation which takes a long time to resolve

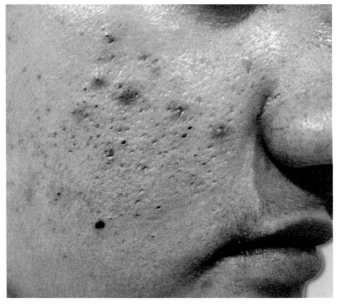

Fig. 22.10: An admixture of blackheads and papules

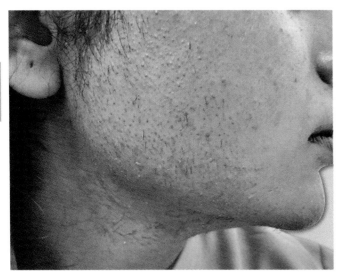

Fig. 22.9: Acne with marked hirsutism in a patient with PCOS

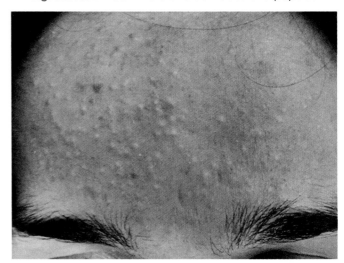

Fig. 22.11: 'Whiteheads' or closed comedones

CLINICAL FINDINGS

Acne is characterized by polymorphic lesions (Box 22.2).

1. **The non-inflamed lesions** in acne are called comedones and are of two types:
   a. *The open comedone or 'blackhead'*, which appears as a dilated pore filled with black keratinous material (not dirt) (Fig. 22.10). The apparent black color is

Box 22.2	Clinical morphology of acne

Noninflammatory lesions:
- Open comedones
- Closed comedones

Inflammatory lesions:
- Papules
- Pustules
- Nodules

thought to be due to melanin deposited within the cellular debris.[Q]

   b. *The closed comedone or 'whitehead'*, which is a small, flesh-colored, dome-shaped papule that often is difficult to see (Fig. 22.11).

   – Missed comedones will be visualized on stretching the skin, and using a good light, at a shallow angle, in about 20% of patients, which would have been otherwise missed and therefore, not treated.

   – 'Sandpaper' comedones consist of multiple, very small whiteheads, frequently distributed on the forehead (Fig. 22.11), which produce a roughened, gritty feel to the skin.

   – 'Macrocomedones' are large whiteheads or occasionally blackheads greater than 1 mm in diameter.

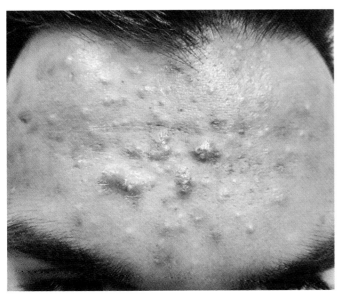

Fig. 22.12: Submarine comedones which are visible on stretching the skin, 'pop out' as nodules on treatment

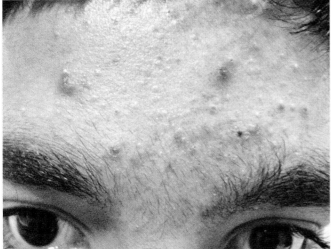

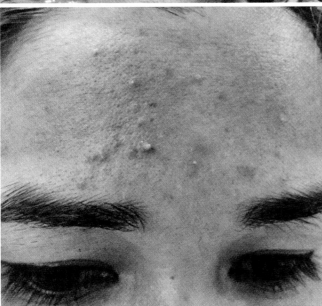

Fig. 22.13: Papules and pustules—inflammatory acne

– 'Submarine' comedones are large comedonal structures greater than 0.5 cm in diameter and are deeply entrenched and lead to inflammatory nodular lesions (Fig. 22.12).

2. **Inflammatory acne** lesions are seen more easily by both patient and physician. They appear as papules, pustules, or nodules, depending on the magnitude of the inflammatory response (Fig. 22.13).

3. **Scarring** is often seen in the more severe types of acne and is of 3 types—ice pick, boxcar and rolling scars.[Q] The raised scars including keloids may also be seen (Fig. 22.14A to E).

4. In Asian and Indian skin, the lesions often leave behind pigmentation called postinflammatory hyperpigmentation (Fig. 22.15).

History

Some important questions that can help elicit the various trigger factors are listed in Table 22.1.

DIFFERENTIAL DIAGNOSIS

The diagnosis of acne is rarely difficult, particularly in teenagers.

1. Milia: Closed comedones may be confused with milia
2. Warts: Occasionally, acne comedones may be confused with flat warts, which are small, flesh-colored, flat-topped papules usually located on the face. On close inspection, the flat wart is seen to have a sharp right-angled edge[Q] and a finely textured surface.
3. Steroid acne is caused by use of corticosteroids and is distinguished from acne vulgaris by its sudden onset[Q] (usually within 2 weeks of starting high-dose systemic or potent topical corticosteroid therapy) and appearance (uniform, 2 to 3 mm, red, firm papules

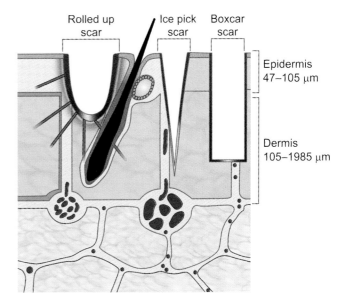

Fig. 22.14A: A depiction of the various types of atrophic acne scar

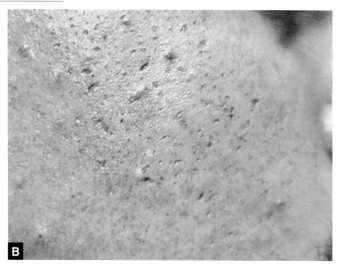

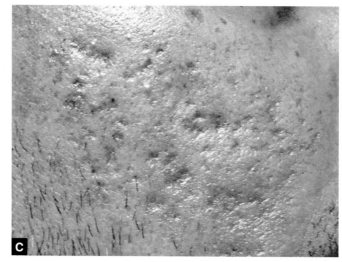

Fig. 22.14B and C: (B) Ice pick scars; (C) Boxcar scars

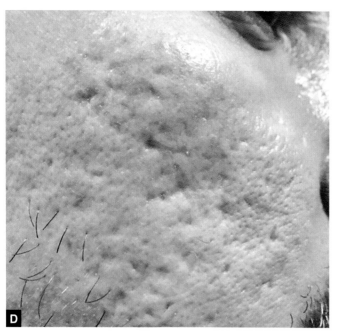

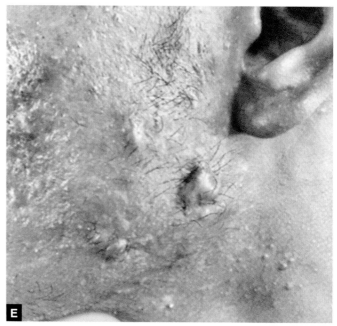

Fig. 22.14D and E: (D) Rolling scars; (E) Keloidal scars

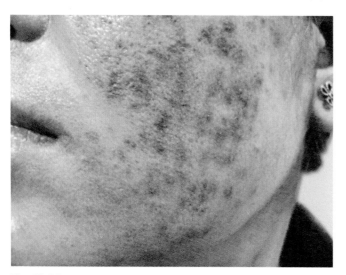

Fig. 22.15: Marked pigmentation after acne lesions have healed

and pustules). Steroid acne caused by topically applied agents occurs most often on the face. With systemic corticosteroids, the eruption is most prominent on the upper trunk.

4. In bacterial folliculitis, hairs are visible in some of the pustules and a bacterial culture is positive, usually for *Staphylococcus aureus* or, less often, a Gram-negative organism.

5. Rosacea is distinguished from acne vulgaris by the presence of a background blush of erythema and telangiectasia,[Q] and the absence of comedones. Rosacea also usually occurs later in life.

INVESTIGATION

The vast majority of patients with acne do not require investigations. Most of the investigations are in females

Table 22.1	Potential factors predicting acne
Questions	Details
Duration/frequency	Waxes and wanes? Cyclical with menses? Chronic?
Current treatment	• All OTC and prescription products • Creams, foundations, sunscreens • Hair-styling gels, moisturizers, cleansing regimen and products used • Makeup • Therapies that worked or did not work
Prescribed medications	Look for drugs that can trigger acne
Females with acne	• Premenstrual flares and menstrual history • Pregnancy • Increase of androgen-dependent hair-hirsutism • Thinning of scalp hair • Hormones/testing/USG-PCOS
Diet	• Dairy products, high glycemic index foods • Gym supplements including whey protein
Triggers or exacerbating factors	• Stress • Seasonal variation • Foods • Topical products

or patients with history suggestive of a hormonal defect. In persistent acne in females, PCOS is common cause.

• DHEAS and free testosterone are good initial screening laboratory studies in evaluating hormonal influences. As free testosterone testing requires highly sensitive parameters, either a calculated free testosterone or a free androgen index[Q] is a better tool. In any case, a testosterone level greater than 5 nmol/L (144 ng/dL) should warrant a detailed evaluation.

• Another condition that needs to be considered from time-to-time is late onset (non-classical) congenital adrenal hyperplasia, for which a test for serum levels of 17-hydroxyprogesterone levels[Q] in the follicular phase around 8 am is done.

• If there is a suspicion of precocious puberty, PCOS, or hyperandrogenism, referral to endocrinology is appropriate.

TREATMENT

Regardless of the severity of the acne, for patients seeking a consult (even those with apparently mild disease), the disease is important and deserves serious attention. The advise that they will eventually 'outgrow' the disease is an ill-advised advise. The disorder can be treated by various topical and systemic measures as

also based on the severity of disease as mild, moderate and severe.

The basic **principles of treatment** are:

• The primary aim of acne treatment is to prevent or minimize scarring, once scarred, the skin will never return to normal.

• Topical preparations containing benzoyl peroxide and/or topical retinoids are an essential part of the treatment. It is important to explain to the patient that such treatments will dry the skin and cause local irritation, in order to reduce adverse effects, patients may wish to start using the treatment 2–3 nights a week and gradually increase the frequency and duration of applications.

> The patient should apply these medications to the entire affected area (e.g. the entire face) rather than just to the individual lesions.[Q]

• There are increasing levels of *Propionibacterium acnes* resistance to antibiotics, especially erythromycin and azithromycin, the use of which should be restricted. The ideal antibiotics are doxycycline and minocycline but they should be used for a maximum of 3 months.[Q]

• The type of acne is important. For example, there are some variants such as sandpaper acne and macrocomedonal acne that respond poorly to conventional treatment.

• For severe cases, isotretinoin is the drug of choice.[Q]

• In hormonal cases, OCP, and spironolactone are given.

• Monitoring response to treatment with serial photography is important.

The various types of medical therapy include topical agents, oral agents and hormonal therapy. Their use depends on the types of acne. The management approach steps up from the milder comedonal acne to the severe acne types. Thus as a dictum a photographic scale can be used to classify acne as mild, moderate and severe (Fig. 22.16A to C), as the therapy would depend on this severely and the predominant type of lesion seen.

Thus for different aspects of the disease, specific therapies are given (Fig. 22.17). Here a step-by-step approach to the treatment of acne is given.

Step 1: Treatment of comedonal acne

First line

• A topical retinoid is needed as this reduces comedonal activity.

• Choices include tretinoin, adapalene, adapalene combined with benzoyl peroxide 2.5%, or isotretinoin (topical).

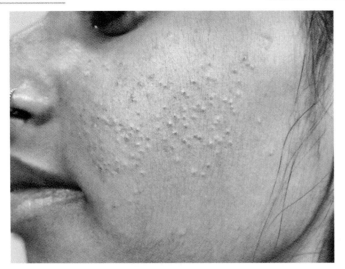

Fig. 22.16A: Mild acne with comedones

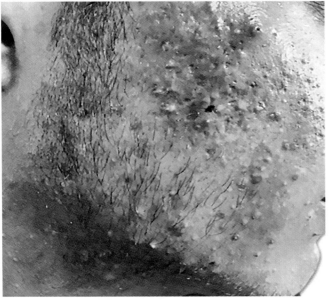

Fig. 22.16B: Moderate acne with predominant papules and pustules

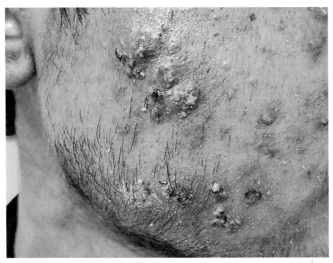

Fig. 22.16C: Severe acne with nodules, cysts, papules and pustules

- Topical retinoids should be avoided in pregnancy, they are safe to use in all other patients including sexually active women.
- Tretinoin is photolabile[Q] and inactivated by BPO[Q] (so generally applied at night, separately from BPO).

Second line: Azelaic acid. It should also be chosen for acne with postinflammatory hyperpigmentation.

A list of topical agents is given in Table 22.2.

Step 2: Treatment of mild to moderate papular/pustular acne: Use a fixed dose combination treatment, ideally containing benzoyl peroxide (BPO), which reduces bacterial resistance[Q], with either a topical retinoid or topical antibiotic.

First line: Adapalene + BPO

Second line: Clindamycin + BPO

- Both BPO and topical retinoids will dry the skin,[Q] hence start alternate nights and gradually increase to a daily evening pattern
- BPO can bleach clothing/bedding and cause contact dermatitis (irritant >allergic)
- Response requires 3–4 weeks (sometimes preceded by pustular flare).

Though expensive, a list of combinations of topical agents is given in Box 22.3. This helps to decrease compliance, but in some the combinations may cause irritation.

Though nadifloxacin combination is prescribed in India, this drug should not be used in acne as this class of drugs has many other medical use and is only approved in Japan for acne.[Q]

Step 3: Not responding to the above and/or more widely distributed: Combine *systemic antibiotics* with an appropriate topical agent, preferably BPO, to reduce bacterial resistance. If patients cannot tolerate BPO, use a topical retinoid.

A list of systemic agents is given in Table 22.3.

First line: Tetracycline group of drugs
Options are lymecycline 408 mg OD, doxycycline 100 mg OD and lastly in failure minocycline.

Box 22.3 | **Topical combination products for acne**

- Adapalene 0.1% and BPO 2.5% gel
- Erythromycin 3% and BPO 5%
- Clindamycin 1% and BPO 5%
- Clindamycin 1.2% and BPO 2.5%
- Clindamycin 1.2% and tretinoin 0.025%
- Clindamycin 1.2% and tretinoin 0.025%

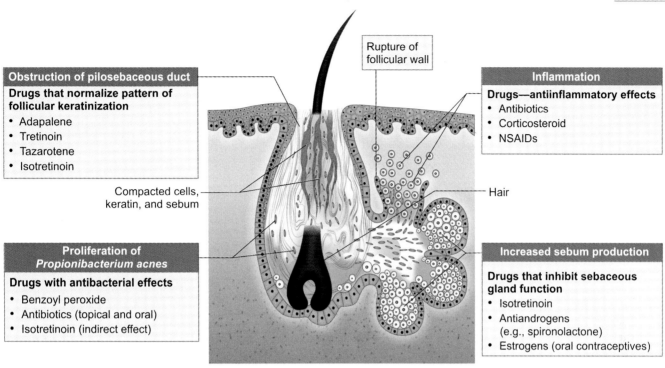

Obstruction of pilosebaceous duct

Drugs that normalize pattern of follicular keratinization
- Adapalene
- Tretinoin
- Tazarotene
- Isotretinoin

Rupture of follicular wall

Inflammation

Drugs—antiinflammatory effects
- Antibiotics
- Corticosteroid
- NSAIDs

Compacted cells, keratin, and sebum

Hair

Proliferation of *Propionibacterium acnes*

Drugs with antibacterial effects
- Benzoyl peroxide
- Antibiotics (topical and oral)
- Isotretinoin (indirect effect)

Increased sebum production

Drugs that inhibit sebaceous gland function
- Isotretinoin
- Antiandrogens (e.g., spironolactone)
- Estrogens (oral contraceptives)

Fig. 22.17: Therapeutic options in acne vulgaris and their mechanism of action

Table 22.2 Topical medical therapy for acne

	Types	Pregnancy	Comments
Cleansers	Mild cleansers (nonabrasive)		• Twice daily • For dry/sensitive skin or irritation from treatment • Antibacterials are drying
	BPO wash	C	Bleaches fabrics, keratolytic, anti-inflammatory, antimicrobial
	Salicylic acid 2%	C	Keratolytic
Antimicrobials	BPO 2.5–10%		• Daily wash or leave on gel • Irritating • Possible allergic contact dermatitis • Bleaches fabric
	Azaleic acid 15% gel	B	• Good for skin of color • Also comedolytic • Decreases hyperpigmentation^Q
Antibiotics	Clindamycin 1% sol, lotion, gel	B	• Daily or twice daily • Rare pseudomembranous colitis • Bacterial resistance*
	Erythromycin 2%	B	• Daily or twice daily • Good for sensitive or dry skin • Bacterial resistance*
	Dapsone 5%	C	• Twice daily but not at same time as using BPO (orange skin) • Decrease inflammation
Retinoids	Tretinoin	C	Irritating^Q, use on dry face
	Adapalene	C	Apply small amount at nighttime
	Tazarotene	X	Start 2–3/wk and slowly increase Use as maintenance

*Combine with BPO or retinoids. Though nadifloxacin gel is prescribed in India, this drug should not be used in acne as this class of drugs has many other medical use and is only approved in Japan for acne, where BPO is not approved.

Table 22.3 List of systemic antibiotic agents

	Types	Pregnancy	Comments
Antibiotics	Doxycycline 50–100 mg Minocycline 50–100 mg Doxycycline 40 mg	X	• Use with BPO to reduce drug resistance[Q] • Do not take with calcium • GI upset, photosensitivity[Q] • Birth control failure risk • Vaginal candidiasis • Daily or twice daily
	Azithromycin 250 mg Erythromycin 250–500 mg	C	• Safe in pregnancy[Q] • High levels of resistance thus they should be avoided • Azithromycin is an antibiotic used for URTI and its use for acne should be restricted specially as tetracyclines are still effective

Table 22.4 Treatment algorithm for management of acne

Rx	Mild acne		Moderate acne	Severe
	Comedonal	Inflammatory		
First line	Topical retinoid	Topical antimicrobial[1] + topical retinoid	Oral antibiotic + topical retinoid ±BPO	Oral isotretinoin (+oral CS for acne fulminans)
Second line	• Azelaic acid • Salicylic acid	• Azelaic acid • Dapsone	Oral isotretinoin, if nodular, scarring or recalcitrant	• Dapsone • Oral antibiotic + topical retinoid ±BPO[2]
Female patients			OCP/antiandrogen	OCP/antiandrogen
Refractory to treatment		• Exclude Gram-negative folliculitis • Female patient: exclude adrenal or ovarian dysfunction • Resistance specially to macrolides including azithromycin		
Maintenance	Topical retinoid	Topical retinoid ±BPO	Topical retinoid ±BPO	

[1]The common antibiotics used include clindamycin and nadifloxacain. Increased effectiveness when used in conjunction with BPO or a retinoid.
[2]BPO ± a topical antibiotic may also be used as monotherapy, especially as an initial treatment in a younger patient.

Tetracyclines are avoided in children <8 years of age and pregnant women.

Second line: Macrolides should generally be avoided due to high levels of *P. acnes* resistance.

They are first line in pregnancy and in children under the age of 12 years (in both groups tetracyclines are contraindicated).[Q]

The systemic antibiotics can be given for **3 months** and, if there is a response, they can be stopped and topical agents can be continued.

Third line: Isotretinoin (1 mg/kg/d—3 months).

Step 4: Severe acne

Isotretinoin: Typically 0.5–1 mg/kg/day (lower initially, especially if acne fulminans) × 4–6 months (cumulative dose 120–150 mg/kg).[Q]

The most common side effects are cheilitis > mucosal dryness (ocular, nasal) and xerosis.[Q] In female patients contraceptions should be ensured during therapy and for 3 months after stopping therapy.

An overview of the therapy based on the severity of acne is given in Table 22.4.

Special Scenarios

1. *Female acne unresponsive to the above therapies*: Hormonal therapy may be necessary; combined oral contraceptives (COCs) are most commonly used. Consideration for hormonal therapy must be made on an individual patient basis. And since many of these patients are young adult females, education and counseling for the patients and their parents are very important.

• Oral contraceptive pills (OCPs) are used in acne to suppress testosterone production.[Q] This can be especially effective in conditions such as PCOS and can reduce the occurrence of acne and excess facial hair. OCPs approved by the Food and Drug Administration (FDA) for the treatment of acne include:
  – Ethinyl estradiol (EE) 35 µg with norgestimate 180/215/250 µg (e.g.Ortho Tri-Cyclenn®)
  – EE 20 µg, drospirenone 3000 µg (e.g.Yaz®)
  – EE 20/30/35 µg, norethindrone 100 µg (e.g. Estrostep®) (EE 20 µg, drospirenone 3000 µg)

• Drospirenone may have increased risk for blood clots compared to pills containing other progestins.

Cyproterone acetate based OCP^Q can be used but they are not FDA approved for acne.

- Another option is spironolactone in a dose of 25 to 50 mg per day for 1 to 2 months and this can then be increased to a maximum of 100 mg BD.

- Cyproterone acetate based OCP can be used but they are not FDA approved for acne.

2. ***Acne in pigmented skin:*** Acne is common in pigmented skin, but postinflammatory hyperpigmentation can be a significant issue and often persists for months to years. As such, early and more aggressive treatment is advocated, including early referral for consideration of isotretinoin.

Secondary acne can be a result of cultural practices—hair oil can induce pomade acne^Q on the forehead and skin lightening products containing topical steroids can cause a steroid-induced acne.

Topical retinoids, benzoyl peroxide and azelaic acid play an important role in the treatment of the comedonal aspects of acne. If used daily, they often cause dryness and irritation, which in pigmented skin can lead to further hyperpigmentation.

Accordingly, these treatments should initially be used for shorter periods of time (e.g. in an evening and washed off before bed) and perhaps less frequently (e.g. every 2nd or 3rd day), if tolerated the duration and/or frequency of treatment can be increased—if used in this way then, apart from treating the comedones, they may help treat hyperpigmentation rather than aggravate it.

3. ***Acne in pregnancy:*** The following are usually regarded as being safe, should the physician and patient feel it necessary, to prescribe during pregnancy:
- Benzoyl peroxide preparations
- 2% topical erythromycin

- If the acne is troublesome and not responding to topical treatments, consider oral erythromycin, 500 mg BD.^Q

4. ***Localized cystic acne:*** Intralesional injections (ILC) with corticosteroids for large stubborn painful cystic lesions can give great relief to the patient and often will achieve resolution of the lesion within 48 hours of injection. Small amounts of triamcinolone (Kenalog 10 mg/mL) diluted 1:1 with lidocaine or normal saline is the treatment of choice (Fig. 22.18).

5. ***The management of scarring:*** Up to 50% of scars (especially smaller scars) may improve naturally over 6–12 months. Treatment of established scars is difficult and while some patients will benefit from treatment others will not.

Management of Acne Scars

Up to 50% of scars (especially smaller scars) may improve naturally over 6–12 months. Treatment of established scars is difficult and while some patients will benefit from treatment others will not.

Atrophic Scars

- The development of ablative lasers combined with appropriate surgical techniques has led to a significant improvement in the way that certain atrophic scars can be treated. Though the images in Fig. 22.19 reveal variably good results, the results take time, require multiple sessions, and are not as dramatic as the cost.

- Punch excision of small atrophic scars which can be very helpful prior to resurfacing.

- For deep scars—scar revision may help.

- Other options include intradermal injections of collagen or compounds, which stimulate collagen synthesis.

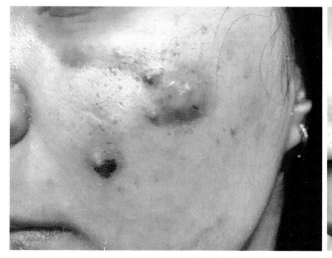 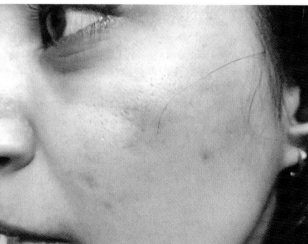

Fig. 22.18: Cystic acne and after IL steroid injection

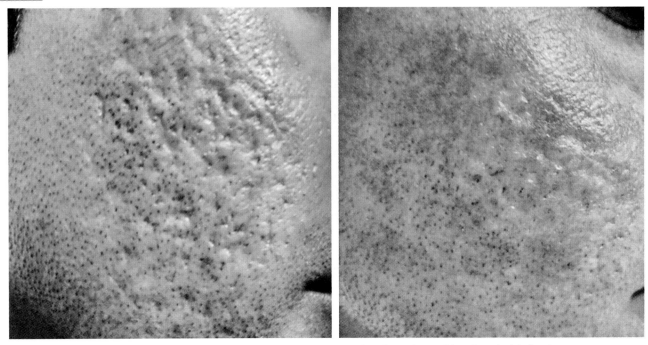

Fig. 22.19A: Before and after images of rolling scars after 7 sessions of fractional ablative lasers

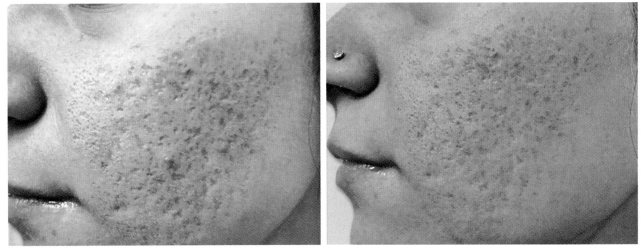

Fig. 22.19B: A case with ice pick and boxcar scars response after 6 sessions. Note that some of the scars still remain

Hypertrophic/Keloid Scars

- Silicone gels applied to scars can be prescribed by general practitioners.
- Local steroids or by using intradermal triamcinolone given for a trial period of two to three months. Look closely for side effects such as skin thinning and telangiectasia.
- Pulsed dye laser can reduce the redness of scars and flatten them. This procedure is only possible through specialized hospital departments.

ROSACEA

Rosacea is a disease of middle-aged adults,[Q] with a peak around 40–50 years.[Q] It is equally common in both sexes, but more severe in men.

Causative factors include dysregulation of facial blood flow, skin type I-ll (fair skin: 'curse of the Celts'),[Q] chronic ultraviolet (UV) exposure, Demodex colonization, and induction of innate antimicrobial peptides. An older connection to gastrointestinal disease has not been substantiated.

Clinical Presentation

The classic features are:

- Facial erythema, flushing and blushing[Q]
- The appearance of papules and pustules[Q]
- Mild edema, telangiectases, and occasionally a disseminated violaceous hue.

Ocular symptoms such as burning and stinging may occur and are often ignored. Sebaceous hyperplasia

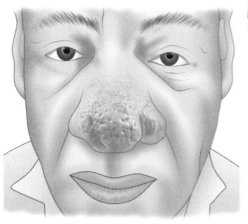

Rhinophyma

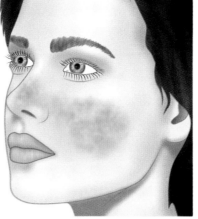

Erythematotelangiectatic
rosacea

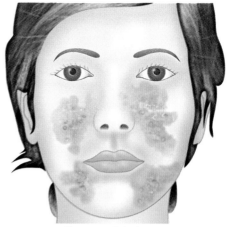

Rosacea fulminans

Fig. 22.20: Depiction of the variants of rosacea

may be observed, and skin thickening, particularly of the nose (rhinophyma)[Q] can occur.

Site: Rosacea often affects the convex surfaces[Q] of the face, including the nose, centrofacial area, and forehead.

Subtypes include erythematotelangiectatic type, papulopustular (Fig. 22.20), phymatous and ocular.

Rosacea-like Dermatoses

Steroid rosacea: Chronic topical corticosteroid use on the face may help resolve underlying dermatitis but eventually causes erythema, telangiectases, and pustules (Fig. 22.21). Bums and flares occur when corticosteroids are discontinued.

Perioral dermatitis: Grouped papules about the mouth (with pale spared zone adjacent to vermilion) or around eye (Figs 22.22 and 22.23).Topical or inhaled corticosteroid use may predispose to perioral dermatitis.

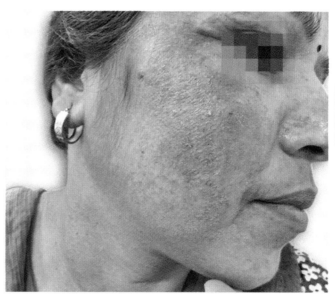

Fig. 22.22: A case of steroid rosacea. The patient had been applying potent steroids for 2 years. Note the papules superimposed on an erythematous background

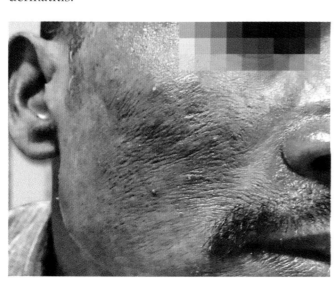

Fig. 22.21: Background erythema with papules and pustules

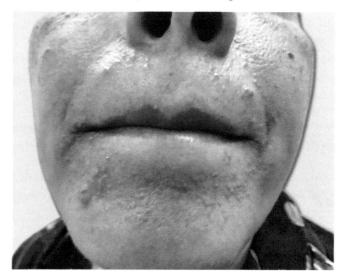

Fig. 22.23: Perioral dermatitis in a female patient

Table 22.5   Therapies of rosacea based on the predominant morphology

	Flushing and fixed erythema	Inflammatory papules and pustules	Ocular
Ivermectin cream 1% (greater efficacy than metronidazole)		+++	
Azelaic acid gel 15%		++	
Metronidazole gel or cream 0.75%		+	
Brimonidine gel 0.33% (effective and fast acting vasoconstrictor, there is a chance of rebound flush)	++		
Doxycycline MR 40 mg (as effective as conventional dose, less chance of resistance)		+++	
• Doxycycline 100 mg • Lymecycline 408 mg caps		++	++
Isotretinoin		++	
IPL, PDL	++		
• Clonidine 25–50 µg • Propranolol 10–40 mg • Carvedilol 3.125–6.25 mg	++		

Demodicosis: Older adults may develop often unilateral grouped papules and pustules with fine scale,[Q] typically involving the cheek, nose, or forehead.[Q] Occasionally, there are deep inflamed nodules. Lesions are full of Demodex mites, which can be seen under the microscope.

Drug-induced rosacea: Antibodies against the epidermal growth factor (EGF) receptor[Q] and inhibitors of the EGF receptor tyrosine kinase used for targeted cancer therapy can cause a rosacea-like dermatosis; the worse the rash, the better the systemic response.

Management

Management of rosacea is driven by the subtype and level of severity. An overview of the various therapies depending on the predominant skin manifestation is given in Table 22.5. There is global agreement on the need for the following:

- *Photoprotection for all subtypes*: A broad-spectrum UVA/UVB sunscreen should be applied daily at appropriate intervals, depending on outdoor exposure and activities.
- *Trigger avoidance*: The most common triggers provided by the National Rosacea Society include: Food (spicy and hot), alcoholic beverages, skin care products (astringents, exfoliants), emotional influences, health conditions, types of physical exertion, and temperature- or weather-related factors.

 Topical products reported to be sources of irritation are alcohol, witch hazel, fragrance, menthol, peppermint, and eucalyptus oil.

- *Demodex eradication*: It has been achieved with use of permethrin cream, lindane, BPO, or sulfur-based lotions,[Q] and is a promising area of clinical trials.

Therapy

- All patients should avoid sunlight and irritating substances.
- Light emollients and camouflage skin care products are beneficial. Topical steroids can exacerbate rosacea and should be avoided.
- Treatment options are directed by the predominant type of rosacea. Flushing and fixed erythema can be helped by topical brimonidine, intense pulsed light (IPL) or pulsed dye laser (PDL). Inflammatory changes (i.e. papules and pustules) can be treated with topical agents (ivermectin, azelaic acid or metronidazole gels or creams)[Q], or oral antibiotics (Table 22.5).
  - *Mild rosacea*: Long-term topical metronidazole 0.75% gel or cream; azelaic acid 15% cream.
  - *Rosacea papulopustulosa*: Systemic doxycycline 40–100 mg daily or isotretinoin 10–20 g daily for 6–9 months.
  - *Rosacea fulminans*: Isotretinoin 10–20 mg plus prednisolone. 5 mg/kg daily for weeks to months, with gradual taper.
  - *Phymatous type*: Surgical measures (dermabrasion, shaving) always combined with standard therapy.
  - *Ocular rosacea*: Doxycycline 40–100 mg daily for 6–9 months; an alternative is isotretinoin 10 mg daily.
  - *Perioral dermatitis, steroid rosacea*: Stop corticosteroids! Doxycycline 40–100 mg daily; consider topical calcineurin inhibitors.

Eccrine and Apocrine Gland Disorders

Eccrine Glands

- Functional from birth[Q] and activated by thermal stimuli via the hypothalamic pre-optic nucleus[Q] sweat center; their major function is thermoregulation by evaporative heat loss.
- Innervated by sympathetic fibers that have acetylcholine[Q] as their major neurotransmitter.
- Generalized distribution, with greatest concentration on the palms and soles.[Q]
- The eccrine duct opens directly onto the skin surface, (merocrine glands) and the excretory product is a clear hypotonic fluid that is mostly water but also contains NaCl.

Apocrine Glands

- Unclear function in humans; functional development requires androgens.[Q] They are under adrenergic control.
- More limited distribution[Q]—primarily *axillae*, *nipples/areolae*, and *umbilical* and *anogenital regions*; modified apocrine glands are found in ear (ceruminous gland) and eyelids (Moll's gland).[Q]
- The apocrine duct drains into the superficial portion of the hair follicle.
- 'Decapitation'[Q] of apocrine gland cells produces an **odorless**[Q] and viscous fluid; however, its degradation by flora on the skin surface can lead to an odor.

HYPERHIDROSIS

Primary Hyperhidrosis

This is a common disorder, especially in younger individuals with up to 100-fold increased parasympathetic stimulation of eccrine sweat.

Clinical Features

Attacks of uncontrollable severe sweating on the hands (Fig. 23.1), feet or axillae, which are aggravated by stress or heat, but often spontaneous.

Therapy

Aluminum chloride hexahydrate in 10–20% concentration is useful for axillary hyperhidrosis and is to be applied at night. Axillary sweat glands can be completely removed by excision or subcutaneous curettage. The ultimate surgery for hands is endoscopic sympathectomy; there is risk of compensatory hyperhidrosis at other sites.

Tap water iontophoresis is best for **palmoplantar hyperhidrosis**, initially daily until improvement, then several times weekly.

Botulinum toxin injections are an effective and safe option for localized hyperhidrosis. The toxin blocks the

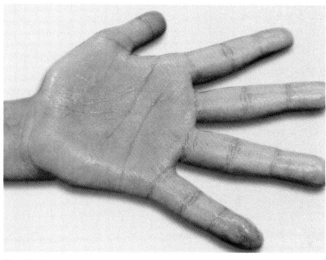

Fig. 23.1: A case of excessive sweating of the palms (hyperhidrosis)

innervation of eccrine glands. It is costly and must be repeated every 6–12 months for the axillae and every 3–6 months for the palms of the hands and soles of the feet. On an average, 100 units are required for each side (palm or sole).

For **generalized hyperhidrosis**, anticholinergic agents can be tried.

Secondary Hyperhidrosis

Increased sweating, especially at night, should raise a suspicion of chronic infections, autoimmune diseases, or malignancies. Sweating is also seen in hot flashes during menopause, along with erythema and warmth. Localized hyperhidrosis may be secondary to nerve damage (carpal tunnel syndrome, cervical rib, neurological disease). Other important syndrome complexes include:

Gustatory hyperhidrosis: Also known as Frey syndrome or auriculotemporal syndrome.[Q] Following facial nerve injury with misdirected regrowth of fibers, chewing stimulates not only parotid gland secretion but also sweating in the distribution of one or more facial nerve branches.

Ross syndrome: Unilateral segmental hypohidrosis of the trunk with compensatory contralateral hyperhidrosis. Unilateral lack of pupil and tendon reflexes.[Q]

HYPOHIDROSIS AND ANHIDROSIS

Reduced sweating with heat intolerance in systemic disorders (renal failure, hypothyroidism, Addison disease, diabetes insipidus) and neurological diseases (leprosy) and with marked dehydration. Anhidrotic and hypohidrotic ectodermal dysplasias are rare syndromes with reduced to absent sweat glands.

BROMHIDROSIS (FOUL-SMELLING SWEAT)

Sweat is usually odorless. It is usually the extraneous influences that give it the odor.

- *Eccrine variant* associated with degradation of sweat by resident microflora; most commonly involves the feet.[Q]
- *Apocrine variant* associated with degradation of odiferous substances (e.g. triglycerides) by skin flora.[Q]
- The smell can be rancid (*Corynebacterium*) or sweaty (*Micrococcus*).
- Occasionally, the food that one takes may give an odor, thus the more smelly foods, line onion, garlic and hing can cause an odor.[Q]
- Rarely, it is a sign of an inherited metabolic disorder.

Chromhidrosis

Discoloration of sweat, usually by drugs or dyes; there are many different colors (blue, green, red, gray-black) (Fig. 23.2).

Intrinsic: Here it is due to the lipofuscin content of apocrine sweat[Q] (yellow, green, black). Most common is black color[Q] (Fig. 23.2).

Extrinsic: Staining of sweat by clothing or chromogenic bacteria (e.g. *Corynebacterium*) or fungi. The former is called pseudochromhidrosis.[Q]

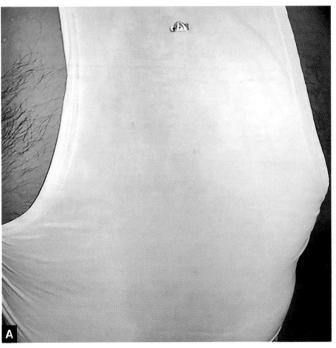
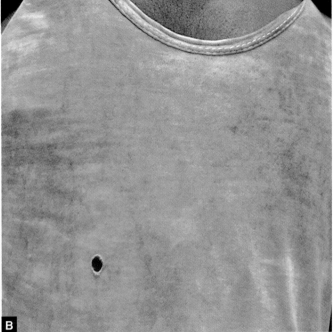

Fig. 23.2A and B: Chromhidrosis: Colored sweat staining the undergarments; (A) Yellow; (B) Black

INFLAMMATORY DISEASES^Q

Miliaria

This results from occlusion of eccrine ducts^Q (Fig. 23.3).

- *Miliaria crystallina*: When the blockage is within the stratum corneum,^Q presents as tiny clear ('dewdrops') vesicles (Fig. 23.4A).
- *Miliaria rubra* (*prickly heat*): Pruritic erythematous papulovesicles and occasionally pustules that favor the upper trunk. Patient has multiple small, discrete, uniform-sized papules not associated with hair follicles (Fig. 23.4B). There is a block in mid-epidermis at the level of the granular cell layer.^Q Most common form is miliaria pustulosa a variant with erythematous pustules (Fig. 23.4C).

Sweating, followed by:
- Itching—cholinergic urticaria.^Q
- Itchy red papules—miliaria rubra.^Q

- *Miliaria profunda* have deeper obstruction with inflammation producing red papules at the dermal-epidermal junction.^Q If extensive, decrease in eccrine function can give rise to hyperpyrexia.

Differential diagnosis: Miliaria rubra and pustulosa may be confused with folliculitis. In miliaria, the pustules are usually smaller and more numerous, and do not have a centrally placed hair. Sometimes, however, the two conditions coexist because they may share the same predisposing factor of occlusion.

The word milia sounds similar to miliaria, but the condition it denotes is different. Milia are small, noninflamed, superficial, epidermal keratin cyst.

Fox-Fordyce Disease^Q

Skin-colored itchy axillary papules due to occluded inflamed apocrine ducts^Q (apocrine miliaria) (Fig. 23.4D).

More common in females, appear after puberty.

Fordyce spots → Ectopic free lying^Q sebaceous glands, duct is connected directly to overlying skin or mucosal surface.
Most common site: Upper lip^Q
No treatment required.

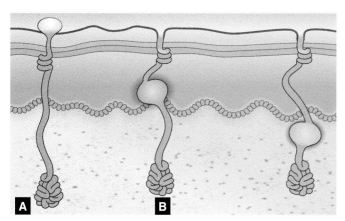

Fig. 23.3: (A) Miliaria cystallina affects the surface of the acrosyringium; (B) Miliaria rubra affects the acrosyringium as it crosses the stratum spinosum

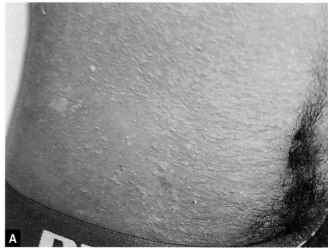
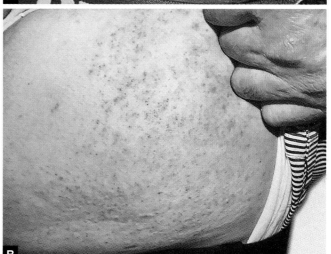
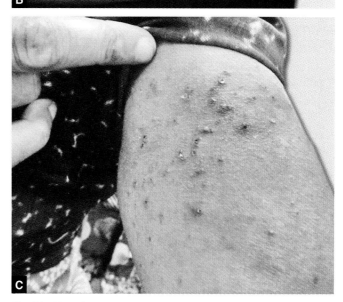

Fig. 23.4A to C: Types of miliaria: (A) Crystallina; (B) Rubra (prickly heat); (C) Miliaria with pustules—miliaria pustulosa

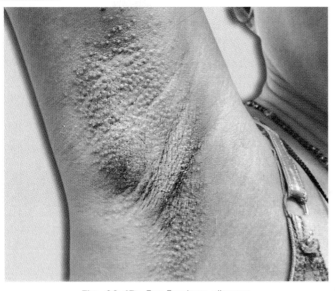

Fig. 23.4D: Fox-Fordyce disease

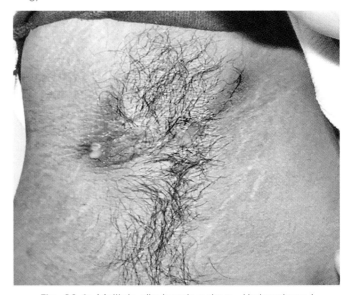

Fig. 23.6: Multiple discharging sinus—Hurley stage I

HIDRADENITIS SUPPURATIVA (HS) OR INVERSE ACNE

HS, also known as acne inversa,[Q] is a persistent disease which most often has its onset after puberty, with a mean age of 38 years.

Pathophysiology

Originally, in 1854, Verneuil believed that HS was a result of apocrine gland dysfunction, but current research has identified blockage of the follicular structure with ensuing rupture of the follicle as the origin of the disorder.

Clinical Features

A diagnosis of HS is made in the presence of key characteristic findings.

Typical lesions that are red, painful papules, nodules, and abscesses; cord-like scarring; double open comedones (Figs 23.5 to 23.9) with secondary staphylococcal infection.

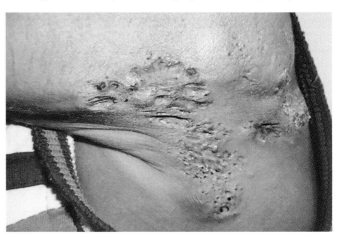

Fig. 23.7: HS cutaneous lesions: inflamed nodules along with cord-like scars from previous flares on the left axilla—Hurley stage II

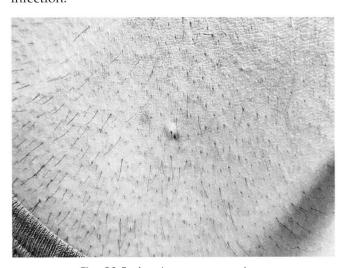

Fig. 23.5: A polyporous comedone

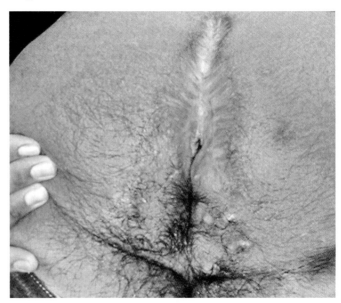

Fig. 23.8: Nodules, sinuses and initial signs of scarring—Hurley stage II

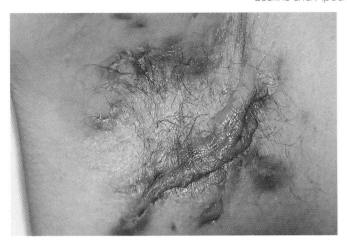

Fig. 23.9: Nodules, sinuses and severe scarring—Hurley stage III

The Hurley staging^Q system is the most widely used HS classification scale in routine clinical practice. This staging system, proposed by Hurley in 1989, classifies patients into three stages (Figs 23.6 to 23.9):

Stage	Abscesses	Sinus tracts	Cicatrization
I	Single or multiple	–	–
II	Recurrent (separated)	+ (separated)	+
III	+++	Multiple, interconnected	++

Recurrent pattern of disease since the age of 10 years, including the presence of one active lesion in the axillae or groin, and a history of at least three draining lesions of those areas.

Distribution: A characteristic distribution common in the axillae, groin, medial thighs, and anogenital region, less commonly in the breasts, perianal and perineal areas (Fig. 23.10).

Complications may include anemia of chronic disease, secondary amyloidosis, lymphedema, fistulas, arthropathy, and the rare development of SCCs within the chronic scars.

Treatment

General Measures
• Weight reduction, if obese or overweight
• Measures to reduce friction and moisture:
  1. Loose undergarments
  2. Absorbent powders
  3. Antiseptic soaps
  4. Topical aluminum chloride
• Warm compresses
• Stop smoking

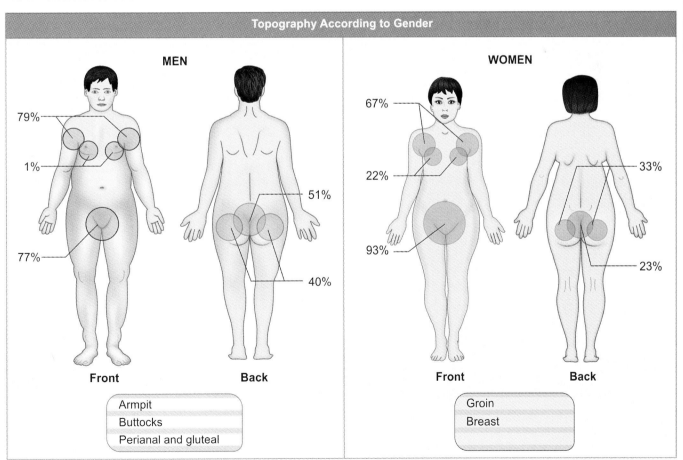

Fig. 23.10: Distribution of HS lesions in men and women

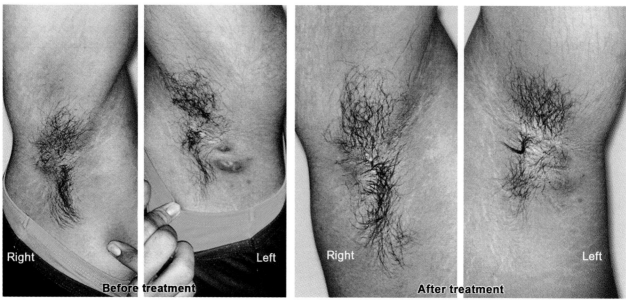

Fig. 23.11: A patient of hidradenitis suppurativa before and after treatment with adalimumab

Table 23.1	Treatment options in HS
Hurley stage I disease • Solitary or multiple isolated abscesses • No scarring or sinus tracts	*Medical therapy* • Intralesional triamcinolone (5 mg/mL) injections into early inflammatory lesions • Topical clindamycin • Eradication of *S. aureus* carriage with topical mupirocin in nose, axillae, umbilicus, perianal regions • Oral antibiotic therapy (alone or in combination) for its anti-inflammatory effect (tetracycline, doxycycline, minocycline, clindamycin, rifampin + clindamycin, dapsone, trimethoprim-sulfamethoxazole) • Oral anti-androgen therapy (e.g. finasteride)
Hurley stage II disease • Recurrent **abscesses** • **Sinus** tract formations • Early scarring	*In addition to the above* • Acitretin • Infliximab • Cyclosporine *Surgical treatment* • Limited local excisions with secondary intention healing • CO_2 laser ablation with secondary intention healing
Hurley stage III disease • Diffuse or broad involvement with multiple interconnected **abscesses and sinus tracts** • More extensive scarring	*Medical treatment* Adalimumab[Q] for 12 weeks *Surgical treatment* • Early wide surgical excision of involved areas

In general, medical treatment is recommended in early stages; surgical treatment should be performed as early as possible once abscesses, fistulas, sinus tracts, and scars develop.

In the early stage, doxycycline 100 mg bid or minocycline 100 mg bid should be prescribed and continued for 3 to 6 months. Topical clindamycin 1% bid can also be used as monotherapy or in combination with systemic therapy.

The ideal drug for severe disease is the biological drug adalimumab, which is given subcutaneously once in 2 weeks for 3 months (Fig. 23.11).

An overview of the therapeutic intervention is given in Table 23.1.

CHAPTER 24

Disorders of Hair

Chapter Outline

INTRODUCTION

Hair follicles form before the ninth week of fetal life when the hair germ, a solid cylinder of cells, grows obliquely down into the dermis. There it interacts with a cluster of mesenchymal cells (the placode) bulging into the lower part of the hair germ to form the hair papilla. The dermal papilla contains blood vessels bringing nutrients to the hair matrix. The sebaceous gland is an outgrowth at the side of the hair germ, establishing early the two parts of the pilosebaceous unit. Adjacent to the sebaceous gland is the region of insertion of the arrector pili muscle called the *bulge*.[Q] This area contains hair *follicle stem cells* which presumably can regenerate the entire hair follicle and sebaceous gland. Damage to this area will cause *permanent hair* loss.[Q]

Melanocytes migrate into the matrix and are responsible for the different colors of hair (eumelanin, brown and black; pheomelanin and trichochromes, red). Gray or white hair is caused by low pigment production, and the filling of the cells in the hair medulla with minute air bubbles that reflect light.[Q]

HAIR ANATOMY

The structure of a hair follicle is depicted in Fig. 24.1.
They can be divided into four parts:
1. Infundibulum, extending from the follicular orifice to the sebaceous gland.
2. Isthmus, extending from the sebaceous gland to insertion of the arrector pili muscle.
3. Suprabulbar area, insertion of the arrector pili muscle to matrix.
4. Bulb, consisting of the dermal papilla and matrix intermixed with melanocytes.

HAIR BASICS

The entire scalp contains around 100,000 pigmented, terminal hair follicles. Hair of people originating from east Asia (China, Korea, and Japan) is usually referred to as, Oriental or Asian hair. It generally shows the greatest diameter, ranging from 100 to 130 µm.

Every hair follicle undergoes an individual recurring cycle with growing and resting periods. The growing period[Q] (anagen) persists for 2–8 years, and the hair grows approximately 1 cm/month or 0.35 mm/day[Q] during this time. During the hair cycle, the middle and upper portions of the hair follicle are the permanent[Q] segment, whereas the lower portion is nonpermanent[Q] (Fig. 24.2).

The root (bulb area) of an anagen terminal follicle reaches deep into subcutaneous fat tissue. The anagen phase is followed by a transition period (catagen) of 2 weeks,[Q] during which the hair follicle undergoes programmed apoptosis. This transitional state is followed by a resting period (telogen) that lasts around 3 months.[Q] During telogen, the hair does not grow longer; the shaft is anchored in the mid-deep dermis.

Unlike most fur-bearing animals, where the hair cycle is synchronous, on the human scalp, there is an asynchronous mixture of hairs actively growing and resting. If many hairs pass into the resting phase (telogen) at the same time, then a correspondingly large number will be shed 2–3 months later (telogen effluvium).[Q]

The scalp consists of almost 90% hairs in anagen, 1% in catagen, and 10% in telogen.[Q] A normal anagen to telogen ratio for the scalp hair is 9:1,[Q] although seasonal variations can be found. The scalp sheds around 100 telogen hairs per day.

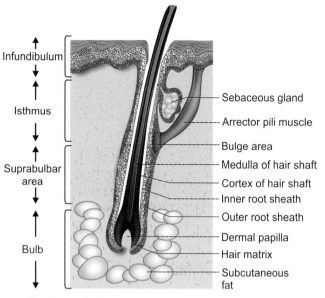

Fig. 24.1: A depiction of the parts of a hair follicle

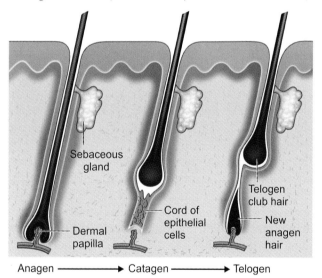

Anagen ⟶ Catagen ⟶ Telogen

Fig. 24.2: Phases of hair cycle

Hairs are classified into three main types:
1. *Lanugo hairs*: Fine long hairs covering the fetus, but shed about 1 month before birth.
2. *Vellus hairs*: Fine short unmedullated hairs covering much of the body surface. They replace the lanugo hairs just before birth.
3. *Terminal hairs*: Long coarse medullated hairs seen, e.g. in the scalp or pubic regions. Their growth is often influenced by circulating androgen levels.

Terminal hairs convert to vellus hairs in male-pattern alopecia, and vellus to terminal hairs in hirsutism.[Q]

ALOPECIA

The term means loss of hair and alopecia has many causes and patterns. One convenient division is into localized and diffuse types. It is also important to decide whether or not the hair follicles have been

Table 24.1	A list of causes of alopecia
Localized nonscarring	• Androgenetic alopecia • Alopecia areata (noninflammatory patchy baldness, exclamation mark hair sign present)[Q] • Tinea capitis (pediatric age scaling, itching, patchy baldness)[Q] • Hair-pulling habit (trichotillomania) (patchy bizarre baldness, broken hair, follicular hemorrhage may be present)[Q] • Traction alopecia • Hair shaft abnormalities • SLE
Scarring	• Lichen planus • Pseudopelade of Brocq • Frontal fibrosing alopecia (Kossard) • Chronic cutaneous lupus erythematosus • More severe or advanced infections (deep tinea capitis, massive folliculitis, zoster) • Physical, chemical or mechanical alopecia • Aplasia cutis congenita • Epidermolysis bullosa—junctional, dystrophic or acquired

replaced by scar tissue; if they have, regrowth cannot occur, this is termed cicatricial alopecia. The presence of any disease of the skin itself should also be noted (Table 24.1).

Localized Nonscarring Alopecia

Amongst the various causes, if localized non-scarring alopecia, tinea capitis has been discussed previously unless it is complicated by inflammation and postulation, is usually non-scarring.[Q] In psoriasis, uncommonly the rough removal of adherent scales can also remove hairs, but here regrowth is the rule.[Q]

Alopecia Areata

Sudden localized hair loss without clinically visible inflammation; variety of clinical patterns.

Pathogenesis: Alopecia areata is most likely an organ-specific autoimmune disorder, with autoaggressive T cells possibly directed against melanocytes in the anagen follicle. Likely association with other autoimmune diseases[Q] such as vitiligo, Hashimoto thyroiditis, and diabetes mellitus; also seen with other thyroid diseases and atopy.

Classification

• *Localized alopecia areata*:[Q] One or several areas of alopecia on scalp or beard (Fig. 24.3A).
• *Alopecia totalis*:[Q] Loss of most or all of scalp hair, sometimes with loss of eyebrows and eyelashes (Fig. 24.3B).
• *Alopecia universalis*: Loss of all scalp and body hair.[Q]

Clinical features: Round to oval sharply circumscribed areas of hair loss without inflammation[Q] (Fig. 24.3C).

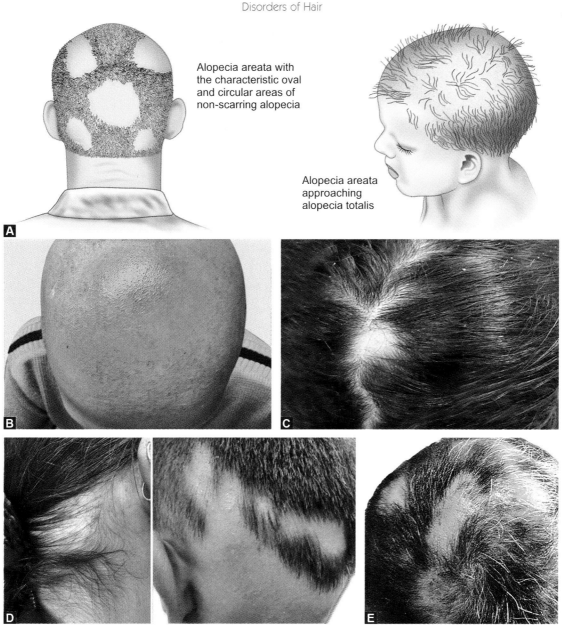

Alopecia areata with the characteristic oval and circular areas of non-scarring alopecia

Alopecia areata approaching alopecia totalis

Fig. 24.3A to E: (A) Localized and generalized alopecia areata on the scalp. This responds readily to IL steroids; (B) Alopecia totalis; (C) Localized alopecia areata; (D) Ophiasis pattern of alopecia areata (bad prognosis); (E) Regrowing hair are usually gray in color

Usually starts as single lesion; most often spontaneous resolution. In others, expansion of lesion or development of new patches. The loss of hair may be preceded by a feeling of itching or burning. Also, the gray hair are spared by the autoimmune attack. Thus, in sudden onset alopecia areata, it is also known as 'going gray overnight' phenomenon.[Q]

Other important aspects of the disorder include:

Ophiasis:[Q] Band-like loss from ear to ear across the nape; poor prognostic sign (Fig. 24.3D).

Focal areas of poliosis (gray hairs) where previous patches have regrown (Fig. 24.3E).

Exclamation point hairs:[Q] Broken-off 1–2 mm hairs at the periphery of the patch; when plucked, look like exclamation point with a thick bulb. These are broken off about 4 mm from the scalp, with the proximal end more narrowed and less pigmented (Fig. 24.4A).

Cadaver hairs: Hairs broken before they reach surface; also sign of activity and progression.

Fine pitted[Q] nails are present in around 20% of adults and up to 50% of children with alopecia areata; association with twenty-nail dystrophy (trachyonychia). The pitting is called geometric pitting or thimble pitting[Q] (Fig. 24.4B).

Associations

- Autoimmune diseases such as vitiligo, Hashimoto thyroiditis, and diabetes mellitus
- Atopy
- Hypertension
- Down syndrome

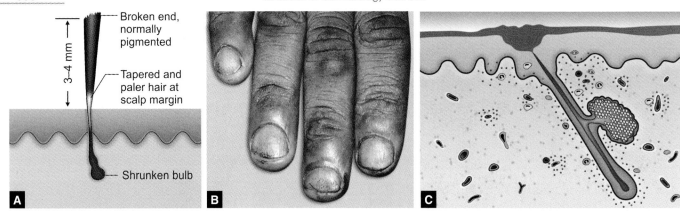

Fig. 24.4A to C: (A) A depiction of exclamation mark hair; (B) Fine pitting in a case of alopecia areata; (C) Small, dystrophic hair structures. A lymphocytic infiltrate surrounds the early anagen hair bulbs like a **'swarm of bees'**

Course: Fifty percent of cases resolve spontaneously without treatment in 1 year, and only 10% go onto develop severe chronic disease. Subsequent episodes tend to be more extensive and regrowth is slower.

Unfavorable signs are:[Q]
- Positive personal or family history for atopy, alopecia areata, or autoimmune diseases
- Onset before puberty
- Rapid progression
- Widespread recurrence
- Persistence for >2 years
- Ophiasis (alopecia areata involving temporal and occipital margins of scalp in a continuous band).
- Involvement of eyelids or eyelashes.

Histology: Only indicated for confirmation of suspected diffuse variant of alopecia areata. In early stage, dense lymphocytic infiltrate about lower follicles (*swarm of bees* pattern around *anagen hair bulb*)[Q] and increased number of catagen follicles (Fig. 24.4C).

Investigations: None is usually needed. The histology of bald skin shows lymphocytes around and in the hair matrix. Syphilis can be excluded with serological tests, if necessary.

Organ-specific autoantibody screens provide interesting information but do not affect management. Check blood pressure. Alopecia areata tends to be more aggressive in young patients from families with high prevalence of hypertension.

Differential diagnosis: Trichotillomania, tinea capitis, syphilitic alopecia, scarring alopecia:
- In alopecia areata, the hair loss is not scaly, unlike T capitis.
- The patches of alopecia are skin colored in contrast to lupus erythematosus and lichen planus.
- In trichotillomania and in traction alopecia, broken hairs may be seen but true exclamation-mark hairs are absent.

Treatment: Tends to self-resolve by 1 year in 50% patients. No curative therapy; two main strategies to alter immune picture around follicles—immunosuppression with corticosteroids and immunomodulation via intentional allergic contact dermatitis.
- The therapy also depends on the extent of disease with localized disease responding to topical agents in which topical steroids and intralesional steroids[Q] are the mainstay.
- Mild irritants, such as 0.1–0.25% dithranol, have been used but with limited success.
- Ultraviolet radiation or even psoralen with ultraviolet A (PUVA) therapy may help extensive cases, but hair fall often returns when treatment stops.
- Topical immunotherapy with contact sensitizers (e.g. diphencyprone and squaric acid dibutyl ester) is another promising treatment for patients with extensive disease.
- Systemic agents including steroids, methotrexate, azathioprine and sulfasalazine have been tried for extensive disease but has variable results.
- Ruxolitinib, janus kinase (JAK 1 and 2) inhibitors, both orally and topically administered, are under investigation.

Trichotillomania

This is a disorder with localized alopecia secondary to plucking, cutting, or rubbing away hairs.

Clinical features: Poorly circumscribed bizarre patterned areas of broken-off hairs of variable length occasionally follicular hemorrhages. Pull test is negative and trichogram shows a few telogen hairs.

'Hallmark sign' is an area of hair loss with *irregular* borders and hairs of *various* lengths present at the same time. It is commonly seen in the easily-reached *frontoparietal* region of the scalp and should always be suspected when there is hair loss of the eyebrows or eyelashes (Fig. 24.5).

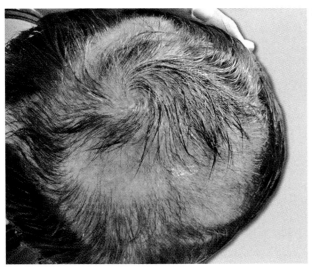
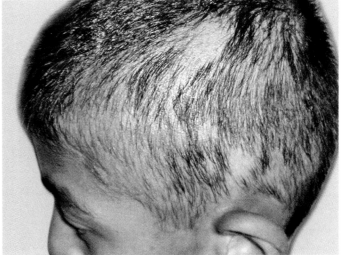

Fig. 24.5: Bizarre, patterns of alopecia with irregular borders with hairs of various lengths on accessible areas of scalp (trichotillomania)

In infants, this is an almost normal habit of no consequence. They may also induce nuchal alopecia simply by rubbing their heads on mattress or pillow. In older children or adults, usually associated with psychiatric disturbances, in the general category of obsessive-compulsive^Q disorder. Clinically, tends to be more diffuse than in small children; sometimes entire scalp is involved (*tonsure pattern*).

Histology: Biopsy shows perifollicular hemorrhage and damaged follicles; useful to exclude alopecia areata.

Therapy: Confronting the patient with the diagnosis may help in mild cases. Most teenagers and adults require psychiatric support and therapy (SSRIs). Often manifestation of conflict between child and parents, making management even more difficult. Recently, N-acetylcysteine (an amino acid) has been shown to be effective at decreasing this compulsive behavior.

Self-induced Alopecia

There are several other forms of self-induced alopecia in which there is no underlying psychological problem:

Traction alopecia:^{Q} Hair loss secondary to tight hair styles, such as corn rows in blacks, tight braids, or long, heavy ponytails. If not interrupted, can progress to scarring and permanent hair loss. In India, it is seen in those who braid their hair tightly.

Clinical features: The changes are usually seen in girls and young women, particularly those whose hair has always tended to be thin anyway. The most common pattern is 'marginal alopecia' in which the hair loss is mainly around the edge of the scalp—at the sides or at the front (Fig. 24.6). The bald areas show short broken hairs, folliculitis and, sometimes, scarring.

Management: Invariably patients do not accept the cause for alopecia and slow to alter their cosmetic

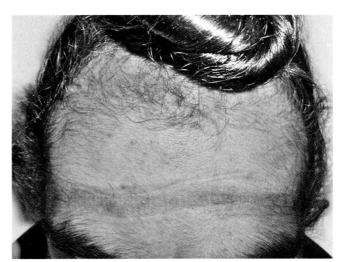

Fig. 24.6: Traction alopecia in a boy who used to braid his hair, due to his religion

practices. If prolonged, the regrowth is often disappointingly incomplete.

Localized Scarring Alopecia

This is also known as cicatricial alopecia and is characterized by areas of hair loss, *without* hair follicles, which means that hair regrowth is difficult. In most cases, there is permanent damage to the follicular stem cell region, or the bulge area.

In some cases, the cause is obvious, like a severe burn, trauma, a carbuncle or an episode of inflammatory scalp ringworm. The other causes are listed in Table 24.2, of which the term pseudopelade^Q applies to a slowly progressive non-inflamed type of scarring which leads to irregular areas of hair loss without any apparent preceding skin disease (Fig. 24.7A to E). But most cases of pseudopelade represent end-stages of lichen planopilaris (most common) or chronic cutaneous lupus erythematosus (less common).

24

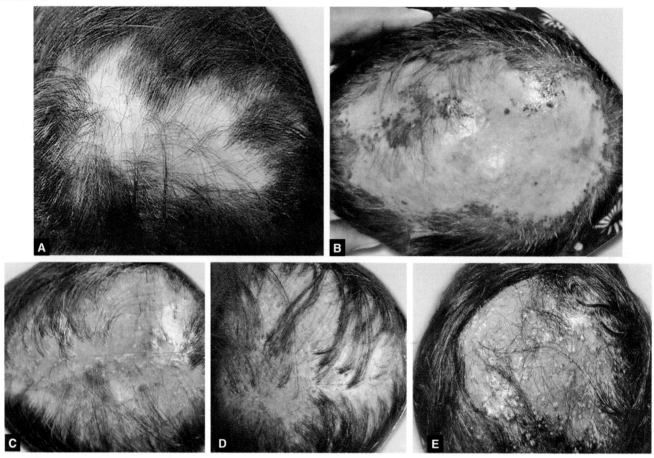

Fig. 24.7A to E: (A) A case of pseudopelade of Brocq with scarring alopecia demonstrating the reticular elongation also known as **'footprints in the snow pattern'**; (B) A late stage of DLE with depigmentation of the scalp with scarring; (C) Lichen planopilaris on the scalp; note the lack of follicular ostia and multiple follicular hyperkeratotic lesions; (D) This can progress to scarring alopecia; (E) Multiple pustules with associated cicatricial alopecia in a case of folliculitis decalvans

Table 24.2   Overview of common causes of cicatricial alopecia (localized)

Dermatoses	Clinical features	Treatment
Discoid lupus erythematosus	Erythema, follicular plugging, and scale; later hypopigmentation, atrophy, and scarring alopecia (Fig. 24.7B). Marginal hyperpigmentation	• High-potency topical or intralesional corticosteroids, corticosteroid pulse therapy or cyclosporine • HCQS for maintenance
Lichen planopilaris	Follicular or perifollicular hyperkeratoses, usually multiple, evolving into atrophic patulous follicles, sometimes with erythematous rim, and then permanent scarring (Fig. 24.7C).	• High-potency topical or intralesional corticosteroids with salicylic acid ointments. • Systemic corticosteroids, perhaps combined with acitretin (0.3–0.5 mg/kg). • Doxycycline or minocycline 100 mg bid for their anti-inflammatory effect
Folliculitis decalvans	Pustules, erythema, scarring and sometimes marked seborrhea (Fig. 24.7D)	*Systemic*: Rifampicin-clindamycin, rifampicin-doxycycline, rifampicin-ciprofloxacin, rifampicin-clarithromycin *Topical*: Mupirocin, clindamycin, fusidic acid
Pseudopelade of Brocq	• Small confluent atrophic scarred areas (footprint in the snow)^Q, usually occipital or parietal (Fig. 24.7A). • Typically bundles of hair remain • Affected areas smooth and glistening, sometimes pruritic.	• Empiric treatment with antibiotics or antimalarials. • Symptomatic treatment with wig/hair transplantation or scalp reduction can be considered, *if* disease is completely *quiescent*.

24

DIFFUSE HAIR LOSS

Androgenetic Alopecia (Most Common Alopecia)[Q]

This is a physiologic process consequent to an increased follicle sensitivity to androgens leading to change from terminal to vellus hair follicles with distinct patterns of alopecia, often associated with telogen effluvium.

Pathogenesis

Polygenic inheritance; variable penetrance. The hair follicles have increased numerous of androgen receptors as well as increased activity of 5-α-reductase type II, leading to increased androgen sensitivity. Dihydrotestosterone also causes shift to telogen hairs. In female-pattern hair loss, there may be an increased sensitivity to circulating androgen, as androgen levels are usually within normal limits.

Clinical Features

Thinning of hair without scalp disease; two classic pattern schemes used for grading (Fig. 24.8):

- Male patterns
- Female patterns

It has been recently suggested that bald men are more likely to have a heart attack and prostate cancer than those with a full head of hair.

History

The process begins at any age after puberty, but temporal recession is often noticed between the ages of 20 and 30 years. Women can note the onset of hair thinning in their 20s and 30s or around menopause. The onset and progression are gradual. Women often report see-through hair where scalp skin is noticed.

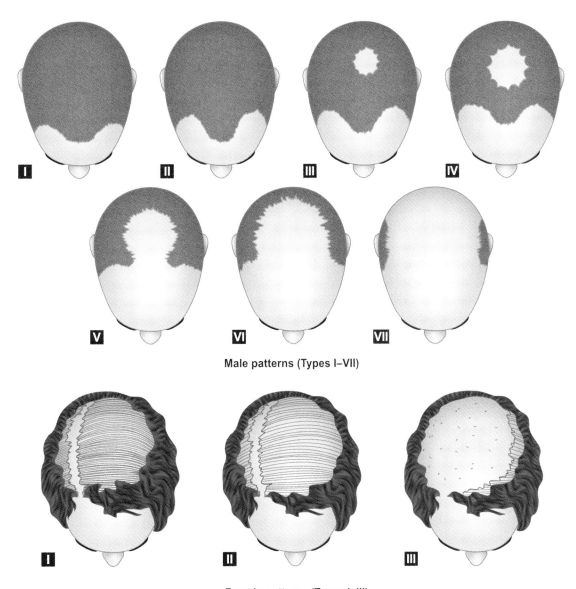

Male patterns (Types I–VII)

Female patterns (Types I–III)

Fig. 24.8: Androgenetic alopecia: Male pattern (after Hamilton)[Q] and female pattern (after Ludwig)[Q]; men can also develop the Ludwig pattern and women the Hamilton pattern. Note: Overlap forms are common in both sexes

Estrogen protects against hair loss and, therefore, FPHL is seen to some degree in all women who are postmenopausal.

Androgens cause scalp baldness but stimulate hair growth on the chest, face, and genital regions. This phenomenon may be explained by regional differences in androgen metabolism.♀ Hair follicles in bald areas of the scalp have increased levels and activity of 5-α-reductase, which causes increased levels of dihydro-testosterone that shortens the hair cycle and miniaturizes scalp follicles.

Diagnostic Approach

- Usually obvious, but many younger patients are skeptical and disappointed in the diagnosis.
- *Site*: In men, usually receding frontal hairline (Fig. 24.9A and B). In women, more diffuse thinning and retention of frontal pattern (Fig. 24.10A and B). Thus in women, FPHL most often is manifested by

diffuse thinning over the top of the scalp (e.g. the crown) (*fir tree pattern*♀).
- Vellus hairs usually prominent in areas of loss; hairs are thinner and remain shorter.
- In women, often associated with telogen effluvium.
- Patients may complain that hairs are finer and grow more slowly, while at other body sites, hair growth may be increased. Often seborrhea more prominent than previously.
- Family history is almost always positive, if one is persistent enough. Many patients initially say that no one in the family was bald, but this typically means only that their father had a relatively full head of hair. Ask about hair loss in grandparents, uncles, aunts.

Investigation

1. Trichogram or phototrichogram reveals reduced anagen/telogen ratio, frontal >occipital.

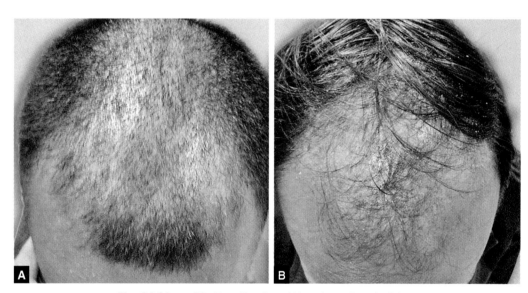

Fig. 24.9A and B: Hamilton I and V male pattern hair loss

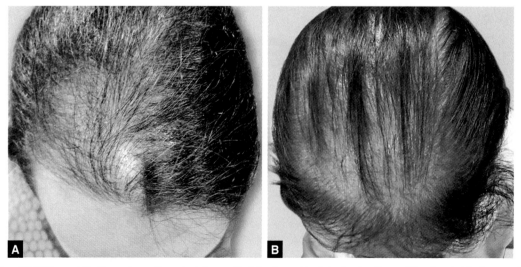

Fig. 24.10A and B: Female pattern hair loss with thinning of hair but retention of the frontal hair margin

2. Hormone levels usually normal. Studies only needed when hirsutism, virilization, menstrual problems, infertility, galactorrhea, or other indications of endocrine abnormalities are present. Hormone studies including DHEAS, free testosterone, SHBG, prolactin, thyroid function; hormone studies should be done on day 3–7 of cycle, after withholding oral contraceptives for 3 months.

Differential Diagnosis

Diffuse alopecia areata, androgen-induced alopecia. In women, there are multiple causes of diffuse hair loss that may have to be excluded, though in some cases, they may overlap with pattern alopecia (Table 24.3).

Therapy

Treatment of men

- Minoxidil is a systemic vasodilator, used for severe hypertension, which causes hypertrichosis. Topical minoxidil 2–5% solution is effective in androgenetic alopecia. Minoxidil can also be compounded, but considerable care is required as it is poorly soluble. After 4–12 months of usage, hairloss may be stabilized and some regrowth of terminal hair shafts seen infrontal and vertex vellus regions. Side effects include hypertrichosis in undesired locations (face, nipples), allergic contact dermatitis and hypotension. When minoxidil treatment stops, the new hairs fall out after about 3 months.

  Minoxidil is applied to the entire affected area (dry scalp) twice daily and should remain on for at least 1 hour. When applied at night, it should be 2 hours before bedtime to prevent transfer of the product to the pillowcase. Touching the face during sleep could result in an increase of facial hair.

- Systemic finasteride[Q] (5-α-reductase type II inhibitor) is the most effective therapy available. 1 mg daily

'forever' is the dosage. It blocks conversion of testosterone into dihydrotestosterone, the active agent in androgenetic alopecia. Side effects during short-term use (1–3 years) are minimal; the inhibitor is highly specific and even effects on libido are quite rare. The long-term effects over 30 years are still unpredictable. Once stopped, there is rapid progression of hair loss at the pretreatment level.

- Be alert to cofactors such as thyroid disease; appropriate endocrinologic management can help slow progression of hair loss.
- Hair transplantation: Effective technique that depends on donor dominance plugs or micrografts of hairs taken from an area where androgenetic alopecia does not occur can be transplanted to bald areas and hairs will continue to grow.

Treatment of women

- Minoxidil also useful; at least 6 months trial, better 12 months; more risk of facial hypertrichosis in women.
- Systemic antiandrogens can be employed, always in conjunction with oral contraceptives in premenopausal women
- Hair transplantation usually not indicated in women because of their more diffuse thinning and the impossibility of reliably determining the border between androgen-sensitive and insensitive hair follicles.
- Same supportive measures as in men; also consider iron, zinc, and biotin supplementation.

A summary of the salient aspects of the two main medications used is given in Box 24.1.

Telogen Effluvium (TE)

This is a non-scarring alopecia with sudden loss of hair consequent to an altered hair growth cycle, with premature shift of hairs into catagen and then telogen phase. This condition is best viewed as a symptom, almost always reflecting an earlier trigger event. These include:

1. *Androgenetic alopecia*: Most common cause is flare of androgenetic alopecia in both men and women.

Table 24.3	Causes of diffuse hair loss
Endocrine causes	• Hypopituitarism • Hypo- or hyperthyroidism • Hypoparathyroidism • High androgenic states
Drug-induced	• Antimitotic agents (anagen effluvium) • Retinoids • Anticoagulants • Vitamin A excess • Oral contraceptives
• Iron deficiency • Severe chronic illness • Malnutrition • Diffuse type of alopecia areata	

Box 24.1	Drug summary
Minoxidil	• Men: After 1 year of treatment, 20 to 40% of men achieve moderate to dense regrowth. Useful for vertex and frontal but not temporal thinning • Women: Up to 60% of women experience hair regrowth with the 2% solution or 5% foam after 6 months of treatment. Useful for vertex, frontal and temporal thinning • Hair growth plateaus after 1 year
Finasteride	Five-year data show that 90% of men maintain their present hair and two-thirds of men experience some degree of hair regrowth.

Telogen effluvium may also be the only sign of a developing androgenetic alopecia where the terminal-to-vellus hair conversion has not yet occurred.

2. *Thyroid dysfunction*: Always check thyroid function tests; sometimes normal values in patients on thyroid replacement can still be associated with unexplained hair loss, requiring more detailed endocrinologic studies.

3. *Sudden drop in estrogen levels*: Delivery,[Q] miscarriage, or discontinuing oral contraceptives.

4. *Inadequate diet*: Always ask about eating disturbances, crash diets, or other peculiarities.

5. *Iron deficiency*: May be first sign of modest iron deficiency[Q] with only abnormal ferritin levels and no laboratory signs of anemia.

6. *Scalp diseases*: Seborrheic dermatitis; less often psoriasis, tinea capitis or allergic contact dermatitis. Any inflammatory scalp disease increases the shift into telogen phase and thus the rate of hair loss; thus prompt and aggressive treatment required.

7. *Medications*:
   - Retinoids (acitretin, isotretinoin)
   - Discontinuation of birth control pills
   - Anticoagulants (especially heparin)
   - Antidepressants
   - Lithium
   - Amphetamines
   - Antithyroid (propylthiouracil, methimazole)
   - Anticonvulsants (e.g. phenytoin, valproic acid, carbamazepine)
   - Heavy metals
   - β-blockers (e.g. propranolol)

   It is not necessary to discontinue these medications as the hair growth cycle will *eventually* adjust itself back.

8. *Other possible causes include*:
   - Severe acute illnesses,[Q] infections, high fever, general anesthesia.
   - Hyperprolactinemia (especially if associated with late-onset acne).
   - Malabsorption and inflammatory bowel disease.
   - Endocrine disorders (Addison disease, Hashimoto thyroiditis).
   - Chronic diseases (connective tissue disorders, chronic infections, malignancies).
   - Psycho-emotional stress.

Clinical Features

Typically patient describes markedly increased diffuse hair loss during hair washing and combing, well above the previously observed level (Fig. 24.11).

> Patients complain, "I am losing my hair" or "I am noticing a lot of hair in the shower drain."

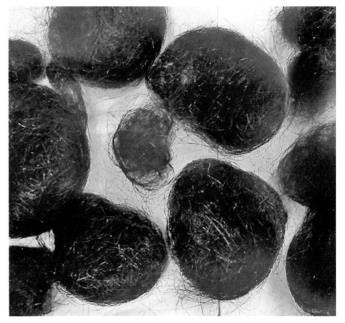

Fig. 24.11: Hair shed each day, brought by a patient with CTE (*Courtesy*: Dr Ananta Khurana)

Chronology of triggers: It takes approximately 100 days for hairs to shed; therefore, the diagnosis of TE depends on the chronology of events and symptoms. The precipitating event is usually identified and precedes the hair loss by approximately 3 to 4 months.[Q] The shedding continues for about 1 to 2 months but may last 4 to 6 months before it subsides.

In *acute TE*, the hair loss can be triggered by any severe illness, particularly those with bouts of fever or hemorrhage, by child birth and by severe dieting. All of these synchronize catagen so that, later on, large numbers of hairs are lost at the same time in the telogen phase. There is a characteristic lag of 2–3 months after the provoking illness (Fig. 24.12).

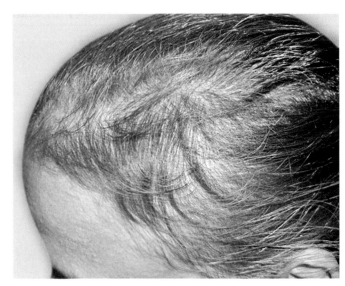

Fig. 24.12: A young girl with acute telogen effluvium. There is hair loss from the frontal and temporal areas

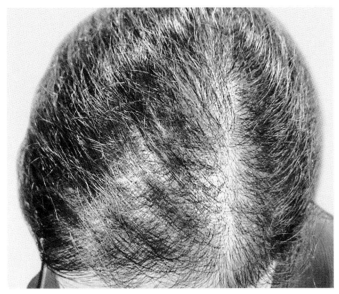

Fig. 24.13: Chronic telogen effluvium. There is diffuse decrease in hair density

In case of *chronic TE*, the hair loss persists for more than 3 months and here the hair loss may represent a flare of underlying androgenetic alopecia (Fig. 24.13).

Patients begin to shampoo less often in hope of preserving hair. They fail to realize that the average number of hairs lost daily is more evident on days they shampoo.

Investigation

- Examine hairs, trichogram shows >25% telogen hairs (in extreme cases, 80–90%). Pulling out more than three hairs consistently from different scalp areas confirms that excessive shedding is present.

  In stress-induced alopecia, the number of telogen hairs is increased from a normal percentage of 10 to 20% to more than 25%. This results in as many as 400 to 500 lost hairs daily. Normally, fewer than 100 hairs are lost daily.
- *Laboratory screening* (complete blood count [CBC], liver function tests, renal status, iron, ferritin).
- In case of *chronic hair loss*, testing for serum free testosterone and dihydroepiandrosterone sulfate levels in women with menstrual irregularities or hirsutism may be warranted.

Differential Diagnosis

1. *Anagen effluvium*: Hairs are damaged and lost during growth phase; bayonet hairs without telogen bulb; usual causes chemotherapy, radiation therapy, sepsis; rarely seen with alopecia areata.
2. In androgenetic alopecia in females, the onset is gradual in mid-adulthood, and hairs remain rather firmly anchored to the scalp. In telogen effluvium, the onset is abrupt and follows acute illness, an opera-

tion or pregnancy by 1–2 months. Hair fall is prominent and lightly pulling on scalp hairs dislodge many.
3. In diffuse alopecia areata, the hair loss is more patchy, and the onset abrupt with waxing and waning. Shedding may be prominent. Exclamation-mark hairs are often present.

Therapy

Usually no therapy is needed. Most patients accept the message that underlying factors must be corrected and nature given time to restore cycle. It is important to rule out androgenetic alopecia specially in females with chronic telogen effluvium.

HIRSUTISM AND HYPERTRICHOSIS

Hirsutism is the growth of terminal hair in a woman, which is distributed in the pattern normally seen in a man. Hypertrichosis is an excessive growth of terminal hair that does not follow an androgen-induced pattern.

Hirsutism

Definition

Increased growth of terminal hairs in women in androgen-dependent areas, producing male-like hair growth pattern (Fig. 24.14). Virilization is the association of hirsutism with other signs of male development, such as voice deepening, clitoral enlargement, increased muscles, loss of breast tissue, acne, and androgenetic alopecia.

Most cases of hirsutism are physiologic; in many ethnic groups, female body hair does not fit the current Western beauty standard, leading to psychosocial problems as people move between cultures. Hirsutism combined with androgenetic alopecia can be a sign of elevated prolactin levels, typically caused by neuroleptic agents, polycystic ovary syndrome, or prolactinoma (usually a small tumor not otherwise symptomatic) (Fig. 24.15).

Investigation

Significant hormonal abnormalities are not usually found in patients with a normal menstrual cycle.

Investigations are needed:
- If hirsutism occurs in childhood;
- If there are other features of virilization, such as clitoromegaly;
- If the hirsutism is of sudden or recent onset
- If there is menstrual irregularity or cessation.

Measurement of the serum testosterone, sex hormone binding globulin, dehydroepiandrosterone sulfate, androstenedione and prolactin will help determine the source of excess androgen (i.e. adrenal cortex, ovaries, pituitary). Ovarian ultrasound is useful, if polycystic ovaries are suspected. An approach to the investigation of a case of hirsutism is given in Fig. 24.16.

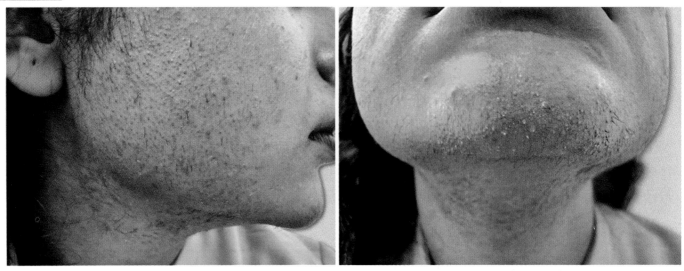

Fig. 24.14: Patient of PCOS with acne and marked hirsutism

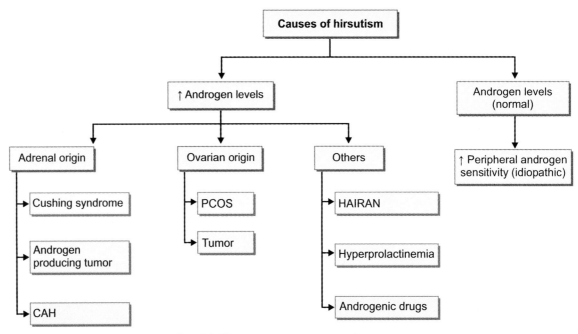

Fig. 24.15: Overview of causes of hirsutism

Table 24.4	Medical therapy for hirsutism	
Premenopausal female	**First-line:** OCP **Second-line:** OCP + spironolactone or CPA (cyproterone acetate)	
Postmenopausal female	**First-line:** Spironolactone or CPA	**Severe or refractory:** Finasteride, flutamide, or GnRH agonist; plus an OCP, if premenopausal
NC-CAH	**First-line:** OCP ± spironolactone or CPA **Second-line** or if seeking ovulation induction: Glucocorticoids	

NC-CAH, nonclassic congenital adrenal hyperplasia.

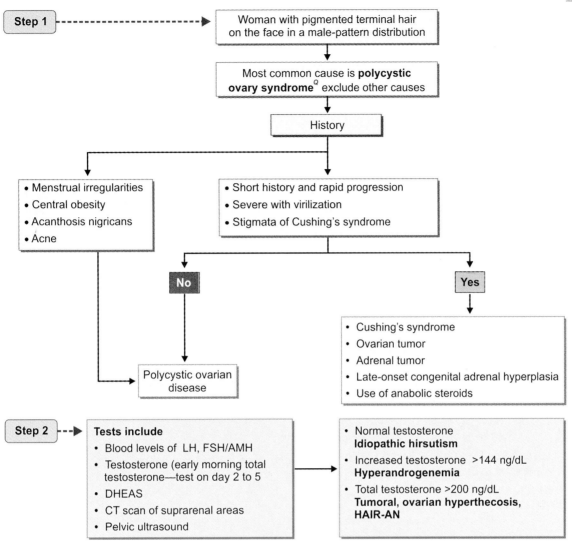

Step 1 - - - - - - - - - - - - - ▶ Woman with pigmented terminal hair on the face in a male-pattern distribution

Most common cause is **polycystic ovary syndrome**[Q] exclude other causes

History

- Menstrual irregularities
- Central obesity
- Acanthosis nigricans
- Acne

- Short history and rapid progression
- Severe with virilization
- Stigmata of Cushing's syndrome

No / Yes

Polycystic ovarian disease

- Cushing's syndrome
- Ovarian tumor
- Adrenal tumor
- Late-onset congenital adrenal hyperplasia
- Use of anabolic steroids

Step 2 - - - ▶ **Tests include**
- Blood levels of LH, FSH/AMH
- Testosterone (early morning total testosterone—test on day 2 to 5
- DHEAS
- CT scan of suprarenal areas
- Pelvic ultrasound

- Normal testosterone
  Idiopathic hirsutism
- Increased testosterone >144 ng/dL
  Hyperandrogenemia
- Total testosterone >200 ng/dL
  Tumoral, ovarian hyperthecosis, HAIR-AN

Fig. 24.16: Approach to diagnosis of the cause of hirsutism

Treatment

Most topical agents are depilatory creams (often containing a thioglycollate). Also used are measures like waxing or shaving, or making the appearance less obvious by bleaching; none remove the hair permanently. Plucking should be avoided as it can stimulate hair roots into anagen. Topical therapy with eflornithine,[Q] an inhibitor of ornithine decarboxylase,[Q] can slow regrowth.

Methods to destroy hair include electrolysis or lasers. Oral antiandrogens (e.g. cyproterone acetate; spironolactone) may sometimes be helpful, but will be needed long-term use for results (usually 6 months).

An overview of medical therapies is given in Table 24.4.

Disorders of Nail

ANATOMY OF THE NAIL (Fig. 25.1)

1. *Epidermis of dorsal nail fold*: Skin at proximal end of nail; folded upon itself.
2. *Cuticle*: Sheet of cells that seals proximal nail fold.
3. *Nail matrix*: Epithelium that keratinizes without granular layer (onycholemmal keratinization);[Q] the lunula is the most distal aspect of the nail matrix, visible through the nail plate.[Q]

   The proximal nail matrix forms the top (surface) of the nail plate. The distal nail matrix forms the underside of the nail plate; therefore, biopsies of the distal matrix are less likely to produce a deformity of the surface of the nail plate.

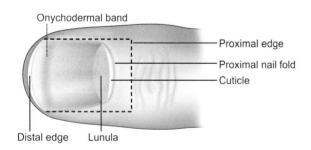

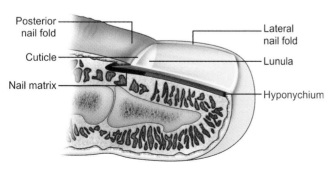

Fig. 25.1: Normal anatomy of the nail

4. *Nail bed*: Produces a thin sheet of parakeratotic keratinocytes attached to deep surface of nail plate; perhaps helps in attachment, which is also facilitated by a system of ridges and furrows (zipper effect).
5. *Hyponychium*: Point of separation of nail plate from nail bed; lacks dermatoglyphics.

The rate at which nails grow varies from person-to-person but is slow:

- Fingernails average 1 mm/week—thus they are replaced in about 6 months.[Q]
- Toenails grow 0.3–0.5 mm/week and are replaced every 12 months.[Q] Nails grow faster in the summer, if they are bitten and in youth.

We will discuss the main disorders affecting the nail and have divided them into discrete sections according to the site of involvement. Also we have summarized the findings of the common disorders in the end.

CHANGES IN THE NAIL PLATE

1. *Lamellar splitting (onychoschizia)*: In this, there is transverse splitting (Fig. 25.2) of the distal part of the fingernails, commonly seen in housewives, and has been attributed to repeated wetting and drying. Also seen in lichen planus and with systemic retinoids.
2. *Onychorrhexis*: The term onychorrhexis describes nail plate brittleness in longitudinal direction (Fig. 25.3).
   - Severe diffuse fissuring with nail thinning[Q] of several nails is typical of nail matrix lichen planus.
   - Other causes include iron and vitamin deficiency.

3. *Onycholysis*: A separation of the nail plate from the nail bed (Fig. 25.4).
   - May be a result of minor trauma
   - Also seen in nail psoriasis

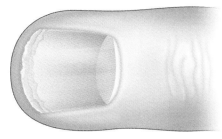

Lamellar splitting—flaking and fragility of the distal end of the nail plate

Fig. 25.2: Onychoschizia

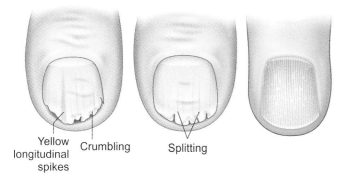

Yellow longitudinal spikes   Crumbling   Splitting

Fig. 25.3: Onychorrhexis

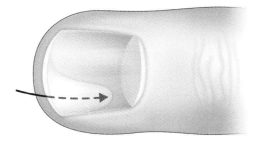

Onycholysis is the separation of the nail plate from the nail bed

Fig. 25.4: Onycholysis

- Phototoxic reactions (photo-onycholysis from tetracyclines)[Q]
- Repeated immersion in water
- After the use of nail hardeners

4. *Beau's line*: It appears as a transverse depression of the nail plate, with a variable depth and length (Fig. 25.5A). It results from a transitory damage to the proximal nail matrix with temporary decrease of the keratinocyte mitotic activity.[Q] The resulting nail plate is thinner than normal and appears as a transverse depression involving the whole nail width.
   Onychomadesis: It represents a more severe degree of Beau's line, where the damage involves the whole matrix, with complete temporary arrest of nail plate production (Fig. 25.5B).

5. *Trachyonychia*[Q] (*20-nail dystrophy*): As the Greek term *trakos* (rough) indicates, the nails are rough and appear as if sandpapered in longitudinal direction (Fig. 25.6A). Despite the name 20-nail dystrophy, trachyonychia does not necessarily involve all the nails.
   Trachyonychia is a sign of mild and diffuse damage to the proximal nail matrix by inflammatory disorders (PALE).[Q]
   Causes:
   - **P**soriasis
   - **A**lopecia areata of the nail
   - **L**ichen planus (Fig. 25.6C)
   - **E**czema
   Alopecia areata or lichen planus >> psoriasis.

6. *Koilonychia* (*spoon nails*): The nail is thin and has an abnormal concavity, resembling a spoon, as can easily be appreciated looking at it from the side (Fig. 25.7).
   Koilonychia is common in the 2nd–4th toenails of children aged from 1 to 3–4 years, where it is physiological and transitory and due to age-related nail plate thinness; in adults, koilonychia is rare and occurs in the fingernails of manual workers in contact with irritants and detergents that damage the nail plate. It is also seen in iron deficiency.[Q]

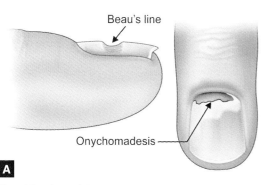

Beau's line

Onychomadesis

A

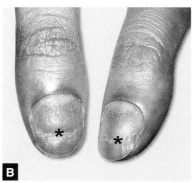

B

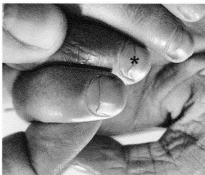

Fig. 25.5A and B: (A) Beau lines and onychomadesis; (B) Left shows pitting with Beau's line. Right shows shedding of nails—onychomadesis

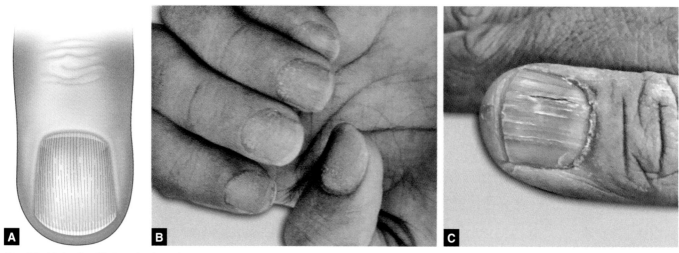

Fig. 25.6A to C: (A) Rough, 'sandpaper' nails, often thin—trachyonychia; (B) A patient with trachyonychia; (C) Onychorrhexis with thinning of nail plate in a case of lichen planus

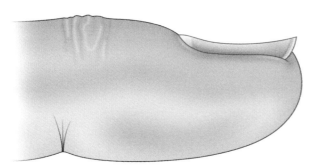

The concave, spoon-shaped nail of koilonychia
(seen in iron deficiency)

Fig. 25.7: Koilonychia

7. *Clubbing* (*watch-glass nails*): This is a bulbous enlarge-ment of the terminal phalanx with an increase in the angle (Schamroth sign/lovibond angle) between the nail plate and the proximal fold to over 180° (Fig. 25.8). Its association with chronic lung disease and with cyanotic heart disease is well known.

8. *Onychogryphosis*: Thickening, over curvature and lateral deviation of nails, especially toe nails. Causes: Chronic trauma, ill-fitting shoes, digital ischemia and old age (Fig. 25.9).

9. *Habit tic nail dystrophy*: The cuticle of the thumbnail is the target for picking or rubbing. This repetitive trauma causes a ladder pattern of transverse ridges and grooves to run up the center of the nail plate causing a midline nail deformity (Fig. 25.10).

10. *Ingrown nail*:Q Growth of nail into the lateral nail fold. Usually in young men, on the medial side of the great toe, caused by tight shoes and incorrect trimming (Fig. 25.11).

11. *Pitting*: It is characterized by several punctate depressions on the nail plate, appearing as small, irregularly round holes (Fig. 25.12). It is rarely seen in the toenails. It is seen in psoriasis, LP, eczema and alopecia areata.

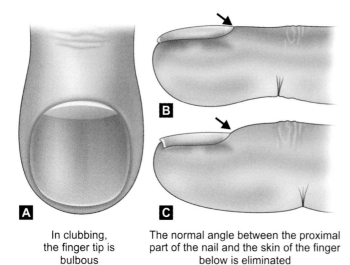

In clubbing,
the finger tip is
bulbous

The normal angle between the proximal
part of the nail and the skin of the finger
below is eliminated

Fig. 25.8: Clubbing

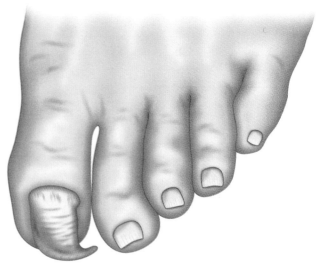

Fig. 25.9: Onychogryphosis (ram horn nails)

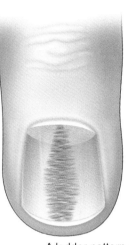 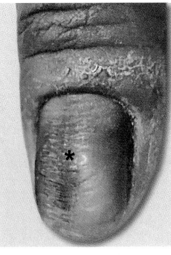

A ladder pattern of transverse ridges and furrow which runs up the center of a thumb nail

Fig. 25.10: Habit tic deformity

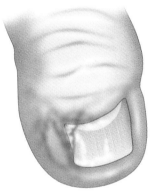 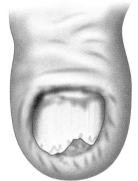

Ingrown toenail.
Lateral nail fold swollen, red and tender

Deformed toenail.
Yellow, thickened nail plate with subungual debris caused by chronic fungal infection

Fig. 25.11: Ingrowing toenail

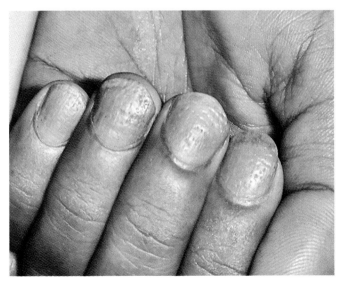

Fig. 25.12: A depiction of pitting in the nail

Pitting results from focal defective keratinization of proximal nail matrix cells, with persistence of groups of nucleated and incompletely keratinized (parakeratotic) cells on the nail plate surface. The parakeratotic cells are shed and the nail plate only show pits.

In psoriasis: Pits are large and irregular in shape and distribution.[Q]

In alopecia areata: The pits are superficial, regular, and homogeneously distributed along geometrical line.[Q]

ALTERATION OF NAIL COLOR

Leukonychia

This refers to a white discoloration of the nail and can be of three types with different clinical features and different pathogenesis:

- *True leukonychia*: The white color moves distally with nail growth. It results from defective keratinization of the keratinocytes of the distal nail matrix,[Q] with persistence of parakeratotic cells within the nail plate. These cells are not transparent and reflect light, causing the white discoloration.

  They are of various types, including, partial, total, punctate and transverse and are mostly consequent to trauma or aggressive pedicure (Fig. 25.13).

- *Apparent leukonychia*: The whitish discoloration fades with pressure, as it is due to nail bed abnormalities (Fig. 25.14A).
  a. Terry's nails,[Q] leukonychia affects the whole nail except for a 1–2 mm pink to brown distal band (seen in *cirrhosis*, cardiac failure, and diabetes mellitus) (Fig. 25.14B).
  b. Half and half nails (Lindsay's nails),[Q] the proximal area is dull white and the distal area (20–60% of the total length) is pink or reddish brown, with a distinct border between the two colors. Seen in patients on *hemodialysis* (Fig. 25.14C).
  c. Muehrcke's lines,[Q] where the nail has multiple transverse[Q] whitish bands (Fig. 25.14D), parallel to the lunula. Initially described in patients with liver *cirrhosis*, *hypoalbuminemia*, they are now commonly seen after *chemotherapy*.

- *Pseudoleukonychia*, where the nail discoloration has an external origin, and it is due to a friable surface of the nail plate with keratin degranulation that induces the white pigmentation.

Longitudinal Melanonychia

The term longitudinal melanonychia describes a longitudinal black-brown-gray band that contrasts with the pink color of the normal nail and is due to the

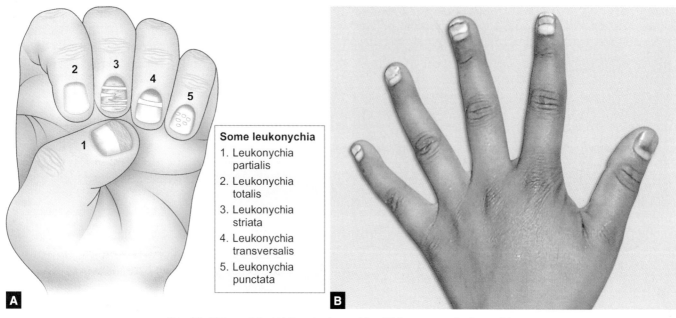

Fig. 25.13A and B: (A) True leukonychia; (B) Transverse leukonychia

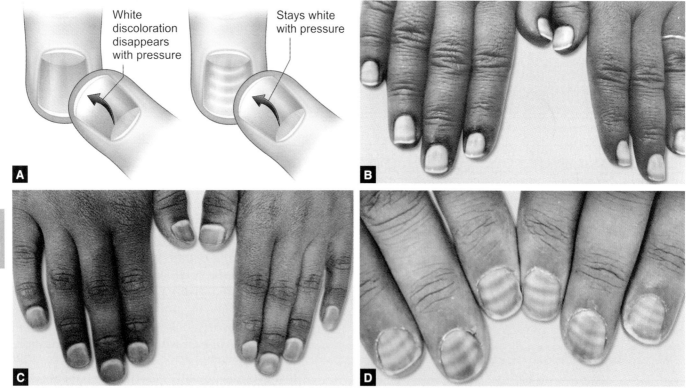

Fig. 25.14A to D: (A) Demonstration of apparent leukonychia and true leukonychia; (B) Leukonychia in a case with liver cirrhosis; (C) Half and half nails—in a case of CRF; (D) Muehrcke's lines: Multiple transverse whitish bands

presence of melanin within the nail plate. The corresponding nail plate can show some changes or be completely normal. The pigmentation may extend to the periungual soft tissues[Q] or may be usable through the transparent cuticle (Pseudo Hutchinson's sign) (Fig. 25.15).

• Multiple bands common in darker skin types (physiologic); also can be due to trauma.
• A single uniform streak suggests a melanocytic nevus

• An irregular streak or nail fold discoloration (Hutchinson's sign) suggests melanoma.[Q]

Yellow Nail Syndrome

A rare triad of yellow nails, pleural effusions and lymphedema.[Q] The nails are thickened and slow growing; chronic pulmonary disease is common (bronchiectasis, bronchitis, rhinosinusitis).

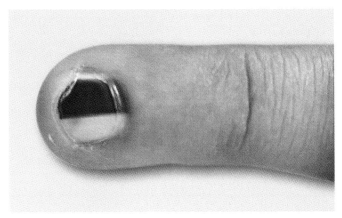

Fig. 25.15: A single uniform black band with the Pseudo Hutchinson's sign

Green Nails

Caused by subungual colonization by *Pseudomonas aeruginosa*, producing green-black pyocyanin. Treat with antibacterial solutions or acetic acid.

Vascular/Traumatic Lesions

1. *Splinter hemorrhages*: They are most commonly seen under the nails of manual workers and are caused by minor trauma (Fig. 25.16).

   They may also be a feature of psoriasis of the nail and of subacute bacterial endocarditis.
2. *Capillary prominence ± cuticular hemorrhages* (Fig. 25.17A).
   • Associated with lupus erythematosus and Osler-Weber-Rendu syndrome.
   • Also associated with dermatomyositis and scleroderma, with a slightly different appearance.
   • Capillary dropout alternating with dilated capillary loops (Fig. 25.17B).
   • Associated with dermatomyositis and scleroderma.
3. *Subungual hematomas*: They are usually easy to identify but the trauma that caused them may have escaped notice and dark areas of altered blood can raise worries about the presence of a subungual melanoma (Fig. 25.18).

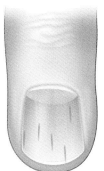
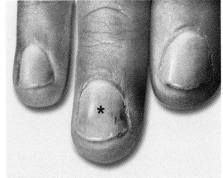

Fig. 25.16: Splinter hemorrhages

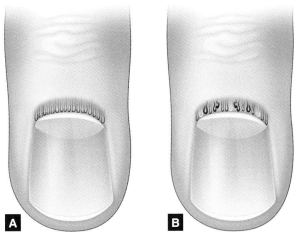

Fig. 25.17A and B: (A) Capillary prominence; (B) Dropout of vessels

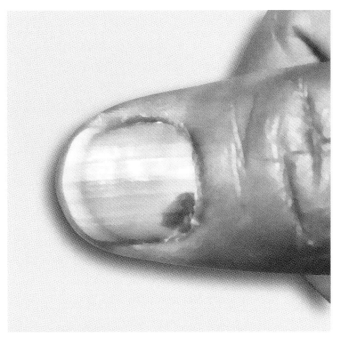

Fig. 25.18: Subungual hematoma

NAIL CHANGES IN COMMON DERMATOSES

Psoriasis

Most patients (50%) with psoriasis have nail changes at some stage; severe nail involvement is more likely (90%) in the presence of arthritis.

Defect in the nail matrix: Surface texture of the nail plate is altered.

Defect in the nail bed: Color defects and onycholysis. Also thickening or lifting of the nail and subungual hyperkeratosis, result from accumulation of scales in psoriatic lesions of the nail bed and hyponychium (Fig. 25.19A and B).

The most classic change[Q] is pitting though the most specific[Q] is the 'oil drop' sign wherein red or brown areas are seen due to psoriasis involving the nail bed

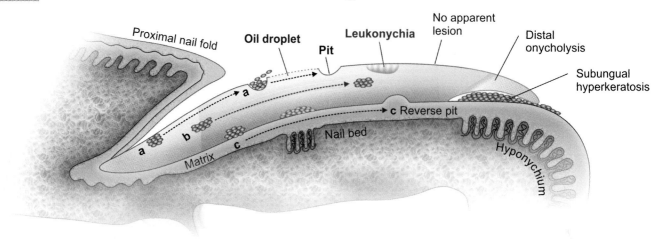

Fig. 25.19A: Overview of nail findings in psoriasis depending on the defect on the (a) proximal, (b) intermediate, (c) distal matrix, and nail bed

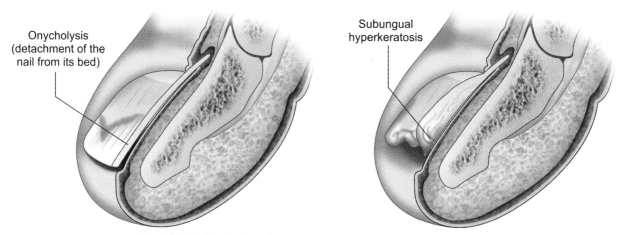

Fig. 25.19B: Depiction of onycholysis and subungual hyperkeratosis

causing onycholysis bordered by obvious discoloration.

a. Onycholysis with erythematous border: It is the most common[Q] sign of psoriasis and seen mainly in the fingernails. It results from psoriatic involvement of the nail bed (Fig. 25.19C).

b. Yellow-brown spot ('oil-drop' sign): Guttate psoriasis of nail bed with serum glycoprotein deposits (Fig. 25.19D).

c. Subungual hyperkeratosis is usually marked in the toenails, as trauma worsens it through the Koebner's phenomenon.

d. Psoriatic pitting is typical of the fingernails and indicates proximal nail matrix involvement by psoriasis. In psoriasis, pits are irregular in depth and distribution on the nail plate[Q] (Fig. 25.19E). Pitting is often the only sign of nail psoriasis in children.

Other signs include:

a. Red spots in lunula: Active psoriasis in distal matrix.

b. Splinter hemorrhages: Bleeding of superficial dilated capillaries in nail bed due to trauma.

Lichen Planus

Some (10 to 15%) of the patients with lichen planus have nail changes.

The most common change is a reversible thinning[Q] of the nail plate with irregular longitudinal grooves and ridges. While the most classic change is pterygium,[Q] in which the cuticle grows forward over the base of the nail and attaches itself to the nail plate (Fig. 25.20).

a. Nail matrix LP is the most common type and presents with nail thinning with longitudinal ridging and fissuring.

b. Dorsal pterygium indicates destruction of a part of the nail matrix, with absent nail plate and adhesion of the dorsal skin to the nail bed, with formation of a V-shaped extension of the proximal nail fold.

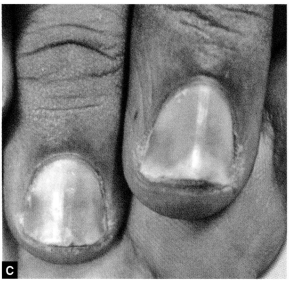
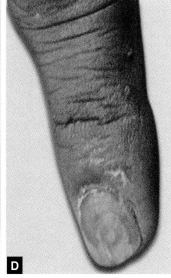
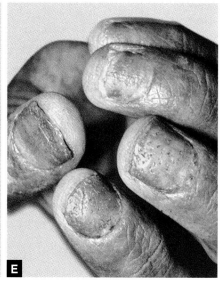

Fig. 25.19C to E: (C) Onycholysis; (D) Oil drop sign; (E) Pitting—large deep pits

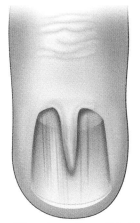

Pterygium—the cuticle is adherent to the nail plate and grows out with it. Seen in lichen planus

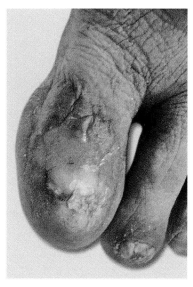

Fig. 25.20: Pterygium is pathognomonic of lichen planus and is associated with thinning and loss of nail plate

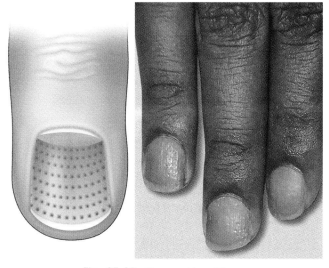

Fig. 25.21: Geometric pitting

Alopecia Areata

The more severe the hair loss, the more likely there is to be nail involvement. A roughness or fine pitting is seen on the surface of the nail plates and the lunulae may appear mottled.

a. *Geometric pitting* ('scotch-plaid'[Q] pattern), extremely characteristic. Pits are regular, small, superficial, and distributed on the nail surface along a geometric grid (Fig. 25.21).

b. *Geometric leukonychia*: Small white spots of leukonychia with regular distribution in the nail.

c. *Trachyonychia*: Nail roughness due to surface abnormalities that seem to be caused by sandpaper run longitudinally on the plate.

INFECTIONS

Acute Paronychia

This is an infection that is usually caused by bacteria, usually staphylococci.[Q] The route of entry is a break in the skin or cuticle as a result of minor trauma. The subsequent acute inflammation, often with the formation of pus in the nail fold or under the nail, requires systemic treatment with cephalexin or erythromycin and appropriate surgical drainage. Recurrent acute paronychia may be related to herpes simplex virus infection.

Chronic Paronychia

Chronic infection of the nail fold.

Cause: A combination of circumstances can allow a mixture of opportunistic pathogens (*Candida albicans*;[Q] secondary infection with *Staphylococcus aureus* and *Pseudomonas aeruginosa*) to colonize the space between the nail fold and nail plate producing a chronic dermatitis.

25

Predisposing factors include a poor peripheral circulation, wet work, working with flour, diabetes, vaginal candidiasis and over-vigorous cutting back of the cuticles.

Clinical feature: Thumb and index finger are most often involved. Usually starts as slight swelling of proximal nail fold, then loss of cuticle and discharge of pus from under the nailfold (Fig. 25.22). Once the cuticle is damaged, water, irritants, and microorganisms all cause trouble.

Treatment: Manicuring of the cuticle should cease. Treatment is aimed at both the infective and dermatitic elements of the condition.

GENETIC NAIL ANOMALIES

- In Darier disease, nails have multiple longitudinal[Q] red and white stripes with distal notches (Fig. 25.23A).[Q]
- Hailey-Hailey disease has more discrete white stripes.
- Patients with ectodermal dysplasia syndrome have combinations of nail, hair, tooth, and sweat gland changes.
- In pachyonychia congenita, the nails are thickened.
- Tuberous sclerosis features subungual angiofibromas[Q] (Koenen's tumors)[Q] (Fig. 25.23B).

TUMORS OF THE NAIL REGION

- Verrucae vulgares are the most common subungual and periungual tumors.[Q]

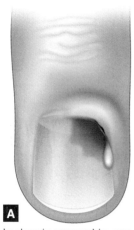
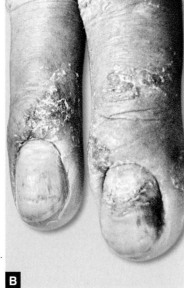

In chronic paronychia, pus exudes from below the bolstered, swollen nail folds. The adjacent nail becomes ridged and discolored

Fig. 25.22A and B: (A) A depiction of chronic paronychia and (B) a patient with paronychia associated with changes of chronic eczema

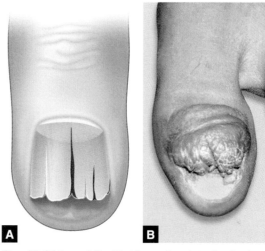

Fig. 25.23A and B: (A) Alternating longitudinal red and white streaks (i.e. erythronychia and leukonychia). Darier's disease; (B) Koenen's tumor in a case of tuberous sclerosis

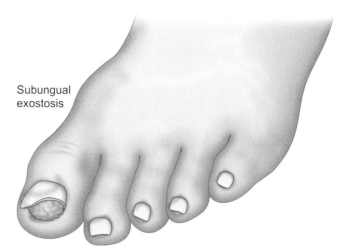

Subungual exostosis

Fig. 25.24: Subungual exostosis lifting up the nail plate

- Bowen's disease and squamous cell carcinoma of the digits are often caused by HPV. They are most common on the thumb, tend to be eroded and damage the nail bed and plate.
- About 3% of melanomas arise in the nail bed, usually of the thumb or great toe.

> Be suspicious of poorly healing nail injuries; think of melanoma (especially amelanotic melanoma) and squamous cell carcinoma.

- Subugual exostosis or chondroma is a slowly growing spur of bone or cartilage arising from the distal phalanx, which pushes up and damages the nail plate (Fig. 25.24).
- Glomus tumors can present as blue subungual masses that are tender to touch or temperature change (Hildreth test/Love's pin test).

25

Systemic Disease and Photoaggravated Disorders

Collagen Vascular Disorders

INTRODUCTION

The collagen vascular disorders (connective tissue disorders) are a complex group, without a unifying pathogenesis. All disorders have arthritis or arthralgias, and most have prominent skin involvement. Though a vast topic, the following entities will be discussed in this chapter, though with varying degrees of emphasis.

1. *Lupus erythematosus*
   - Chronic cutaneous lupus erythematosus[Q]
   - Subacute cutaneous lupus erythematosus
   - Systemic lupus erythematosus
   - Drug-induced lupus erythematosus
   - Antiphospholipid syndrome
2. *Dermatomyositis and polymyositis*
3. *Localized scleroderma*
   - Morphea
4. *Systemic sclerosis*
5. *Pseudoscleroderma*
6. *Mixed collagen vascular disorders and other overlap syndromes*
7. *Other rheumatologic diseases*
8. *Raynaud syndrome*

DIAGNOSIS OF AN AUTOIMMUNE DISORDER

Patients frequently present initially with non-specific features of an autoimmune rheumatic disease but do not fulfil criteria for any specific disorder. Thus they are frequently misdiagnosed. Less than one-third of patients with undifferentiated autoimmune rheumatic diseases evolve clinically to fulfil classification criteria for a classifiable autoimmune rheumatic disease.

The Antibody Profile—ANA

Most of these disorders are characterized by the formation of autoantibodies against various antigens, which is the reason that they are classified as autoimmune disorders.

However, their occurrence does not necessarily indicate the presence of any specific disease—they are thus **sensitive but not specific**. Serology is of particular value in situations where clinical expression of the autoimmune rheumatic disease is *incomplete*.

- The indirect immunofluorescence test, using the HEp2 cell substrate, is the gold standard for detecting antinuclear antibodies.[Q]
- The individual pattern is of limited diagnostic value.
- It is not cost-effective to test specific antibodies immediately.

In patients suspected of having an autoimmune rheumatic disease, the indirect immunofluorescence test is enough as a screening test for antinuclear antibodies. In systemic lupus erythematosus and scleroderma, antinuclear antibodies (ANA) can be detected in 95%[Q] or more of untreated patients with active disease by this method. It is **not cost-effective** to test automatically for anti-dsDNA or other antibody specificities. The individual antinuclear antibody fluorescent patterns are of **limited diagnostic utility** but are detailed in Fig. 26.1.

Examples of the limited utility of ANA include:

1. A false negative anti-nuclear antibody test result sometimes occurs, if either the antigen is outside the nucleus (e.g. anti-Jo-1 and anti-ribosomal P protein antibodies, both often categorized under the umbrella term 'antinuclear antibodies').

Peripheral (rim)	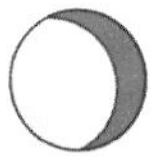	Anti-DNA (not on HEp-2)	SLE
Homogeneous (diffuse)		Anti-DNA Anti-histone Anti-DNP (nucleosomes)	RA and SLE Misc. disorders (anti-ssDNA)
Speckled	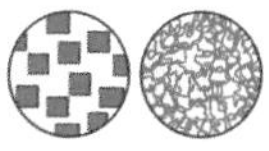	Anti-Sm and RNP Anti-Ro and La Anti-Jo-1 and Mi-2 Anti-Sci-70	SLE and SS PM/DM PSS (systemic)
Centromere	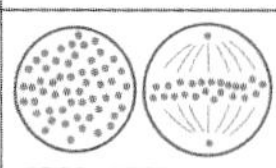	Anticentromere	PSS (CREST)
Nucleolar	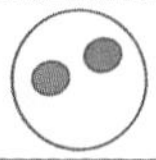	Antinucleolar	SLE and PSS

Fig. 26.1: A depiction of ANA patterns

2. Anti-Ro is directed exclusively to determinants on the native Ro molecule and is not expressed in cultured HEp2 cells.

Specific Antibodies

Specific antinuclear antibody tests are often helpful in stratifying patients into clinical subsets, which may be useful in the further management of specific clinical manifestations and prognostication (Table 26.1).

Other Syndromes

Three different terminologies are stated in literature (Box 26.1).

A distinctive type of overlap syndrome is that of 'mixed connective tissue disease'. Here patients have an overlap of puffy fingers of early scleroderma, systemic lupus erythematosus, polymyositis, and a characteristic serological profile that includes high levels of antibodies to U1RNP. However, there is controversy as to whether this is a distinct systemic rheumatic disease.

The concept of 'undifferentiated connective tissue disease', as opposed to 'mixed connective tissue disease', was coined by LeRoy and represent a sizeable proportion (25–50%) of patients presenting to autoimmune rheumatic disease clinics. Only a minority of these patients, about 30% evolve into a defined connective tissue disorder. This is characterized by 3 important features:

Table 26.1	List of autoantibodies seen in various collagen vascular disorders		
Systemic lupus erythematosus	Double-stranded DNA	70%	Lupus nephritis[Q]
	Anti-nucleosome	70%	Early disease, lupus nephritis, drug-induced lupus
	Antiribosomal P protein	15%	Neuropsychiatric lupus[Q] (psychosis or depression)
	Sm antigens	10–25%	Vasculitis, CNS
Drug-induced lupus	Histone		
Subacute cutaneous lupus	SS-A(Ro) SS-B(La)	50–70% 20–30%	• Photosensitive rash • Neonatal lupus[Q] • Congenital heart block • Sjögren's syndrome
Dermatomyositis	Jo-1	20–30%	• Antisynthetase syndrome: a. Mechanic's hands b. Interstitial lung disease
	Mi-2	10%	Dermatomyositis
	Anti-SRP	4%	Severe necrotizing myositis
Systemic sclerosis	SCL-70 (topoisomerase 1)	20–30%	• Diffuse cutaneous disease[Q] • Interstitial lung disease
	Centromere	20–30%	• Limited cutaneous disease[Q] • Microvascular or macrovascular disease • Telangiectasia • Pulmonary hypertension[Q]
	Anti-RNA polymerases	20	• Rapidly progressive diffuse cutaneous disease • Scleroderma renal crisis[Q]
	Antifibrillarin (anti-U3RNP)[Q]	5–20	Diffuse cutaneous disease in blacks, pulmonary hypertension
Mixed connective tissue disease	U1-RNP[Q]	100%	

Modified from ABC of Rheumatology, Fifth Edition. Edited by Ade Adebajo and Lisa Dunkley.
© 2018 John Wiley & Sons Ltd. Published 2018.

Box 26.1	Terminology of CTDs with overlap
Undifferentiated connective tissue disease	Rheumatic symptoms and signs with autoantibodies, but not meeting the criteria for a specific systemic auto-immune rheumatic disease
Overlap syndrome	Patients meet criteria for two or more systemic autoimmune rheumatic diseases
Mixed connective tissue disease	Specific overlap syndrome of rheumatoid arthritis like systemic lupus erythemato-sus, scleroderma and inflammatory myositis with antibodies to U1RNP

1. In the majority of patients, the undifferentiated connective disease state persists.
2. Spontaneous remission occurs in 5–10% of patients
3. Importantly, major organ involvement is rare in these patients.

LUPUS ERYTHEMATOSUS (LE)

Lupus → 'wolf-like' or lupine facial rash.
This is a disease featuring autoimmune phenomena that may involve one or multiple organs, which has characteristic skin findings, and runs an acute or chronic course.

Classification

The combination of history, clinical findings, and laboratory values can be used to classify LE as follows, (Fig. 26.2A). Cutaneous LE is classified into specific and nonspecific skin lesions, based on the histopathologic presence (specific) or absence (non-specific) of an 'interface dermatitis'.

There are exceptions to this division as specific entities (e.g. LE tumidus, lupus panniculitis) do not demonstrate an interface dermatitis and other, non-lupus entities may display an 'interface dermatitis' on histopathology (e.g. dermatomyositis).

The three specific subtypes are (Fig. 26.2B):
1. *Chronic cutaneous LE*: Almost exclusively skin findings.
2. *Subacute cutaneous LE (SCLE)*: Predominantly skin findings, mild systemic involvement.
3. *Systemic LE (SLE)*: Primarily systemic involvement.

Pathogenesis

LE is a multifactorial disease with genetic and immunopathologic abnormalities. The release of nuclear antigens because of enhanced apoptosis (FAS-FAS-L)

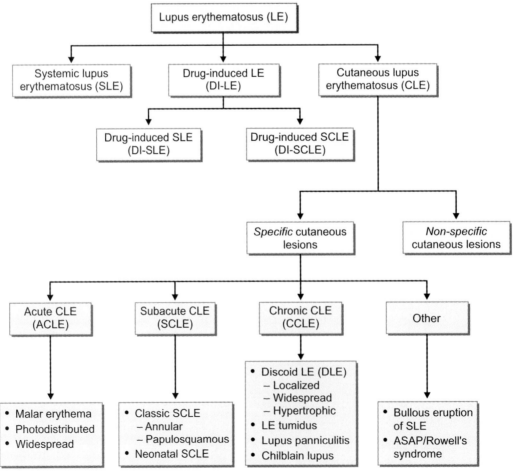

Fig. 26.2A: Classification of LE (Gillian classification)

is a key factor. Variations in the major histocompatibility complex (MHC) is the most important genetic risk factor for the development of SLE, and a number of non-MHC genetic variants also play a part. Exposure to sunlight and artificial ultraviolet radiation (UVR) may precipitate the disease or lead to flare ups, probably

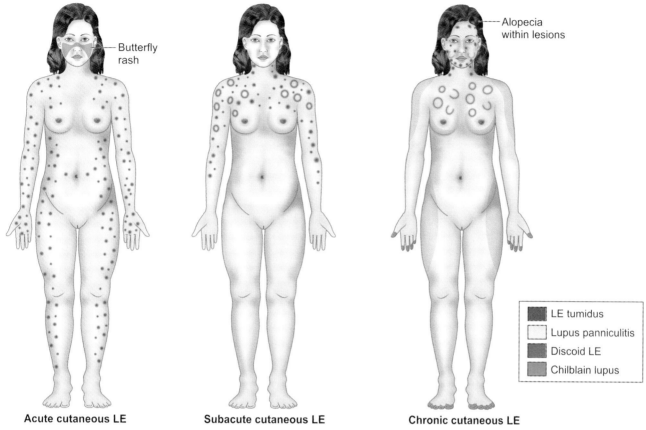

■	LE tumidus
□	Lupus panniculitis
■	Discoid LE
■	Chilblain lupus

Acute cutaneous LE   **Subacute cutaneous LE**   **Chronic cutaneous LE**

Fig. 26.2B: Depiction of the morphology of LE

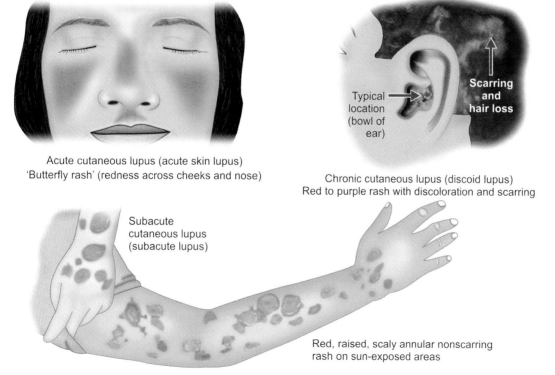

Acute cutaneous lupus (acute skin lupus)
'Butterfly rash' (redness across cheeks and nose)

Chronic cutaneous lupus (discoid lupus)
Red to purple rash with discoloration and scarring

Subacute cutaneous lupus (subacute lupus)

Red, raised, scaly annular nonscarring rash on sun-exposed areas

Fig. 26.2C: Depiction of the malara rash of acute LE, scarring seen in DLE and annular rash of subacute LE

26

by exposing previously hidden nuclear or cytoplasmic antigens to which autoantibodies are formed. Such autoantibodies to DNA, nuclear proteins and other normal antigens are typical of LE, and immune complexes formed from these redeposited in the tissues or found in the serum.

Chronic Cutaneous Lupus Erythematosus (CCLE)

This is the most common[Q] skin manifestation of LE; the terms CCLE and DLE are often used interchangeably, but CCLE encompasses all the clinical types.

This variant of LE presents with chronic scarring erythematosquamous lesions primarily in sun-exposed skin and frequently leads to *scarring alopecia*.[Q] Some groups refer to all chronic cutaneous LE as discoid LE (DLE) but here we are using the term for a specific type of lesion, which may also be seen in SCLE or SLE. Overall, 5–10%[Q] of patients will go onto develop SLE.

Epidemiology: More common in women (2–3:1); usually appears 15–60 years of age.

Clinical Features

Erythematous well-circumscribed persistent plaques with follicular hyperkeratoses, telangiectases; heals with scarring, peripheral hyperpigmentation and central hypopigmentation[Q] (Fig. 26.3A to C).

Sites: Chronic sun-exposed areas: Scalp, forehead, cheeks, ears, nose, upper lip, and chin. In some patients, the lesions are seen below the neck, wherein it is called the disseminated variety (Fig. 26.3C).

Histology: The histologic findings (Fig. 26.4) exactly match the clinical picture: Epidermal atrophy with vacuolar degeneration of basal cells, telangiectases, follicular plugs, lymphocytic infiltrate in dermis. Valuable clues are widened periodic acid-Schiff (PAS)-positive basement membrane and deposition of mucin.

Investigation

1. Skin biopsy (Fig. 26.4)
2. Direct immunofluorescence: Deposits of IgG and C3 along the basement membrane in affected skin in up

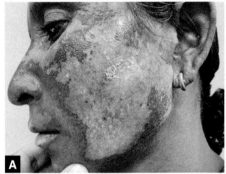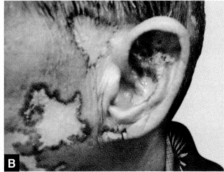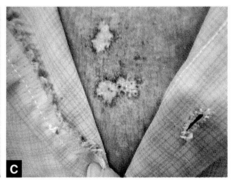

Fig. 26.3A to C: Discoid lupus erythematosus: (A) Plaque with central depigmentation and scarring with involvement of the ear; (B) The lesions are classically surrounded by hyperpigmented border; (C) Discoid lesions of DLE on the chest—disseminated variant of DLE

Follicular plug of keratin

— Thick stratum corneum

— Thin epidermis

— Destruction of basal cells

— Destruction of hair follicle

— Perivascular and peri-appendageal T lymphocyte infiltrate

Fig. 26.4: A depiction of the histology of DLE

26

to 80%, but normal, nonexposed skin is always negative (lupus band test).[Q]

3. Laboratory: Negative or low-titer ANA; sometimes higher titer in disseminated lesions.

Differential Diagnosis

Tinea faciei (KOH examination), granuloma faciale (brown color, no scarring), psoriasis (silvery scale), lupus vulgaris (diascopy), sarcoidosis (diascopy, no prominent follicles), rosacea (pustules, ears spared). In each case, histology is most helpful.

Therapy

Sun avoidance and high-potency sunscreens (UVA, UVB).

1. **Topical agents:** Short-term high-potency topical corticosteroids (TCS) and topical immunomodulators (pimecrolimus, tacrolimus). DLE is one of the few indications where it is justifiable to use steroids on the face, as the risk of scarring is worse than that of atrophy.[Q] Topical steroids should be applied twice daily until the lesions disappear or side effects, such as atrophy, develop. Weaker preparations can then be used for maintenance.

   • Topical retinoids such as tretinoin or tazarotene may be used for hyperkeratotic lesions
   • Cryotherapy or intralesional corticosteroids can be used for stubborn lesions.

2. **Systemic therapy (for widespread, recalcitrant disease)**

   • Antimalarials: Hydroxychloroquine sulfate (HCQS) 200–400 mg daily or chloroquine 250 mg daily[Q]; rarely need to go higher for skin findings alone; monitoring by ophthalmologist required every 6–12 months.
   • Dapsone 50–100 mg daily.
   • Thalidomide 50–200 mg daily (contraception, watch for neuropathy).
   • Corticosteroids should generally be avoided; if disease is recalcitrant, then perhaps prednisolone 40 mg daily for 5 days a month.

The description above refers to the common classic variant of CCLE (DLE), a summary of the other variants is given in Table 26.2.

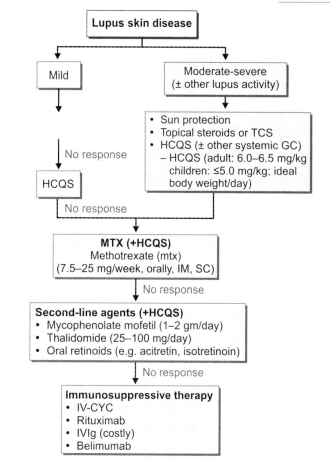

Fig. 26.5: A summary of the therapy of lupus skin disease (from treatment of systemic lupus erythematosus: Kelly Textbook of Rheumatology, 10th edition.)

A summary of the treatment of CCLE is given in Fig. 26.5 and specific treatment of the variants is given in Table 26.2.

Subacute Cutaneous Lupus Erythematosus (SCLE)

This is a less severe form of LE, than acute SLE with involvement of the skin but with systemic disease. Autoantibodies to SSA (Ro)[Q] are particularly common in subacute cutaneous LE, which can activate complement. Antibody-dependent cellular cytotoxicity and autoantibody binding to SSA (Ro) are enhanced by estradiol, perhaps accounting for the increased prevalence of subacute cutaneous LE in women.

26

Table 26.2	Variants of CCLE	
Lupus tumidus	Erythematous papules and nodules on face and upper trunk; very light-sensitive; histology shows abundant mucin[Q]	Intralesional corticosteroids or antimalarials
Lupus panniculitis	LE with deep inflammation involving subcutaneous tissue; overlying skin rarely shows sign of LE; 1/3rd of patients develop SLE[Q]	Dapsone
Chilblain lupus	Blue-red plaques, acral plaques that resemble perniosis but are persistent without history of cold exposure; up to 1/3rd develop SLE	Dapsone
Verrucous lupus erythematosus	Hyperkeratotic plaques, especially on hands and feet	Retinoids

Unusually, drugs may cause subacute cutaneous LE, producing a more widespread rash than in the idiopathic disease.

Clinical Features

1. Symmetrical widespread nonscarring erythematous patches and plaques with tendency to confluence (psoriasiform); usually in light-exposed areas such as trunk and arms (Fig. 26.6). Interestingly, often spares the mid-face.
2. Sometimes the lesions may be annular or target-like (Rowell syndrome).[Q]
3. Drug-induced SCLE: Clinical features similar to SCLE. Typically no systemic symptoms (Anti-Ro/SSA antibodies).

   Causative drugs: HCTZ, terbinafine, calcium channel blockers (e.g. diltiazem), ACE inhibitors (e.g. enalapril), TNF-α inhibitors (e.g. infliximab), proton pump inhibitors (e.g. lansoprazole), interferons.

- About 60% of patients fulfill ACR criteria for SLE; often arthralgias, rarely renal disease. As in SLE, the course is prolonged. The skin lesions are slow to clear but, in contrast to discoid LE, do so with little or no scarring.
- 10–15% of patients transition into SLE[Q], usually with renal or central nervous system (CNS) disease.
- SSA (Ro)[Q] can cross the placenta and children born to mothers who have, or have had, this condition are liable to neonatal LE with transient annular skin lesions (Fig. 26.7) and permanent *heart block*.[Q]

Investigation

1. Skin biopsy.
2. DIF: Deposits of IgG and C3 along the basement membrane in lesional lesion in 50–60%; in normal skin in 10–20%.
3. Laboratory: 20–30% have low titer anti-dsDNA antibodies.

   Often positive for anti-SS-A and anti-SS-B (ANA-negative LE). Occasional complement defects.

Therapy

Same as for discoid LE; emphasis on sun avoidance and sunscreens. Antimalarials usually necessary, for either skin or arthritis. Also NSAIDs for joint pain.

Neonatal LE (NLE)

It occurs in infants whose mothers have anti-Ro/SSA autoantibodies that are passively transferred to the fetus.

Serology: Anti-Ro/SSA[Q] antibodies (>98%),[Q] but may also have anti-La/SSB or anti-U1RNP antibodies.

Approximately 1–5% of mothers[Q] with anti-Ro/SSA antibodies will have infants with NLE, with risk increasing to 10–25% with subsequent pregnancies.

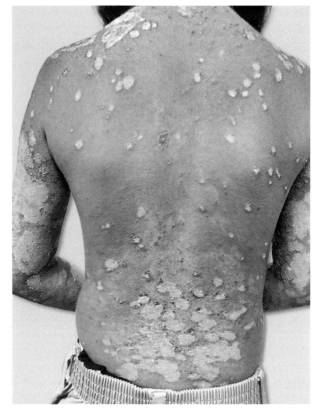

Fig. 26.6: Annular, psoriasiform lesions in a child with subacute LE

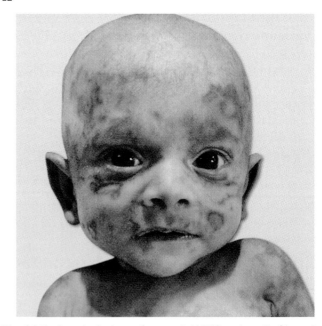

Fig. 26.7: Annular lesions of neonatal LE (*Courtesy*: Dr Chanchal Singh, MD, MRCOG)

Clinical features: Cutaneous lesions are similar to adult SCLE but favor the face and periorbital areas (Raccon sign/owl eye) and may be atrophic (Fig. 26.7).[Q]

New lesions typically cease to develop by 6–9 months[Q] of age, i.e. once the antibodies are cleared; however, there may be residual changes such as dyspigmentation and telangiectases.

Systemic

1. Congenital heart block (60%) (±associated cardio-myopathy). Heart block, if it is going to occur, is almost always present at birth and a pacemaker is often required.
2. Hepatobiliary disease
3. Thrombocytopenia (20%) > neutropenia or anemia
4. Macrocephaly or skeletal dysplasia.

Investigation: If skin signs of NLE are present, an evaluation including physical examination, ECG ±echocardiogram, CBC, and liver function tests, is indicated; the latter laboratory tests should be repeated periodically over the first 6 months of life.

Systemic Lupus Erythematosus (SLE)

Typically, but not always, the onset is acute. SLE is an uncommon disorder, affecting women more often than men (in a ratio of about 8:1). The findings can be divided into cutaneous and systemic (Fig. 26.8).

Cutaneous Lesions

About 40–50% of patients have cutaneous disease at the time of diagnosis.

- *Butterfly rash*[Q]: Classic lesion of SLE; mid-facial circumscribed erythema following sun exposure (Fig. 26.9A); initially waxes and wanes; later permanent.
- There may also be diffuse erythema of scalp, ears, lips, upper trunk, forearms—sun-exposed areas—as also palmoplantar erythema.

On the dorsal hands, there is sparing of the knuckles.

Some have transient exanthems, resembling drug eruption or erythema multiforme.

- *Discoid lesions*: Many patients have hyperkeratotic scarring lesions.

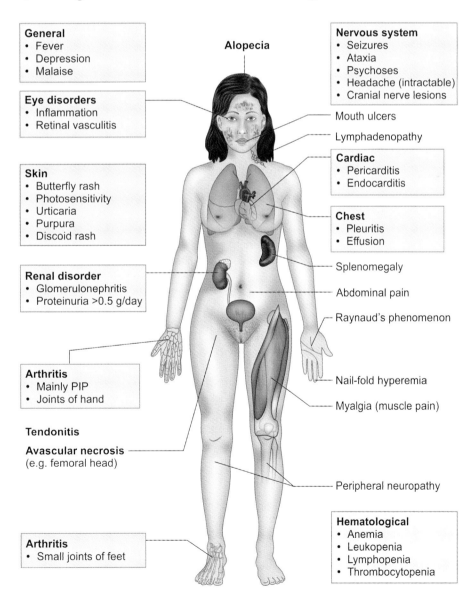

Fig. 26.8: An overview of the organ involvement in SLE

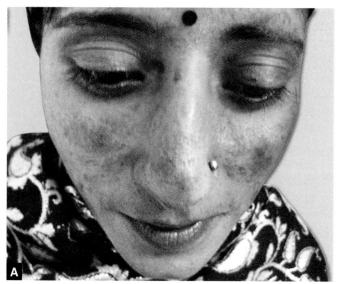
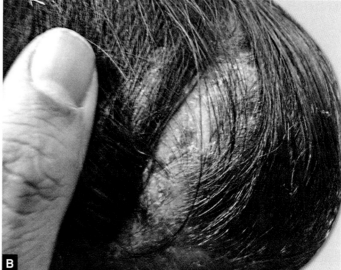

Fig. 26.9A and B: (A) The malar rash seen in a fair skin individual; (B) A case of SLE with associated scarring alopecia

- Rarely there may be bullous lesions.
- *Vasculitis may take many forms*: Typical leukocyto-clastic vasculitis, necrotic infarcted papules on digits, peripheral gangrene, subcutaneous nodules (nodular vasculitis) and livedo racemosa (antiphospholipid syndrome).
- *Alopecia*: SLE per se manifests as a non-scarring alopecia[Q]—lupus hair, alopecia areata and chronic telogen effluvium. Scarring alopecia seen in lesions of DLE (Fig. 26.9B).
- *Oral lesions*: Palatal erythema or erosions; less often elsewhere. Painless ulcers.[Q]
- *ASAP syndrome (Rowell's syndrome)*: The term ASAP[Q] stands for **a**cute **s**yndrome of **a**poptotic **p**an-epidermolysis and is seen in apoptotic injury of the epidermis from various causes.

  Rowell's syndrome and TEN-like ACLE are seen in acute LE or SCLE and can be associated with significant internal organ involvement (e.g. kidney and CNS).

Systemic Lesions

The American Rheumatology Association's 1982 classification criteria for systemic lupus erythematosus were revised in 1997 (Box 26.2). The ACR criteria were designed to identify patients in clinical studies; individuals with four or more criteria were accepted as having SLE. Although they were *never* intended as *diagnostic* criteria, they are widely so employed.

A diagrammatic depiction of the manifestations of SLE are depicted in Fig. 26.8 and Table 26.3. *The same can be remembered by the mnemonic (SOAP BRAIN MD)* (Fig. 26.10). Recently though the Systemic Lupus International Collaborating Clinics (SLICC) revised and validated the American College of Rheumatology

Box 26.2	American College of Rheumatology (previously American Rheumatology Association) revised classi-fication criteria for systemic lupus erythematosus

Malar rash	Renal disorder
Discoid rash	Hematological disorder
Photosensitivity	Immunological disorder
Mucosal ulcers	Positive antinuclear antibodies
Arthritis	
Serositis	
Neurological disorder (psychosis, seizures)	

(ACR) SLE classification criteria (Table 26.3). The SLICC criteria for SLE classification require:

1. Fulfilment of at least four criteria, with at least one clinical criterion and one immunological criterion, OR
2. Lupus nephritis as the sole clinical criterion in the presence of ANA or anti-dsDNA antibodies.

Remember drug-induced SLE does NOT have skin findings,[Q] but presents with systemic features including constitutional features and serositis. Anti-histone anitibodies are seen.[Q] (Drugs—hydralazine, procaina-mide, isoniazid, minocycline, TNF-α inhibitors.)[Q]

Course

The skin changes may be transient, continuous or recurrent and they correlate well with the activity of the systemic disease. Acute SLE may be associated with fever, arthritis, nephritis, polyarteritis, pleurisy, pneumo-nitis, pericarditis, myocarditis and involvement of the central nervous system. Internal involvement can be fatal, but about three-quarters of patients survive for 15 years. Renal involvement suggests a poorer prognosis.

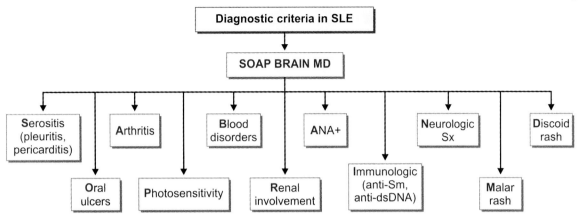

Fig. 26.10: Mnemonic to remember the diagnostic criteria of SLE

Table 26.3	Systemic Lupus International Collaborating Clinics (SLICC) revised (ACR) SLE classification criteria
Clinical criteria	*Immunological criteria*
Acute cutaneous lupus: Malar rash, maculopapular rash, photosensitive rash and non-indurated psoriasiform rash	ANA
Chronic cutaneous lupus: Discoid lupus, lupus panniculitis, mucosal lupus and chilblain lupus	Anti-dsDNA antibodies
Oral ulcers	Anti-Sm antibodies
Non-scarring alopecia, diffuse thinning or hair fragility with broken hairs	Antiphospholipid antibody
Synovitis: Swelling or effusion or tenderness in 2 or more joints and 30 minutes or more of morning stiffness	Low complement
Serositis: Pleurisy for more than 1 day (symptoms/pleural effusions/rub) Pericardial pain for more than 1 day/pericardial effusion/rub/ECG evidence)	Direct Coombs test (in absence of hemolytic anemia)
Renal: Urine protein/creatinin (or 24 h urine protein) representing 500 mg of protein/24 hr or red blood cell casts	
Neurological: Seizures, psychosis, myelitis, mononeuritis multiplex, peripheral or cranial neuropathy, acute confusional stage	
Hemolytic anemia	
Leukopenia (<4000/mm^3 at least once) Or lymphopenia (<1000/mm^3 at least once)	
Thrombocytopenia (<100 000/m^3 at least once)	

*See text for criteria.

Investigation

- Indicators of an increased risk for SLE in patients presenting with CLE include fever, weight loss, fatigue, myalgia, lymphadenopathy, and nonspecific skin findings.
- It is important to exclude drug-induced SLE.
- A negative ANA is helpful because it is highly unlikely that a patient with a negative ANA has SLE.
- A positive ANA is *less helpful*, as it may occur in normal individuals (usually at low titers) and in patients with CLE.
- Specific antibodies to SLE include dsDNA and Sm.

The list of investigations with the common findings is given in Table 26.4.

Treatment

The treatment of this disorder depends largely on the major involvement of skin or systemic organs, the latter of which usually warrant the use of immunosuppressants depending on the severity along with oral corticosteroids. The adjuvant drugs used for systemic involvement include cyclophosphamide (renal involvement), azathioprine and MMF. The newer drugs include the biologicals that work on B cells. For skin involvement apart from sun avoidance, therapy revolves around the use of antimalarials, methotrexate and thalidomide. A basic overview of therapy is given here.

26

Table 26.4	Investigations in a case of SLE
Hematology	Anemia, raised ESR, thrombocytopenia, decreased white cell count
Autoantibodies[Q]	**Anti-dsDNA (60%):** Specific for SLE; fluctuates with disease activity; associated with glomerulonephritis.[Q]
	Anti-Smith (20–30%): Specific for SLE; associated with anti-U1RNP antibodies.
	Anti-U1RNP (30%): Antibody associated with mixed connective tissue disease.[Q]
	Anti-Ro/SSA[Q] (30%): Associated with Sjögren's syndrome, photosensitivity, SCLE, neonatal lupus, congenital heart block
	Antihistone[Q] (70%): Drug-induced lupus
	Antiphospholipid
Urine analysis	Proteinuria or hematuria, often with casts, if kidneys involved
KFT, LFT	Look for involvement of major visceral organs

1. Drugs used in the treatment of systemic lupus erythematosus

- *Steroids* are indicated for systemic involvement and when combined with immunosuppressive agents, the GC dose should rarely exceed 0.5 to 0.6 mg/kg prednisone due to concerns for infections and other toxicities. Tapering of GC dose starts after the first 4 to 6 weeks of therapy, targeting a dose of 0.25 mg/kg every other day at 2 to 3 months. In severe, rapidly progressing disease, intravenous (IV) pulses of methylprednisolone (MP) (250 to 1000 mg daily for 1 to 3 consecutive days) are used.
- *Azathioprine (AZA)* is effective as an induction agent and in a maintenance regimen in mild to moderate SLE including nephritis.
- The combination of high-dose glucocorticoids with pulses of intravenous CYP (cyclophosphamide) remains the standard of care for severe SLE with major organ involvement, specially kidney involvement.
- *Mycophenolate mofetil (MMF)* is at least equally efficacious and has a better toxicity profile than CYP in the treatment of moderately severe kidney disease.

- *Antimalarials* are effective for skin and mucocutaneous manifestations. Their use has been associated with reduced organ damage.
- *Biologic treatments* currently used in lupus.

Belimumab:[Q] Monoclonal antibody that inhibits B lymphocyte stimulation and has been shown to be effective in lupus patients, especially those with high dsDNA antibodies and low complement. Usually given 4 weekly by intravenous infusion.

Rituximab (RTX): This monoclonal antibody targets CD20 and causes B cell depletion. It has been used successfully in refractory lupus nephritis and cerebral lupus. Given as two infusions 15 days apart which may be repeated after 6–12 months, if necessary.

2. Treatment based on severity (Table 26.5): For major organ involvement, the treatment plan is based on an induction and maintenance steps. The severity of disease is based on subjective criterion.
- *Mild systemic diseases:* Arthritis, fever, headache, and other minor systemic complaints.
- *Moderate systemic disease:* Serositis, pneumonitis, hematologic problems, vasculitis.

Table 26.5	Recommended immunosuppressive therapy for major organ involvement in systemic lupus erythematosus	
Disease severity	*Induction therapy*	*Maintenance therapy*
Mild	**High-dose GC** (0.5–1 mg/kg/day prednisone × 4–6 wk, tapered to 0.125 mg/kg every other day within 3 mo) alone or in combination with **AZA** (1–2 mg/kg/day)	**Low-dose GC** (prednisone ≤0.125 mg/kg on alternative days) alone or with **AZA** (1–2 mg/kg/day)
Moderate	**MMF** (2 g/day) (or **AZA**) with **GC** as above	**MMF** tapered to 1.5 g/day for 6–12 mo and then to 1 g/ day; consider further tapering at the end of each year in remission
Severe	**Pulse IV-CYP** alone or in combination with **pulse IV-MP** for the first 6 mo (background GC 0.5 mg/kg/day for 4 wk, then taper) If no response, consider adding **RTX** or switch to **MMF**	Quarterly pulses of **IV-CYP** for at least 1 year beyond remission Alternative: **AZA** (1–2 mg/kg/day), **MMF** (1–2 g/day)

GC—Glucocorticoid , MMF—Mycophenolate mofetil, CYP—Cyclophosphamide, AZA—Azathioprine, RTX—Rituximab

• *Severe systemic disease*: Renal, pulmonary, and CNS disease require aggressive therapy.

3. Organ specific therapy: Skin manifestations in SLE usually respond to sun exposure prophylaxis, topical glucocorticoids, and systemic antimalarials (Fig. 26.5 above).

Moderately severe lupus nephritis[Q]: Mycophenolate mofetil[Q] may be preferred as induction regimen, especially when gonadal toxicity is a concern.

Severe lupus nephritis[Q]: Combination of monthly pulses of intravenous CYC and pulse intravenous methylprednisolone is the treatment of choice.

CNS: Glucocorticoids alone or in combination with immunosuppressive agents.

Antiphospholipid syndrome: Antiplatelet and/or anticoagulation therapy is recommended.

SYSTEMIC SCLEROSIS

There is a spectrum of disorders that come under the umbrella of sclerosing disorders (Fig. 26.11). We will focus on systemic sclerosis.

Scleroderma (Progressive Systemic Sclerosis)

This is a multiorgan disease with diffuse sclerosis of connective tissue favoring skin, lungs, gastrointestinal tract and kidneys. There is marked patient-to-patient variability in clinical and laboratory manifestations, disease course, and molecular signatures, suggesting the existence of distinct disease subsets.

Epidemiology

Peaks between third and fifth decades; increases with age; female: male ratio 5:1, but men have worse prognosis; considerable geographic and ethnic variation.

Pathogenesis

Systemic sclerosis features small-vessel vasculopathy, fibrosis, immune activations and tissue sclerosis. Probably vessel damage is the most likely primary event.[Q]

Autoreactive T cells appear, as in graft-versus-host disease and this leads to production of types **I, III,** and **IV** collagen as well as fibronectin and proteoglycans with deposition in affected connective tissue (Fig. 26.12).

The altered balance between T helper (Th)1 and Th2 cytokines in fibrosis favors Th2 pattern that secrete abundant IL-4, IL-5, and IL-13, and these cytokines are profibrogenic because they can directly stimulate collagen synthesis. TGF-β (transforming growth factor-β) is the main cytokine implicated in fibrosis.

Diagnostic Criteria

A subcommittee of the American College of Rheumatology (ACR) established diagnostic criteria based on a consensus of experts who evaluated a multicenter survey of scleroderma patients compared with other patient groups (Table 26.6). The single finding of thickening of the skin typical of scleroderma proximal to the metacarpophalangeal (MCP) joints of the hands is considered a major criterion confirming the

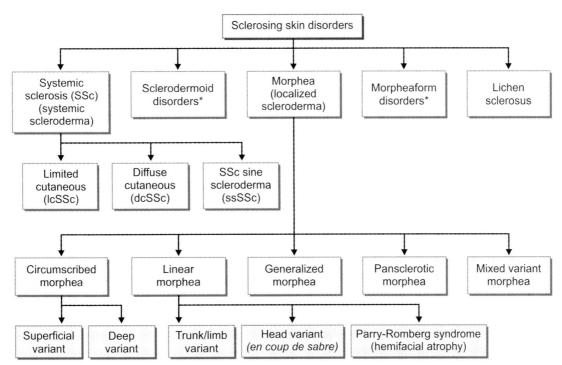

*Disorders with a clinical presentation similar to systemic sclerosis are referred to as sclerodermoid, while those reminiscent of morphea are referred to as *morpheaform*. As with any disease spectrum, there can be overlapping clinical features.

Fig. 26.11: The spectrum of sclerosing skin disorders

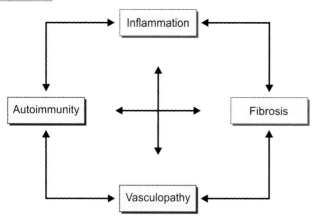

Fig. 26.12: The pathophysiologic quartet underlying systemic sclerosis. Autoimmunity and vasculopathy generally precede the onset and contribute to the progression of fibrosis

Table 26.6	Criterion for diagnosis of scleroderma
Must have (a) or **two** of (b), (c), or (d)	a. Proximal sclerosis (proximal to MCP/MTP) b. Digital pits c. Sclerodactyly d. Pulmonary fibrosis (CXR; HRCT)
CREST criteria must have **three** of the five features	• Calcinosis • Raynaud's phenomenon • Esophageal dysmotility • Sclerodactyly • Telangiectases

diagnosis. This includes changes on the face, arms, legs, or trunk. If skin thickening is found only distal to the MCP joints, then two of three minor criteria (digital pits, sclerodactyly, and pulmonary fibrosis on chest radiograph) must be present to confirm the diagnosis.

This has been modified and the latest criteria are given in Table 26.7.

Classification

Scleroderma is divided into two subsets—limited and diffuse (Figs 26.13 and 26.14). The classification has profound prognostic implications (Fig. 26.14).

Diffuse cutaneous systemic sclerosis (dcSSc): Patients are considered to have diffuse skin disease (dcSSc), if skin changes are found proximal to the elbows and/or knees or on the trunk, excluding the face.Q This form of systemic sclerosis shares some features with lcSSc such as Raynaud phenomenon and sclerodactyly, but the onset of disease is more rapid, and Raynaud's phenomenon occurs concurrently with sclerodactyly.Q Anti-DNA topo I (anti-Scl-70) antibodies are found. These patients tend to have higher risk of multisystem disease and poor survival (Fig. 26.14).

Limited cutaneous systemic sclerosis (lcSSc): Patients are considered to have limited disease (lcSSc), if skin changes occur distal to the elbows and/or knees and

Table 26.7	American College of Rheumatology/European League against Rheumatism classification criteria for the classification of systemic sclerosis	
Item	*Sub-item (s)*	*Weight/score*
Skin thickening of the fingers of both hands extending proximal to the metacarpophalangeal joints (*sufficient criterion*)	—	9
Skin thickening of the fingers (*only count the higher score*)	Puffy fingers Sclerodactyly of the fingers (distal to the MCPs but proximal to the proximal inter-phalangeal joints)	2 4
Fingertip lesions (only count the higher score)	Digital tip ulcers Fingertip pitting scars	2 3
Telangiectasia	—	2
Abnormal nailfold capillaries	—	2
Pulmonary arterial hypertension and/or interstitial lung disease (*maximum score 2*)	Pulmonary arterial hypertension Interstitial lung disease	2 2
Raynaud's phenomenon	—	3
SSc-related autoantibodies (maximum score is 3)	ACA Scl-70 RNA Pol	3

*The total score is determined by adding the maximum weight (score) in each category. Patients with a total score of ≥9 are classified as having definite SSc.
ACA, Anticentromere; MCPs, metacarpophalangeal joints; RNA Pol, anti-RNA polymerase III, Scl-70, antitopoisomerase 1; SSc, systemic sclerosis.
Modified from van den Hoogen F, Khanna D, Fransen J, et al: 2013 classification criteria for systemic sclerosis: an American College of Rheumatology/European League against Rheumatism collaborative initiative. *Arthritis Rheum* 65:2737–2747, 2013.

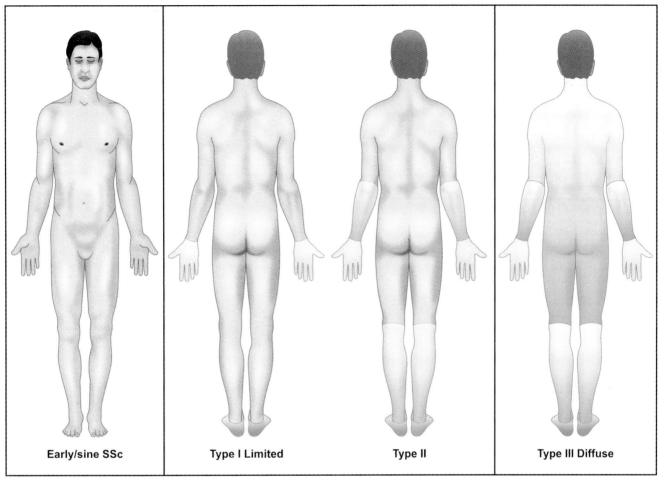

| Early/sine SSc | Type I Limited | Type II | Type III Diffuse |

Fig. 26.13: Types of scleroderma

not on the trunk. Facial skin thickening can be present in the limited group. In lcSSc, the skin disease is usually confined to the extremities and face, and onset is slow. Raynaud's phenomenon often precedes the skin changes in contrast with dcSSc. Some argue that the term CREST syndrome should be eliminated, and that these patients should be classified in the limited skin group (Fig. 26.14).

LcSSc and dcSSc can also occur with other AI-CTD (called 'overlap syndrome'), most notably polymyositis and SLE; another minor form is pre-SSc, in which the full extent of the patient's cutaneous sclerosis has not been reached.

Clinical Features

The essential symptom is Raynaud's phenomenon (95%).[Q] The other symptoms are described below.

1. Skin: Cutaneous involvement in scleroderma begins with clinical signs of inflammation. This is called the *edematous* phase because it is characterized by nonpitting edema of affected body areas. In limited scleroderma, this event is mild and is restricted to the digits; however, in the diffuse form of the disease, cutaneous swelling and edema can be widespread and so impressive in the limbs as to mimic a fluid overload state such as congestive heart failure.

During the *fibrotic* phase, acute inflammation is clinically less obvious, and deposition in the dermis of excessive collagen and other extracellular material thickens the skin, making it inflexible and causing further loss of skin appendages (Fig. 26.15A).

In late stages of the disease, skin actually thins with *atrophy* and has a noninflammatory bound-down appearance. Deeper tissue fibrosis causes permanent contractures around joints or may involve underlying muscle, causing a myopathy.

 a. *Hands*: Fingers initially puffy and edematous; later sclerodactyly (Fig. 26.15B), with loss of finger pads, tightening, reduced motion; painful fingertip ulcers; loss of cuticle with telangiectases; peripheral calcinosis, often with ulceration of overlying skin and extrusion of calcified debris.

 b. *Face*: Mask-like facies[Q] (due to reduced expression lines), microstomia with tightening of frenulum, hyperpigmentation and prominent telangiectases (Fig. 26.15C).

26

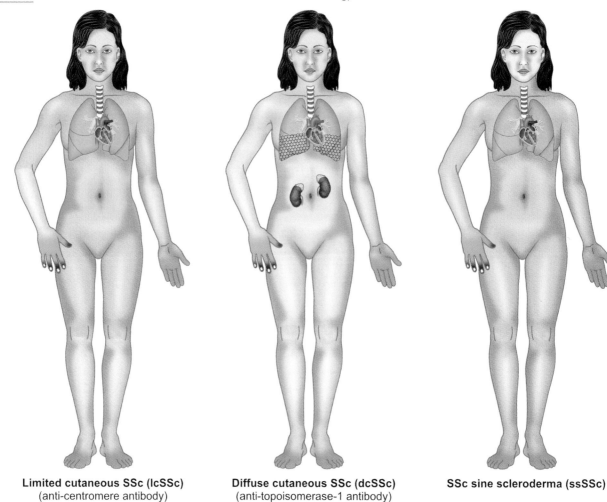

Limited cutaneous SSc (lcSSc)
(anti-centromere antibody)

Diffuse cutaneous SSc (dcSSc)
(anti-topoisomerase-1 antibody)

SSc sine scleroderma (ssSSc)

- Formerly called **CREST** syndrome
- **Long** preceding history of **Raynaud's phenomenon**
- Slower development of limited cutaneous sclerosis
- **Late**r onset of **internal organ** involvement (after 10–15 years)
- Pulmonary arterial hypertension
- More favorable long-term prognosis
- Constitutional symptoms—fatigues are common, exclude hypothyroidism and malnutrition
- Skin involvement is generally mild but vascular complications can be severe.

- **Rapidly progressive**, more widespread cutaneous sclerosis (usually peaks within 12–18 months)
- >90% demonstrate **internal organ**^{Q} involvement within the **first 5 years**
- Interstitial lung disease (ILD), pulmonary arterial hypertension
- Kidney disease—presence of **anti-RNA polymerase III**^{Q} pattern of ANA or tendon friction rubs—renal crisis
- Weight loss is common in early disease which is also associated with severe skin itching
- Otherwise similar to lcSSc

26

| | Cutaneous sclerosis | | Raynaud's phenomenon | | Nail fold capillary abnormalities |

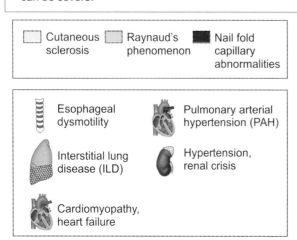

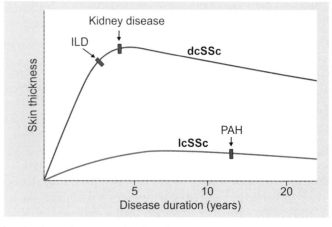

Fig. 26.14: A depiction of clinical variants and course of scleroderma

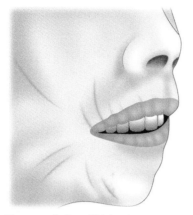

Characteristics: Thickening, tightening, and rigidity of facial skin, with small, constricted mouth and narrow lips, in atrophic phase of scleroderma

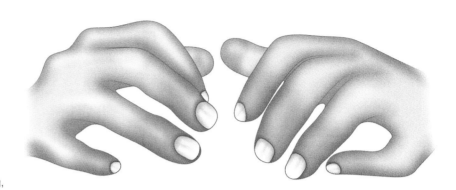

Sclerodactyly: Fingers partially fixed in semiflexed position; terminal phalanges atrophied; fingertips pointed and ulcerated

Fig. 26.15A: A depiction of the classic facial and acral findings of scleroderma

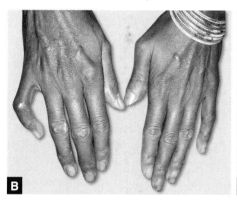

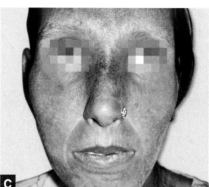

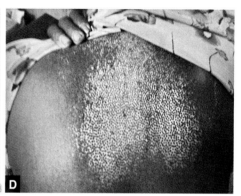

Fig. 26.15B to D: (B) Note the thinned tapered fingers with calcinosis cutis on the joint and contracture of the fingers; (C) **Mask-like facies**—taut bound down skin, lack of supraorbital furrowing, thin nose and pursed lip and pigmentation on the face; (D) **Salt and pepper** pigmentation seen on the back

c. Characteristic confetti-like hypopigmentation: Focal hypopigmentation with follicular repigmentation (Fig. 26.15D).

d. Diffuse sclerosis of skin may sometimes restricts respiratory motion.

> • The degree of skin sclerosis does not predict the degree of internal organ involvement.
> • Survival is dependent on the type and degree of internal organ involvement.

2. Systemic findings

- *Gastrointestinal tract*: Sclerosis of lingual frenulum reduces tongue motility; often sicca syndrome; swallowing problems; impaired esophageal motility; with more diffuse involvement, impaired transit and ileus.

- *Lungs*: Skin fibrosis restricts motion and pulmonary fibrosis interferes with oxygen diffusion.

> Pulmonary disease (interstitial lung disease (ILD) > pulmonary arterial hypertension (PAH)) is the most common cause of mortality.[Q]

- *Kidneys*: Hypertension and progressive renal failure because of nephrosclerosis.

- *Heart*: Subtle and late, but can develop myocardial fibrosis and cor pulmonale. Pericardial effusions common, but usually asymptomatic.

- *Liver*: 15% have associated primary biliary cirrhosis[Q] and positive antimitochondrial antibodies.

- *Musculoskeletal*: Many present with arthralgias and muscle pain: Later main problem is muscle atrophy. Overlap syndrome with polymyositis (anti-PM-Scl antibodies).

- *Bones*: Acro-osteolysis.

- *Teeth*: Widening of periodontal membrane (useful in radiologic diagnosis, but of little clinical significance).

- SSc overlap syndrome (20%) → most common myositis (42.8%) > RA (32%) > SJS (16.8%) > SLE (8.4%)

Investigation

- *Lungs*: Chest radiograph, pulmonary diffusion studies, bronchoalveolar lavage (to assess inflammatory cells; prognostically useful).

- *Skeleton*: Radiologic documentation of osteolysis, calcification.

26

- *Gastrointestinal tract*: Esophageal manometry and functional scintigraphy.
- *Heart*: EKG, echocardiogram, cardiac catheterization, if cor pulmonale is present.
- *Kidneys*: Renal function, urine status.
- *Serology*:
  - More than 90% have positive ANA.
  - Anti-Scl-70 positive in 30–70%; usually with severe course.[Q]
  - Rarely anti-RNA polymerase I-II; poor outlook.
  - Anti-centromere antibodies present in type I systemic sclerosis and CREST syndrome.

A summary of the serological markers and their significance is given in Table 26.8.

Differential Diagnosis

1. Pseudoscleroderma: Table 26.9.
2. Other collagen vascular disorders:
   - Mixed collagen vascular disorders and overlap syndromes.
3. Graft-versus-host disease.
4. Others: Generalized morphea. Puffy hands can be confused with early stage of acrodermatitis chronica atrophicans.

Treatment

The treatment of this disorder is difficult specially as there is no known medicine that can halt the fibrosis, except if it undergoes natural resolution. Thus optimal therapy is based on understanding the shortcomings of current therapy, not getting locked into 'traditional' therapy, focusing on an organ-specific approach, and defining the disease subtype and level of disease activity are most important in establishing optimal management protocols.

Table 26.8 Autoantibody profile of scleroderma

Antibody target	Prevalence	Comments
Centromere	60% lcSSc	Associated with typical CREST pattern of disease[Q]
Scl-70 (topoisomerase-1)	40% dcSSc 15% lcSSc	Predictive of interstitial lung involvement in both SSc subsets[Q]
RNA polymerase III	20% SSc	Anti-RNA polymerase III associated with diffuse skin disease, scleroderma renal crisis and malignancy
U1-RNP	10% SSc	Associated with overlap features
U3-RNP (fibrillin)	5% SSc	Poor outcome, cardiac disease and pulmonary arterial hypertension[Q]
PM-Scl	3% SSc	Myositis overlap
Th/to	5% SSc	Lung fibrosis in lcSSc[Q]
Anti-M2	5–10% SSc	Especially in lcSSc with primary biliary cholangitis

Although no good studies have been conducted to prove the effectiveness of this approach, it seems reasonable to use combination therapy with rapid control of the inflammatory immune process early on, followed by maintenance immunosuppression for an extended time.

A. Cutaneous disease

1. *Raynaud phenomenon*: This has been discussed previously and calcium channel blockers are treatment of choice: Nifedipine 5 mg tid; if orthostatic hypotension is problem, try diltiazem 60–120 mg daily or verapamil 240–360 mg daily.

Table 26.9 A List of common conditions that constitute the entity pseudoscleroderma

Diabetes mellitus	Stiff hand syndrome, sclerodactyly in juveniles
Graft-versus-host disease	Chronic stage often features cutaneous sclerosis, usually depigmented
Nephrogenic fibrosing dermopathy	Resembles scleromyxedema but found as complication of renal dialysis
POEMS syndrome	Polyneuropathy, organomegaly, endocrinopathy, monoclonal gammopathy (plasma cell dyscrasia), skin changes (sclerosis)
Porphyria cutanea tarda	Sclerotic areas, usually on chest, coupled with skin fragility on hands and facial hirsutism
Premature aging syndromes	Both Werner syndrome and progeria may be confused with scleroderma initially
Scleredema	Usually sclerosis of back; extensive mucin; associated with diabetes mellitus
Scleromyxedema	Sclerosis associated with gammopathy
Stiff skin syndrome	Fibrillin mutation leads to sclerodermoid changes, restriction of motion; neurological changes; hypertrichosis[Q]
Toxin exposure	- Eosinophilia-myalgia syndrome: Ingestion of contaminated tryptophan led to pulmonary disease, hypereosinophilia, and cutaneous sclerosis - Toxic oil syndrome: Ingestion of contaminated rapeseed oil caused similar picture - Drugs: Bleomycin, administered locally or systemically, can cause sclerosis

26

2. *Calcification*: Surgery sometimes required; low-dose coumarin may reduce inflammation.

3. *Ulcers*: Occlusive dressings and skin equivalents are helpful for distal ulcers.

4. *Sclerosis*: Neither penicillamine nor extracorporeal photophoresis has been proven definitely effective. For rapidly progressive disease, immunosuppressive drugs are often tried.

   Immunosuppressive agents: Systemic corticosteroids (prednisolone 0.5 mg/kg daily), perhaps combined with azathioprine 1–2 mg/kg daily. Methotrexate 20–30 mg weekly, cyclosporine 3–5 mg/kg daily, or cyclophosphamide 2 mg/kg daily or as pulse therapy (500–800 mg once monthly) can be tried; none is overwhelmingly useful.

5. In the early active stage of diffuse scleroderma, pruritus can be one of the most distressing symptoms. Antihistamines, analgesics, or tricyclic antidepressants (e.g. doxepin) are often used but usually provide only partial benefit. Dryness of the skin surface results from damage to the exocrine structures caused by decreased or absent natural oil (sebum) production. Thus emollients are essential for application.

B. Internal organ involvement: Though the details of the varied therapeutic interventions are beyond the scope of this book, an overview of various system specific therapies are enlisted in Table 26.10 based on latest guidelines.

- Kidney: Scleroderma renal crisis (SRC) is a life-threatening condition that occurs in 5 to 10% of scleroderma patients. Angiotensin-converting enzyme (ACE) inhibitors are treatment of choice to control and reverse renal hypertension.
- Proton pump inhibitors (omeprazole 20–40 mg daily) indicated for esophageal dysfunction.
- Lung disease is a major cause of morbidity and mortality in scleroderma patients.
  - *Pulmonary hypertension* is best treated with endothelin-1 inhibitors, phosphodiesterase inhibitors, or prostacyclin analogues, given alone or in combination.
  - *Interstitial lung disease* may respond best to an induction phase of cyclophosphamide (6 to 12 months; daily oral or monthly IV therapy) followed by maintenance (several years) with mycophenolate or azathioprine.

Physical therapy: Infrared light may help increase circulation by raising body temperature; physical therapy can help avoid contractures and retain function.

Table 26.10	Current recommendations for treatment of scleroderma	
Disorder	*Primary therapy^Q*	*Secondary therapy*
Raynaud's phenomenon	Vasodilators (CCB) PDE-5 inhibitors Fluoxetine	Intravenous iloprost Endothelin antagonists Antiplatelet agents
Digital ulcers	PDE-5 inhibitors Bosentan	Intravenous iloprost
Hypertensive renal disease	ACE inhibitors, ARBs	CCB, prostacyclin, renal transplant (wait at least 24 mo)
GI involvement	*Upper GI* Dental/periodontal care, lifestyle modifications, proton pump inhibitors, prokinetics *Lower GI* Probiotics, rotational antibiotics	
Skin	Methotrexate	Phototherapy (UVA-1:340–400 nm phototherapy for affected skin in systemic sclerosis)
Interstitial lung disease	Cyclophosphamide	Mycophenolate mofetil, azathioprine
Pulmonary arterial hypertension	• ERA (ambrisentan, bosentan and macitentan) • PDE5 inhibitors (sildenafil, tadalafil) • Riociguat	• Intravenous epoprostenol • Iloprost, treprostinil
Cardiac involvement	Heart failure therapy, diuretics, CCB	Immunosuppression (myocardial inflammation)
Joints/muscles	Prednisone, methotrexate, TNF inhibitors	IVIg

Update of EULAR recommendations for the treatment of systemic sclerosis. Kowal-Bielecka O, et al. *Ann Rheum Dis* 2017;76:1327–1339.

MORPHEA

Cutaneous sclerosis without systemic involvement with several clinical variants. Morphea does not progress to SSc, except for a few rare case reports.

Epidemiology: Uncommon disease; female: male 3:1.

Pathogenesis: Poorly understood. Association with *Borrelia burgdorferi* not substantiated. Circulating autoantibodies support immune role.

Clinical Features

- Plaque (circumscribed) form: Starts as ≤3 discrete indurated plaques erythematous patch that slowly spreads. Most importantly, it feels indurated.
- Early lesions have a lilac border, indicating inflammatory activity, and a whitish center (Fig. 26.16A and B). Mature lesions are hyperpigmented. Most often affect the trunk, except for the linear variant, which usually involves the head or an extremity. Its prognosis is usually good, and the fibrosis slowly clears leaving slight depression and hyperpigmentation.

- Generalized form: Presents with >3 indurated plaques larger than 3 cm and/or involving ≥2 body sites; spares the face and hands.

Variants

- *Linear*: Lesion involving limb, usually leg, in children with bone loss and shortening of limb, as well as loss of function (Fig. 26.16C).
- *En coup de sabre*:[Q] Lesion on forehead resembling scar from saber blow; may involve orbit and its content (Fig. 26.16D).
- *Hemifacial atrophy (Parry-Romberg syndrome)*: Extreme form of linear morphea, distortion of one side of face with alopecia and abnormal pigmentation, sometimes with seizures or trigeminal neuralgia. Deeper involvement then en coup de sabre. Some do not recognize it as morphea variant.

Investigation

1. Skin biopsy can confirm diagnosis, but not distinguish between morphea and systemic sclerosis. Must rely on clinical findings.

Morphea (localized scleroderma)

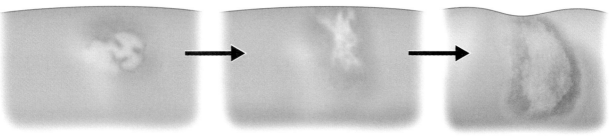

Typical progression of skin lesions
Affected skin begins as a discolored area (red or purple) that hardens and thickens

The area spreads into a thickened oval plaque and develops a whitish center

Gradually the area thins and tightens, leaving the skin darker

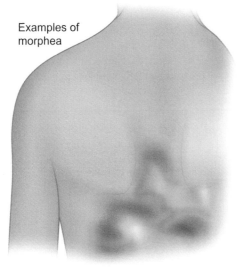

Examples of morphea

Circumscribed (few patches) or generalized (many patches) on trunk, arms or legs

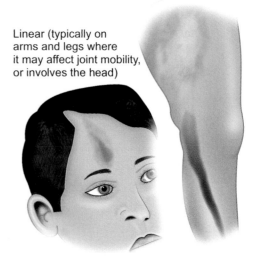

Linear (typically on arms and legs where it may affect joint mobility, or involves the head)

Fig. 26.16A: Depiction of the course of morphea and the common variants

26

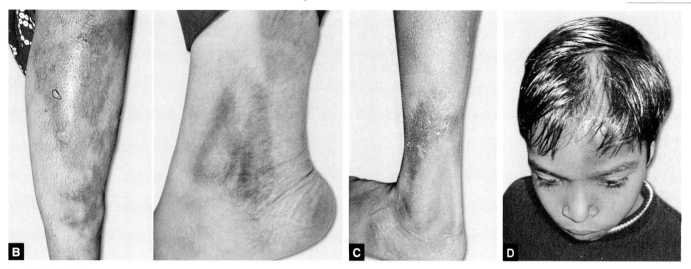

Fig. 26.16B to D: (B) Localized plaque form of morphea; (C) Linear morphea on the leg; (D) Linear morphea with scarring alopecia—**En coup de sabre** variant

Collagen bundles are increased in number and thickness, and appear more eosinophilic on hematoxylin and eosin staining. These changes are most marked in the lower two-thirds of the dermis and extend into the subcutaneous fat. Inflammation is present in the early stages, when the diagnosis is easily missed histologically. In later stages, the sclerotic process entraps, and finally obliterates, the dermal appendages with an end result that may resemble a scar (Fig. 26.17).

2. ANA and anti-ss-DNA are positive in linear and widespread morphea.
3. With widespread disease, evaluate joints and esophagus.

Therapy

Plaque form: High-potency topical corticosteroids, also under occlusion or intralesional.

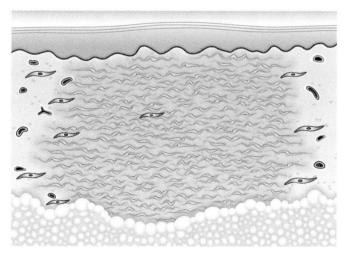

Fig. 26.17: Scleroderma. Epidermis—normal. Dermis—thickened; fibroblasts are increased in number; collagen bundles are increased in thickness and number

Generalized morphea/pansclerotic and linear morphea: In addition to the treatment for plaque form, the following options have been tried:
- Bath PUVA or UVA1.
  (NB-UVB more effective for superficial lesions and UVA1 more effective for deeper lesions.)
- Weekly methotrexate doses: Adults, 15–25 mg/week; children, 0.3–0.4 mg/kg/week.
- Systemic steroids.

DERMATOMYOSITIS AND POLYMYOSITIS

These are an uncommon group of autoimmune diseases with loss of muscle strength secondary to autoimmune muscle damage.

Polymyositis: No cutaneous involvement.

Dermatomyositis: Both muscular and cutaneous abnormalities.

In adult patients >50 years, it may be associated with an underlying malignancy.

Pathogenesis

There is a strong link with autoimmunity which is linked to the presence of circulating autoantibodies, (Table 26.11) both myositis-specific and overlapping. Most common suspected trigger is viral infections.

Table 26.11	Autoantibodies seen in DM/PM
Antisynthetase autoantibodies	More common in polymyositis than dermatomyositis; **interstitial lung disease,** arthritis, Raynaud's phenomenon, fevers, **mechanic's hands**[Q]
Signal recognition particle (SRP)	Polymyositis; possible **severe disease** and cardiac involvement
Anti-Mi2 (helicase)	Dermatomyositis; **good outlook**

In the case of polymyositis, the reaction appears primarily cellular with CD8 cytotoxic T cells damaging muscles while in dermatomyositis, humoral mechanisms are predominant and the CD4 cells are involved.[Q]

Classification

The latest updated classification is given in Table 26.12.

Important Aspects of Various Types

DM with malignancy: In up to 25% of adults; ovarian, colon, breast, lung, gastric, pancreatic carcinomas (nasopharyngeal in southeast Asian populations), and lymphoma; risk decreases to normal after 2–5 years.

Juvenile onset: Calcinosis cutis (panniculitis/ lipoatrophy) is more common in juvenile-onset dermatomyositis.[Q] Associated with delay in Rx or Rx-resistant disease.

Overlap syndrome: Systemic sclerosis > SLE, Sjögren's syndrome, rheumatoid arthritis.

Amyopathic DM: Provisional = cutaneous findings without muscle weakness and with normal muscle enzymes for >6 months; confirmed = for 24 months (MIDA-5 antibody).

The diagnosis of these disorders is traditionally based on the criteria proposed by Bohan and Peter,[Q] wherein skin rash plus at least 3 criteria can help in diagnosis of dermatomyositis (Table 26.13).

Clinical Features

An overview of the features is given in Fig. 26.18.

Skin: Skin changes in 80–100% of cases; presenting sign in 25% (Fig. 26.19). The condition is markedly pruritic.

The most specific skin manifestations are Gottron's papules and the heliotrope rash.[Q] Gottron's papules are considered to be pathognomonic of DM (Fig. 26.19).[Q]

- Scalp: May resemble seborrheic dermatitis, very itchy, involves posterior > anterior scalp.
- Lichenoid papules over the finger joints and knuckles (Gottron papules, Fig. 26.20A).[Q] These

Table 26.13	Bohan and Peter criteria for polymyositis and dermatomyositis

1. Symmetric proximal *muscle weakness*.
2. Increase in serum *muscle enzymes*, such as CK, AST, ALT, aldolase, and LDH.
3. Abnormal *electromyographic* findings, such as short, small, polyphasic motor units; fibrillations; positive sharp waves; insertional irritability; and bizarre high-frequency repetitive discharges.
4. Abnormal *muscle biopsy* findings such as mononuclear infiltration, regeneration, degeneration, and necrosis.
5. *Skin rashes*, such as heliotrope rash, Gottron's sign, and Gottron's papules.

papules may also occur over the extensor side of the wrist, elbow, or knee joints.

- A macular rash (without papules) with the same distribution as Gottron's papules is called Gottron's sign[Q] (Fig. 26.20B).
- Periorbital and eyelid edema with violet tint to eyelids; known as heliotrope lids (sun-pointing lids)[Q]; sometimes associated with reduced facial expression (Fig. 26.20C).
- Pink-violet patches of the lateral thighs (holster sign).[Q]
- Erythematous macules and plaques on forehead, chin, shoulders and upper arms (shawl sign)[Q] (Fig. 26.20D) or anterior neck and upper chest (V sign).
- Raynaud phenomenon: Children frequently have distal sclerosis.
- Nail fold telangiectases and atrophy, cuticular dystrophy (Ragged cuticles)
- Fissures and ulcers on tips of fingers and toes (mechanic's hands).[Q] This rash is often associated with the presence of antisynthetase autoantibodies and can be seen in both PM and DM. The rash is a hyperkeratotic, scaling, fissuring of the fingers, particularly on the radial side of the index fingers.

> Both SLE and DM have erythematous rash on the hand. However, the erythema in DM is present in a linear pattern on the fingers involving interphalangeal areas and knuckles (also Gottron papules). But in SLE, only the interphalangeal area is involved, knuckles spared.

Mucosa: 10–20% have oral ulcers.

Calcinosis: Distinctive feature of juvenile dermatomyositis; can be very extensive; soft tissue, vessel and muscle calcifications. Often most disturbing sequelae.

Arthritis: Most common at onset of disease; usually peripheral; 25% have morning stiffness.

Table 26.12	Revised classification system for the idiopathic inflammatory dermatomyopathies	
Dermatomyositis (DM)	Adult-onset	<ul><li>Classic DM</li><li>Classic DM with malignancy</li><li>Classic DM as part of an overlapping connective tissue disorder</li><li>Clinically amyopathic DM</li></ul>
	Juvenile-onset	<ul><li>Classic DM</li><li>Clinically amyopathic DM</li></ul>
Polymyositis		<ul><li>Isolated polymyositis</li><li>Polymyositis as part of an overlapping connective tissue disorder</li></ul>
Inclusion body myositis		

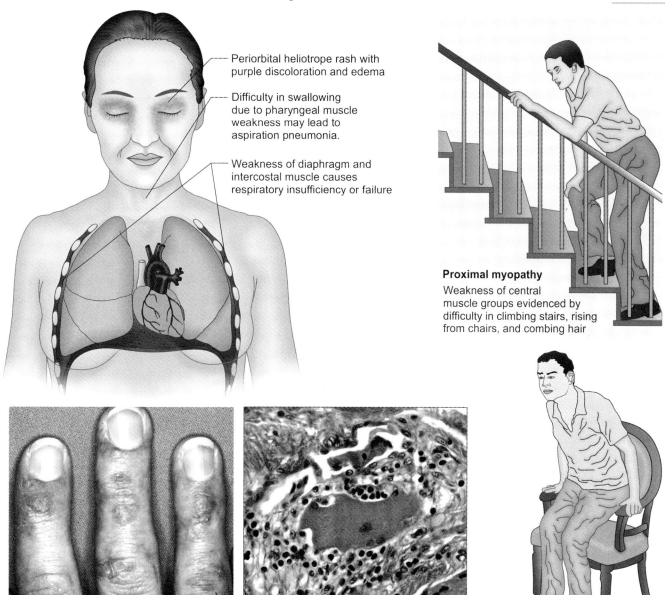

Periorbital heliotrope rash with purple discoloration and edema

Difficulty in swallowing due to pharyngeal muscle weakness may lead to aspiration pneumonia.

Weakness of diaphragm and intercostal muscle causes respiratory insufficiency or failure

Proximal myopathy
Weakness of central muscle groups evidenced by difficulty in climbing stairs, rising from chairs, and combing hair

Gottron's paules. Erythematous or violaceous, scaly papules on dorsum of interphalangeal joints

Longitudinal section of muscle showing intense inflammatory infiltration plus degeneration and disruption of muscle fibers

Difficulty in arising from a chair is often an early complaint.

Fig. 26.18: A depiction of the major manifestations of dermatomyositis including the features of proximal myopathy

Systemic Features

A depiction of the systemic affliction is given in Fig. 26.21 and the main involvements include.

Muscles: Pain and then weakness in shoulder and hip girdle muscles (Fig. 26.18). Typical problems include difficulty in combing hair, getting out of chair, getting up from horizontal position, climbing stairs, or leaving a car. Difficulty in swallowing and ptosis or strabismus can also occur. Early disease often associated with fever and malaise.

- *Lungs*: More common in patients with anti-Jo-1 antibodies[Q]; 20% have pulmonary fibrosis.

- *Gastrointestinal tract*: Children have vasculitis and frequent gastrointestinal ulcerations and hemorrhage. In adults, motility problems may occur.

- *Heart*: Asymptomatic EKG changes common; occasionally myocarditis or myopathy.

Serum tests such as CK-MB to detect cardiac involvement are unreliable in patients with inflammatory myopathies because CK-MB can be released from regenerating skeletal muscle fibers, a common feature in biopsies from patients with PM or DM. The CK-MB/total CK ratio is greater than 3%, a threshold value that is used to define myocardial damage.

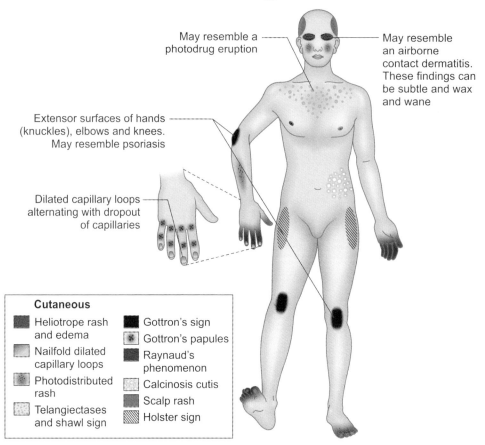

Fig. 26.19: A depiction of cutaneous features of dermatomyositis

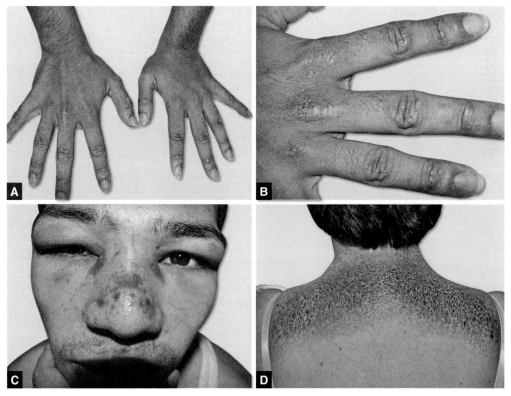

Fig. 26.20A to D: (A) **Gottron's papules:** Flat-topped papules develop on the knuckles and they may become atrophic; (B) Also note the macular erythema in a linear fashion—**Gottron's sign**; (C) **Heliotrope sign:** Pink-violet color is seen with involvement of the hairline, lower forehead, upper eyelids, and cheeks—the edema is striking and involves the nasal root as well as the eyelids; (D) Erythematous rash on the upper back **'shawl sign'**

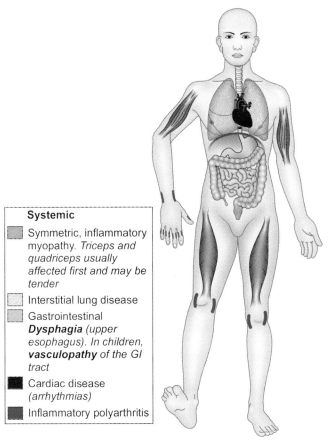

Systemic

- Symmetric, inflammatory myopathy. *Triceps and quadriceps usually affected first and may be tender*
- Interstitial lung disease
- Gastrointestinal *Dysphagia (upper esophagus). In children, vasculopathy of the GI tract*
- Cardiac disease (arrhythmias)
- Inflammatory polyarthritis

Fig. 26.21: A depiction of systemic features of dermatomyositis

Investigation

- *Electromyogram (EMG)*: Characteristic changes in affected muscles in 70%

  DM → Fibrillations, +ve sharp curves

  Myopathy → Multiple, small amplitude, short duration motor unit action potentials
- *MRI*: Displays inflamed muscles; superior to sonography or CT.
- *Muscle biopsy*: Most reliable diagnostic text; shows varying stages of necrosis and regeneration with inflammatory infiltrate. In polymyositis, CD8 cells; in dermatomyositis, CD4 cells, vasculitis, and perifascicular atrophy[Q] (almost diagnostic). Also helps exclude trichinosis.

Always biopsy muscle that EMG or MRI shows to be affected. Preserve muscle in solution provided by special muscle pathologist and keep under tension with muscle clamp. Otherwise, the procedure is worthless.

Laboratory

- Creatine kinase (CK) is the best marker; it is elevated at some point in disease. But there can be marked variations with normal CK being more common in DM than in PM.
- 24-hour urine creatine (not creatinine-common error) level >200 mg is diagnostic.[Q] In children

and pregnancy, more marked spontaneous variation.

Serology

Certain muscle specific antibodies (MSAs), such as anti-Jo-1, are more frequently associated with **PM**; others such as Mi-2 are more frequent in **DM**.

- **Anti-Jo-1**[Q] (antisynthetase): Present in 20%, correlates with lung disease and Raynaud phenomenon.
- **Anti-SRP** (signal recognition protein): Acute disease, *poor outlook*.
- **Anti-Mi2** (helicase): Dermatomyositis, *good outlook*.
- Others: Rheumatoid factor (10%), ANA (20%); no anti-DNA antibodies.
- Anti-PM-SCL (anti-PM1): Marker for polymyositis/systemic sclerosis overlap.
- General evaluation: Chest radiograph, EKG, echocardiogram pulmonary function.
- Search for underlying tumor in patients >50 years of age or with suspicious history. It is important to undertake a pelvic examination as ovarian carcinoma is one of the more commonly associated tumors.

Treatment

1. *Corticosteroids:*[Q] Start with 20 mg prednisolone bid; if needed, increase to 40 mg tid or use pulse therapy. In children with dermatomyositic vasculitis, tid regimens are recommended to suppress disease rapidly.

   As soon as CK starts to drop, switch to single dose in morning and start tapering in 2-week intervals, checking clinical status and CK before each dose reduction. After several months, switch to alternate-day therapy for its adrenal-sparing role. Often long-term low-dose corticosteroids are needed, but a try at discontinuation is warranted.

2. *Second-line/adjuvant agents*:
   - Methotrexate 5–15 mg p.o. or 15–50 mg IV weekly or azathioprine 1–3 mg/kg daily; either can be combined with corticosteroids.
   - Cyclophosphamide and cyclosporine are less effective.
   - Intravenous immunoglobulins: 2 g/kg daily for 2 days; repeat every 4 weeks for 6–12 months; indicated for resistant cases, children with vasculitic component, and in those with steroid-induced diabetes mellitus.

3. *Skin*: Antimalarials may help cutaneous lesions, as do topical corticosteroids. Sunscreens essential.

4. *Other measures*: Bed rest during flares; physical therapy when stable; absolutely essential to avoid loss of function, especially for children, but if too strenuous, can trigger relapse. Watch for pneumonia—common complication.

26

Skin in Systemic Disease

This topic tends to encompass textbooks and it is not the aim of this book to focus extensively on this topic. Our aim thus will be to focus on the common and important conditions, and to give an overview wherever possible with pictoral depiction of the clues that can be encountered on skin examination that represent an underlying disorder.

SKIN AND INTERNAL MALIGNANCY

A *paraneoplastic sign* is one that is associated with a malignancy but does not involve direct extension or metastasis. It must fulfil the following criteria:

- No other explanation for the disease
- Statistical connection is shown
- Skin changes appear at about the same time as the malignancy or they may precede any clinical manifestations of the underlying cancer
- Skin changes improve with cancer treatment and may reappear, if cancer recurs:
  1. *Acanthosis nigricans*: This is a velvety thickening and pigmentation of the major flexures and is commonly seen consequent to obesity (Fig. 27.1), metabolic syndrome (including type 2 diabetes^Q with insulin resistance), or due to drugs such as nicotinic acid^Q used to treat hyperlipidemia. It is caused by stimulation of epidermal or fibroblast growth factor receptor by insulin, tumor products, or other unknown triggers.

     When an adult who is *not overweight* presents with acanthosis nigricans, he must be investigated for underlying GI malignancy. Amongst malignancies, it is seen with adenocarcinoma^Q localized to the abdominal cavity.

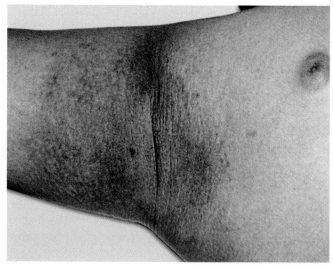

Fig. 27.1: Thickened velvety pigmented appearance of skin in acanthosis nigricans

  2. *Erythema gyratum repens:*^{Q} This is a shifting pattern of waves of erythema that look like the grain on wood. It may precede the onset of bronchial or esophageal neoplasms.
  3. *Acquired hypertrichosis lanuginosa (malignant down)*: This is an excessive and widespread growth of fine lanugo hair. It is more common in women, when it is usually associated with colorectal, lung and breast malignancies.
  4. *Necrolytic migratory erythema:*^{Q} An annular scaly migratory erythema coupled with severe periorificial and periungual erosions (often confused with candidiasis).

     If associated with anemia, stomatitis, weight loss and diabetes, it signals the presence of a glucagon-secreting tumor of the pancreas. It is occasionally seen with other pancreatic disease or zinc deficiency.

5. *Bazex syndrome*: This is a psoriasiform papulo-squamous eruption of the fingers and toes, ears and nose, seen with some tumors of the upper respiratory tract.

6. *Dermatomyositis*: In 20% of adult patients with dermatomyositis, an underlying malignancy may be seen. The antibody anti-P155 may be helpful in discriminating between idiopathic and malignancy-associated cases. Onset in adulthood should always prompt a thorough search for an underlying malignancy specially in the ovaries.[Q]

7. *Generalized pruritus*: Though uncommon, some-times a lymphoma may present with generalized itching.

8. *Superficial thrombophlebitis*: The migratory type has traditionally been associated with carcinomas of the pancreas. Also known as Trousseau sign.[Q]

9. *Acquired ichthyosis*: This may result from a number of underlying diseases including Hodgkin's[Q] lymphoma (70–80% of cases) and other hemato-logical neoplasms.

10. *Genetic conditions*: Muir-Torre syndrome is characterized by sebaceous adenomas accompa-nied by surprisingly non-aggressive visceral malignancies.

11. *Acute febrile neutrophilic dermatosis (Sweet's synd-rome)*: This disorder is a neutrophilic dermatoses, composed of red edematous plaques, with fever, a raised erythrocyte sedimentation rate (ESR) and a raised blood neutrophil count. Approximately, 20% of cases are associated with an underlying malignancy. The most important internal association is with myeloproliferative disorders.[Q]

12. *Paraneoplastic pemphigus*: This mimicks pem-phigus vulgaris but has in addition extensive and persistent mucosal ulceration. The blisters on the palms and soles can look like erythema multiforme. It is associated with lymphoma or Castleman tumor.[Q]

ENDOCRINE DISORDERS

Thyroid Gland

Hyperthyroidism

This presents with warm, moist skin, sweaty palms, onycholysis (Plummer nail), and diffuse alopecia. The most common cause is Graves' disease,[Q] which features orbital disease with exophthalmos, acropachy, and pretibial myxedema. The latter shows sharply demarcated plaques on the shins, often with 'orange-peel' surface. Biopsy shows massive deposits of mucin.

Hypothyroidism

The most common cause in adults is autoimmune or Hashimoto thyroiditis.[Q]

Symptoms are dry puffy skin, alopecia, and loss of the lateral one-third of the eyebrows (Hertoghe sign).[Q] The skin is yellow from carotinemia, but the sclerae are unaffected.[Q] Biopsy reveals discrete mucin deposits.

Diabetes Mellitus

About 30 to 70% of patients with diabetes mellitus have cutaneous changes, which can be divided into 3 groups:

1. Skin infections

- *Candida albicans* is the most common pathogen,[Q] causing perlèche, vulvitis, balanitis and paronychia. Patients also have more tinea pedis, particularly because of the peripheral vascular disease.
- The common bacterial infections include staphylo-coccal and streptococcal pyodermas, and erythrasma.[Q] Recurrent folliculitis and necrotizing fasciitis and gangrene can occur more commonly.
- Less common but more serious infections are mucormycosis, clostridial gangrene, and malignant otitis externa (*Pseudomonas aeruginosa*).

2. Specific disorders of diabetes mellitus

- *Diabetic dermopathy*: Small atrophic hyperpigmented patches on the shins are seen in 25–30% and reflect vessel damage and leakage (Binkley spots).[Q]
- *Necrobiosis lipoidica*: Over 50% of patients with necrobiosis lipoidica have or develop diabetes mellitus, but less than 1% of diabetics have this skin change (female: male 3:1). Thus non-diabetic necrobiosis patients should be screened for diabetes as some will have impaired glucose tolerance or diabetes, and some will become diabetic later.

  The lesions appear as discolored areas on the fronts of the shins. The early plaques are violaceous, but later on they atrophy and leave behind shiny, atrophic and brown-red lesions. The underlying blood vessels are easily seen through the atrophic skin and the margin may be erythematous or violet (Fig. 27.2).

- *Disseminated granuloma annulare*: An association with diabetes mellitus is seen in a few adults with extensive superficial granuloma annulare. The classic lesions of granuloma annulare often lie over the knuckles and are composed of dermal nodules that form a rough ring shape (Fig. 27.3).
- *Sclerotic disorders*: Adults with scleredema present with firm hard skin, usually of the back. There is an increase in both collagen fibers and mucin. Diabetic stiff skin typically involves the fingers.
- *Signs of insulin resistance*: Acanthosis nigricans, lipodystrophy.

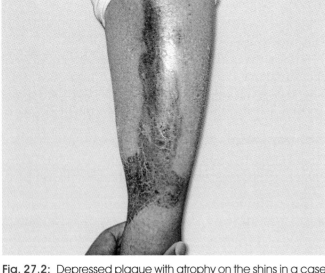

Fig. 27.2: Depressed plaque with atrophy on the shins in a case of necrobiosis lipoidica

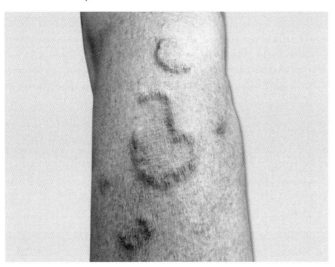

Fig. 27.3: Annular plaques with peripheral papules in a case of granuloma annulare

- *Others*: These include, vitiligo, pruritus, facial erythema, eruptive xanthoma, perforating disorders and rarely diabetic bulla.

3. Complications of diabetes

- *Macroangiopathy*: Cutaneous atrophy, especially on soles, dry skin, hypothermia, nail dystrophy, hair loss.
- *Microangiopathy*: Binkley spots: Tiny brown macules on shins.
- *Diabetic stiff skin syndrome*
- *Neuropathy*: Hyperhidrosis, malum perforans.

Every patient with a painless or slow-to-heal foot ulcer (malum perforans) requires an investigation for DM.

Pituitary Gland

- **Prolactinoma** is caused by a pituitary adenoma and the main effects are delayed puberty in either sex, galactorrhea-amenorrhea in women, and decreased

libido in men. It can also be caused by drugs (including haloperidol, trifluoperazine, metoclopramide), hypothyroidism and other tumors in or near the pituitary gland. Treatment consists of bromocriptine or cabergoline as well as neurosurgery.

- **Acromegaly** results from over secretion of growth hormone by pituitary tumors, in adolescents or adults resulting in excessive bone growth of the face, hands and face with coarsening of facial features, thickening of the skin, seborrhea, hyperhidrosis, hypertrichosis, and acanthosis nigricans.
- **Cushing disease** is the result of hyperadrenocorticism caused by excessive pituitary secretion of ACTH, usually because of a pituitary adenoma.

Adrenal Glands

Cushing syndrome

Cushing's syndrome is an illness resulting from excess cortisol secretion, which has a high mortality, if left untreated. There are several causes of hypercorti-solemia which must be differentiated, and the commonest cause is iatrogenic (oral, inhaled, or topical steroids). Endogenous or exogenous excess amount of corticosteroids leads to steroid acne, hirsutism, hyperpigmentation, striae, telangiectases, hypertrichosis and purpura (weakened vessels) (Fig. 27.4).

It is important to decide whether the patient has true Cushing's syndrome rather than pseudo-Cushing's associated with depression or alcoholism. Secondly, ACTH-dependent Cushing's must be differentiated from ACTH-independent disease (usually due to an adrenal adenoma or, rarely, carcinoma). Once a diagnosis of ACTH-dependent disease has been established, it is important to differentiate between pituitary-dependent (Cushing's disease)[Q] and ectopic secretion.

> - *Cushing disease* is a neurosurgical problem, as the hyperadrenocorticism results from a pituitary tumor in most cases (**DPT: D**isease, **P**ituitary, **T**umor).
> - *Cushing syndrome* is the result of hyperadrenocorticism from any other cause.

A list of causes of Cushing's syndrome is given in Box 27.1.

Addison Disease

Characterized by hypoadrenalism, Addison disease is usually caused by autoimmune adrenal damage or tuberculosis.[Q] Autoimmune is the commonest cause in the developed world (approximately 70% cases). In tuberculosis, the medulla is more frequently destroyed than cortex.

Diffuse bronze hyperpigmentation that darkens with light exposure with darkening of scars, and reduced sebum flow (Fig. 27.5).

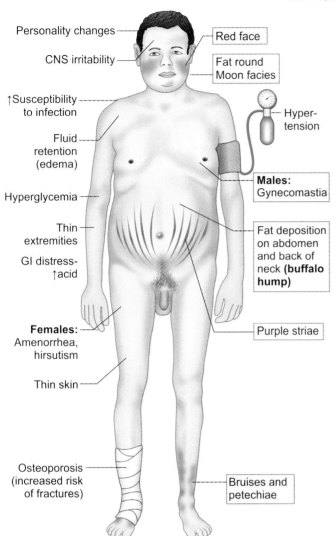

Fig. 27.4: A depiction of the varied manifestations of skin in Cushing's disease or syndrome

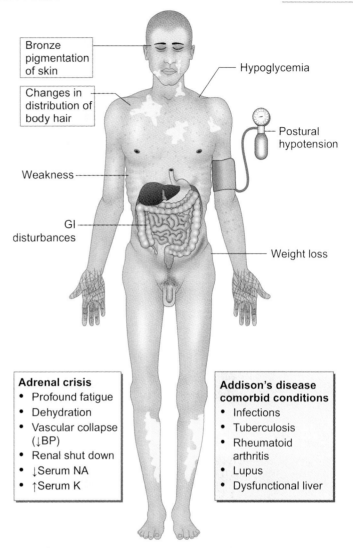

Fig. 27.5: An overview of skin features of Addison's disease

Sudden withdrawal of systemic corticosteroids after weeks of therapy leads to systemic features of hypoadrenalism (hypotension, hypothermia) but no cutaneous findings.^{Q} This is referred to as adrenal crisis.^{Q}

Box 27.1	Causes of Cushing's syndrome

- Pseudo-Cushing's syndrome:
  - Alcoholism <1%
  - Severe depression 1%
- ACTH-dependent:
  - Pituitary adenoma 68% (*Cushing's disease*)
  - Ectopic ACTH syndrome 12%
  - Ectopic CRH secretion <1%
- ACTH-independent:
  - Adrenal adenoma 10%
  - Adrenal carcinoma 8%
  - Nodular (macro- or micro-) hyperplasia 1%
  - Carney complex
- Exogenous steroids, including skin creams, e.g. clobetasol

Hyperandrogenism

This is primarily a problem in women. After the testes and ovary, the adrenal glands are the other major source of androgens. Excessive production leads to acne, hirsutism, virilization, and bitemporal hair recession (Fig. 27.6). Congenital adrenal hyperplasia should be excluded in adults with therapy-resistant acne.^{Q}

SARCOIDOSIS

This is a multisystem granulomatous disease that favors the lungs, lymph nodes, and skin.

- It is believed that in predisposed individuals, an infectious or environmental antigen (as yet unknown) stimulates a predominantly Th1 immune-mediated response, resulting in the clinical manifestations. The Th1 cells in turn release interferon (IFN-γ). TNF-producing macrophages are activated and the fact that TNF antagonists improve sarcoidosis without provoking disseminated infections, argues against an infectious cause.

27

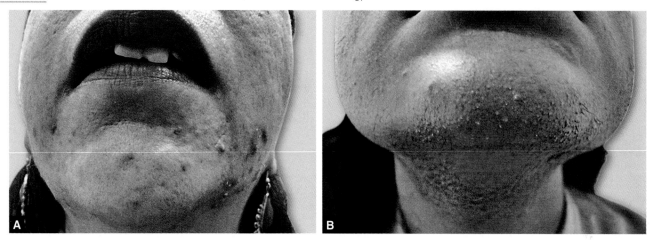

Fig. 27.6A and B: Hyperandrogenism in females: (A) Persistent acne in a 32-year-old female with acne on the jawline and hirsutism; (B) Acne with hirsutism in a 23-year-old female

- About one-third of patients with systemic sarcoidosis have skin lesions; it is also possible to have cutaneous sarcoidosis without systemic abnormalities.

Clinical Features

Systemic findings: Any organ can be involved, but most commonly affected are the hilar lymph nodes, lungs, joints, and skin (Fig. 27.7).

Cutaneous findings: Sarcoidosis can mimic almost any skin lesion. They can be specific or non-specific with the former showing the classic 'naked granuloma'[Q]

- *Erythema nodosum* (*non-specific*): Usually associated with fever, arthralgias; appears in 10% of patients and is good prognostic sign.[Q]

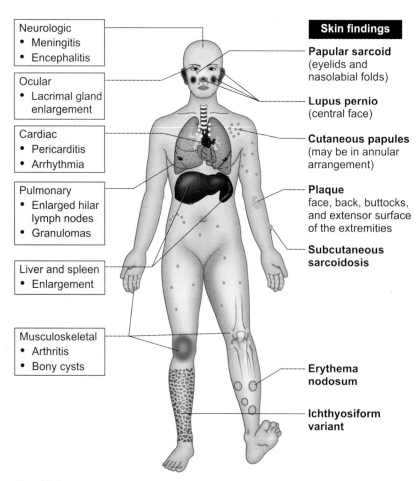

Fig. 27.7: Depiction of systemic and cutaneous involvement in sarcoidosis

- *Lupus pernio (specific)*: Red-violet chronic infiltrate on tip of nose. It is often associated with chronic pulmonary involvement and digital bone cysts.[Q]
- *Nodular sarcoidosis (specific)*: Red-brown plaques and nodules, often symmetrical, favor the thighs; associated with hilar lymphadenopathy and splenomegaly.
- *Maculopapular sarcoidosis (specific)*: Transient red-brown papules, appear early in disease and may reappear, heralding disease flares. Favor trunk, but may appear on face and extremities. Can be annular, especially in blacks.
- *Scar sarcoidosis (specific)*: Nodular changes in scars may be early sign of sarcoidosis. Sometimes subtle trauma, such as venipunctures, is sufficient trigger.
- *Darier-Roussy sarcoidosis (subcutaneous variant-specific)*: Painless, firm, mobile nodules or plaques.

Diascopy: It is helpful in the diagnosis of cutaneous sarcoid. Pressure with a glass slide over the lesion may reveal the characteristic 'apple jelly nodules'.[Q]

Special variants of sarcoidosis include:

Lofgren syndrome:[Q] Ill patient with fever, malaise, arthritis, erythema nodosum, and bilateral hilar lymphadenopathy.

Mikulicz syndrome:[Q] Swelling of the salivary or lacrimal glands.

Heerfordt syndrome:[Q] A triad of facial nerve palsy, parotid swelling, and iridocyclitis, sometimes with CNS findings.

Parinaud syndrome: Conjunctivitis with papillary nodules, lacrimal gland involvement, and ipsilateral lymphadenopathy.

Investigation

- Skin biopsy: Reveals multiple non-caseating naked granulomas
- Chest and hand radiographs.
- Serum calcium level (granulomas produce 1,25-dihydroxycholecalciferol) and serum angiotensin-converting enzyme (ACE)[Q] level may both be elevated, as are urine hydroxyproline and calcium levels.

Therapy

Treatment based on general condition of patient.

- Topical corticosteroids usually helpful for cutaneous lesions; if not, consider PUVA for maculopapular disease.
- Methotrexate is the best choice for severe cutaneous and systemic disease.
- Systemic agents tried include hydroxychloroquine, cholorquine, minocycline, TNF-α inhibitors, and thalidomide.

CUTANEOUS MANIFESTATIONS OF LIVER DISEASE

1. *Pruritus*: This is related to obstructive jaundice and may sometimes precede the obstructive pathology.
2. Hair loss and generalized asteatotic eczema may occur in alcoholics with cirrhosis who have become zinc deficient.
3. *Pigmentation*: The bile pigments and sometimes melanin may increase in patients with liver disorders.
4. *Spider naevi*: These benign vascular disorder may be seen in large numbers in chronic liver disease.
5. *Palmar erythema*
6. *White nails*: This is consequential to hypoalbuminemia.
7. Lichen planus can be seen associated with hepatitis C infection.
8. Polyarteritis nodosa is associated with hepatitis B infection.
9. *Porphyria cutanea tarda*
10. *Xanthomas*: Seen in primary biliary cirrhosis.

CUTANEOUS MANIFESTATIONS IN RENAL DISEASE

The main changes are associated with chronic renal failure are as follows.

1. *Pruritus and generally dry skin*: The only cutaneous symptom reliably associated with renal disease is pruritus. Prior to the introduction of renal dialysis and renal transplantation, prurigo nodularis was considered a marker for chronic renal failure.

> Nephrogenic pruritus responds well to broad-spectrum ultraviolet (UV) B, but not to UVB 311 nm.

2. *Pigmentation*: A yellowish sallow color and pallor from anemia.
3. *Half-and-half nail*:[Q] The proximal half is white and the distal half is pink or brownish.
4. *Perforating disorders*: Small papules in which collagen or elastic fibres are being extruded through the epidermis.
5. *Pseudoporphyria*
6. *Calciphylaxis*:[Q] Patients in renal failure with secondary hyperparathyroidism may develop sudden vessel calcification. This calciphylaxis may be an analog to anaphylaxis but the exact cause is unknown.

   Early lesions are characterized by non-inflammatory reticulate purpura, while the late stage has necrosis with black eschar, and painful ulcerations.
7. Nephrogenic systemic fibrosis:[Q] Cutaneous and systemic (often retroperitoneal) fibrosis in dialysis patients, caused by exposure to contrast material containing gadolinium.[Q] It may improve with transplantation.

METABOLIC DISORDERS

Xanthomas

They are deposits of fatty material in the skin and subcutaneous tissues and can provide the first clue to important disorders of lipid metabolism.

They are classified into two types:

1. *Primary hyperlipidemias* are usually genetic. They fall into six groups, classified on the basis of an analysis of fasting blood lipids and electrophoresis of plasma lipoproteins. All, except type I, carry an increased risk of atherosclerosis.
2. *Secondary hyperlipidemia* may be found in a variety of diseases including diabetes, primary biliary cirrhosis, the nephrotic syndrome and hypothyroidism.

Not all xanthomas are associated with lipid abnormalities; sometimes normolipemic xanthomas are seen.

Clinical Features

The cutaneous consequence of elevated plasma lipoprotein levels is the uptake of lipids by macrophages following leakage through vessels, leading to the formation of xanthomas and xanthelasma. The difference types of xanthoma include (Fig. 27.8):

- *Plane xanthoma*: Irregular yellow-tan macules and flat-topped papules.
- *Tuberous xanthoma*: Larger red-brown or yellow nodules on pressure points—elbows, knees, hands, feet.
- *Tendon xanthoma*: Large subcutaneous nodules over Achilles' or digital tendons.
- *Eruptive xanthoma*: Numerous small yellow papules, often with red border, that appear suddenly. It is a marker for familial hypertriglyceridemia.[Q]
- *Palmar xanthoma*: Yellow streaks (striate) or papules in the palmar creases.
- *Xanthelasma*: Most common xanthoma;[Q] yellow flat-topped papules and plaques on lids, especially upper lid; no clear association with lipid abnormalities.

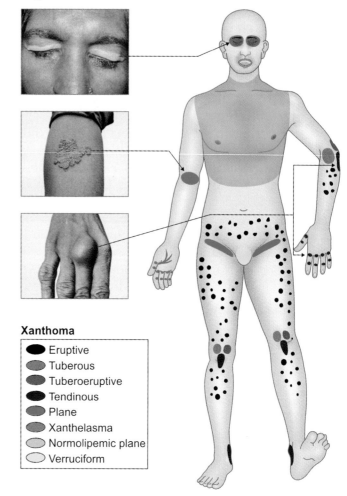

Xanthoma

- ● Eruptive
- ● Tuberous
- ● Tuberoeruptive
- ● Tendinous
- ● Plane
- ● Xanthelasma
- ○ Normolipemic plane
- ○ Verruciform

Fig. 27.8: Typical distribution of different types of xanthoma

The clinical patterns of xanthoma correlate well with the underlying cause (Table 27.1).

Management

The role of the dermatologist is to identify a lesion as a xanthoma. Then the patient must evaluated first for abnormalities of cholesterol and triglyceride metabolism and treated according to the latest guidelines.

Table 27.1	Correlation of clinical types of xanthoma with underlying defect	
Types	*Clinical features*	*Types of hyperlipidemia*
Xanthelasma palpebrarum	Soft yellowish plaques on the eyelids	None or type II, III or IV
Tuberous xanthomas	Firm yellow papules and nodules, most often on points of knees and elbows	Types II, III and secondary Marker for familial hypercholesterolemia, familial defective apolipoprotein B-100, and familial dysbetalipoproteinemia
Tendinous xanthomas	Subcutaneous swellings on fingers or by Achilles tendon	Types II, III and secondary
Eruptive xanthomas	Sudden onset, multiple small yellow papules	Types I, IV, V and secondary
Plane xanthomas	Yellow macular areas at any site	
Yellow palmar creases	Type III and secondary	
Generalized plane xanthomas	Yellow macules lesions over wide areas	Myeloma

27

DERMATOLOGICAL MANIFESTATIONS OF NUTRITIONAL DISORDERS

Malnutrition occurs because of poverty, alcoholism, child or elder abuse, eating disorders, or chronic disease. Nutritional disorders constitute an important problem even today in India and though these disorders usually present to physicians and pediatricians, some of them have marked dermatological manifestations.

Many vitamins and trace elements can influence skin disorders. Vitamin D analogs are used topically to treat psoriasis, while vitamin A analogs (retinoids) are used both topically and systemically for treating acne, disorders of keratinization, and other problems.

An overview of the varied manifestations of nutritional disorders is given in Fig. 27.9 and Table 27.2.

Protein Malnutrition

This has two different spectrum of skin manifestations—kwashiorkor and marasmus (Fig. 27.10).

Marasmus: This is a severe caloric defect, with growth retardation, wasting of subcutaneous fat and loss of muscle mass, known as starvation in adults. Dry skin, hair and nail growth disturbances, and follicular hyperkeratoses may develop. Marasmus patients have a characteristic 'old man' look.

Kwashiorkor: This is severe protein deficiency but with adequate to low caloric content; there is growth and mental retardation, marked edema, and thickened darkened skin with scales (flaked paint sign).[Q] Changing bands of light and dark hair color reflect varying nutritional levels is characterized by alternating bands of light and dark bands in the hair (flag sign).[Q]

Metal Deficiency

Zinc Deficiency

Acrodermatitis enteropathica[Q] (dermatitis of hands, feet, perioral/anal areas).

Though Zn deficiency can be acquired, the term acrodermatitis enteropathica refers to a disorder where there is a defect in intestinal zinc transport gene SLC39A4(ZIP4); autosomal recessive inheritance.

Clinical features: Acral, well-circumscribed, erythematous weeping plaques; most prominent around mouth, nares, anogenital region (Fig. 27.11). When not moist, such as on the hands, can be psoriasiform. Also telogen effluvium loss of eyebrows and eyelashes.

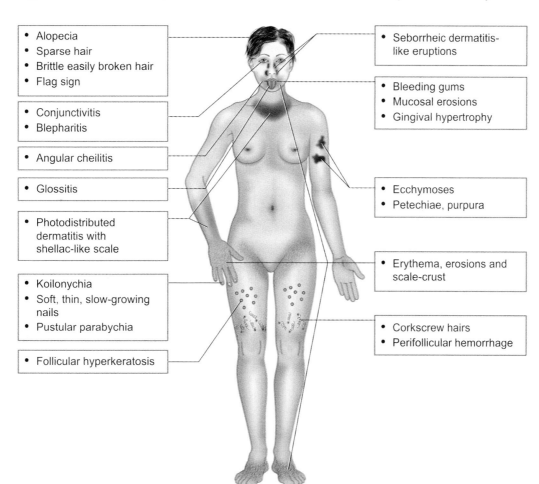

- Alopecia
- Sparse hair
- Brittle easily broken hair
- Flag sign

- Conjunctivitis
- Blepharitis

- Angular cheilitis

- Glossitis

- Photodistributed dermatitis with shellac-like scale

- Koilonychia
- Soft, thin, slow-growing nails
- Pustular parabychia

- Follicular hyperkeratosis

- Seborrheic dermatitis-like eruptions

- Bleeding gums
- Mucosal erosions
- Gingival hypertrophy

- Ecchymoses
- Petechiae, purpura

- Erythema, erosions and scale-crust

- Corkscrew hairs
- Perifollicular hemorrhage

27

Fig. 27.9: Mucocutaneous clues that suggest a posible nutritional disorder

Table 27.2 Physical signs of selected nutritional deficiency states

	Signs	Deficiencies
Hair	Alopecia	Severe undernutrition, zinc deficiency
	Brittle	Biotin, severe undernutrition
	Color change	Severe undernutrition
	Dryness	Vitamins E and A
	Easy pluckability	Severe undernutrition
Skin	Acneiform lesions	Vitamin A
	Follicular keratosis	Vitamin A
	Xerosis (dry skin)	Vitamin A
	Perioral and perianal bullous dermatitis (wet, red plaques)	Zinc
	Ecchymosis	Vitamin C or K
	Intradermal petechiae	Vitamin C or K
	Erythema (especially where exposed to sunlight)	Niacin
	Hyperpigmentation	Niacin
	Seborrheic dermatitis (nose, eyebrows, eyes)	Vitamin B_2, vitamin B_6, niacin
	Scrotal dermatitis	Niacin, vitamin B_2, vitamin B_6
Eyes	Angular palpebritis[Q]	Vitamin B_2
	Corneal revascularization[Q]	Vitamin B_2
	Bitot's spots	Vitamin A
	Conjunctival xerosis, keratomalacia[Q]	Vitamin A
Mouth	Angular stomatitis[Q]	Vitamin B_2, vitamin B_6, vitamin B_{12}
	Atrophic papillae	Niacin
	Bleeding gums	Vitamin C
	Cheilosis	Vitamin B_2, vitamin B_6
	Glossitis	Niacin, folate, vitamin B_1 (thiamine), vitamin B_2, Vitamin B_6, vitamin B_{12}
	Magenta tongue	Vitamin B_2
Extremities	Genu valgum or varum, metaphyseal widening	Vitamin D
	Loss of deep tendon reflexes of the lower limb	Vitamins B_1 and B_{12}

- Frequent secondary infections, usually with *Candida albicans*.
- Diarrhea, photophobia, loss of smell.
- Most common causes of acquired zinc deficiency are inflammatory bowel diseases.

> The differential diagnosis of severe periorificial and acral dermatitis when nutritional problems are suspected includes zinc, biotin-dependent carboxylases, free fatty acid deficiency, cystic fibrosis, and mixed deficiencies, as well as glucagonoma syndrome.

Investigation: Serum for determination of zinc level must be obtained using zinc-free needles and collecting system; marked diurnal variation, so always draw in a.m.

Iron Disorders

Iron deficiency is the most common cause of anemia.

Cracks at corner of mouth (perleche), glossitis, and diffuse alopecia may result.

Other rare findings are:
- Koilonychia
- Plummer-Vinson syndrome[Q]—esophageal webs and dysphagia.

Iron excess: Increased iron absorption and tissue stores result in hemochromatosis.

Copper

Deficiency: Abnormal intestinal absorption of copper is seen in Menkes syndrome[Q] (kinky hair syndrome), inherited in an X-linked recessive fashion and caused by a mutation in the ATP7A gene encoding a copper-transporting ATPase.

Infants have severe mental retardation, are floppy, and have striking kinky hair.

27

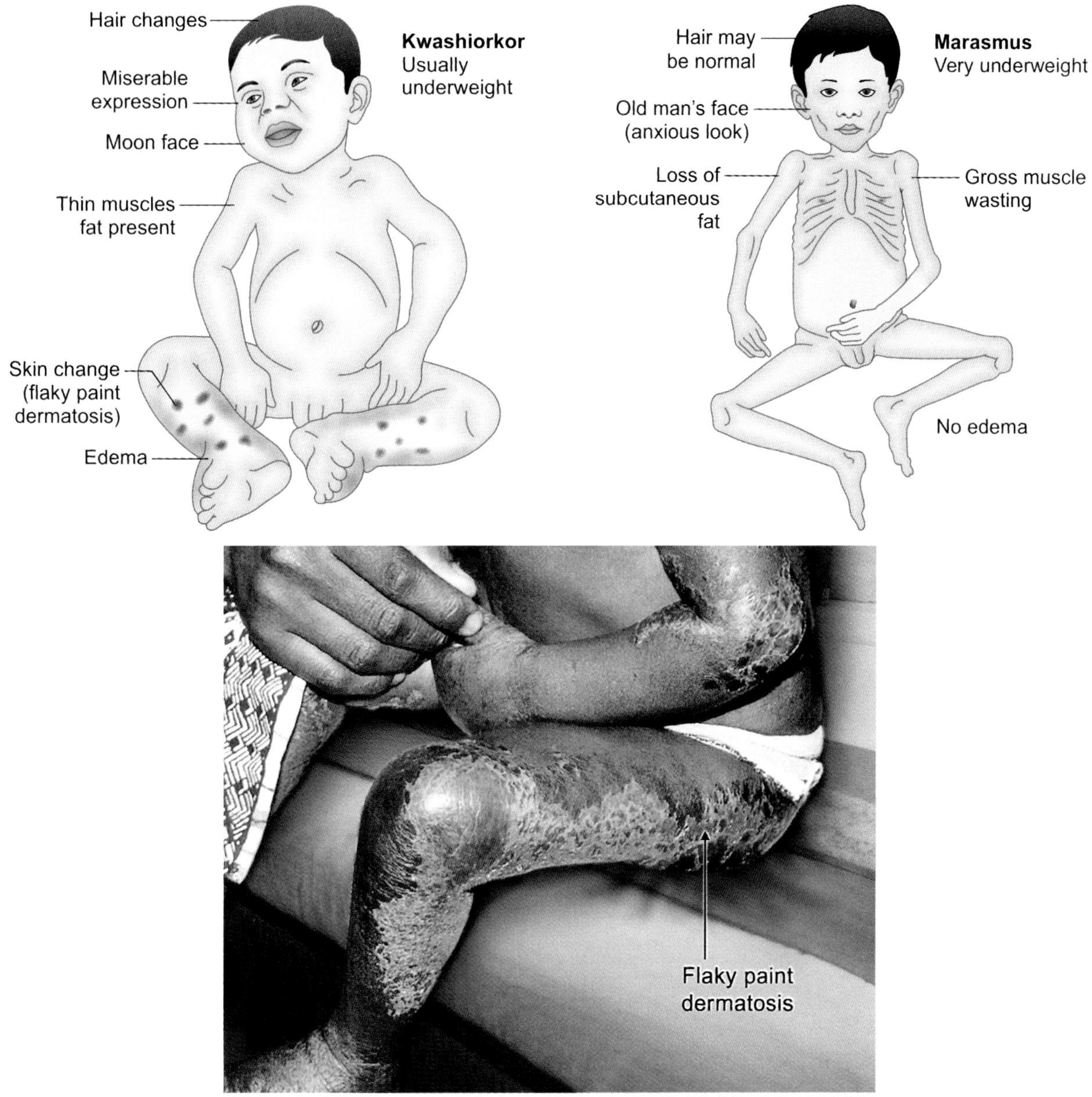

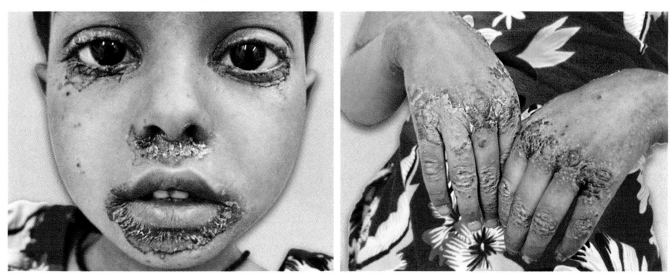

Hair changes

Miserable expression

Moon face

Thin muscles fat present

Skin change (flaky paint dermatosis)

Edema

Kwashiorkor
Usually underweight

Hair may be normal

Old man's face (anxious look)

Loss of subcutaneous fat

Marasmus
Very underweight

Gross muscle wasting

No edema

Flaky paint dermatosis

Fig. 27.10: Comparison of kwashiorkor and marasmus

Fig. 27.11: Periorifacial eczematous eruption with involvement of the extremities—zinc deficiency

27

Copper excess: In Wilson syndrome, patients are unable to normally excrete copper, and thus build up high tissue levels, with Kayser-Fleischer[Q] corneal ring, blue lunulae, and occasionally pretibial hyperpigmentation.

It is treated with penicillamine which often causes elastosis perforans serpiginosa, a peculiar dennatosis where abnormal dermal elastic fibers are discharged through the epidermis.

Vitamin Deficiency

Vitamin A

Vitamin A deficiency, also known as phrynoderma, is a multisystem disorder caused by a deficiency of vitamin A, either from lack of intake or from a decrease in normal absorption (Fig. 27.12A).

Clinical findings:

- *Night blindness* is one of the earliest findings in vitamin A deficiency. Vitamin A is crucially important for proper functioning of the retinal rods, through production of rhodopsin (Fig. 27.12B).

Xerophthalmia (dry eyes) often precedes the night blindness and is typically the first sign of vitamin A deficiency,[Q] although this sign is neither sensitive or specific. As the deficiency progresses, the xerophthalmia may result in corneal dryness, abrasions, ulceration, and keratomalacia, which leads

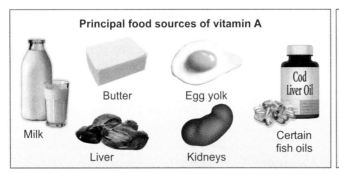
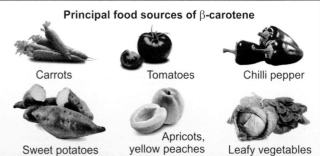

Fig. 27.12A: Food sources of vitamin A and β-carotene

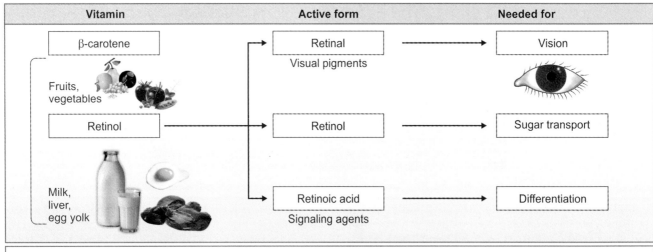

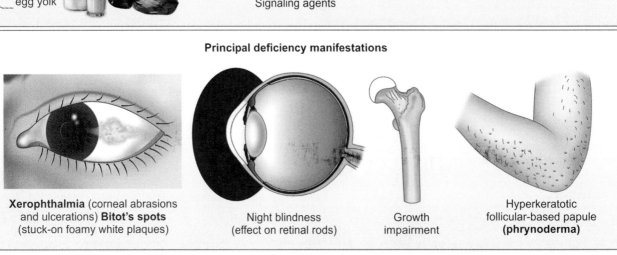

Fig. 27.12B: Role of vitamin A derivatives and deficiency states of vitamin A

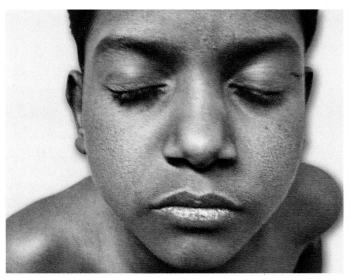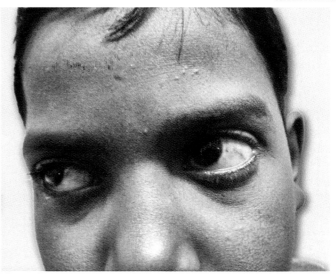

Fig. 27.12C: Dry skin with **Bitot spots**—vitamin A deficiency

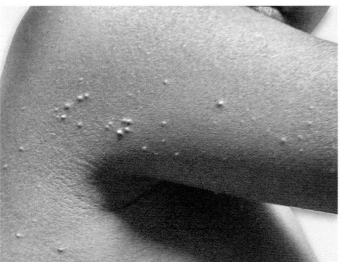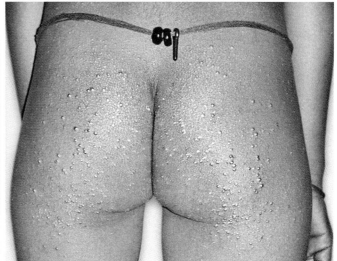

Fig. 27.12D: Phrynoderma—follicular keratotic papules—vitamin A deficiency

to blindness. Bitot's spots can be seen on the lateral conjunctiva of the eye. These are highly specific[Q] for vitamin A deficiency and appear as stuck-on foamy white papules and plaques that cannot be removed by swabbing (Fig. 27.12C).

- *Phrynoderma*[Q] is the name given to the skin findings in vitamin A deficiency. Phrynoderma literally means 'toad-like' skin,[Q] and it is manifested by hyperkeratotic follicle-based papules. The skin is dry and rough (Fig. 27.12D).
- Patients with vitamin A deficiency may also have cheilitis and glossitis. These latter two conditions are nonspecific and can be seen in a variety of vitamin deficiencies.

Vitamin B₁ (Thiamine) Deficiency: Beriberi Edema

Beriberi is a nutritional deficiency state that is caused directly by a lack of thiamine (vitamin B₁) in one's diet or by a lack of proper absorption of the vitamin. It is seen in those whose diet is composed of polished rice or are alcoholics. Thiamine deficiency has been reported in cases of short gut syndrome and after bariatric surgery. Other cases are seen in some people taking long-term furosemide therapy without adequate thiamine intake. Another common cause is alcoholism (Fig. 27.13A).

Clinical findings: The organ systems most commonly involved are the central nervous system (CNS) and the muscular system. Two major forms of beriberi occur, although there is much overlap.

- *Dry beriberi* is a form of the disease in which the CNS symptoms predominate this includes Wernicke's syndrome (Fig. 27.13B and C).
- *Wet beriberi* is the form in which the predominant symptoms are salt retention and congestive heart failure (Fig. 27.13D).

27

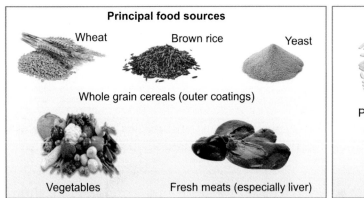

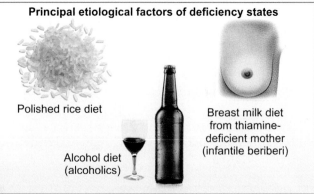

Fig. 27.13A: Sources of thiamine and the cause of the deficiency state

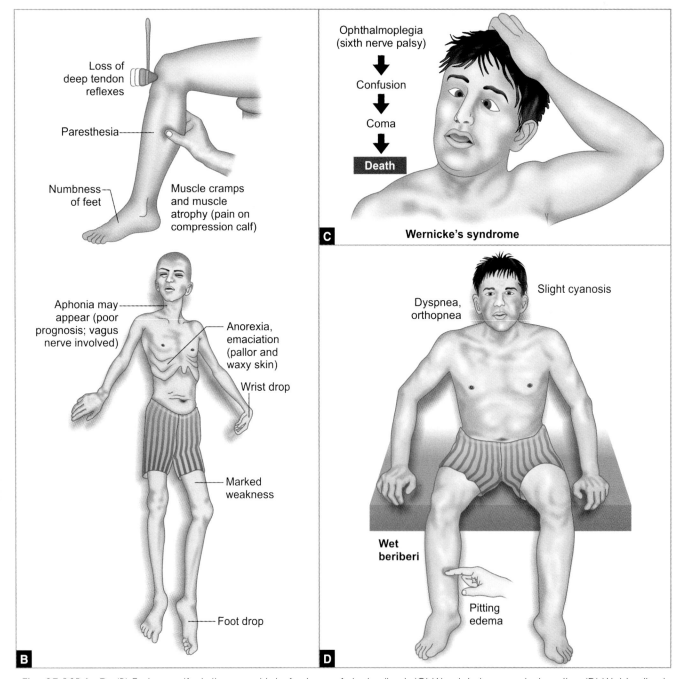

Fig. 27.13B to D: (B) Early manifestations, and late features of dry beriberi; (C) Wernicke's encephalopathy; (D) Wet beriberi

- Infantile beriberi is rare but is manifested by a combination of dry and wet beriberi with severe CNS depression, heart failure, and sudden death.
- *Therapy* consists of supplementation of the patient's diet with 50 mg/day intramuscularly of thiamine until the symptoms resolve.

Vitamin B₂ (Riboflavin) Deficiency

Angular stomatitis, smooth purple tongue (Fig. 27.14), seborrhoeic dermatitis-like eruption.

Vitamin B₃ (Niacin) Deficiency

Pellagra[Q] is caused by inadequate dietary intake of niacin (nicotinic acid, vitamin B₃)[Q] or its precursor amino acid, and tryptophan. Pellagra has been dominant in regions of the world that rely heavily on corn as the main dietary staple (Fig. 27.15A and B).

Clinical features: These unique clinical findings seen in pellagra can be simplified by the oft-quoted mnemonic, '4Ds': *Dermatitis, Diarrhea, Dementia, and Death*[Q] (Fig. 27.15C).

The clinical cutaneous hallmark of pellagra is a severe dermatitis. The dermatitis is photosensitive,[Q] and exposure to the sun often brings out the rash or exacerbates it. The head, neck, and arms are the most involved regions. The dermatitis along the anterior neck and upper thorax has been termed Casal necklace.[Q] Non-sun-exposed areas can also be involved, and the intertriginous regions are almost universally affected, including the perineum, axillae, and inframammary skin folds (Fig. 27.15D).

As time progresses, the dermatitis begins to desquamate. This process begins in the central portions of the dermatitis and spreads outward in a centrifugal manner. As the skin desquamates, it leaves behind red, eroded patches and plaques.

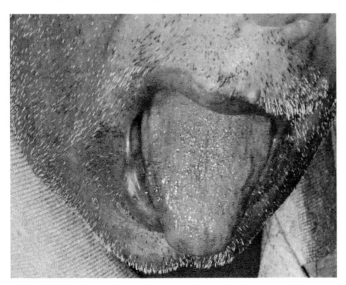

Fig. 27.14: Glossitis is a feature of most vitamin deficiency

Mucous membrane involvement is common with, angular cheilitis, red, shiny, edematous tongue with atrophied papillae.

Excess niacin (used for hyperlipemia) causes flushing.

Vitamin B₆ (Pyridoxine) Deficiency

Deficiency may cause cheilitis, glossitis, and seborrheic dermatitis.

Vitamin B₇ (Biotin) Deficiency

Periorificial macular rash, seborrheic dermatitis, brittle hair and alopecia.

Vitamin B₁₂

The main sign of deficiency is pernicious anemia; the classic signs is severe glossitis. Also seen are a wide array of neurological problems.

Vitamin C Deficiency

Scurvy is a well-known nutritional disease that results from a lack of the water-soluble vitamin, ascorbic acid (vitamin C). Scurvy has a well-documented history.

Clinical findings: Most cases are the result of abnormal dieting, psychiatric illness, or alcoholism (Fig. 27.16).

Scurvy has an insidious onset with nonspecific constitutional symptoms such as generalized weakness, malaise, muscle and joint aches, and easy fatigability with shortness of breath. These symptoms may be related to the macrocytic anemia that is frequently seen in patients with scurvy and is believed to be caused by a coexisting folic acid deficiency.

The first clinical findings are often in the mucous membranes and the skin.

- Early in the course of disease, skin becomes dry and rough, in association with a dulling of the skin tone.
- Small, hyperkeratotic papules may be noticed and resemble those of keratosis pilaris (Fig. 27.16B).
- More specific and sensitive skin findings then develop, including perifollicular hemorrhage and 'corkscrew hairs'.[Q] The corkscrew hairs are most noticeable on the extremities (Fig. 27.16B).
- Swan-neck deformity of the extremity hair may also occur due to abnormal bending of the hair; this is less common than corkscrew hair (Fig. 27.16B).
- The nail bed shows splinter hemorrhages. All cutaneous findings appear to be more common on the lower extremities.
- The mucous membranes may show the first sign of the disease. The main finding is edematous, bleeding gums. As the disease progresses, the gums become friable and peel away from the teeth.

27

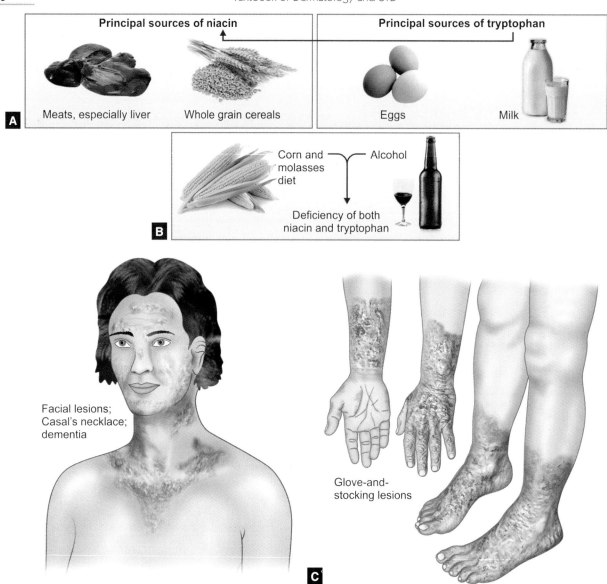

Fig. 27.15A to C: (A) Dietary sources of niaicn and tryptophan; (B) Causes of pellagra; (C) Manifestations of pellagra

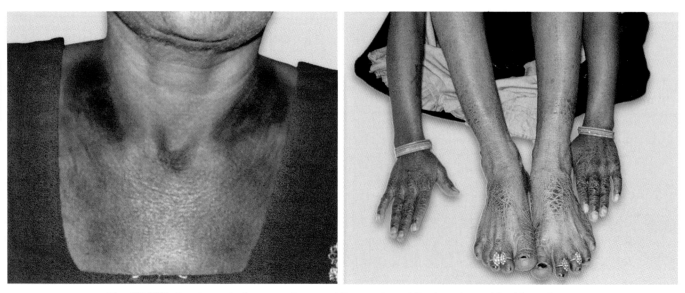

Fig. 27.15D: Involvment of exposed area of the neck and the hands and feet in pellagra

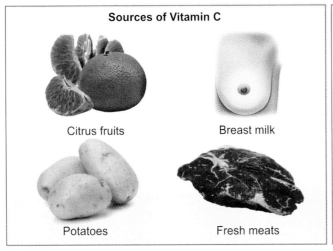

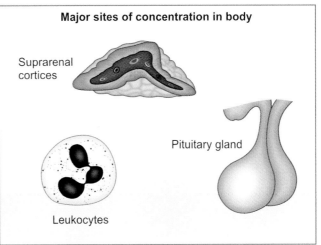

Fig. 27.16A: Sources of vitamin C

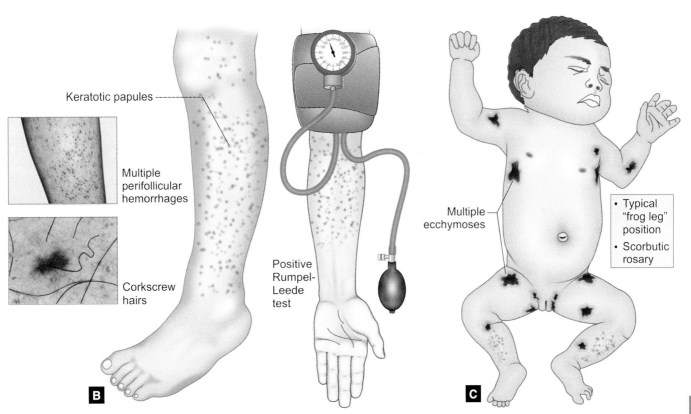

Fig. 27.16B and C: (B) Skin manifestations; (C) Pediatric scurvy

The teeth may develop dental calculi at the base. This may result in loose teeth and pain. Teeth eventually become disrupted from their attachments and fall out.

- Compared with scurvy in adults, congenital scurvy and scurvy during early childhood have unique manifestations related to bony development. Scorbutic rosary[Q] (Fig. 27.16C) is a term given to the prominence of the costochondral junctions. Infants with scurvy develop 'frog legs' due to subperiosteal hemorrhage. Radiographs of the long bones reveal the classic white line of Frankel,[Q] which represents the abnormal calcification of the cartilage within the epiphysial-diaphysial juncture.

Breast milk contains adequate amounts of vitamin C, so infantile scurvy is more likely to occur in children who are not breastfed and are given a diet devoid of vitamin C.

Treatment: Therapy requires the replacement of vitamin C at a dosage of 300 to 500 mg daily until the symptoms resolve.

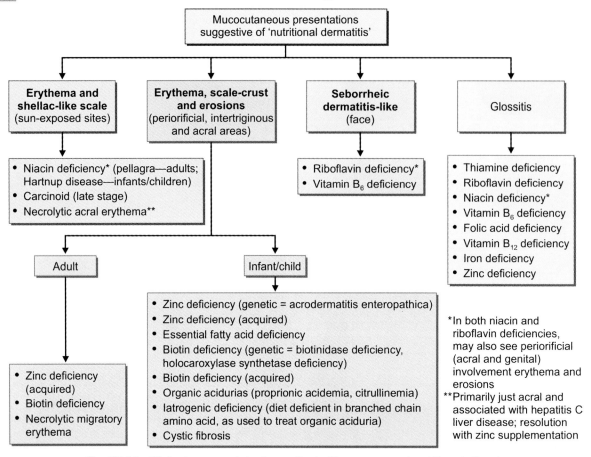

Fig. 27.17: Clinical approach to the patient with a presumed nutritional disorder

Vitamin D Deficiency

This is seen in children as rickets, with impeded growth and bone deformities. The ends of the ribs, where they join the costal cartilages, may become enlarged, giving rise to the 'rickety rosary.' In adults, osteomalacia is the result.

Vitamin D_3, is synthesized in skin by the action of light on 7-dehydrocholesterol. Though commonly believed, it is unlikely that sunscreens reduce vitamin D synthesis, and lead to increase the risk of fractures in the elderly.

Vitamin H (Biotin)

This is often prescribed for nail problems, but its exact role is unclear. Lack of biotin-dependent carboxylases may lead to periorificial dermatitis in infants, mimicking zinc deficiency.

Vitamin K

The most common deficiency is iatrogenic, produced by coumarin and leading to bruise ability and hemorrhage.

As most of the disorders can overlap in their manifestations, an approach is given in Fig. 27.17 to arrive at the likely diagnosis.

PRURITUS

Pruritus or itching is the most common cutaneous symptom. Patients with pruritus may complain of sleep loss or inability to concentrate. They may scratch or rub their skin inducing excoriations or even erosions and ulcers.

Diagnosis

1. The first step is to decide whether skin lesions are present or not (pruritus sine mareria). The common *skin disorders* are atopic dermatitis, lichen planus, arthropod assault, and urticaria.
2. When no skin findings are present, a systemic cause should be sought.
3. When no cutaneous or systemic disease is identified, the diagnosis is idiopathic pruritus, but one should still keep looking for a possible cause, which frequently is xerosis.

An approach to the diagnosis of pruritus is given in Fig. 27.18A.

Localized Pruritus

- Notalgia paresthetica[Q] is localized intrascapular pruritus, sometimes associated with sensory nerve entrapment. Damage to keratinocytes by chronic scratching may lead to localized amyloidosis.

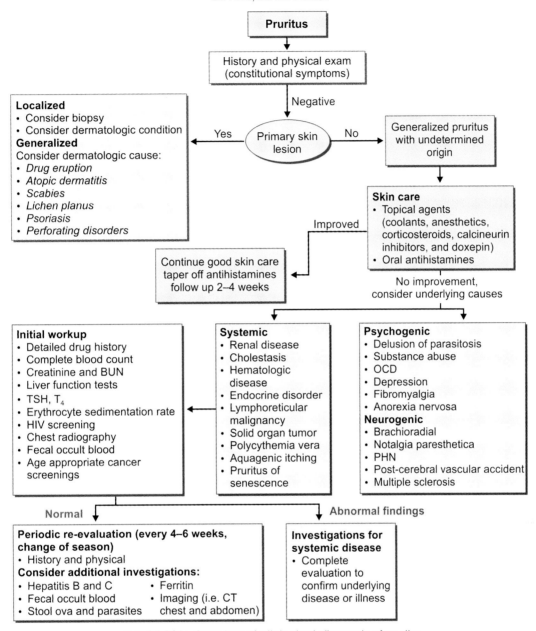

Fig. 27.18A: Overview of etiological diagnosis of pruritus

- Pruritus ani may also be caused by improper hygiene, pinworms, or ingestion of spicy foods.
- Both pruritus vulvae and scroti are more common in atopic patients, but usually have a significant psychological component and are difficult to treat.
- Both diabetes mellitus and iron deficiency may also play a role in anogenital pruritus.

Treatment

To manage pruritus effectively, it is necessary to identify the underlying etiology which requires a intensive relook at the patient's medical history focusing on the pruritus (Fig. 27.18A).

The initial treatment or first-line therapeutic approach for all patients should include good skin care as xerosis can contribute to severity of pruritus and

should always be included in the management of pruritus (Box 27.2).

If the underlying cause has not been identified, a stepwise approach should be initiated the overview of which is given in Fig. 27.18B.

Systemic Therapy

- Oral glucocorticoids should be limited to controlling acute severe forms of pruritus.
- Renal and neuropathic pruritus—gabapentin and pregabalin have been effective for treating pruritus caused by CKD as well as neuropathic pruritus. Also broad-spectrum UVB light and activated charcoal have been tried.
- Hepatic pruritus can be treated with ursodeoxycholic acid or cholestyramine.

First-line topical therapies
- Good skin care
- **Emollients**—petrolatum, ceramide-based creams, coconut oil
- **Cooling agents**—menthol, camphor, phenol
- **Topical anti-inflammatory**—corticosteroids, calcineurin inhibitors
- **Topical anesthetics**—capsaicin, pramoxine, lidocaine/prilocaine (use with caution)
- **Topical antihistamine**—doxepin

If little or no improvement, add

Systemic: Antihistamines
- **Low dose**—nonsedating drugs *daily*
- **High dose**—nonsedating drugs **bid–qid,** or combination with sedative drugs at bedtime

First-generation, sedative	**Second-generation, nonsedative**
Hydroxyzine	Cetrizine
Diphenhydramine	Levocetrizine
	Fexofenadine
	Loratidine
	Desloratidine

If little or no improvement

Other systemic agents

First choice	**Second choice**	**Third choice**
• Gabapentin	• Mirtazapine	• Naltrexone (especially
• Pregabalin	• Tricycline and tetracyclic	for renal or liver
• Selective serotonin reuptake	antidepressant	dysfunction)
inhibitors (SSRI), (paraneoplastic,	• Phototherapy: Narrow-	• Lidocaine 5% patch
polycythemia vera, or depression)	band UVB	

Fig. 27.18B: Treatment protocol for pruritus

Box 27.2 | Basic care of pruritic skin

- Avoid hot water.
- Bathe or shower in tepid/lukewarm water for 20 minutes.
- Avoid washing with soap. When cleanser is needed, use a gentile, nondrying, fragrance-free one. Use mild soap only on the under-arms, genitalia, and soles or the feet.
- Apply topical emollients/moisturizers immediately after bathing to skin that has been gently patted dry.
- Moisturizers with ceramides and lipids are preferred. If cost is an issue, petrolatum (petroleum jelly) may be used.
- Moisturize an additional one to two times daily. Apply gently in the direction of hair growth. *Caution:* Heavy emollients or occlusion can cause folliculitis.
- Topicals with menthol and camphor may be utilized. Refrigeration may aid in the calming effect.
- Avoid fragrance and dyes.

- Selective serotonin reuptake inhibitors have also been reported to be beneficial for various forms of chronic pruritus. Mirtazapine, a noradrenergic and specific serotonergic antidepressant, may relieve nocturnal itch.
- Tricyclic antidepressants are sometimes utilized despite randomized trials for pruritus.
- Opiate agonists and antagonist may also aid in relief of resistant chronic pruritus.

ARSENICOSIS

Arsenicosis is a chronic multi-system disorder arising out of high level of the metalloid arsenic (As) in body. It has been defined by the World Health Organization (WHO) working group as "a chronic health condition arising from prolonged ingestion (not less than six months) of arsenic above a safe dose, usually manifested by characteristic skin lesions, with or without involvement of internal organs."

Arsenicosis is a global problem but the magnitude of problem is mostly confined to Bangladesh, India (primarily the state of West Bengal), Argentina, Chile, Mexico, China/Taiwan, Mangolia and Thailand (in decreasing order of population affection).

The metalloid Arsenic can exist in four different valence states (–3, 0, +3 and +5) but the problem of arsenicosis originates from the uptake of trivalent (arsenite) and pentavalent (arsenate) forms. Drinking water is the chief source of arsenic intake and various geo-chemical processes, industrial pollution and agricultural source (pesticides) are responsible for its presence in ground water.

Chronic arsenicosis predominantly involves the skin in the form of pigmentary changes, hyperkeratosis, and skin cancers. Peripheral vascular disease (Blackfoot disease), non-cirrhotic portal hypertension, hepato-megaly, hepatic cirrhosis, peripheral neuropathy, respiratory and renal involvement hypertension, ischemic heart disease, bad obstetrical outcome, hematological disturbances (e.g. anemia), diabetes mellitus, etc. are also reported with chronic exposure to arsenic.

The pigmentary change can take the form of diffuse pigmentation, fine freckle-like spotty pigmentation (*rain-drop pigmentation*) or macular areas of depigmentation on normal/hyperpigmented skin (*leukomelanosis*) (Fig. 27.19). Mucous membrane (undersurface of the tongue or buccal mucosa) may also involved by blotchy pigmentation. Arsenical hyperkeratosis symmetrically affects the palms and soles and can range from minute papules (<2 mm) giving gritty sensation (*mild*), punctuate, wart-like papule of 2–5 mm (*moderate*) or diffuse hyperkeratosis (*severe*) (Fig. 27.20). Malignant changes are the major cause of morbidity and mortality associated with chronic arsenicosis and involves skin (Bowen's disease, squamous cell carcinoma, and basal cell epithelioma) (Figs 27.20 and 27.21), lung, bladder, kidney, prostate, liver, uterus, and sometimes lymphatic tissues.

Diagnosis of chronic arsenics relies mostly of classical clinical manifestations (clinically confirmed) and if

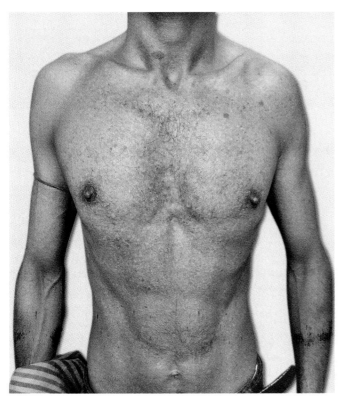

Fig. 27.19: Dispigmentation of chronic arsenicosis (leuko-melanosis)

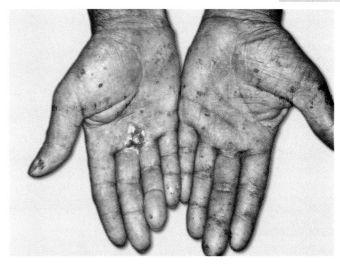

Fig. 27.20: Arsenical keratosis symmetrically affecting the palms with malignant change (squamous cell carcinoma arising over the keratotic lesion causing ulceration)

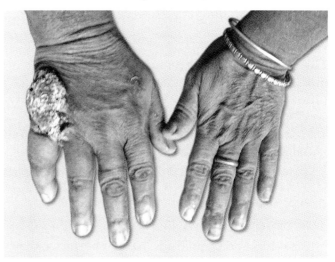

Fig. 27.21: Squamous cell carcinoma in a case of chronic arsenicosis

infrastructure permits, then further confirmed by arsenic estimation in hair (>1 mg/kg of dry hair), nail (>1.5 mg/kg of nail) and drinking water (>10 µg/L by WHO guideline).

Management of chronic arsenicosis depends primarily on prevention and symptomatic management; since there is no established therapy for the condition available yet. Cessation of exposure to arsenic contami-nated water, removing arsenic from the contaminated water and administration of nutritional supplement are the preventive modalities available to fight the menace. Deep wells, traditional dug wells (mordenized as applicable), treatment of surface water (arsenic removal unit) and rain-water harvesting are the methods of obtaining arsenic-free safe water. Counselling and edu-cation to those residing in areas having arsenic in ground water about the hazard is of paramount importance.

27

Genetic Disorders of Skin

ICHTHYOSES

The ichthyoses (ichthys = fish) are widespread disorders featuring prominent scales. There are many different types with varying pathogenesis and clinical features. These are of two main types:

1. Defects in keratin or intercellular substances (lipids, filaggrin) limited to the skin.
2. Metabolic disease with involvement of other organs.

Congenital

Ichthyosis Vulgaris

This is the most common^Q ichthyosis, with an incidence of 1:300 (AD).

Clinical features: There is a defect in filaggrin,^{Q} so scales are retained (retention hyperkeratosis). It appears during the first year of life. Patients have diffuse pale polygonal scales, typically sparing the flexural areas; it is often associated with atopic dermatitis (Fig. 28.1).

X-Linked Ichthyosis

This only occurs in **males**.^{Q}
    The defect is in steroid sulfatase.

Clinical features: Patients have **dirty thick scales** and also corneal defects (50%) and cryptorchidism (20%). It is associated with steroid sulfatase deficiency and premature delivery in carrier females (Fig. 28.2).

Lamellar Ichthyosis

There are several forms, with mutations in transglutaminase, lipoxygenase, and other genes. The most common type is inherited in an autosomal-recessive

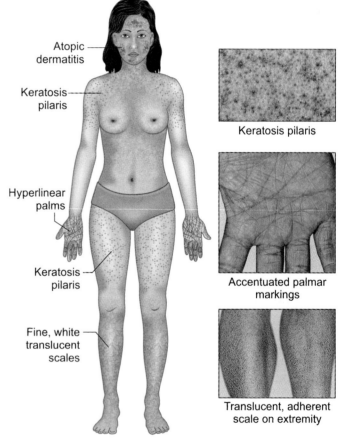

Atopic dermatitis

Keratosis pilaris

Hyperlinear palms

Keratosis pilaris

Fine, white translucent scales

Keratosis pilaris

Accentuated palmar markings

Translucent, adherent scale on extremity

Fig. 28.1: Fine, white, adherent scale in ichthyosis vulgaris in depiction of the features of ichthyosis vulgaris

manner with mutation in transglutaminase and thus a defect in the cornified envelope.

Clinical features: It is likely to present as collodion baby^Q with large sheets of scales and fissures at birth (Fig. 28.3A). The **flexures**, face, and scalp are generally

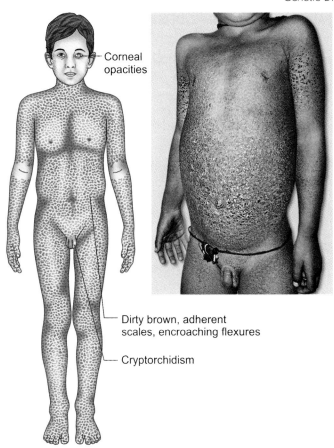

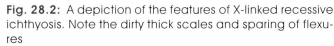

Fig. 28.2: A depiction of the features of X-linked recessive ichthyosis. Note the dirty thick scales and sparing of flexures

involved. There is also a risk of ectropion and sweat gland occlusion, causing heat intolerance (Fig. 28.3B). Some collodion babies resolve entirely.

Harlequin Ichthyosis

Extremely thick armor-like scales are present at birth and it is often fatal in infancy. There is a massive defect in keratinization caused by mutations in ABCA 12, an ATP-binding cassette protein (Fig. 28.4).

Congenital Ichthyosiform Erythroderma (CIE)

Autosomal recessive; mutation in transglutaminase gene.

Clinical features: Collodion baby at birth.

After infancy: Generalized erythroderma with fine, white scale, flexures involved (Fig. 28.5); extensor legs. with large, platelike, dark scale; palmoplantar keratoderma; hypohidrosis with heat intolerance.

Congenital Bullous Ichthyosiform Erythroderma (BIE)

Caused by mutations in keratins 1 or 10, inherited in autosomal dominant fashion.

Clinical features: Patients have bullae at birth, later develop thick scales and spiny hyperkeratoses; increased in flexures (Fig. 28.6).

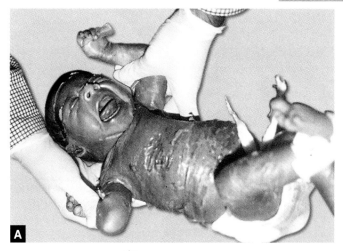

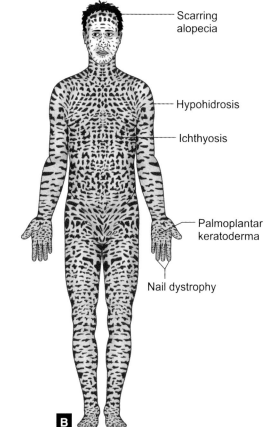

Fig. 28.3A and B: (A) Collodion baby with a translucent membrane encasing the body; (B) Depiction of lamellar ichthyosis

Clumps of keratin with vacuolar degeneration produce the typical histologic picture (epidermolytic hyperkeratosis)[Q].

Therapy

There is no curative therapy available:

Topical: Keratolytic agents (lactic acid 5–10%), humectants (urea 5–12%), or lubrication.

Systemic: Systemic retinoids are helpful for severe cases, but are required for life.

28

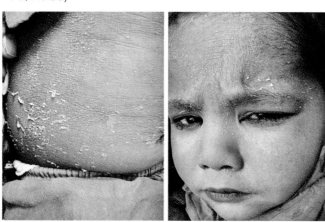

Fig. 28.4: Harlequin ichthyosis: Massive hyperkeratotic plates with deep fissures encasing a newborn (*Courtesy*: Dr Bharat M Tiwari, ESIC, Noida)

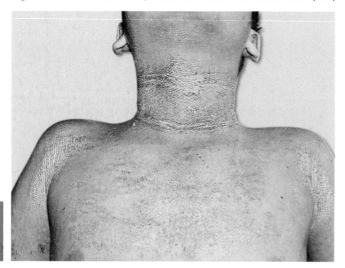

Fig. 28.5: Generalized erythroderma with fine, white scale (CIE)

Fig. 28.6: Dark, warty scales with spiny ridges, pronounced in the flexures; BIE

Acquired Ichthyoses

Caused by drugs interfering with lipid metabolism (nicotinic acid), underlying tumors (myeloproliferative malignancies), sarcoidosis, and malnutrition.

PALMOPLANTAR KERATODERMAS

These are disorders with mutations in keratin or other genes expressed in the palmoplantar skin.

Vörner Type

This type is the most common; it is caused by mutations in keratin 1 or 9, the main components of the palmoplantar stratum corneum.

Clinical features: Patients have thick noninflamed plaques that do not extend onto the lateral aspects of the extremities (Fig. 28.7A and B).

Histology shows epidermolytic hyperkeratosis.

Greither Type

This is a classic (AD) transgrediens type with gradual progression from the palms of the hands and soles of the feet to the sides and backs of the hands and feet, as well as the ankles, knees, and elbows.

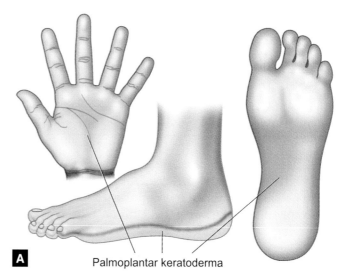

A   Palmoplantar keratoderma

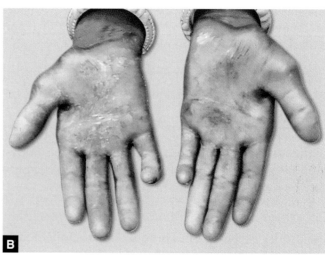

B

Fig. 28.7A and B: (A) Diffuse bilateral, symmetric hyperkeratosis of palms and soles with white-yellow hue; well-demarcated with erythematous border; (B) Diffuse thickening of palms with early contractures of the fifth finger

Mal de Meleda

It is caused by mutations in SWRP1.

Patients are most commonly from an isolated population on the Adriatic island Meleda; it is a transgrediens type of keratoderma, with neonatal erythema, then hyperkeratosis, hyperhidrosis, and nail dystrophies. There is sometimes perioral and perinasal disease.

DYSKERATOTIC-ACANTHOLYTIC DISORDERS

Two disorders are important with abnormal keratinization (dyskeratosis) and loss of adhesion between keratinocytes (acantholysis). Hailey-Hailey disease has been discussed in Chapter 18.

Darier's Disease

Mutation in the ATP2A2 gene, coding for a calcium pump protein. It is inherited in autosomal dominant fashion.

Clinical features: The presentation is pruritic brown follicular plugs that are most common in seborrheic areas, warty papules of the hands (acrokeratosis verruciformis), dystrophic nails (alternating red or white bands), and cobblestoning of the oral mucosa (Fig. 28.8A and B).

Patients are susceptible to secondary infections, such as widespread herpes simplex. It is also worsened by ultraviolet (UV) light.

Histopathology: Dyskeratosis with modest acantholysis; a hallmark is individual cell keratinization (corps ronds and grains).

Therapy: Topical or systemic retinoids, disinfectants or antibiotics for secondary infections.

MOSAICISM

Definition: A mosaic is an organism with genetically different populations of cells arising from a homogenous zygote. In contrast, a chimera results when two genetically different zygotes fuse.

Pathogenesis: While mosaicism can involve any organ. It is especially easy to see in the skin. When mutations occur in the 8–32-cell embryo, a somatic mosaic results.

When such mutations the genes that are important in skin differentiation, a mosaic pattern following Blaschko lines results. These lines reflect the distortions that occur as a round early embryo is converted into a human form. The best examples are epidermal nevi (Fig. 28.9).

- **Epigenetic mosaicism:** All females are epigenetic mosaics because of the Lyon hypothesis and random inactivation of one X chromosome.
- Often, a mutation may be fatal in males but, because of mosaicism, is compatible with life in a female.

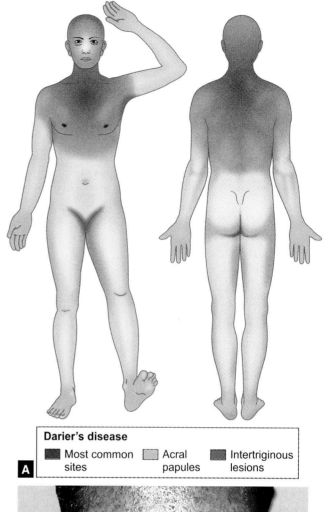

Darier's disease
- Most common sites
- Acral papules
- Intertriginous lesions

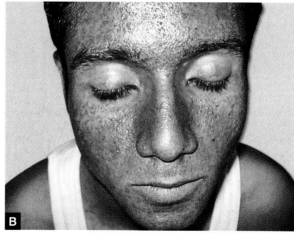

Fig. 28.8A and B: (A) A depiction of the distribution of lesions in Darier's disease; (B) Greasy papules on the face

Congenital

Incontinentia pigmenti

X-linked dominant^Q

This is caused by a mutation in the NEMO (nuclear factor xB essential modulator) gene which controls apoptosis. It presents at birth and goes through four stages (Fig. 28.10):
- Vesicular: Linear vesicles rich in eosinophils
- Verrucous: Verrucous lesions

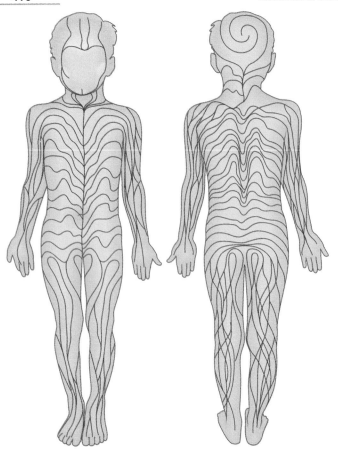

Lines of Blaschko. Epidermal nevi often follow these embryological lines.

Fig. 28.9: Blaschko's lines

- Hyperpigmented postinflammatory hyperpigmentation
- Hypopigmented atrophic scars, especially on legs.

Patients may have dental, ocular, and central nervous system (CNS) problems.

Pigmentary Mosaicism (*Hypomelanosis of Ito*)

Hypopigmentation along Blaschko lines with a variety of systemic defects, depending on the nature of mosaic.

Acquired Dermatoses

Some acquired dermatoses are linear and appear to follow Blaschko lines. One explanation might be a silent mosaic, with a population of cells that are capable of reacting to a stimulus (infection, trauma) differently from the rest of the body.

- *Lichen stratus*^{Q}: This usually occurs in children, with linear lichenoid papules usually running down the limb; it appears suddenly, and resolves spontaneously. It may be confused with epidermal nevus or linear lichen planus. Usually no therapy is needed; if pruritic, topical corticosteroids are used.
- *Others*: Linear psoriasis, linear lichen planus, linear porokeratosis, and linear atrophoderma are all examples of possible mosaicism.

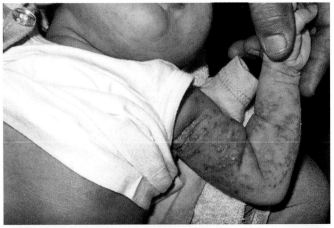

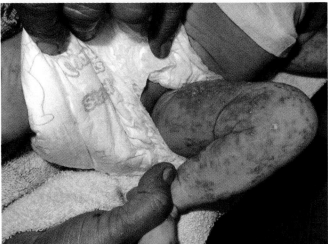

Fig. 28.10: Stage I vesicular (birth to 1 to 2 weeks): Vesicles and bullae in a linear arrangement on extremities

NEUROCUTANEOUS SYNDROMES

Neurofibromatosis

There are several variants of neurofibromatosis (NF); we will only discuss NF1 (von Recklinghausen's disease).

> Neurofibromatosis type 2: AD; cutaneous and bilateral vestibular schwannomas; meningiomas, spinal tumors; NF2 gene, chromosome 22.^{Q}

Epidemiology: Common; prevalence 4:10 000.

Pathogenesis: Inherited in an autosomal dominant^Q fashion; caused by mutations in neurofibromin^Q which controls cell growth chromosome 17.^{Q}

Clinical features: The NIH diagnostic criteria for NF1 (Table 28.1) are met in 97% of patients by age 8 years. The salient features are depicted in Fig. 28.11A.

Cutaneous Findings

1. **Café au lait macules (CALMs)**^{Q}
   - (>90%; often evident within first year of life)
   - Most patients have ≥6 by early childhood (Fig. 28.11B)

28

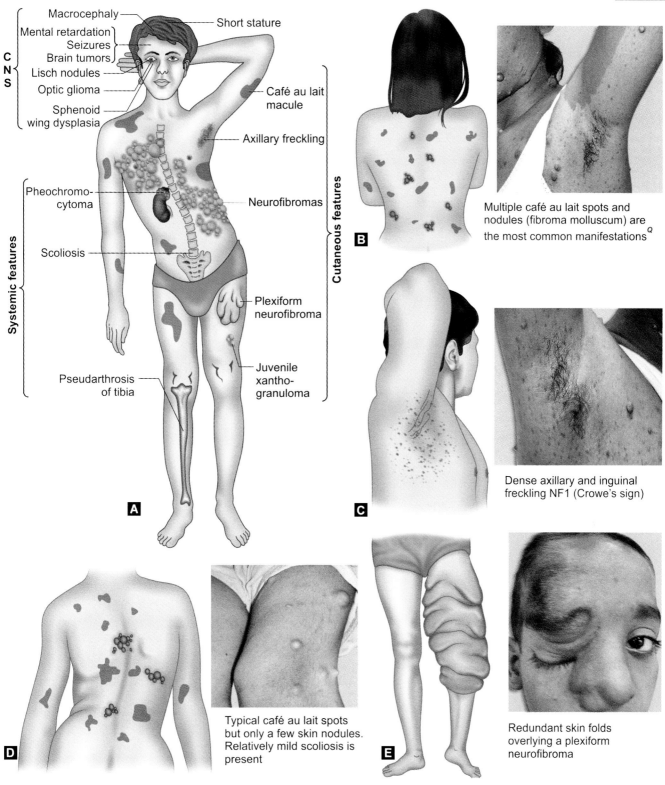

Fig. 28.11A to E: (A) A depiction of the manifestations of neurofibromatosis; (B) Café au lait macule; (C) Axillary freckling–Crowe's sign; (D) A depiction of neurofiromas; (E) Plexiform neurofibroma

- Also can be seen in McCune-Albright syndrome, Noonan syndrome, LEOPARD syndrome, TSC, idiopathic.

2. Axillary and/or inguinal freckling (Crowe's sign):[Q] ~80%; usually present by 4–6 years of age (Fig. 28.11C).

3. Cutaneous neurofibromas
- 70–90%; typically begin to appear around puberty
- Skin-colored to pink-tan, soft papulonodules that invaginate with gentle pressure ('buttonhole' sign)[Q] (Fig. 28.11D).

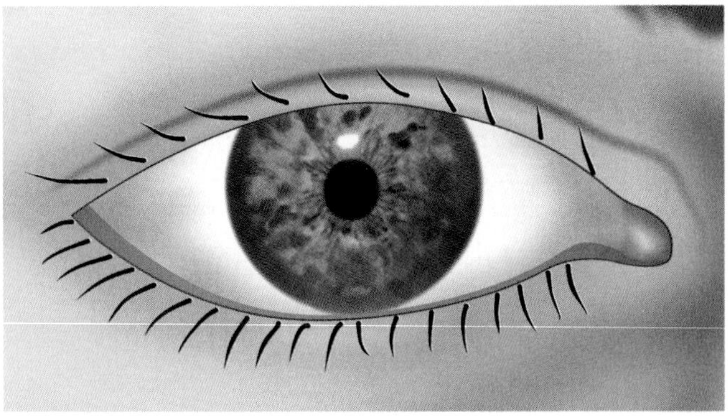

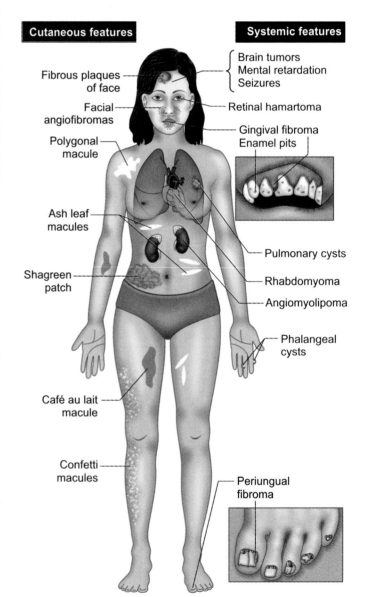

Fig. 28.11F: Lisch nodules are hamartomas of the iris. They are raised and frequently pigmented

Table 28.1	Diagnostic criteria for neurofibromatosis type 1 (NF1)

Two or more of the following must be present:
- Six or more café au lait macules (>5 mm, if prepubertal; >15 mm, if postpubertal[Q])
- Two or more neurofibromas of any type or one plexiform neurofibroma
- 'Freckling' in the axillary or inguinal regions
- Optic gliomas
- Two or more Lisch nodules[Q]
- Typical osseous lession, e.g. sphenoid wing dysplasia, thinning of long bone cortex ± pseudarthrosis
- First-degree relative (parent, sibling, or offspring) with NF1 by the above criteria.

4. **Plexiform neurofibromas (PNF)**
   - 25%; congenital origin, enlarge during first 4–5 years of life.
   - Deeper nodules or masses resembling a 'bag of worms' upon palpation[Q] (Fig. 28.11E).

Systemic: The major findings are depicted in Fig. 28.11A.

Ocular lesions: Lisch nodules (iris hamartomas)[Q] (Fig. 28.11F):
- >90% by 20 years of age; begin to appear at ~3 years of age.
- Hypertension (~30%) essential > from renal artery stenosis (~2%) or pheochromocytoma (1%).

Complications

Optic glioma: Acoustic neuroma, learning deficits, malignant peripheral nerve sheath tumors, hypertension, pheochromocytoma.

Therapy

Genetic counseling: Antihistamines for pruritus, individual lesions excised, dose attention to complications.

Tuberous Sclerosis

Also known as Bourneville-Pringle disease.[Q]

Epidemiology: Common; prevalence 1:10 000.

Pathogenesis: Inherited in an autosomal dominant fashion; caused by mutations in two different tumor suppressor genes (hamartin and tuberin).

These genes regulate the **m**ammalian **t**arget **of r**apamycin (mTOR) pathway that promotes cell growth.

Clinical features: Characteristic skin findings include (Fig. 28.12A):
- Ash leaf macules—depigmented[Q] ellipsoid macules (Fig. 28.12B) present at birth.
- Collagenoma[Q] connective tissue nevi—pebbly plaque on the back (shagreen patch[Q]); also facial plaques (Fig. 28.12B).

Fig. 28.12A: A depiction of the manifestation of tuberous sclerosis

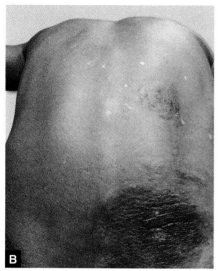
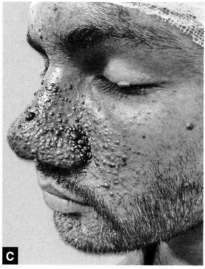
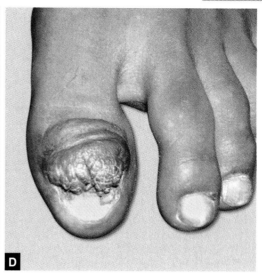

Fig. 28.12B to D: (B) Ash leaf macules with a shagreen patch; (C) Adenoma sebaceum and (D) Koenen's tumor

- Angiofibromas[Q]—multiple facial papules concentrated about the nose, erroneously called adenoma sebaceum;[Q] the periungual version is known as Koenen's tumor[Q] (Fig. 28.12C and D).

> Multiple facial angiofibromas can occur in multiple endocrine neoplasia type 1 (MEN1) and Birt-Hogg-Dubé syndrome.

- *CNS*: Subependymal nodules or cortical tubers (found in ≥80% of TS patients <2 years of age). MRI is more sensitive than CT for tubers
- *Eye*: Retinal hamartomas or achromic patches

The criterion of diagnosis is listed in Table 28.2.

Complications: Systemic problems are protean but a major concern is CNS involvement with seizures and mental retardation.[Q] Other complications are renal angiomyolipomas, cardiac rhabdomyomas with conduction defects, and pulmonary lymphangiomas.

Therapy: Genetic counseling. Anticonvulsants as needed; facial lesions can be laser ablated; regular imaging to monitor for systemic tumors.

Systemic administration of mTOR inhibitors (rapamycin or sirolimus, everolimus)[Q] for astrocytomas, renal angiomyolipomas, and pulmonary lymphangioleiomyomas; topical rapamycin, lasers (pulsed dye or ablative), and electrosurgery to treat angiofibromas.

LIGHT-SENSITIVE GENODERMATOSES

Porphyria

Porphyria is a group of diseases characterized by defects in hemoglobin metabolism and clinically presenting with varying degrees of photosensitivity and neuropsychiatric problems (Fig. 28.13A).

Table 28.2	Revised diagnostic criteria for tuberous sclerosis complex
Major features	
Cutaneous	• Hypomelanotic macules (≥3, each ≥5 mm in diameter) (≥90%) • Facial angiofibromas (≥3) (~80%) or fibrous cephalic plaque (~20%) • Nontraumatic ungual fibromas (≥2) (30–60%) • Shagreen patch (40–50%)
Systemic	• Eye: Multiple retinal nodular hamartomas (~40%) • CNS: Cortical dysplasias (>90%), subependymal nodules (>80%), subependymal giant cell astrocytoma • Renal: Angiomyolipomas (≥2) (75–90%) • CVS: Cardiac rhabdomyoma (~80% during infancy, with subsequent involution) • Lung: Pulmonary lymphangioleiomyomatosis (~30% of women)
Minor features	
Cutaneous	'Confetti' hypopigmented skin lesions (~5%)
Systemic	• Dental enamel pits (≥3) (>90%) • Intraoral fibromas (≥2) (up to 70%) • Retinal achromic patch (~40%) • Multiple renal cysts • Nonrenal hamartomas

Definite clinical diagnosis: Either two major features or one major feature plus two minor features.
Possible clinical diagnosis: One major feature or two minor features.
Definite genetic diagnosis: Identification of a pathogenic mutation in either TSC1 or TSC2 in DNA from normal tissue.

Pathogenesis

Acute attacks of porphyria are a life-threatening emergency. They are triggered by drugs, alcohol, hormones, diet, and infections, but often unexplained. Photosensitivity is caused by the ability of many

28

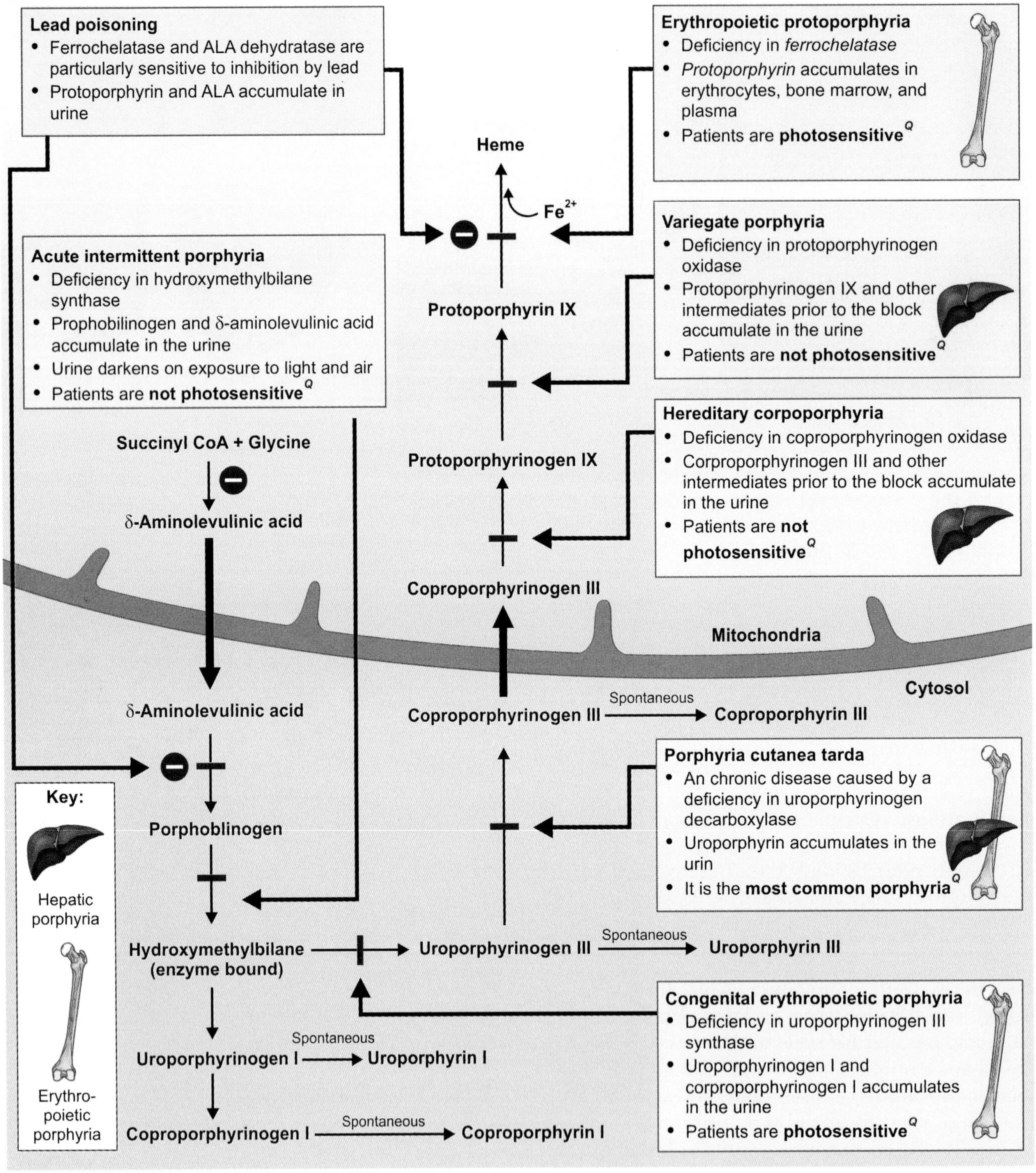

Lead poisoning
- Ferrochelatase and ALA dehydratase are particularly sensitive to inhibition by lead
- Protoporphyrin and ALA accumulate in urine

Erythropoietic protoporphyria
- Deficiency in *ferrochelatase*
- *Protoporphyrin* accumulates in erythrocytes, bone marrow, and plasma
- Patients are **photosensitive**[Q]

Acute intermittent porphyria
- Deficiency in hydroxymethylbilane synthase
- Prophobilinogen and δ-aminolevulinic acid accumulate in the urine
- Urine darkens on exposure to light and air
- Patients are **not photosensitive**[Q]

Heme

Fe^{2+}

Protoporphyrin IX

Variegate porphyria
- Deficiency in protoporphyrinogen oxidase
- Protoporphyrinogen IX and other intermediates prior to the block accumulate in the urine
- Patients are **not photosensitive**[Q]

Protoporphyrinogen IX

Hereditary corpoporphyria
- Deficiency in coproporphyrinogen oxidase
- Corproporphyrinogen III and other intermediates prior to the block accumulate in the urine
- Patients are **not photosensitive**[Q]

Succinyl CoA + Glycine

δ-Aminolevulinic acid

Coproporphyrinogen III

Mitochondria

δ-Aminolevulinic acid

Coproporphyrinogen III — Spontaneous → Coproporphyrin III

Cytosol

Key:

Hepatic porphyria

Porphoblinogen

Porphyria cutanea tarda
- An chronic disease caused by a deficiency in uroporphyrinogen decarboxylase
- Uroporphyrin accumulates in the urin
- It is the **most common porphyria**[Q]

Hydroxymethylbilane (enzyme bound) —→ Uroporphyrinogen III — Spontaneous → Uroporphyrin III

Erythro-poietic porphyria

Uroporphyrinogen I — Spontaneous → Uroporphyrin I

Coproporphyrinogen I — Spontaneous → Coproporphyrin I

Congenital erythropoietic porphyria
- Deficiency in uroporphyrinogen III synthase
- Uroporphyrinogen I and corproporphyrinogen I accumulates in the urine
- Patients are **photosensitive**[Q]

Fig. 28.13A: A depiction of the enzymatic defects that determine porphyria subtypes

porphyrins to absorb 408 nm ultraviolet (UV) light in the skin (Soret Band).[Q]

Pseudoporphyria refers to patients who clinically resemble porphyria patients but have normal porphyrin levels. Patients with chronic renal disease, often on dialysis, develop lesions on their hands that resemble porphyria, but have normal porphyrin values. Some patients with epidermolysis bullosa acquisita may also mimic porphyria.

Porphyria Cutanea Tarda (PCT)

Inheritance/enzyme defect: AD (familial form) or acquired. Uroporphyrinogen decarboxylase (UD).

*PCT-**UD**: **U**rine **D**azzles pink (fluorescence with Wood's light)*

Clinical features: This is the most common form.[Q] Presents with photosensitivity, fragile skin, milia and blisters on the backs of hands, hirsutism, scleroderma-like changes and facial hyperpigmentation[Q] (Fig. 28.13B and C).

There is often a history of alcoholism, hepatitis C infection, HIV or hormone use.

Treatment: Treated with blood letting (phlebotomy) or low-dose antimalarials.

> Hepatoerythropoietic porphyria—a variant of PCT presenting in childhood with more severe photosensitivity.

Acute Intermittent Porphyria (AIP)

Inheritance/enzyme defect: AD, porphobilinogen deaminase (PBD).

AIP-PBD: Abdomen Is Painful, Progesterone Barbiturates Drugs

Clinical features: No cutaneous findings; only neuro-psychiatric emergencies with nausea, vomiting, and poorly explained signs like paralysis or severe unexplained pain, which are often misdiagnosed (Fig. 28.13C).

Triggers[Q]: Drugs (barbiturates, sulfonamides, griseofulvin), stress, fasting, alcohol, hormonal changes (progesterone) and infection.

Treatment: Remove trigger, glucose loading, hematin infusion.

> Variegate porphyria and coproporphyria combine features of PCT and AIP.

Erythropoietic Protoporphyria

Inheritance/enzyme defect: AD, ferrochelatase.

Clinical features: Photosensitivity, and often solar urticaria, in childhood. Later there is typical waxy or cobblestone scarring on the nose and dorsal hands.

Systemic: Gallstones, hepatic damage (Fig. 28.13D).

Treatment: UVA blockers and beta-carotene (must take enough to get discolored skin: 120–180 mg daily).

Congenital Erythropoietic Porphyria

Inheritance/enzyme defect: AR, uroporphyrinogen III cosynthase.

CEP: Colorless (anemia), Erythrodontia, Photosensitivity
UTC (uro three cosynthase): Ur Teeth r Colored

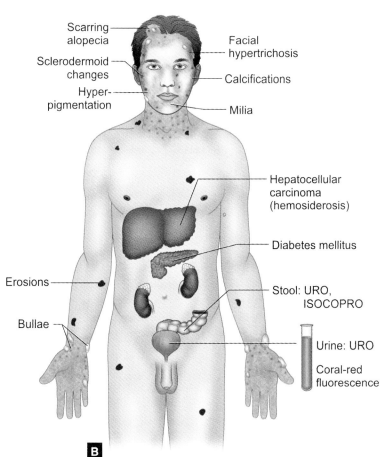

Scarring alopecia
Sclerodermoid changes
Hyper-pigmentation
Facial hypertrichosis
Calcifications
Milia
Hepatocellular carcinoma (hemosiderosis)
Diabetes mellitus
Erosions
Bullae
Stool: URO, ISOCOPRO
Urine: URO
Coral-red fluorescence

B

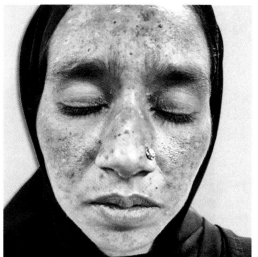

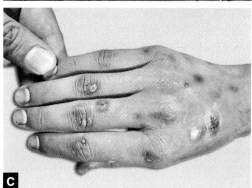

C

Fig. 28.13B and C: (B) A depiction of the manifestaions of porphyria cutanea tarda; (C) Small vesicles and healed lesions on the face and exposed aspects of the hand in PCT

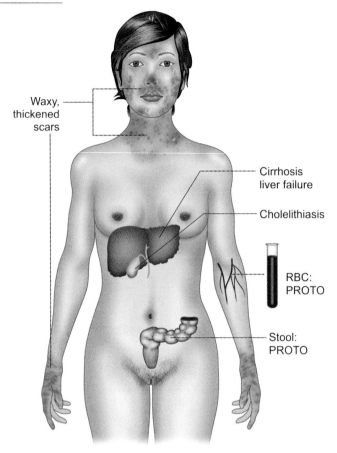

Fig. 28.13D: A depiction of the manifestations of EPP

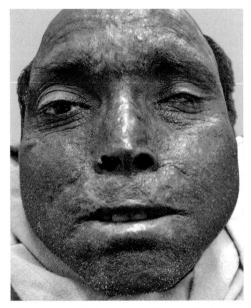

Fig. 28.13E: CEP—mutilated scarred face, with deformed nose, hyper- and hypopigmentation and sclerodermoid changes

Clinical features: Probably represents the were wolves of legend.

Patients have extreme photosensitivity mandating night-time activity, as well as blisters with marked scarring, hirsutism, and even fluorescent teeth (erythrodontia), hemolysis, red urine (stains diapers) (Fig. 28.13E).

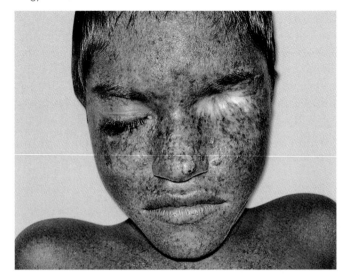

Fig. 28.14: Pigmented macules, achromic macules, dry, scaly, atrophic skin, actinic keratosis with surgical excision of damaged left eye in a case of XP

Treatment: Light avoidance, transfusions for anemia, ± bone marrow transplantation (BMT), ± splenectomy.

Xeroderma Pigmentosum (XP)

Inheritance/defect: AR,^{Q} due to defect in DNA repair.^{Q}

Seven complementation groups (A–G) and one XP variant described, each encoding different proteins in the nucleotide excision repair (NER) pathway (except XP variant).

Clinical features: Presents with marked photosensitivity,^{Q} early onset of all major skin malignancies, exaggerated sunburn following minimal sun exposure, solar lentigines by age of 2, ocular abnormalities (photophobia, keratitis, corneal opacification, vascularization), neurologic abnormalities (progressive deafness) (Fig. 28.14).
- XP variant (mutation in DNA polymerase): No neurologic abnormalities.
- De Sanctis-Cacchione syndrome: Severe neurologic abnormalities (MR, deafness, ataxia).

Differential diagnosis: There are some overlaps with Cockayne syndrome and trichothiodystrophy, which involve the same genes, but have no increased risk of skin cancer. Other childhood diseases with photosensitivity include erythropoietic protoporphyria, Bloom syndrome, and Hartnup syndrome.

Therapy: The mainstay is absolute sun avoidance, becoming night people, and maximum protection sunscreens. Actinic keratoses are treated with topical 5-fluorouracil or imiquimod. Monitoring and prompt excision of tumors is essential. Routine ophthalmologic care is also important bacterial DNA repair enzyme in a topical liposome-containing preparation may reduce the number of new actinic keratoses and basal cell carcinomas.

28

Skin Disorders due to Light

These are skin disorders caused or exacerbated by exposure to light.

PHOTOBIOLOGY

Almost all cutaneous light reactions are caused by UV radiation of wavelength 290–400 nm (Fig. 29.1).

UVC (<290 nm): Shorter wavelengths are filtered out by the atmosphere.[Q]

UVB (290–320 nm): The B wavelengths (UVB) cause sunburn and carcinogenic and are effectively screened out by window glass.[Q]

UVA (320–400 nm): This penetrates more deeply, and is most responsible for skin aging;[Q] it passes through window glass, causes most photo-induced drug reactions and may promote skin cancers (Fig. 29.1).

Depth of penetration (Fig. 29.2): It depends on wavelength; the longer wavelengths penetrate deeper. Virtually, all of the UVB is absorbed in the epidermis, whereas some 30% of UVA reaches the dermis. The UVA reaches deeper into the dermis, while lasers designed to selectively reach and interact with dermal vessels or pigment are all in the visible light spectrum or longer.

UV protection: The main natural protective agent is melanin. In addition, the stratum corneum provides protection. Appropriate clothing and sunscreens are the best additional protections, along with avoidance.

Sunscreens: Sunscreens can either be blockers, simply reflecting sunlight or active chemicals that absorb solar radiation. The individual chemical sunscreens tend to be more effective in either the UVA or UVB range so a combination is usually needed. Solar protection factor[Q]

(SPF) gives a rough guide to the degree of protection;[Q] SPF of 20 suggests that someone who can normally stay in the noonday sun for 15 minutes can now stay for 300 minutes. In Indian skin, an SPF of 25 is sufficient for protection due to the natural melanin.

Though in the tropics the skin is adapted to sunlight, for those who are fair skinned, have photodermatoses or history of ageing, preventive measures (reducing exposure to UVR) are advisable and a list of such measures is given in Table 29.1.

Advantages of Sunlight

The kind of pigmented skin varies across geographical borders and it must be emphasized that the rich pigment in Indian skin is a effective protection against carcinogenesis and thus the use of 'fairness creams' in Indian skin is an attempt to play against nature's

Table 29.1	Advise for basic protection against UV light

- Apply sunscreen daily to all exposed parts—usually in a normal environment, reapply every 4 hours.
- Do not leave areas as SPF calculations are based on 2 mg/cm² coverage. Most people underuse.
- Use a sunscreen with a protective factor (SPF) of at least 15, preferably 30.
- Choose a sunscreen that screens out both UVA and UVB.
- Wear wide-brimmed hats.
- Wear dense weave clothing. If you can see through it, it is not protective.
- Target outdoor activities for early morning or late afternoon (avoid sun between 11 am and 3 pm).
- Wear cosmetics, including lipstick.
- Advise similar protection measures for children.

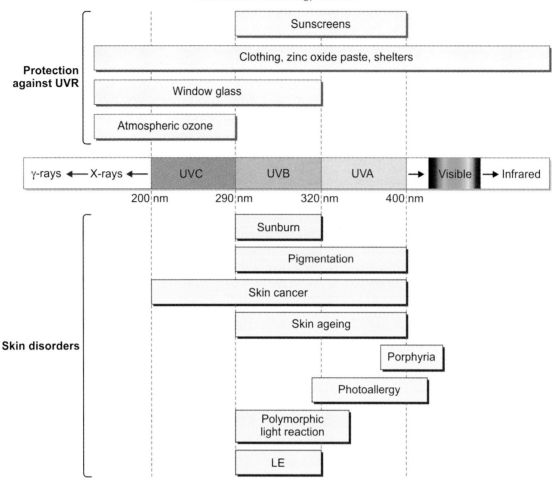

Fig. 29.1: Spectrum of light and their effect on the skin and the various protective UVR factors

Photodermatoses

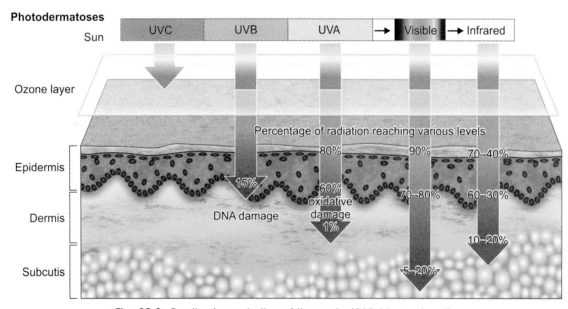

Fig. 29.2: Depth of penetration of the major UV light wavelengths

mechanism of skin protection and thus invariably fails to have a lasting effect. Thus though we need a pale enough skin to synthesise vitamin D, our skin also needs enough eumelanin to protect from carcinogenesis and neural tube defect-inducing folate destruction.

Observational studies show that subjects with high levels of circulating vitamin D are less likely to have cardiovascular disease, hypertension, type 2 diabetes, multiple sclerosis and rickets than those with low levels. A newly identified alternative

Table 29.2	Fitzpatrick skin types	
Type	Definition	Description
I	Always burns but nerver tans	Pale skin, red hair, freckles
II	Usually burns, sometimes tans	Fair skin
III	May burn, usually tans	Darker skin
IV	Rarely burns, always tans	Mediterranean
V	Moderate constitutional pigmentation	Latin American, middle eastern
VI	Marked constitutional pigmentation	Black

mechanism is mediated by the vasodilator nitric oxide. The skin contains large stores of nitrate and nitrite, which are converted by sunlight to the nitric oxide from where it enters the circulation and lowers blood pressure.

The skin types are detailed in Table 29.2 and Indian skin types vary from types I to VI.

CUTANEOUS EFFECTS OF UVR EXPOSURE

Acute

The visible short-term effects of UVR include:
- Sunburn and tanning: Tanning occurs as a biphasic response:
  - 'Immediate pigment darkening' occurs during and immediately after exposure and is most prominent with UVA (Meirowsky phenomenon)[Q]
  - 'Delayed tanning' persistent pigment darkening usually results from UVB[Q] exposure and peaks about 3 days
- Vitamin D synthesis
- Epidermal hyperplasia
- Proinflammatory responses
- Immunosuppression.

Sunburn

This is defined as acute sun damage to skin, caused primarily by UVB.[Q]

Lack of natural protection (no tan), excessive exposure, reflecting surfaces (water, sand, snow), altitude (degree of filtration of light), and latitude (angle of light) all play a role.

When UVB penetrates the epidermis and superficial dermis, it tends to stimulate the production and release of prostaglandins, leukotrienes, histamine, interleukin-1 (IL-1) and tumor necrosis factor-α (TNF-α). These cause pain and stimulate the production of the inducible nitric oxide synthase (iNOS) enzyme. This generates very high local inflammation.

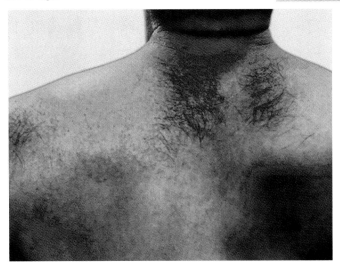

Fig. 29.3: A patient with an acute sunburn involving the upper back following exposure to sunlight while on a beach holiday

Clinical features: There are painful, *sharply demarcated* areas of erythema limited to areas of sun exposure (Fig. 29.3.); if severe, blister formation; later, peeling. The redness is maximal after 1 day, which parallel the peak levels of the iNOS enzyme, and then settle over the next 2–3 days. A widespread blistering sunburn is comparable to a second-degree burn and requires similar treatment.

Histology: Apoptotic keratinocytes (sunburn cells),[Q] widened vessels, marked edema, lymphocytic infiltrate.

Therapy: Immediate use of NSAIDs[Q] may help. Lubricate the skin and await natural healing. Potent topical corticosteroids can be used early and briefly. Oral aspirin (a prostaglandin synthesis inhibitor) relieves the pain.

Chronic Effects

UV is the single most important environmental hazard for humans. It is responsible for almost all extrinsic aging. DNA damage and elastosis, as well as many skin cancers, although genetic and other environmental factors also play a role. The effects tend to be cumulative over many years (Fig. 29.1).

SUNLIGHT-INDUCED SKIN DISEASES

Some patients react to UV exposure in an abnormal way leading to disorders which are listed in Table 29.3.

Phototoxic and Photoallergic Reactions

An interaction of light and certain topical or systemic agents can lead to an enhanced reaction to UV light. The clinical distribution of the dermatoses is depicted below, and depends largely on the clothing of the patient (Fig. 29.4).

29

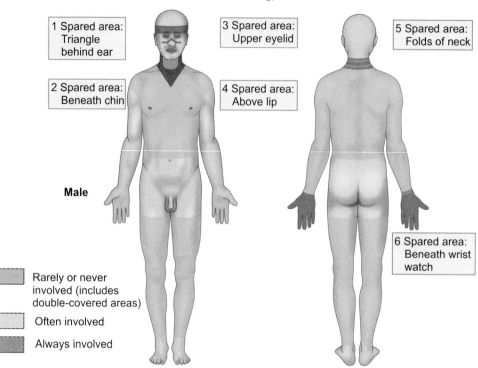

1 Spared area: Triangle behind ear

2 Spared area: Beneath chin

3 Spared area: Upper eyelid

4 Spared area: Above lip

5 Spared area: Folds of neck

6 Spared area: Beneath wrist watch

Male

☐ Rarely or never involved (includes double-covered areas)

☐ Often involved

☐ Always involved

Fig. 29.4: A depiction of the sites of involvement in phototoxic and photoallergic reactions

Table 29.3	Classification of photodermatoses
Genetic diseases	
• Xeroderma pigmentosum	• Bloom syndrome
• Cockayne syndrome	• Trichothiodystrophy
• Porphyria (several forms)	
Phototoxic and photoallergic reactions	
Mediators include:	
• Medications (tetracyline)	
• Plants (giant hogweed, meadow grass)	
• Chemicals (psoralens, eosin, acridine)	
Idiopathic diseases	
• Polymorphic light eruption	
• Solar urticaria	
• Hydroa vacciniforme	
Photo-provoked diseases	
• Lupus erythematosus	• Pemphigus
• Pellagra	• Porphyria cutanea tarda
• Albinism	
Occasionally photo-provoked diseases	
• Atopic dermatitis	• Lichen planus
• Psoriasis	• Mycosis fungoides

Phototoxic reactions are far more **common** than photoallergic reactions. Some substances, such as psoralens, cause a phototoxic reaction[Q] in almost everyone exposed to them and the appropriate wavelength of light. Photoallergic reactions are difficult to distinguish; the more so as the same drugs can often cause both photoallergic and phototoxic reactions.

Phototoxic Reaction

A phototoxic reaction is an exaggerated sunburn; the photosensitizers make the skin sensitive to light, often by causing the production of free oxygen radicals. A phototoxic reaction can occur the first time the patient uses the medication or product (Table 29.4).

UVA light is the commonest UV trigger (UVA > UVB).[Q] Every patient who takes enough medication and gets enough sun is at risk; a classic example is systemic doxycycline.[Q] PUVA therapy for psoriasis is also a 'mini-phototoxic reaction.' The likelihood of reaction is dose-related. As most of the drugs absorb UVA as well as UVB, window glass, protective against sunburn, does *not* protect against most phototoxic drug reactions.

Phytophotodermatitis (PPD)[Q] is a phototoxic reaction that may occur at any time, without prior sensitization to the offending agent. It occurs when the

Table 29.4	Common agents that can cause a phototoxic reaction
Tars	Acridine or Anthracene
Dyes	Bengal red, eosin, fluorescin, methylene blue, riboflavin, acridine, thiopyronine
Medications[Q]	Amiodarone, furosemide, NSAIDs (especially piroxicam, diclofenac), psoralens, phenothiazines, tetracyclines (especially doxycycline).
Furocoumarins	Celery, parsley, turnip, citrus fruits
Berloque dermatitis	Bergamot oil

29

| Box 29.1 | Plants containing psoralen compounds |

- Angelica
- Carrot (wild)
- Celery
- Cow parsley
- False bishop's weed
- Fig (wild)
- Hogweed

- Meadow grass (agrimony)
- Parsnip (wild parsnip)
- Persian limes
- Rue
- Sweet orange
- Wild angelica

skin comes in contact with a plant or fragrance containing furocoumarin.[Q] Furocoumarins are chemical compounds which occur naturally in a variety of plants and vegetables commonly ingested. The common plants that can trigger this dermatitis are listed in Box 29.1.

Treatment

- First, identification and avoidance of the photosensitizing agent must be done.
- Topical and systemic corticosteroids may provide relief to the erupted skin.
- Cool compresses are helpful in relieving discomfort.

> Nonsteroidal anti-inflammatory drugs (NSAIDs)[Q] are not recommended, as they may potentiate the phototoxic reaction.[Q]

- As phototoxic reactions are primarily triggered by UVA, patients should use sunscreens that contain UVA-protective ingredients such as avobenzone, titanium dioxide, and zinc oxide.

Photoallergic Reaction

A photoallergic reaction requires previous exposure, the development of sensitization and then a repeated exposure with the right combination of sensitizer and light exposure. Sometimes a different wavelength of light is required for the sensitization and the re-elicitation of the dermatitis, which can lead to variable morphology ranging from exanthem to urticaria.

Common causes are systemic phenothiazine, topical halogenated salicyl-anilides in soaps and disinfectants. Organic UV absorbers in sunscreens and non-steroidal anti-inflammatory drugs are other topical agents to lead to photoallergic reactions[Q] (Table 29.5).

The areas exposed to UVR are affected, but the morphology is eczematous, appears later and lasts

Table 29.5	Common agents that can cause a photoallergic reaction
Medications	Benzodiazepines, nalidixic acid, NSAIDs, phenothiazines, sulfonamides, sulfonyl-ureas, thiazides
Antimicrobial agents	Halogenated salicylanilides added to deodorant soaps
Sunscreens	Para-amino benzoic acid, benzophe-none

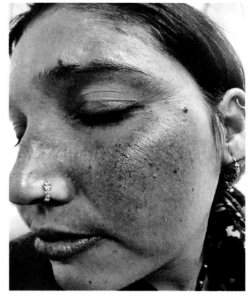
Fig. 29.5: Allergic contact dermatitis with photoaggravation

longer. The eruption is on the exposed areas such as the hands, the V of the neck, the nose, the chin and the forehead (Fig. 29.5). There is also a tendency to spare the upper lip under the nose, the eyelids and the submental region, axillae, bathing suit area, buttocks, inframammary folds (Fig. 29.4). If a photo-eruption is suspected, examine the unexposed areas for diagnostic clues as they should be uninvolved. As it is an allergic response, the eruption does not occur on the first exposure to ultraviolet, but only after a second or further exposures.

Investigation: Photopatch testing is required to confirm the diagnosis.

Treatment

- Identification and avoidance of the allergen and sun protection are crucial.
- Unless sunscreens are the suspected cause of the photoallergy, they should be used. As photoallergic reactions are primarily triggered by UVA, patients should use sunscreens that contain UVA-protective ingredients such as avobenzone, titanium dioxide, and zinc oxide.
- Topical steroids provide relief to the inflamed skin. Oral corticosteroids should only be used in severe cases.

Chronic Actinic Dermatitis (CAD)

Synonyms: Persistent light reaction, actinic reticuloid (when histology shows atypical lymphocytes).

This is a persistent photoallergic dermatitis which follows sensitization but without further antigen exposure. As most patients have positive patch or photo-patch tests, contact allergy presumably plays a part.

UVR: UVB > UVA; occasionally visible light.

29

Pathogenesis: Poorly understood; presumably photohaptens induce autoimmune response including persistent lymphocytic infiltrates.

Clinical features: Pruritic chronic dermatitis in light-exposed areas, most commonly on the exposed sites (Fig. 29.6). There is lichenified skin with multiple excoriations and erosions.

Course: These patients may be exquisitely sensitive to UVR. They are usually middle-aged or elderly men who react after the slightest exposure, even through window glass or from fluorescent lights. Affected individuals are also become allergic to a range of contact allergens, especially oleoresins in some plants (e.g. chrysanthemums), like parthenium in India.

Histology: Acanthosis, dermal fibrosis, lymphocytic infiltrates on some instances may show marked atypia (actinic reticuloid). Progression to lymphoma most uncommon.

Diagnostic approach: Clinical examination, biopsy. Photo-provocation (UVA, UVB, and visible light) as well as photopatch testing.

Differential diagnosis: Atopic dermatitis, mycosis fungoides, Sézary syndrome.

Airborne allergic contact dermatitis may be confused, but does not require sunlight for its manifestation. Sometimes the diagnosis is difficult as exposure both to sunlight and to the airborne allergen occurs only out of doors. Airborne allergic contact dermatitis also affects sites that sunlight is less likely to reach, such as eyelids and under the chin (Fig. 29.7).

Therapy: Patients must protect themselves from UVR (UVA and UVB) coming through windows or from fluorescent lights.

Azathioprine 50 mg daily followed by 3 times weekly can be almost miraculous; PUVA hardening also helpful. In severe cases, cyclosporine can be used.

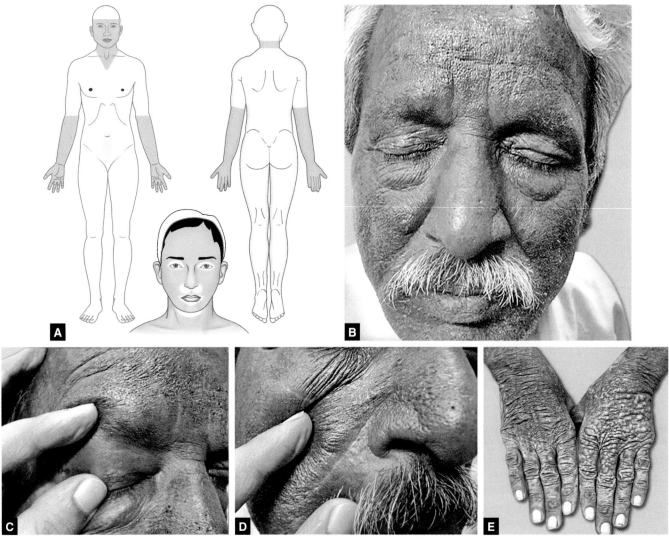

Fig. 29.6A to E: (A) Distribution of lesions in a classic case of CAD; (B to D) Lichenified appearance of CAD sparing the upper eyelid and the skin folds; (E) Marked involvement of dorsum of hand

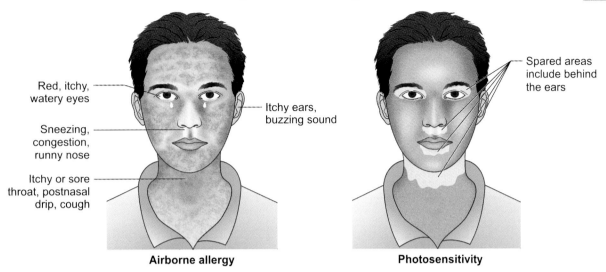

Fig. 29.7: A comparison of airborne allergy and photosensitivity

Labels (left, Airborne allergy): Red, itchy, watery eyes; Sneezing, congestion, runny nose; Itchy or sore throat, postnasal drip, cough; Itchy ears, buzzing sound

Labels (right, Photosensitivity): Spared areas include behind the ears

IDIOPATHIC DISORDERS

Polymorphous Light Eruption (PMLE)

This is an idiopathic eruption caused by UV exposure which appears in hours to days with a morphology varying considerably between patients.

PMLE is triggered by **both** wavelengths UVA and UVB.[Q]

The eruption is usually most prominent following the first UVA exposure in the spring, thus often a feature of a winter trip to sunny climes. Some degree of hardening over the summer and recurrences each year are to be expected.

Epidemiology

It is believed to be the most common photodermatosis,[Q] with an estimated prevalence of 10–20%. Usually starts in adolescents or young adults. It is believed to be consequent to type IV/DTH response to damaged keratinocytes where UVR causes a natural skin constituent to change into an allergen, to which an immune response is activated similar to drug photoallergy.

Clinical Features

The lesions in any one patient are relatively uniform and remain so over the life of the disease. The term polymorphous refers to the different patterns in different patients.

The eruption is itchy and usually confined to sun-exposed areas, but other areas may be involved as some UVR passes through thin clothing. The most common type is the papular type, in which small erythematous dermal papules appear on a patchy erythematous base (Fig. 29.8A). The second most common type is the plaque type (Fig. 29.8B), where superficial urticarial plaques are seen. The least common type is the

papulovesicular type, where urticarial plaques develop into vesicles. 'Juvenile spring eruption' is a clinical variant seen most often in boys, presenting as papulovesicles on the helices of the ears.

Histology

Dermal edema, lymphocytic perivascular infiltrates and minimal epidermal damage; no mucin (in contrast to lupus erythematosus).

Therapy

- Avoidance of sunlight via sunscreens and protective clothing; gradual increases in light exposure rather than intensive exposure on first day.
- Use of antioxidant for 1 week before exposure.
- Hardening with UVB or PUVA before exposure.
- If lesions develop, topical corticosteroids and oral antihistamines.
- Hydroxychloroquine 400 mg per day[Q] for the first month, then 200 mg per day throughout the summer is effective.
- Severe, persistent disease: Consider azathioprine 50–100 mg daily to 3 times weekly for 3 months.

Actinic Prurigo

Onset: Childhood; flares within hours of sun exposure.

Duration: Lesions are chronic and persistent throughout childhood, but often fade in adolescence.

Clinical features: Pruritic, erythematous papules and nodules with hemorrhagic crusts and lichenification. The lesions may persist through the winter. They frequently are misdiagnosed as excoriated acne, insect bites, eczema, erythropoietic protoporphyria or neurotic excoriations.

29

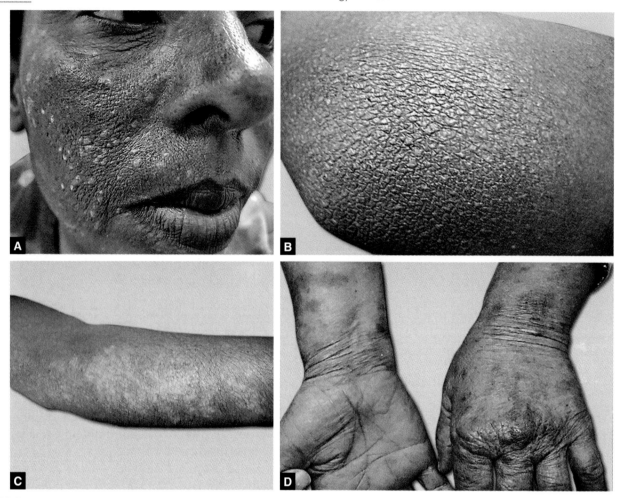

Fig. 29.8A to D: Variants of PMLE. (A) Papular PMLE on the face; (B) Papular PMLE on the elbows; (C) Plaque form on the extensor aspect of arms; (D) Edematous plaque on the exposed aspects

Table 29.6 Effects of UVR on various dermatoses	
Helps	*Worsens*
• Atopic eczema	• Albinos
• Cutaneous T cell lymphoma	• Darier's disease
• Parapsoriasis	• Herpes simplex
• Pityriasis lichenoides	• Lupus erythematosus (exaggerated sunburns and can develop renal failure following such an event)
• Pityriasis rosea	
• Pruritus of renal failure, liver disease	
• Psoriasis	• Pemphigus vulgaris and folioceus (both are usually very photosensitive; probably mediated by urokinase release)
	• Pellagra
	• Porphyrias
	• Xeroderma pigmentosum

Solar Urticaria

Rare patients develop hives with sun or light exposure;[Q] always exclude erythropoietic protoporphyria and photoallergic reactions.

Hydroa Vacciniforme

This rare peculiar eruption in children presents with large facial blisters and smallpox-like scars. In Japan and Mexico, it is associated with cutaneous lymphoma.

SUNLIGHT EXACERBATED DISEASES

Though there are various other disorders, including genodermatoses and metabolic disorders, associated with sunlight exposure, they are beyond the purview of this book. UVR is useful in the treatment of many skin diseases, but it can also make some worse and a list of the same is given in Table 29.6.

29

HIV and STD

HIV, Skin Manifestations and Management

INTRODUCTION

Acquired immunodeficiency syndrome (AIDS) is caused by HIV (human immunodeficiency virus) which is a retrovirus^Q of the lentivirus genus which has two subtypes HIV-1 and HIV-2, the former being the most common and of global distribution.

The number of patients with HIV/AIDS who will develop some type of cutaneous manifestation varies according to the series but around **80–95%** of HIV-infected patients have skin manifestations at any time in the course of infection.

EPIDEMIOLOGY

In Africa and Asia, heterosexual transmission of HIV dominates, in contrast to the situation in Western Europe where most patients are homosexual men, prostitutes, or intravenous drug users (Fig. 30.1A).

PATHOPHYSIOLOGY

HIV is a retrovirus in the lentivirus family. It has an affinity for CD4+ helper T cells, macrophages, and microglia.^{Q} HIV can be found in all body fluids.

The most important methods of transmission include (Fig. 30.1B):

- Contact of semen or blood with damaged mucosa, especially if genital ulcers (syphilis, herpes) are present.
- The second main way is via infected blood. While transfusions are so carefully controlled that the risk today is infinitesimal, drug abusers continue to contaminate one another via shared needles.
- Mother–infant transmission is possible at several levels—intrauterine, intrapartum, and while nursing.

It is significantly diminished by antiretroviral therapy.

The steps in the invasion of the virus and actions of ART drugs are depicted in Fig. 30.2.

The dermatological manifestations do not only occur due to the decrease in CD4 T lymphocytes, but also due to a change in the profile of cytokines towards a profile predominantly T helper 2 (Th2), molecular mimicry and over-expression of superantigens. The change in the cytokine profile from T helper 1 (Th1) to Th2 may explain the appearance or exacerbation of non-infectious diseases such as atopic dermatitis.

CLINICAL CLASSIFICATION

- **Acute HIV infection:** Often overlooked or confused with other viral illnesses, this presents with fever, night sweats, maculopapular exanthema, and sometimes oral ulcers 2–8 weeks after transmission of HIV. Later there may be neurological problems such as meningoencephalitis and facial nerve palsy, as well as a period of generalized lymphadenopathy (Fig. 30.3).
- **HIV-associated, non-AIDS defining illnesses:** There are several illnesses that are often seen with-HIV infection but are not regarded as AIDS defining; like bacillary angiomatosis, therapy-resistant oropharyngeal candidiasis, and zoster taking a normal course for healing. These suggest count a CD4 count <500/mm.^{3}
- **AIDS:** The AIDS-defining illnesses are detailed in Box. 30.1.

There are two ways of classifying the manifestations, the first one is through staging as proposed by WHO which has 4 stages, while the other is CDC classification which is given in Fig. 30.4.

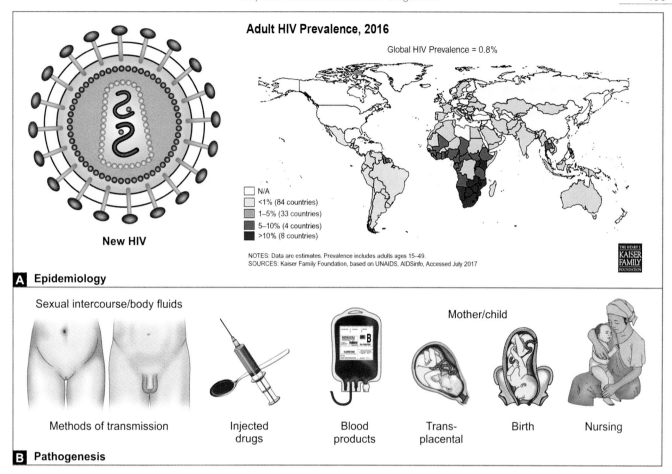

Fig. 30.1A and B: Epidemiology and pathogenesis of HIV

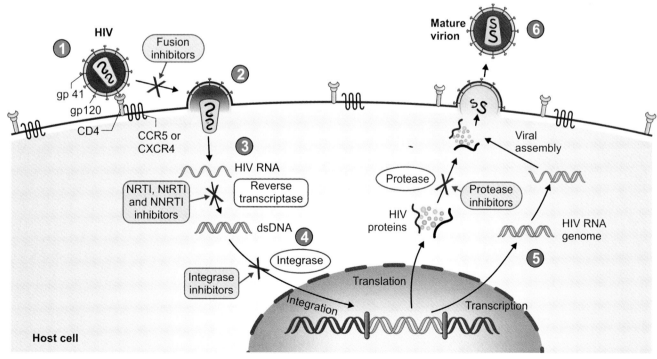

Fig. 30.2: Pathogenesis of HIV and site of action of various drugs: (1) Fusion of HIV to the host cell; (2) HIV RNA and other viral proteins enter the host cell; (3) Viral DNA is formed by reverse transcription; (4) Viral DNA is transported across the nucleus and integrated into the host DNA; (5) New viral RNA is used as genomic RNA and to make viral proteins; (6) The virus matures releasing individual HIV proteins

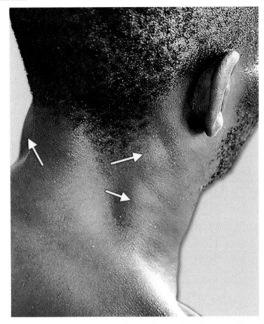

Fig. 30.3: Persistent generalized lymphadenopathy (PGL)—Swollen, firm, painless glands (>1 cm) in two or more areas outside the groin, >3 months

CD4+ lymphocytes		Clinical stages			A: Asymptomatic, acute retroviral syndrome, lymphadenopathy syndrome
		A	B	C	
>500	1	Stage 1		Stage 3	B: HIV-associated but not AIDS-defining illnesses
200–499	2				C: AIDS-defining illnesses
<200	3		Stage 2	AIDS	

Fig. 30.4: CDC staging of HIV

CUTANEOUS MANIFESTATIONS

Cutaneous manifestations of HIV/AIDS infection can be divided into non-infectious (inflammatory, drug induced or neoplastic) and infectious.

The latter can be subdivided according to their etiology into bacterial, viral, fungal and parasitic. The grouping of cutaneous manifestations in this way facilitates the systematization of possible etiologies and helps when facing patients (Table 30.1).

INFLAMMATORY MANIFESTATIONS

Seborrheic Dermatitis

Seborrheic dermatitis (SD) occurs with increased prevalence in patients with HIV/AIDS infection (around 85%). Its appearance and severity are related to the CD4 counts of the patient. In all extensive or atypical SD or non-responsive cases HIV testing should be considered.

Box 30.1 | AIDS defining illness^Q

Protozoal infections
- Toxoplasmosis of the brain
- Cryptosporidiosis, chronic gastrointestinal disease (>1 month)
- Isosporiasis, chronic intestinal infection (>1 month)

Fungal infections
- Candidiasis of the bronchi, trachea, lungs, or esophagus
- *Pneumocystis jiroveci* pneumonia^Q (formerly *Pneumocystis carinii*)
- Coccidiomycosis: Disseminated or extrapulmonary
- Cryptococosis: Extrapulmonary
- Histoplasmosis: Disseminated or extrapulmonary

Bacterial infections
- *Mycobacterium avium complex*,^Q *Mycobacteria*, other species or unidentified, disseminated or extrapulmonary
- *Mycobacterium tuberculosis*: Any site (pulmonary or extrapulmonary)
- Pneumonia, recurrent (>2/year)
- *Salmonella* septicemia, recurrent

Viral infections
- Cytomegalovirus retinitis and involvement other than the liver, spleen, or lymph nodes
- Herpes simplex virus: Chronic ulcers (>1 month) or bronchitis, pneumonitis, or esophagitis
- Progressive multifocal leukoencephalopathy (JC virus)

Others
- Cervical cancer, invasive
- Anal cancer
- Encephalopathy: HIV related
- Kaposi sarcoma^Q
- Lymphoma: Burkitt, immunoblastic or CNS
- Wasting syndrome

Table 30.1 | Classification of cutaneous manifestations of HIV/AIDS

Infections

Bacterial: Impetigo, ecthyma, tuberculosis, atypical mycobacteria, syphilis, bacillary angiomatosis.

Fungal: Oral candidiasis, tinea capitis, corporis, cruris and unguium cryptococcosis, histoplasmosis, sporotrichosis.

Viral: Herpes labialis and genitalis, herpes zoster, chickenpox (varicella), warts, molluscum contagiosum, oral hairy leukoplakia, HHV-8.

Parasitic: Scabies (crusted), leishmaniasis.

Inflammatory

Eczema: Seborrheic eczema, pruritus, xerosis, eosinophilic folliculitis, papular pruritic eruption of HIV.
Aphthous ulcers, psoriasis, urticaria, vasculitis, panniculitis.

Drug eruptions: Morbilliform eruption, erythema multiforme, Stevens-Johnson syndrome, toxic epidermal necrolysis.

HAART related: Drug eruptions, immune reconstitution syndrome.

Tumors: Kaposi sarcoma, non-Hodgkin lymphoma, Hodgkin lymphoma.

Psoriasis

Psoriasis tends to be more intense, acral, extensive, destructive and recalcitrant in seropositive patients with higher frequency of psoriatic arthritis. The initiation of ART can help in the treatment of psoriasis and produce a better response to topical treatments. Phototherapy and retinoids (use with caution in protease inhibitors) are treatment of choice in these patients.[Q]

Atopic Dermatitis and Xerosis

Atopic dermatitis (AD) an xerosis occurs in 20 to 50% of patients with HIV infection compared to 2–20% of the seronegative population and are one of the important causes of pruritus in this group.

Photodermatosis

Photosensitivity is more frequent and severe in patients with HIV infection and worsens directly with the degree of immunosuppression. It presents as lichenoid or eczematous eruption in exposed areas.

Photosensitivity associated with HIV infection usually occurs with lower CD4 counts <50 cells/mm³. Rarely cutaneous porphyria tarda may occur in the context of co-infection with hepatitis C virus and pellagra type reactions due to malnutrition and vitamin B_3 deficiency.

Eosinophilic Folliculitis and Papulopruritic Rash of HIV

Pruritus is one of the prominent symptoms of patients infected with HIV and pruritus without an explained cause in patients with risk factors should raise the suspicion of HIV infection.

Eosinophilic folliculitis (EF) is a chronic skin disease of unknown cause that occurs in patients with advanced HIV infection. It presents as follicular and non-follicular papules and pustules on the face, neck, scalp, upper trunk (in the midline) and proximal region of the extremities (Fig. 30.5A and B).

The disease usually appears at CD4 counts less than 200–250 cells/mm³.[Q] Mild cases of disease respond to antihistamines, topical corticosteroids and scabicides. In more severe cases, oral antifungals, systemic retinoids or phototherapy may be used.

Papular pruritic rash (PPE) is seen in 11 to 46% of patients with HIV especially in the tropics. It is characterized by discrete, intensely pruritic papules. Unlike EF, it has a more distal distribution (extremities) and less truncal involvement. It may represent an exaggerated response to arthropod bites. The disease worsens with low counts of CD4 and improves with the restitution of immunity.

IMMUNE RECONSTITUTION SYNDROME (IRS)

It occurs after the start of ART because of regained capacity to develop an immunological response and recognize multiple microorganisms.

It occurs in 25% patients especially during the first 8 weeks of ART initiation in those with a low CD4 count (<200 cells/mm³) and those with subclinical infections at the time of initiating therapy.[Q] The inflammatory response can be to infectious agents such as mycobacteria, opportunistic fungi and different types of viruses (herpes simplex, human papillomavirus) present at the time of antiviral initiation, resulting in a paradoxical worsening of the patient despite the increase in the CD4 count. There can be worsening of inflammatory pathologies such as sarcoidosis, eosinophilic folliculitis and atopic dermatitis.

NEOPLASMS

Kaposi's Sarcoma

Kaposi's sarcoma (KS) caused by human herpesvirus 8 is classified into four types, with the epidemic variant being the one associated with HIV. The incidence of KS in HIV-infected patients may be as high as 30–40%, especially in homosexual men.[Q] It presents as bright, asymptomatic, erythematous-violaceous macules, plaques or nodules, classically distributed in the Langerhans' lines (Fig. 30.5C and D).

Early stage of KS: KS limited to the skin with minimal involvement of oral mucosa only on the hard palate; CD4 >200/mm³; without opportunistic infections; without oral candidiasis and without symptoms B. In these cases, treatment can be performed only with ART that includes Protease inhibitors.

Late stage of KS: Pulmonary or gastrointestinal KS; excessive oral involvement; tumor ulcerations; CD4 <200; patient with a history of opportunistic infections or B symptoms. Treatment should be administered with antiretroviral therapy along with liposomal anthracyclines such as doxorubicin.

Cutaneous Neoplasms

Patients with HIV infection have a higher incidence (2.1 times) of non-melanoma skin cancers including squamous cell carcinoma and basal cell carcinoma (risk is inversely proportional to CD4 counts for squamous cell cancers). Similarly, the risk of melanoma is also increased and is 26% higher than the general population.

Intraepithelial Anal Cancer; Cervical and Penile Cancer

One of the main risk factors for developing anal cancer in patients with HIV infection is chronic high-risk HPV. Approximately 50% of large anal condylomas may contain high-grade anal intraepithelial neoplasia (which may be clinically nonpalpable) or anal squamous cell cancer in high-risk patients.

INFECTIOUS MANIFESTATIONS ASSOCIATED WITH HIV

Acute Necrotizing Ulcerative Gingivitis

Chronic mixed infection with fusobacteria and spirochetes is facilitated by immunodeficiency and poor hygiene; it is known as trench mouth.

Bacteria

The main group of bacteria that causes skin infections are Gram-positive *Staphylococcus aureus* especially methicillin-resistant *S. aureus* (MRSA). Folliculitis, impetigo and cellulitis are the most common forms of presentation. It can also manifest as ecthyma, boils, carbuncles and abscesses. They are located more frequently in the lower extremities, buttocks and scrotum than the upper extremities and face. The recurrence of these pyoderma is high (41%) in these patients.

Pseudomonas aeruginosa can cause primary infections such as infection of catheters or in the anogenital and axillary regions. In addition, it can cause secondary infection of other dermatoses such as Kaposi's sarcoma or hematogenous spread to the skin, e.g. ecthyma gangrenosum.

Mycobacteria

Tuberculosis (TB) is a common opportunistic infection in HIV disease[Q] especially in endemic countries like India. Cutaneous TB (1 to 2% of TB cases) occurs with increased prevalence in HIV patients. The clinical expression is diverse and can present as papules and crusted indurated plaques or as disseminated lesions (generalized cutaneous miliary TBC). There is usually associated systemic involvement.

Atypical mycobacteria infection (*M. avium* complex, *M. kansasii, M. marinum, M. ulcerans, M. chelonae, M. fortuitum* and *M. abscessus*) incidence is increasing, partly due to the spread of HIV.

Bacillary Angiomatosis

Bacillary angiomatoses are caused by *Bartonella henselae* and *B. quintana* and occur more commonly in advanced stages of AIDS (CD4 <200/mm³).[Q]

They are characterized by angioproliferative lesions that resemble cherry hemangiomas, pyogenic granulomas, or Kaposi's sarcoma, such as papules, nodules, or red to violaceous plaques, most often disseminated. The antimicrobials of choice are macrolides or doxycycline.

Syphilis

There is an epidemiological synergy between ulcerative STDs like syphilis and HIV infection, both favoring the transmission of each other. Clinically, it can present atypically as primary syphilis with more severe and painful chancre, in unusual locations; as multiple chancres in 25% of patients, or even reaching aggressive cankers with perforations of the labia majora or foreskin and a greater delay in the healing.

Secondary syphilis can manifest as malignant syphilis[Q] in 7% of patients coinfected with HIV. The condition is characterized by diffuse papules—squamous papulosquamous eruption with pustules, nodules and ulcers and presence of necrotizing vasculitis. In seropositive patients, primary and secondary syphilis lesions or even primary and tertiary syphilis may coexist.

There may be difficulty in diagnosis as well leading to false negative serologies or "seronegative syphilis" (non-treponemal and false-negative treponemal tests) due to "prozone phenomena" (high antibody titres). Even follow up with serology is difficult as these patients take longer to normalize their titres even after receiving appropriate treatment.

It is important to perform a lumbar puncture in seropositive patients with syphilis who present neurological signs and symptoms; evidence of active tertiary disease; fail treatment without clear evidence of reinfection and in patients with syphilis and HIV who are asymptomatic neurologically but have high titres of VDRL/RPR> 1:32 or low CD4 <350 cells/mm³.

Benzyl-penicillin remains the antimicrobial of choice in these patients and there are reports of resistance to alternative antibiotics like azithromycin.

Viral Infections

- HIV-associated infections often occur in the wrong age group, at an uncommon site or are unexpectedly severe.
- Ulceration—persistence, and dissemination suggest more advanced disease.

Herpes Simplex Virus (HSV) Types 1 and 2

HSV in patients with HIV infection can occur atypically or extensively, in an ulcerative or hypertrophic-tumor form and chronically with frequent relapses. In advanced HIV infection (CD4 <100/mm³), there is an increase in the number and size of the lesions (up to 20 cm), atypical presentations, located in the lower back, buttocks and perianal regions, more frequent and serious recurrences, more painful and deep vesicles and ulcers, which heal more slowly and even have warty, chronic lesions, with or without ulceration.

Chronic herpetic infections (last more than a month) are AIDS defining illness[Q] (Fig. 30.5E).

In patients with chronic skin conditions such as contact dermatitis, atopic dermatitis or psoriasis, a disseminated herpetic eruption known as 'herpetic eczema' or 'varicelliform Kaposi eruption' may occur especially by HSV type 1.

Varicella Zoster Virus Infection (VVZ)

Herpes zoster (HZ) is one of the main and first manifestations in HIV seropositive patients. Episodes of herpes zoster (HZ) VZV reactivation occur 10 times more frequently in patients with HIV infection. Unlike other viral infections; HZ occurs in early stages of HIV infection and complications such as disseminated HZ and Ramsay Hunt syndrome occur even with elevated CD4 counts.

Clinical manifestations may include severe varicella with multidermatomal involvement (more than 20 lesions outside the dermatome or with involvement of associated dermatomes), necrotic/hemorrhagic HZ (Fig. 30.5F), chronic recurrent HZ and systemic dissemination.

Human Papillomavirus (HPV)

HPV infection, manifesting as warts and condylomata a cuminata, is very frequent in patients seropositive for HIV. Their early diagnosis and treatment is important to decrease the risk of associated cancer. More aggressive treatment and a longer duration of therapy may be needed in such patients.

Acquired Verrucous Epidermodysplasia

Verruciform epidermodysplasia (EV) is a rare autosomal dominant genodermatosis caused by HPV 5 and 8. In HIV patients (especially young patients with vertical transmission) with HPV infection, similar presentation with hypopigmented macules (pityriasis versicolor) on the trunk, extremities and face during childhood and lesions similar to flat warts in exposed areas may occur and is known as acquired EV.

Molluscum Contagiosum

MC (caused by poxvirus) occurs approximately in 10 to 20% of patients with HIV infection and is a clinical sign of progression of HIV infection and lower CD4 counts.

- There is a dose correlation between immune status and clinical findings.
- Widespread infections or giant lesions, usually on the face, indicate CD4+ count <200/mm³.

The lesions may be multiple and extensive, larger (diameter greater than 1 cm), confluent, disfiguring, warty, present on atypical location (head and neck)[Q] and resistant to different treatments (Fig. 30.5G and H).

The differential diagnosis of umbilicated papules classically includes fungal infections such as cryptococcosis, histoplasmosis, blastomyces, coccidioides, paracoccidiodes, Sporothrix, atypical mycobacteria, B. hensenlae, and Kaposi sarcoma.

Epstein-Barr Virus

Apart from OHL, it is also a factor in Castleman disease and lymphomas, especially pleural.

Oral Hairy Leukoplakia (OHL)

It is characterized by the appearance of asymptomatic, asymmetric, bilateral, whitish, non-detachable plaques with corrugated surface and hairy projections, usually located on the lateral edges of the tongue[Q] and caused by EBV especially in male patients with low CD4 counts and high viral loads (Fig. 30.5I). The treatment can be done with podophyllin and ART. Other treatments which may be tried include oral and intravenous antivirals and surgery.

Cytomegalovirus Infection (CMV)

The most common presentation of CMV in seropositive patients are extensive perineal ulcers with granulation tissue. Isolated cutaneous involvement is rare and presents as maculopapular eruption and morbilliform rash secondary to the administration of amoxicillin.

Fungal Infections

Candidiasis

Candidiasis is the most frequent opportunistic infection (90% prevalence) in seropositive patients especially with near normal CD4 counts.[Q] It is caused mainly by *Candida albicans* but also by *C. glabrata*, *C. tropicalis*, *C. krusei* and *C. parapsilosis* (Fig. 30.5J).

Clinical presentations include onychomycosis with paronychia, onychodystrophy, intertrigo and chronic recurrent vaginal candidiasis. Disseminated candidiasis is very infrequent and occurs in intravenous drug users.

If patients have complaints of pain on swallowing or heartburn, gastroscopy is needed to exclude candidial esophagitis. Treat is fluconazole or itraconazole in doses up to 400 mg po daily for 1–2 weeks.

Dermatophytosis

It is caused by *Trichophyton* (majority of cases), *Microsporum* and *Epidermophyton* species. In patients with HIV infection, dermatophyte infection can be extensive, atypical, disseminated, involvement of multiple nails and poor response to treatment.

It may present as multiple ulcerations and fluctuating nodules. Majocchi granuloma (nodular granulomatous perifolliculitis) characterized by the presence of firm erythematous–violaceous nodules associated with onychomycosis, tinea corporis or tinea pedis may occur in seropositive patients.

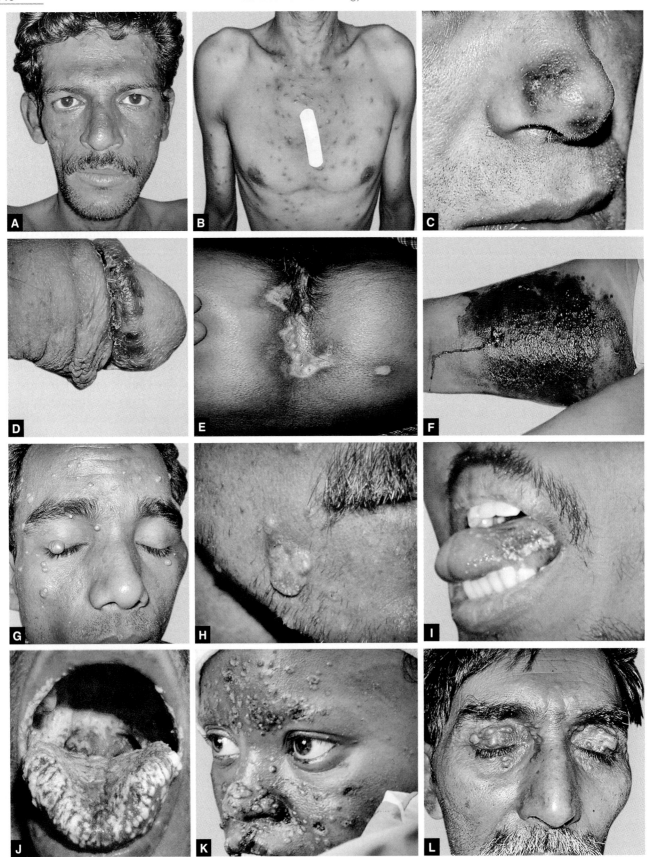

Fig. 30.5A to L: (A and B) Eosinophilic pustular folliculitis seen on the face and above the nipple line; (C and D) Kaposi sarcoma seen on the nose and genitalia; (E) Persistent erosions in a case of herpes in an HIV patient; (F) Hemorrhagic herpes zoster; (G and H) Facial molluscum contagiosum. Note the larger lesions and plaque forms; (I) Oral hairy leukoplakia; (J) Severe oral and pharyngeal candidiasis; (K) Disseminated cutaneous cryptococcosis—note the molluscoid lesions; (L) Disseminated histoplasmosis

Non-dermatophyte fungal infections such as *Fusarium, Acremonium, Aspergillus,* scopulariopsis can occur and cause systemic invasive mycoses (pulmonary, endophthalmitis) thus needing aggressive treatment.

Invasive Fungal Infections

Cryptococcosis, Histoplasmosis, Penicillium, Coccidioidomycosis, Sporotrichosis and Aspergillosis

Cutaneous lesions occur in patients with systemic involvement (secondary to hematogenous seeding from pulmonary foci) or occupational exposure to soil (Asia). The lesions are more frequently located in the head and neck but may be generalized. Oral involvement or systemic dissemination may occur. Infect cryptococcosis is one of the most common fatal subcutaneous mycoses in patients with HIV/AIDS infection (Fig. 30.5K and L).

The most frequent cutaneous morphology is molluscum contagiosum like (skin colored umbilicated papules or nodules) with necrosis or central ulceration. There may be pustules, cellulitis, ulceration, panniculitis, palpable purpura, subcutaneous abscesses, vegetative plaques, and pyoderma gangrenous lesions.

The treatment of choice is intravenous amphotericin B associated with oral flucytosine followed by oral fluconazole.

Parasitic Infections

Scabies

It presents atypically in seropositive patients with disseminated papular or nodular or hyperkeratotic lesions ('Norwegian scabies') and scalp involvement. The Norwegian form occurs more frequently when the CD4 count is <200 cells/mm³. It may also be a manifestation of IRS. Treatment is with repeated doses of ivermectin; permethrin and keratolytic agents like sulphur.

Leishmaniasis

It may present in either of the three forms: Cutaneous or mucocutaneous (2/3rd cases) and visceral (kala-azar, from Hindi 'black fever'). They may present as disseminated lesions (>10 pleomorphic lesions in more than two noncontiguous body sites) or diffuse forms (primary cutaneous or spread in hematogenous form). There is also higher risk of developing mucosal involvement.

However, more than cutaneous forms of leishmaniasis, HIV infection confers an increased risk of presenting forms of visceral leishmaniasis which is also included in AIDS defining illness.

Conclusion

The importance of skin findings in HIV are two fold. Firstly there is a correlation of the skin findings and the CD4 count as seen in Table 30.2 and Fig. 30.6. More importantly a good clinician can make an early diagnosis if the conditions listed in Fig. 30.6 are diagnosed early, specially the disorders that correlate with a CD4 count <200 cells/mm³ which largely constitute the AIDS defining dermatoses. With the

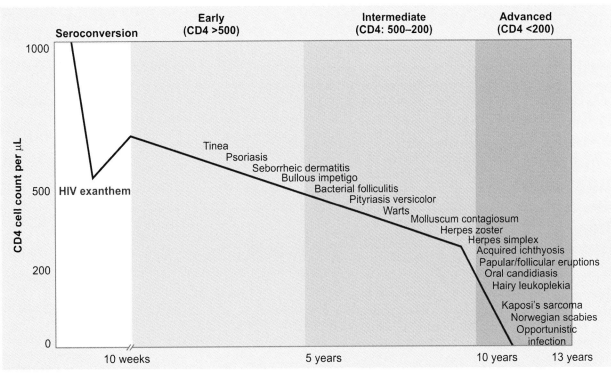

Fig. 30.6: A depiction of the correlation between skin findings and CD4 counts

Table 30.2   Correlation of CD4 counts with the cutaneous manifestations

Stage of HIV/AIDS	Characteristic skin disorders
CD4 >500 cells/mm³	Herpes zoster
CD4 200–400 cells/mm³	Candiadiasis; Dermatophyte infection—oral hairy leukoplakia; Varicella-zoster infection—Seborrheic eczema
CD4 <200 cells/mm³	Persistent herpes simplex infection for >1 month; Cytomegalovirus (CMV retinitis)—Kaposi sarcoma; Atypical mycobacterial infection—histoplasmosis, Cryptococcosis, drug reactions, Papular eruptions
AIDS	Kaposi sarcoma, Persistent herpes simplex viral infection (>1 month), Cryptococcosis, Histoplasmosis, Atypical mycobacterial infection

Table 30.3   Diagnosis of HIV*

Retesting prior to enrollment in care	• Retest all clients diagnosed HIV-positive with a second specimen and a second operator using the same testing strategy and algorithm before enrolling the client in care and/or initiating ART, regardless of whether or not ART initiation depends on CD4 count. • Retesting people on ART is not recommended.
In settings with greater than 5% HIV prevalence	A diagnosis of HIV positive should be provided to people with two sequential reactive tests.
In settings with less than 5% HIV prevalence	A diagnosis of HIV positive should be provided to people with three sequential reactive tests.

*Consolidated guidelines on the use of antiretroviral drugs for treating and preventing HIV infection: Recommendations for a public health approach-2nd ed. WHO.2016.

effective ART therapy many patients can benefit from an early disease control (Table 30.2).

DIAGNOSIS OF HIV

HIV-positive means presence of antibodies against HIV.

- Direct identification of HIV uses the p24 antigen test or polymerase chain reaction (PCR). While indirect methods to identify antibodies include enzyme-linked immunosorbent assay (ELISA) (screening) and Western blot (confirmation).
- Only an unequivocal positive test (two positive screening tests, ELISA; and a confirmatory test, western blot) should be reported to the patient. In doubt testing should be repeated at 6–12 weeks (Table 30.3).

Once the diagnosis is made (Table 30.3), the viral load and CD4 count are most useful in monitoring the course of the disease.

TREATMENT

HAART (highly active antiretroviral therapy) is initiated and is based on the combination of two nucleoside reverse transcriptase inhibitors (NRTIs) and a protease inhibitor (PI) or a non-nucleoside reverse transcriptase inhibitor (NNRTI).

Antiretroviral Drugs Act at various stages of the life cycle of HIV in the body and work by interrupting the process of viral replication. Theoretically, ARV drugs can act in any of the following ways during different stages of viral replication (Fig. 30.2).

    i. Block binding of HIV to target cell (fusion inhibitors)

    ii. Block viral RNA cleavage and one that inhibits reverse transcriptase (reverse transcriptase inhibitors)

    iii. Block the enzyme, integrase, which helps in the incorporation of the proviral DNA into the host cell chromosome (integrase inhibitors)

    iv. Block the RNA to prevent viral protein production

    v. Block the enzyme protease (protease inhibitors)

    vi. Inhibit the budding of virus from host cells.

The various classes of ART drugs are listed in Table 30.4.

Table 30.4   Classes of drugs available

Nucleoside reverse transcriptase inhibitors (NRTI)	Non-nucleoside reverse transcriptase inhibitors (NNRTI)	Protease inhibitors (PI)
Zidovudine (AZT/ZDV)*	Nevirapine* (NVP)	Saquinavir* (SQV)
Stavudine (d4T)*	Efavirenz* (EFV)	Ritonavir* (RTV)
Lamivudine (3TC)*	Delavirdine (DLV)	Nelfinavir* (NFV)
Didanosine (ddI)*	Fusion inhibitors (FI)	Amprenavir (APV)
Zalcitabine (ddC)*	Enfuviritide (T-20)	Indinavir* (INV)
Abacavir (ABC)*	Integrase inhibitors	Lopinavir/Ritonavir (LPV)*
Emtricitabine (FTC)	Raltegravir	Fosamprenavir (FPV)
(NtRTI)	CCR5 entry inhibitor	Atazanavir (ATV)*
Tenofavir (TDF)*	Maraviroc	Tipranavir (TPV)

*Available in India

Table 30.5	Clinical guidelines: Antiretroviral therapy
When to start **ART** in adults (>19 years old)	ART should be initiated in **all adults living** with HIV, **regardless** of WHO clinical stage and at any CD4 cell count
Timing of ART for adults and children with **TB**	• TB treatment should be initiated first, followed by ART as soon as possible within the first 8 weeks of treatment • HIV-positive TB patients with profound immunosuppression (e.g. CD4 counts less than 50 cells/mm^3) should receive ART within the first two weeks of initiating TB treatment

What to start: First-line ART	First-line ART for adults should consist of 2 nucleoside reverse-transcriptase inhibitors (NRTIs)
	plus
	1 non-nucleoside reverse-transcriptase inhibitor (NNRTI) or an integrase inhibitor (INSTI):
	• **TDF + 3TC (FTC) + EFV** as a fixed-dose combination is recommended as the preferred option to initiate ART
	• Alternative options recommended
	  – AZT + 3TC + EFV
	  – AZT + 3TC + NVP
	  – TDF + 3TC (FTC) + NVP

Pregnant women	ART should be initiated in all pregnant and breastfeeding women living with HIV, regardless of WHO clinical stage and at any CD4 cell count and continued lifelong
Infant feeding in the context of HIV	Mothers known to be infected with HIV should exclusively breastfeed their infants for the first 6 months of life, introducing appropriate complementary foods thereafter, and continue breastfeeding for the first 12 months of life
Laboratory monitoring before and after initiating ART	• Viral load monitoring can be carried out at 6 months, at 12 months and then every 12 months thereafter if the patient is stable on ART • CD4 of any value and on ART-every 6 months

Zidovudine (AZT/ZDV), Lamivudine (3TC), Efavirenz (EFV), Tenofavir (TDF), Nevirapine (NVP), Emtricitabine (FTC).
(Consolidated guidelines on the use of antiretroviral drugs for treating and preventing HIV infection: Recommendations for a public health approach 2nd ed. WHO.2016; NACO OM-5th may 2017).

Table 30.6	Antiretroviral drugs for HIV prevention*
Oral pre-exposure prophylaxis for preventing the acquisition of HIV	Oral pre-exposure prophylaxis (PrEP) containing TDF
Post-exposure prophylaxis (a full 28-day prescription)	Post-exposure prophylaxis ARV regimens for adults and adolescents: TDF + 3TC (FTC) is recommended as the preferred backbone 2 regimen for HIV postexposure prophylaxis in adults and adolescents LPV or ATV is recommended as the preferred third drug

TDF Tenofavir, Lamivudine (3TC), Lopinavir/Ritonavir (LPV)
*Consolidated guidelines on the use of antiretroviral drugs for treating and preventing HIV infection: recommendations for a public health approach-2nd ed. WHO.2016.

The method of treatment is complex but a summary of the latest guidelines of NACO and WHO is given in Table 30.5 as a quick reference.

Emergency Measures Following HIV Exposure

The risk of transmission from an infected patient to healthcare worker following needle injury is 1:200–400. The patient's HIV status should be determined after any needle injury. The wound should be encouraged to bleed for 1–3 minutes and then disinfected.

If the patient is HIV positive, then prophylaxis for the healthcare worker should ideally start in the first 2 hours and always before 72 hours. It is usually continued for 28 days. Zidovudine alone has an 80% protective effect. The standard regimen today includes two NRT and a PI (Table 30.6).

Sexually Transmitted Infections

STDs are an important class of infections, more so as they are associated with the enhanced transmission of HIV. The term 'sexually transmitted disease (STD)' is being replaced in some circles by sexually transmitted infection (STI).

The term STD refers to disorders spread by the sexual route and affecting the genitalia, while STI refers to disorders that are transmitted sexually but affecting the systemic organs as well[Q] (like hepatitis B and C). The older term venereal disease refers in a more limited way to diseases such as gonorrhea that are almost exclusively transferred by sexual contact. The most common STDs are listed below, but we will be primarily focusing on the major STDs and not on the STIs.

For the sake of simplicity, all common sexually transmitted infections can be conveniently divided in the following manner (Flowchart 31.1).

ULCERATIVE STIs

SYPHILIS (Lues)

Word origin: Latin, from the poem Syphilis, *Sive Morbus Gallicus* which had a character named Syphilus, presumably the first sufferer of the disease.

Causative agent: *Treponema pallidum*

- The causative agent is a spirochete with characteristic motility described as translation, rotation, flexion and distortion (older description for easy remembrance was **a:** angulation, **b:** bending, **c:** corkscrew, **d:** darting).[Q]

- It is a slender organism (length-5–15 µm, width-0.2 µm), therefore cannot be viewed by light microscopy and requires dark ground microscopy, immunofluorescence or Fontana, Levaditi stain.[Q]

It is important to note that there are saprophytic treponemes too, both in the genital mucosa[Q] (*Treponema refringens*, *Treponema balanitis* and *Treponema gracilis*) as well as oral mucosa (*Treponema microdenticum* and *Treponema macrodenticum*).

Incubation period: 9–90 days,[Q] after sexual exposure.

Average: 3–4 weeks.

The stages of syphilis are depicted in Flowchart 31.2.

Acquired Syphilis

A summary of the salient features are given in Box 31.1 and details are given below.

Primary Syphilis

Clinical features

- After inoculation, about 3 weeks after contact[Q] the first change to appear is a red colored macule, which forms a papule and thereafter an ulcer.
- This ulcer is called hard chancre or Hunterian chancre.[Q] It is single, painless, *indurated* and well defined[Q] and oozes clear serious fluid (Fig. 31.1A).
- After about a week of the ulcer uni- or bilateral, painless lymphadenopathy appears (Fig. 31.1B). The lymphadenopathy is often referred to as rubbery or shotty[Q] in consistency. It is non-suppurative.

Flowchart 31.1: Classification of sexually transmitted disorders

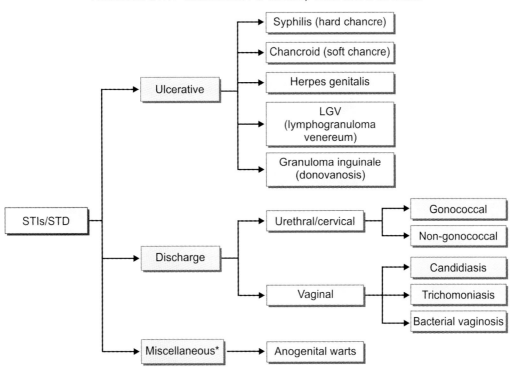

*HIV, hepatitis B, hepatitis C, scabies, pediculosis, candidal balanitis

Flowchart 31.2: Course of syphilis

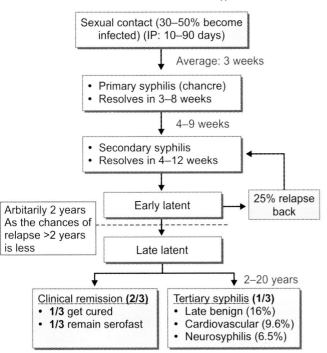

- Chancre resolves spontaneously in 3–8 weeks (average 6 weeks).^Q Only half^Q of affected individuals have the classical *Hunterian chancre*.
- 10% of chancres are extragenital; then they are usually found in the anus, mouth, or nipples.^Q
- In 60–70% of patients, the disease heals spontaneously at this stage.

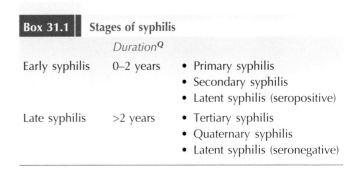

Box 31.1	Stages of syphilis	
	Duration^Q	
Early syphilis	0–2 years	• Primary syphilis • Secondary syphilis • Latent syphilis (seropositive)
Late syphilis	>2 years	• Tertiary syphilis • Quaternary syphilis • Latent syphilis (seronegative)

Diagnosis (Box 31.2)

- A specific diagnosis can be made using the smear from the chancre by dark ground microscopy.
- It is important to note that serological tests will take 3–4 weeks to become positive.
- Generally, the first test to become positive is EIA (IgM)/19S IgM-FTA-Abs^Q followed by Rapid plasma reagin/Venereal Disease Research Laboratory (RPR/VDRL) and then by *Treponema pallidum* hemagglutination (TPHA) tests.

Secondary Syphilis

Clinical features: After 12 weeks of primary infection, or 8 weeks of the appearance of the chancre, the patient passes into the secondary stage. It is possible to pass into secondary syphilis without suffering from primary chancre, when the disease is transferred by other means like transfusion of infected blood.

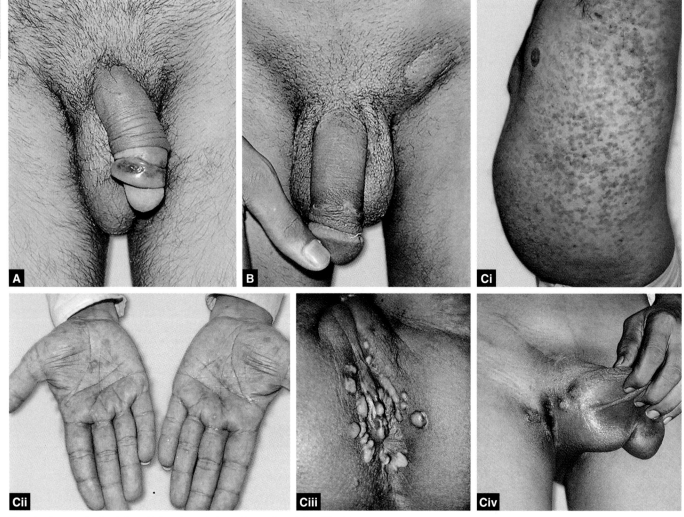

Fig. 31.1A to C: Syphilis: (A) Single painless ulcer of syphilis; (B) Unilateral enlarged lymph node after healing of primary chancre; (Ci to iv) (i) Macular rash of secondary syphilis; (ii) The rash classically involves the palms and soles; (iii and iv) Flat-topped papules in the flexures (condylomata lata)

Box 31.2	Overview of the diagnostic tests in syphilis

Most specific test: DG microscopy
Most specific blood test: TPHA/TPPA
Most sensitive blood test: IgM-FTA-Abs/EIA
Test for monitoring Rx: VDRL
Time taken for seropositivity in primary syphilis
- EIA (IgM)/IgM-FTA-Abs—3 weeks
- VDRL/RPR—4 weeks
- TPHA/TPPA—4–6 weeks

- Constitutional symptoms set in like fever, headache, myalgia and arthralgia.
- There is widespread lymphadenopathy out of which epitrochlear is the characteristic,[Q] besides which cervical, occipital, axillary and inguinal lymph nodes are also involved.
- The secondary stage is considered widely as 'the great mimicker' as the condition can mimic most

dermatoses. The generalized lesions are called 'syphilides'[Q] (Fig. 31.1Ci to iv).
- These are *asymptomatic* and mostly *bilateral* as well as symmetrical and involve the *palms* and *soles* (Fig. 31.1Cii).[Q] An overview of the exanthems is listed in Box 31.3, while the systemic features are listed in Box 31.4.

Box 31.3	Important aspects of cutaneous rash
Most common rash	Macular/roseolar rash
Rash rarely seen[Q]	Bullous (except in infants)
Papular rash	Involving genitalia: Condylomata lata—most infectious lesion of syphilis[Q] (Fig. 31.2Ciii and iv)
Alopecia	Non-scarring-moth-eaten hair loss[Q]
Mucous lesions	Mucous patches and snail track ulcer
HIV or immuno-compromised	Ulcerated (malignant syphilid) or crusted (rupial syphilis)

Box 31.4	**Systemic manifestations of secondary syphilis**
Liver	Acute hepatitis
Kidneys	Acute membranous glomerulonephritis
CNS	Meningitis or meningoencephalitis; it has been estimated that about 25% of patients with secondary syphilis have abnormal CSF, with increased cells, protein and presence of *T. pallidum*, but are largely asymptomatic[Q]
Spleen	Enlarged in almost 100% of cases.
Musculoskeletal abnormalities	Periostitis, polyarthritis, tenosynovitis

Course: Even in the absence of treatment, all lesions resolve and many patients never develop further manifestations. Skin lesions heal within 2 weeks to 2 months, leaving behind dyspigmentation. But if untreated, the lesions can recur episodically for up to 2 years.

Systemic features of secondary syphilis are listed in Box 31.4.

Diagnosis

- All serological tests are usually *positive* in *high titres* in secondary syphilis.
- Additionally, one can detect treponemes from smears made from lesions like condylomata lata.

Latent Syphilis

After 1–3 months, the secondary stage passes into latency, meaning there are no overt signs of the disease but the patient remains capable of transmitting the infection. During this phase patient is serologically positive for tests of syphilis.

This phase is divided into two types:
- Early latent—first 2 years of infection, and
- Late latent—after 2 years of infection.

Diagnosis: EIA is the most sensitive[Q] followed by FTA-Abs and then by TPHA/TPPA.

Tertiary Syphilis

This stage is arrived at after 3–10 years of infection, in an untreated case. This is gradually becoming rare because of the availability of effective medications.

It is important to note here that only 1/3rd out of late latent stage patients, actually get tertiary syphilis.[Q] In itself, tertiary syphilis is further subdivided into late benign, cardiovascular and neurosyphilis (Fig. 31.2).

Late benign: Sometimes referred to as late benign syphilis, as these changes are much less serious and much more responsive to therapy than the other late manifestations. The classic skin lesion described is the

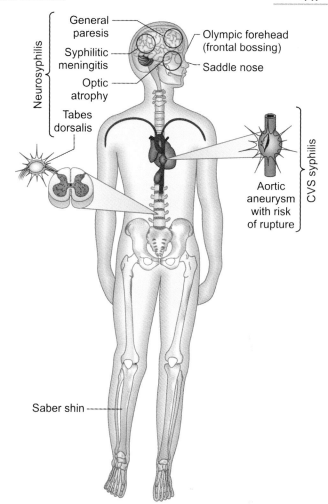

Fig. 31.2: An overview of the various organs involved in tertiary syphilis

gumma[Q] which is a firm 1–3 cm subcutaneous nodules that is painless and usually solitary.

Cardiovascular disease: About 10% of untreated patients develop cardiovascular syphilis in which the vasa vasorum (vessels nurturing the aorta) is affected leading to aneurysm formation and aortic insufficiency and is a frequent cause of death.[Q]

CNS disease: In late syphilis, most neurological symptoms are caused by chronic vessel inflammation. Spontaneous resolution can occur during the tertiary inflammatory phase, but not in the quaternary phase.

1. *Asymptomatic neurosyphilis:* CNS involvement is only detected by examination of CSF; no signs or symptoms.
2. *Meningovascular neurosyphilis:* Main finding in meningeal inflammation, usually with prominent headache. Also CNS thromboses cause a variety of neurological and psychiatric symptoms.
3. *Quaternary syphilis:*[Q] The most devastating complications of syphilis are the late parenchymal problems, which are not generally reversible.

General paresis: Formerly known as general paresis (paralysis) of the insane; about 2% of untreated patients advance to this stage; onset of signs and symptoms is 20–25 years after initial infection.

Tabes dorsalis: About as common as general paresis. Changes involve the dorsal roots and posterior columns of spinal cord. The patients have paresthesias, shooting pains, and a peculiar foot-slap walk.[Q]

Diagnosis

- *For tertiary syphilis*: Most sensitive is FTA-Abs, followed by TPHA/TPPA.
- *Neurosyphilis*: CSF-VDRL is the investigation of choice and a positive test is considered highly specific for neurosyphilis.[Q]
- CSF- FTA-Abs is the most sensitive.[Q] Thus, if the CSF-VDRL is nonreactive, and neurosyphilis is suspected, a CSF FTA-ABS can be ordered and neurosyphilis is highly unlikely with a negative CSF FTA-ABS test.

Congenital Syphilis

If primary infection accompanies conception, many spirochetes cross the placenta, the fetus is damaged, and it usually aborts at 7–8 months.[Q] If the mother has secondary syphilis at conception, a viable infant is born but with a spectrum of clinical findings resembling stages II or III disease. Finally, infection may occur via a spirochete-laden birth canal when the newborn develops a chancre, usually on the presenting part. A mother can transmit syphilis to her child at any stage of the disease. It is divisible into 2 stages.

- Early congenital syphilis—within the first two years of life. It is equivalent to adult secondary syphilis and is infectious.[Q]

 The fetus' immature immune response allows syphilis to run a rapid and damaging course. Prognosis is especially poor, if signs and symptoms are present at birth. The features are listed in Box 31.5.

Box 31.5	Features of early congenital syphilis
Present at birth	Low birth weight, abnormally large placenta, hepatosplenomegaly, blisters and erosions mainly on palms and soles (*pemphigus syphiliticus*),[Q]
First months in untreated infants	• *Snuffles* (chronic runny nose, often bloody), periorificial rhagades[Q] • *Hepatosplenomegaly* with fibrosis and jaundice (flint store liver).[Q] • Periosteitis and osteochondritis involving mainly long bones with so much pain that infants do not move limbs (*parrot pseudo-paralysis*—epiphyseal dislocation of the ulna, leaving a useless forearm)[Q]

- Late congenital syphilis—this takes place after 2 years of life and resembles adult tertiary syphilis but CVS involvement is rare. It is non-infectious:
  - Interstitial keratitis: Affects about 10%, usually bilateral; appears at age 10–30. Initially iritis, then corneal neovascularization and clouding.
  - Sensory deafness: Develops at 10–20 years of age in 10–30%; usually bilateral.
  - Neurosyphilis: Late onset but affects 30–50%.[Q]
- Stigmata-remnants or scars of congenital syphilis (Fig. 31.3A to C).

These are listed in Box 31.6.

Diagnosis: Maternal IgG crosses the placenta, but IgM does not. Finding antitreponemal antibodies in the newborn with the 19S-lgM-FTA-ABS[Q] (IgM fluorescent treponemal antibody-absorption) test proves that in utero infection has occurred.

Investigation of Syphilis

The diagnosis of syphilis can be confirmed using two types of tests:

a. Dark-ground illumination microscopy for visualisation of the organism.

b. Serological tests: Specific and non-specific to detect antibodies against the organism (Fig. 31.4).

 Non-specific also known as non-treponemal

 - VDRL and RPR toluidine red unheated serum test (TRUST)
 - VDRL remains the investigation of choice for monitoring response to therapy in syphilis.[Q]
 - A titre <1: 8 is taken to be false positive[Q] and a four fold decline[Q] in titre over a period of 6 months in primary and secondary and 12–24 months in latent and tertiary syphilis is taken to be successful

Box 31.6	Stigmata of congenital syphilis[Q]

1. **Saddle nose** (75%)
2. **Frontal bossing** (hot cross bun or buttocks skull). Maxillary hypoplasia (85%)
3. **Higouménaki sign:** Thickening of medial end of clavicle
4. **Saber shins**
5. **Clutton joints:** Effusions into large joints
6. Gothic palate (high arched palate): 75%
7. Periorificial furrowed scars (**parrot lines**)
8. **Dental changes:**[Q]
   - Mulberry molars: First molars with complex surface; 65% (Fig. 31.3B)
   - Hutchison incisors: Incisors shaped like tip of a screwdriver, often notched; 65% (Fig. 31.3C)

Note: The Hutchinson **triad**[Q] consists of Hutchison incisors, sensory deafness, and interstitial keratitis.

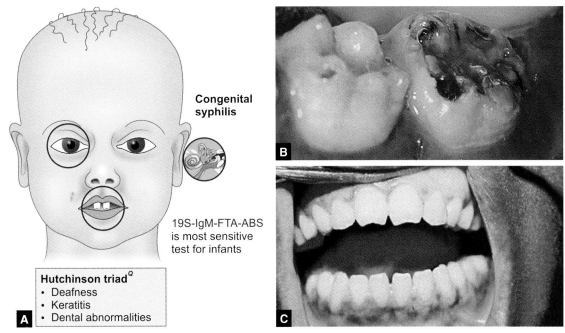

Fig. 31.3A to C: (A) Depiction of the **Hutchinson triad**; (B) Mulberry molars; (C) Upper and lower middle incisors shaped in the form of the head of a screwdriver, known as Hutchinson's teeth

Key Points in Syphilis

- Dory-flop sign[Q]—chancre on the prepuce, being cartilaginous in consistency flips back suddenly on retraction of prepuce
- Rash, generalized lymphadenopathy, condylomata lata (most classical, most infectious), snail track ulcers, moth-eaten alopecia are all features of secondary syphilis.
- Buschke-Ollendorf sign[Q]—pressure with a blunt instrument on the lesions over palms and soles elicits tenderness.
- Pseudochancre redux—gumma occurring over site of chancre
- Chancre redux[Q]—inadequate treatment leading to formation of chancre at the site of healed chancre.
- Cardiovascular syphilis—aortitis of the ascending aorta.
- CNS involvement can occur at any stage of syphilis and manifest as asymptomatic, general paralysis of insane and tabes dorsalis.
- Jarisch-Herxheimer reaction[Q]—Inj. benzathine penicillin given in a state of heavy bacterial load results in mass destruction of the treponemes and symptoms of high fever, lymphadeno-pathy and prostration especially in secondary syphilis.
- Snuffles[Q]—earliest and most common sign[Q] in congenital syphilis
- Bullae (syphilitic pemphigus)[Q]—most classical feature of congenital syphilis
- Parrot's pseudoparalysis[Q]—infant's refusal to move due to diaphyseal epiphysitis and osteochondritis
- Wimberger's sign—bilateral destruction of metaphysis of proximal tibia[Q]
- Clutton's joints—painless, symmetrical swelling of the knees, a feature of late congenital syphilis
- Saddle nose[Q]—another feature of late congenital syphilis
- Hutchinson's triad—in congenital syphilis Hutchinson's tooth (peg shaped upper incisor with a notch) + 8th nerve deafness + interstitial keratitis.
- Mulberry molars—another stigmata of congenital syphilis.

treatment (there are 2 types of false positive VDRL—acute and chronic. While the most common cause of chronic false positive VDRL are, autoimmune diseases; malaria, active pulmonary tuberculosis, leprosy, SABE chickenpox pregnancy is a cause of acute false positive VDRL).

Specific also known as treponemal

- Fluorescent treponemal antibody absorption (FTA-ABS)
- Microhemagglutination test for antibodies to *T. pallidum* (MHA-TP)
- *T. pallidum* particle agglutination assay (TPPA)
- *T. pallidum* enzyme immunoassay (TP-EIA)

TPHA: It is a highly specific test and becomes positive around 4 week and remains positive for life of patient.[Q] As it is expensive, it is used to confirm a positive VDRL test.

FTA-ABS test[Q]: It is also a confirmatory, test and becomes positive around 4th–6th week and remains so forever. It is both sensitive and specific. Which remain positive lifelong, also after therapy, as they recognize IgG antibodies.

The IgM-FTA-ABS test (positive at 3 weeks), test is a modification to identify fetal IgM and clarify the diagnosis of congenital syphilis or a re-infection. IgM antibodies indicate a new infection and have almost 100% specificity.

It is important to understand while generally speaking the titres of non-specific tests of syphilis

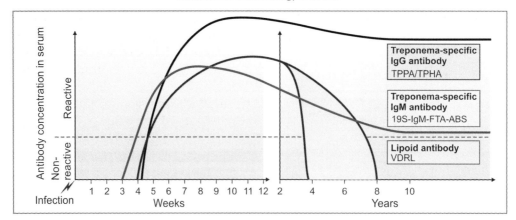

Fig. 31.4: A depiction of the serological response of tests in syphilis (CDC, USA)

lower with treatment and can become negative, the specific tests once positive do not attain negativity throughout life.

Testing Protocol

a. Traditional method—VDRL/RPR and if positive in significant titre ≥1: 16, then perform TPHA/TPPA for confirmation.

b. Reverse testing protocol—first EIA is done. Positive EIA signifies infection, but can be past as well as present. VDRL/RPR is performed, and if it is positive in significant titre (titer >1: 64) it is believed to be an active infection. If VDRL/RPR is negative then it is taken to be a discordant sample and a tie-breaker third test is taken. That test is TPHA/TPPA. When this test is positive, treatment for late latent syphilis is administered.

Treatment

The basic principles are:

1. Early syphilis (first 2 years of infection)—benzathine penicillin G 2.4 million units IM in a single dose.

2. Late syphilis (after 2 years of infection)—benzathine penicillin G 2.4 million units IM, 3 doses in weekly intervals.

3. For penicillin allergic non-pregnant patients—doxycycline 100 mg bd for 14 days.

4. For penicillin sensitive pregnant patient—penicillin after desensitization. Erythromycin is not an effective drug even though it might be safer

5. For neurosyphilis—aqueous crystalline penicillin is the drug of choice[Q] as benzathine penicillin does not cross the blood–brain barrier.

6. In HIV positive patients, the treatment remains the same.

   Since HIV patients with secondary syphilis have an increased risk of neurosyphilis, the approach must be modified slightly. Benzathine penicillin G is only used with a negative CSF serology and then once weekly for 3 weeks. If a CSF diagnosis is not possible,

then the patient should be treated as though they have neurosyphilis.[Q]

8. Rarely, the lesions of syphilis may become worse after treatment, this is called the **Jarisch-Herxheimer** reaction.[Q] This is characterised by acute febrile illness with fever, headache, myalgia and joint pain which occurs within the first 24 hours after therapy. Most commonly seen in secondary stage and it might induce early labor or cause fetal distress in pregnant women.[Q]

A summary of the treatment is given in Table 31.1.

CHANCROID

Synonyms: Soft chancre, soft sore, soft ulcer and ulcus-molle.

Chancroid is an acute, painful, autoinoculable ulcerative STI caused by *Haemophilus ducreyi*.

It is commoner in warm climatic regions, like tropics and subtropics.

It is also commoner in young males in the age group of 20–30 years and is associated with poor hygiene.

Causative agent: *Haemophilus ducreyi*.

It is a facultative anaerobe, pleomorphic gram-negative bacillus. Under the microscope, after Gram staining, it shows the characteristic **'school of fish'** or **'railroad track'**[Q] appearance. It grows best on **Müller-Hinton agar**.

Incubation period: 3–7 days.

Clinical Features

• After a brief incubation period, patient reports with multiple, soft, painful, small, superficial, necrotic (pus on ulcer base) ulcers of variable sizes with undermined and ragged margins. There is purulent discharge and ulcers bleed on touch[Q] (Fig. 31.5A).

• The common sites of affliction are the under surface of the prepuce, preputial orifice, coronal sulcus, frenulum and shaft of penis. In the females, the ulcers are observed over labia majora, labia minora, fourchette and vestibule. Extragenital sites include the thighs, perianal areas, abdomen, fingers, breast and mouth.

Table 31.1	Treatment of syphilis	
Early syphilis	Benzathine penicillin 2.4 million IU IM (1.2 million IU in each buttock)—**single dose**	*Alternatives* Doxycycline 100 mg bid p.o. 14 days Ceftriaxone, 1 g IM or IV daily for 10–14 days
Late syphilis	Benzathine penicillin 2.4 million IU IM (1.2 million IU in each buttock)—**three doses at weekly interval**	Doxycycline 100 mg bid po 28 days Ceftriaxone, 2 g IM or IV daily for 10–14 days
CNS (CNS-CP)	Crystalline Penicillin 3–4 million units IV every 4 hours or continuous infusion for 10–14 days	*Alternative non-penicillin regimens* Ceftriaxone 2g IM or IV daily for 10–14 days Oral doxycycline 100 mg twice daily for 28 days
Congenital syphilis (C-CP)	Crystalline Penicllin 50, 000 IU/kg IV 12 hrly—1st 7 days 50, 000 IU/kg IV 8 hrly next 3 days	
Pregnancy	Benzathine penicillin 2.4 million units IM weekly for two doses	In the case of penicillin allergy • Desensitization to penicillin or alternative regimens • Erythromycin (WHO) • Azithromycin 500 mg daily for 10 days or • Ceftriaxone 1 g IM or IV daily for 10–14 days

- An important feature is a 'kissing ulcers' formed like mirror images due to autoinoculation.^{Q} This ulcerative STI has one of the highest potential to transmit human immunodeficiency virus (HIV) infection.
- *Course:* Spontaneous healing after 4–6 weeks in men, many months in women.
- It has a number of clinical variants like transient, follicular, giant, dwarf, serpiginous, mixed, papular, pseudogranuloma inguinale and phagedenic forms.

Complications

1. A phagedenic ulcer is characterised by a rapidly spreading necrotic ulceration and tissue destruction caused by superimposed secondary anaerobic bacteria.
2. Inguinal lymphadenopathy (bubo) may develop and is characteristically unilateral, unilocular and tender.^{Q} They develop in 50% after 1–2 weeks. Typically forms abscesses that rupture forming fistulas (Fig. 31.5B).
3. Balanoposthitis, phimosis, paraphimosis and urethral stricture are additional complications.

Investigation

- A Gram, Giemsa's or Wright stain is done on a specimen taken from an ulcer or bubo aspitrate. Gram negative coccobacilli are found in small clusters or in parallel chains as described the 'school of fish' and 'railroad track appearance' (Fig. 31.5C).
- Culture requires special media (Mueller-Hinton agar); check with local lab. In best hands, 75% sensitivity.
- Ideally PCR confirmation.
- Other investigations include fluorescent labelled antibody detection and histopathology.
- *Ito test:* It is an historical test, which was an intra-dermal test for the diagnosis of infection.^{Q}

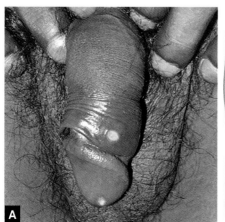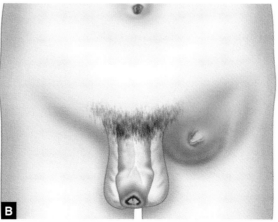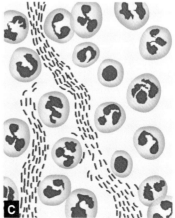

Fig. 31.5A to C: Chancroid: (A) Painful muiltiple ulcers, necrotic base, with a red halo and bleeds on touch; (B) A depiction of the bubo that is classically unilateral painful and unilocular; (C) A depiction of the Gram-negative coccobacilli arranged in a linear 'school of fish' pattern

Treatment

- Azithromycin 1 gm orally in a single dose *or*
- Ceftriaxone 250 mg in a single dose *or*
- Ciprofloxacin 500 mg orally bd for 3 days *or*
- Erythromycin base 500 mg orally tds for 7 days

Inguinal lymphadenopathy (bubo) can be aspirated with a wide-bore needle from a non-dependent area and the surrounding healthy skin.

Key Points in Chancroid

- Multiple, soft, tender genital ulcers with irregular, undermined edges, bleeds to touch and associated with unilateral, painful bubo is characteristic of chancroid.
- Kissing ulcers
- 'School of fish' or 'railroad track appearance' on Gram stain

GENITAL HERPES

It is important to note that herpes simplex viral infection is one of the most common sexually transmitted infection in the world (WHO, August 2015), along with trichomoniasis and chlamydial infections.[Q]

Herpes genitalis is a chronic viral infection, described first by French physician Jean Astruc in 1736. It is characterised by recurrences occurring due to reactivation of the virus.

Much like chancroid, herpes is also commoner in males in the age group of 15–40.

Causative agent: Herpes simplex virus 1 and 2 (HSV-1 and 2).

Ordinarily, it was believed that HSV 1 is responsible for herpetic infections above the waistline and HSV-2 below it, but with change in sexual practices no such demarcation can be considered accurate.

The virus can be acquired by genital as well as orogenital contact, although qualitatively the nature of disease is subtly different.

Most of the infection is spread by asymptomatic shedders of the virus.[Q]

Incubation period: 2 days–2 weeks.

Clinical Features

The course of illness is characterised by a primary illness, which is considered to be very symptomatic, followed by unpredictable recurrences and asymptomatic shedding in between.

- Prior infection with HSV-1 modifies the symptoms of 1st infection by HSV-2.
- After the 1° infection, the virus establishes in local sensory ganglia, reactivating periodically and appearing subsequently at the skin surface (where it may or may not produce symptoms).
- HSV replication occurs much more frequently then previously thought, with the virus trickling down the sensory nerve thus accounting for recurrence.
- This viral replication explains the concept of asymptomatic viral shedding.

Types: Primary, recurrent, asymptomatic shedders (Fig. 31.6A).

Why most people do not realise they have herpes?
- Infections (acquired and transmitted) are often asymptomatic.
- Symptoms can be subtle—not identified as herpes by patient (clinician!)
- HSV is not on clinician's radar, therefore, not tested for.

Primary Episode

- The primary episode has classic herpetic lesions that is grouped vesicular lesions or vesicular papules. These breakdown to form multiple, bilateral, superficial, painful ulcers. These are close set, so noticing a coalesced or even polycyclic ulcer,[Q] should raise a suspicion of genital herpes (Fig. 31.6B).

- Typically the lesions are ulcers, but they may be innocuous fissures, abrasions, or even mild erythema.
- It is important to note that chronic non-healing ulcer (>1 month) in the anogenital region, should raise the suspicion of HIV infection.

- Constitutional: Malaise-febrile flu-like illness lasting 5 to 7 days. More common in 1° infection. Less common in non-primary infection. There may be tingling/neuropathic pain in genital area, buttocks or legs (sacral dermatomes).

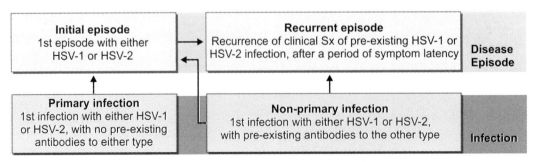

Fig. 31.6A: Classification of herpes virus infection

- Tender inguinal lymphadenitis
- Untreated, a first episode may last 3 weeks or so

Complications

1. 2° infection of lesions (*Candida*, *Streptococcus*)
2. Autoinoculation to fingers and adjacent skin
3. Urinary retention (may be 2° to severe local pain, or may rarely be due to autonomic neuropathy)
4. Aseptic meningitis: Characterized by headache, neck stiffness and photophobia.
5. In the background of immunosuppression, even a relatively immunosuppressed physiological condition of pregnancy, patient may have features of dissemination, resembling chickenpox.

Recurrent

Once the primary illness subsides, the patient suffers an unpredictable course of recurrences. This takes place due to reactivation of virus, present in the sacral dorsal root ganglia.[Q] These recurrences can be triggered by stress (physical and emotional), menstruation, any co-infection, immunosuppression.

Clinical features: Symptoms are milder. A prodrome (local skin tingling, sciatic nerve pain) occurs in 50% of cases up to 48 hours before lesions appear.

Lesions are similar to initial episode, and range from vesicles and erosions unilateral, and lesions heal more quickly (Fig. 31.6C and D).

Asymptomatic Shedding

Subclinical shedding refers to the detection of virus in the absence of visible lesions and most cases of herpes are transmitted without symptoms (asymptomatic viral shedding).

About 50% occur around the episode, while 50% occur after 7 days of the episode.[Q] The importance lies in the fact that if patients are counselled about the mild signs and symptoms of recurrent outbreaks, they can avoid sexual contact during these periods and prevent transmission to their partners.

Investigation

1. **Tzanck smear:** Reveals multinucleate giant cells[Q] (Fig. 31.6E)
2. **Serological testing:** Must be type-specific and needs careful interpretation (IgM detection is an unreliable indicator of recent infection).

   Thus, test based on HSV glycoprotein G[Q] are the most important and reliable diagnostic tool for chronic HSV infection. Antibody tests based on complement fixation, indirect immunofluorescence or neutralisation technologies cannot reliably distinguish antibodies to HSV-1 from those to HSV-2. While a negative result of an antibody test can be reassuring in that it excludes the diagnosis in a patient who has symptoms suggestive of long-standing or recurrent herpes but a positive result on a test that is not HSV glycoprotein G based is of little diagnostic value, because these serologic assays do not reliably distinguish between type 1 and type 2 infections.
3. **Herpes simplex viral culture:** High specificity (100%), sensitivity varies from 75% in primary infection to 50% in recurrences.
4. **Polymerase chain reaction (PCR)** is highly sensitive (gold standard).[Q]

Treatment

Primary Episode

- Acyclovir 400 mg orally TDS for 7–10 days *or*
- Acyclovir 200 mg orally 5 times a day for 7–10 days *or*

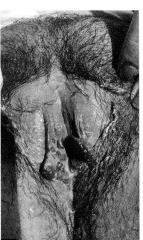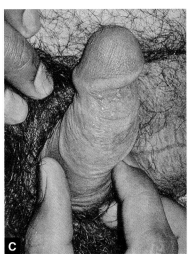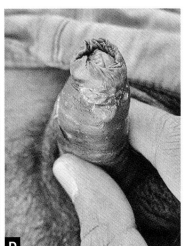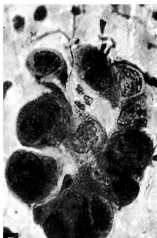

Fig. 31.6B to E: (B) Polycyclic, bilateral and symmetrical erosions seen in herpes primary—first episodic; (C) Recurrent herpes with a few vesicles or (D) Isolated erosions; (E) Multinucleat giant cell with nuclei arranged in a 'jig-saw' puzzle[Q] pattern

- Famciclovir 250 mg orally tds for 7–10 days or
- Valacyclovir 1 gm orally bd for 7–10 days

Treatment can be extended in case of incomplete healing of the ulcer.

Recurrence

- Acyclovir 400 mg orally tds for 5 days or
- Famciclovir 250 mg orally tds for 5 days or
- Valacyclovir 1 gm orally bd for 5 days

Suppressive Therapy

- Acyclovir 400 mg orally bd
- Famciclovir 250 mg orally bd
- Valacyclovir 500 mg orally bd (for <10 episodes/year 500 mg od)

Suppressive Rx should be discontinued after a maximum of 12 months to reassess symptom episode frequency (maximum duration is 6 years).

Special Scenarios

- *Disseminated disease*: I/V acyclovir 10 mg/kg IV every 8 hours for 10–14 days.
- *Treatment of drug-resistant genital herpes*[Q]: Resistance is consequential to a mutation in the gene encoding HSV thymidine kinase (TK).[Q] TK-deficient strains are susceptible to **foscarnet** and **cidofovir** which do not depend upon TK but which inhibit viral DNA polymerase. Systemic therapy may be given with foscarnet (40 mg/kg body weight IV every 8 hours until clinical resolution) or cidofovir (5 mg/kg body weight weekly IV infusion over 1 hour for 2 weeks)

Pregnancy: If you have a pregnant woman with herpes, ask yourself:

- Is this a 1st episode or a recurrence? But this may be difficult to establish
- Which trimester?

Management of first episode HSV in pregnancy

i. 1st and 2nd trimesters: Manage *patients according to clinical need*

- Consider acyclovir orally for 5/7 days, if needed
- Anticipate vaginal delivery at term
- Inform midwife. Vigilance for HSV lesions will be needed at delivery.
- Daily suppressive Rx (acyclovir 400 mg po tds) from 36 weeks may be considered

ii. 3rd trimester: (*Beware!—risk of neonatal infection*)

- If in labor—admit to labor ward and inform admitting doctor. LSCS likely to be needed.
- If not in labor, LSCS may still be needed, especially if within 6 hrs of delivery (can still be shedding virus at delivery, even if no visible lesions).

- Continuous oral acyclovir in the last 4 weeks of pregnancy reduces risks of HSV recurrences at term.

Management of HSV recurrences in pregnancy

- Obstetrician should be informed if Hx of recurrent genital HSV-need to be vigilant for vulval lesions at delivery.
- Symptomatic recurrences are likely to be brief, so aim for vaginal delivery if no lesions at labor.
- Continuous oral acyclovir in last 4 weeks of pregnancy may be beneficial.
- If vaginal delivery was undertaken whilst HSV lesions were present at birth, then community midwife and GP should be informed look out for signs of neonatal HSV in baby subsequently.

 Key Points in Genital Herpes

Recurrent, multiple, painful, superficial, genital ulcers following grouped vesicular eruption with painful bilateral lymphadenopathy and heals without pigmentation.

LYMPHOGRANULOMA VENEREUM

Synonyms: Lymphogranuloma inguinale, climatic/tropical bubo, sixth venereal disease, silent disease.

Lymphogranuloma venereum (LGV) is a sexually transmitted infection with a characteristic transient, herpetiform genital lesion followed by suppurative, multilocular inguinal lymphadenopathy (bubo)[Q] and anal syndrome (Fig. 31.7A).

LGV is commonly seen in males in the age-group 20–40 and is seen like chancroid in unhygienic, promiscuous setting.

Causative agent: Chlamydia trachomatis serovars L1, L2, L2a or L3.[Q] It is an obligate intracellular pathogen.

Incubation period: 3–30 days (usually 10–14 days).

Clinical Features

The disease is characterised by features that are dependent on site of entry and stage of illness (Table 31.2).

Investigation

1. Giemsa stain helps to identify the characteristic inclusion bodies.
2. Culture: Culture on McCoy cell line followed by identification with labeled antibodies.
3. Intradermal Frei's test[Q] (Fig. 31.7B)—now obsolete.
4. Biopsy of the lymph node shows characteristic stellate abscess, surrounded by a palisading arrangement of epithelioid cells.[Q]

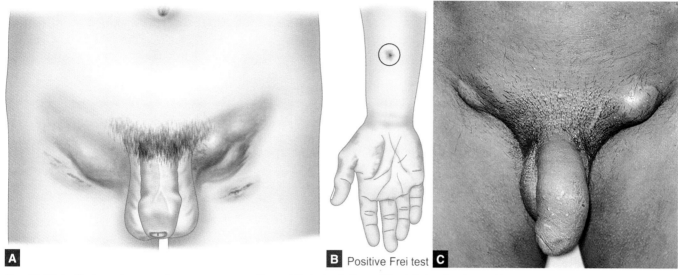

A
B Positive Frei test C

Fig. 31.7A to C: Lymphogranuloma venereum: (A and B) A depiction of the bilateral enlarged lymph node, with positive skin test; (C) 'Sign of groove'

Table 31.2	Clinical stages of lymphogranuloma venereum
Primary stage	• Transient erosion or ulcer • Herpetiform vesicle • Nonspecific urethritis or cervicitis
Secondary stage* (inguinal syndrome)	• Lymphadenopathy is prominent, painless, unilateral in 70% of cases, and both above and below inguinal ligament (sign of groove)^Q (Fig. 31.7C). • Occasionally in 30% of cases multilocular abscesses (buboes)^Q may be seen • These abscess can rupture to form multiple sinuses draining purulent or seropurulent discharge
Tertiary stage (genitoanorectal syndrome)	• Late complications include destruction of lymphatics with elephantiasis of the penis ram-horn ('ramrod penis' and the saxophone penis), scrotum, or vulva (esthiomene), accompanied by fistulas.^{Q} • The anorectal syndrome is characterized by multiple fissures and fistulae in the perianal region • Rectal carcinoma has been observed at later stages of LGV.
Systemic symptoms	• Acute phase, patient usually ill with fever, headache, myalgias; may even get aseptic meningitis or hepatitis. • Skin findings include erythema nodosum, exanthems, and photosensitivity

*Occurs 2–6 week after primary stage.

5. Serology-complement-fixation test and microimmuno-fluorescent test, which picks up type specific antibodies (L1, L2 or L3).

Key Points in LGV

1. • Asymptomatic (ulcer stage)
   • Bubo
   • *Chlamydia trachomatis* is the causative agent
   • Doxycycline is the drug of choice
   • Esthiomene is a known complication
   • Frei's test was done in the past
   • Groove sign of Greenblatt
2. Nucleic acid amplification test (NAAT) is the test of choice.

Treatment

Doxycycline 100 mg 1 cap bd for 21 days.

Alternative and in case of pregnancy:
• Erythromycin base or tetracycline 500 mg qid for 21 days
• Aspiration of bubo and surgical interventions are needed for esthiomene and strictures.

DONOVANOSIS (GRANULOMA INGUINALE)

Synonyms: Granuloma venereum, granuloma inguinale tropicum, fourth (4th alphabet is D = Donovanosis) venereal disease.^{Q}

Donovanosis is a chronic, autoinoculable slowly progressive infection characterized by formation of granulomatous ulceration of genitalia.

Just like LGV, donovanosis too is common in the age-group of 20–40. It is commonly seen in lower socio-economic status and people with poor hygiene.

Causative agent: *Calymmatobacter granulomatis* or *Klebsiella granulomatis.*[Q]

First described by Donovan. These organism are intracellular and give a 'closed safety pin'[Q] appearance (this happens due to clumping of chromatin at the periphery).

Incubation period: 8–80 days.

Clinical Features

- The skin lesion starts as painless papule at the point of entry. It then ulcerates and slowly evolves to form a, large, beefy-red ulcer with profuse granulomatous base which bleeds easily on touch[Q] (Fig. 31.8A).
- This can spreads locally or by autoinoculation to form a pseudobubo,[Q] wherein the skin overlying the lymph node is involved.

Complications

- Complications massive scarring causing pseudo-lymphadenopathy, lymphedema and elephantiasis
- Squamous cell carcinoma—it is the dreaded, long term complication of donovanosis.

Investigation

1. Demonstration of Donovan bodies by Gram's, Wright's, Giemsa or Leishman stain in crush tissue smears.[Q]

   Donovan bodies are intracytoplasmic, vacuolated, mature organism with coccoid, coccobacillary or bacillary forms, classic finding is 'safety pin sign'—bipolar staining bacteria within macrophages[Q] (Fig. 31.8B).

2. Histology shows granulomas in which the organisms can sometimes be identified with Giemsa or silver stains.
3. Culture very difficult; can be tried on McCoy cell lines.

Treatment

Recommended**
- Doxycycline 100 mg PO bid

Alternative**
- Trimethoprim-sulfamethoxazole, 1 double-strength (160 mg/ 800 mg) tablet PO bid *or*
- Ciprofloxacin 750 mg PO bid *or*
- Erythromycin base 500 mg PO qid *or*
- Azithromycin 1 g PO once weekly

Duration for all regimens: Until all lesions completely healed (at least 3 weeks)

**For any of the regimens, the addition of an aminoglycoside (e.g. gentamicin 1 mg/kg iv q 8 h) should be considered, if lesions do not respond within the first few days of therapy.

Key Points in Donovanosis

- Genital ulcer with exuberant granulation tissue on floor, bleeds to touch
- Beefy red genital ulcer
- No lymphadenopathy, pseudobubo
- Crushed smears show Donovan bodies—closed safety-pin appearance

URETHRITIS AND CERVICITIS

Urethritis is usually due to a sexually transmitted infection although a UTI (uncommon in young) may produce similar symptoms. The inflammation may sometimes be due to non-infective causes, but STIs must always be excluded, if the history (i.e. sexual contact, including oral sex) is suggestive.

Urethritis is diagnosed on the basis of any of the following signs or laboratory tests:

- Mucopurulent or purulent discharge on examination.
- Gram stain of urethral secretions demonstrating ≥5 WBC per oil immersion field (>2 according to CDC 2015).

The sexually transmitted infections that cause urethral discharge can be conveniently divided into 2, gonococcal and non-gonococcal, though its difficult to reliably distinguish between these clinically

1. Chlamydia
   - Diagnosed on 1st pass urine (an NAAT test)
   - Common cause of urethritis
2. Gonorrhea (also known as 'Gonococcus' or 'GC' for short)
   - Less common than Chlamydia

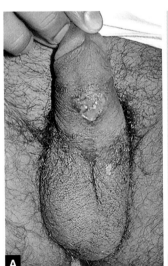
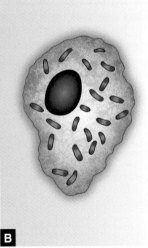

Fig. 31.8A and B: (A) Beefy red ulcer with autoinoculation on the scrotum—donovaniosis; (B) A depiction of the safety pin appearance

3. Non-specific urethritis (NSU)
   - This is really a diagnosis of exclusion after GC and Chlamydia have been ruled out.
   - Lots of different organisms can cause this, such as *Mycoplasma genitalium*, TV, yeasts, herpes, and adenoviruses (the latter is often seasonal and associated with oral sex).
   - Sometimes, there is not an infective cause at all.

The most common STI causes include *N. gonorrhoeae* (purulent discharge) or *C. trachomatis* (mucoid discharge), although it can also accompany *T. vaginalis*, *Candida* or *M. genitalium* infections. Diagnosis is made by clinical examination, microscopy/NAAT of cervical/vaginal samples.

The main diagnostic signs include:
- Purulent/mucopurulent endocervical exudate
- Sustained endocervical bleeding on passing a swab through cervical os.
- Leukorrhea (>10 WBC/hpf) on Gram stain of vaginal discharge. Gram-negative diplococci in gonorrhea infection.

GONORRHEA (Clap)

Latin *gonos* means seed; *rrhea* means flow.

It is a sexually transmitted infection which is an acute catarrhal inflammation of the genital mucosa, resulting into pain, burning during micturition and copious, urethral discharge.

It is frequently seen in males of the age group 20–30, but of late its incidence is declining and is taken over by non-gonococcal urethritis caused among others by chlamydia trachomatis.

In the female, it is notoriously silent, clinically.

Causative agent: *Neisseria gonorrhoeae*

It is a Gram-negative, kidney-shaped diplococcus which is found both intra- as well as extracellularly in neutrophils.

Incubation period: 1–4 days

Clinical Features

Male: It is an acute STI. Within days, the male complaints of burning micturition and copious purulent discharge from the urethra (urethral discharge in >80%, dysuria in >50%). In the early stage, the diagnosis is easy with the characteristic, copious, yellowish discharge[Q] soiling the undergarments (Fig. 31.9).

Female: Endocervical infection is often asymptomatic (up to 50%) but may present as abnormal vaginal discharge.

The infection is surprisingly asymptomatic in females. The reasoning is that the vaginal mucosa is

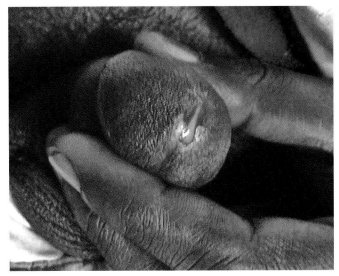

Fig. 31.9: Purulent discharge—gonorrhea

resistant to infection and the infection remains hidden in the cervix.[Q] The infected females remain as silent carriers of the illness with only mild complaints like pain, hesitancy, burning and frequent micturition.

Complications: If not treated early enough, then constitutional symptoms like fever, malaise, dizziness and headache.

Complications (uncommon, but can be serious): PID, epididymo-orchitis, prostatitis, local abscesses, disseminated spread, neonatal infection.

From the infected mother the disease can result into neonatal ophthalmic infections (ophthalmia neonatorum).

Investigation

1. Gram stained urethral smear—obtained with or without milking of the urethra.

   It is a highly sensitive (more than 95%) and specific (more than 99%) tool. When positive, it reveals gram-negative diplococci, typically kidney or bean shaped, found both intra- as well as extracellularly.[Q]

   Also >5 PMN per high power field can be seen.

2. Culture—the organism can be cultured on Thayer-Martin medium with Stuart's medium acting as transport media.

   Pros:
   - Antibiotic susceptibility testing can be carried out
   - Resistance can be monitored

   Cons:
   - Not as sensitive as NAATs
   - Delicate organism swabs require prompt transport to the lab. May not be viable if delay in reaching lab (false negative result)
   - Requires a swab-urine is not suitable

3. Nucleic acid amplification techniques (NAATs)
   Pros:
   • Generally more sensitive than culture
   • Some specimens can be non-invasive, e.g. 1st pass urine can be used in men and self-taken vaginals wabs in women (NB: Urine is not optimal in women).
   • Can also detect Chlamydia on the same specimen
   Cons:
   • Antibiotic susceptibility testing cannot be carried out
   • Because they are so sensitive, may get false +ves from contamination or non-gonococcal *Neisseria* species
   • Lower sensitivity in female urine (thus it is not an optimal specimen in women; vulvovaginal swabs or endocervical swabs are better).

Treatment

1. Uncomplicated gonococcal infections of the urethra, cervix or rectum
   • Injection ceftriaxone 250 mg IM stat[Q] (additional treatment with azithromycin 1 g as single dose or doxycycline 100 mg bid for 7 days).
   • Ceftriaxone 500 mg as a stat im injection *plus* azithromycin 1 g orally stat (azithromycin is given regardless of any Chlamydia results, to boost the ceftriaxone).

   Alternative treatment
   • Cefixime, 400 mg PO as single dose (additional treatment with azithromycin 1 g as single dose or doxycycline 100 mg bid for 7 days) (cefixime and other oral cephalosporins have demonstrated repeated Rx failures and should only be used if im injection is contraindicated or refused.)
   • Inj. spectinomycin 2 gm in a single dose.

2. Disseminated gonococcal infection
   • Recommended regimen
   • Ceftriaxone 1 g IM or IV q24h until 24–48 hours after improvement begins, then cefixime 400 mg PO bid to complete at least 1 week of therapy.

Follow up and Test of Cure

Test of cure is needed in all patients:
• If using NAATs, test 2 weeks after Rx. If +ve send culture
• If using culture, test >72 hours after Rx

NON-GONOCOCCAL URETHRITIS/ NON-SPECIFIC URETHRITIS

Urethritis where *Neisseria gonorrhoeae* is not involved, is referred traditionally as non-goncoccal urethritis, clubbing together multiple agents that can possibly infect the urethral mucosa. They can often co-exist with gonorrheae. Though many different causes are listed below, the most common cause is Chlamydia.[Q]

Causative agents

• *Chlamydia trachomatis* (D–K) (*C. trachomatis* is an obligate intracellular pathogen with a life cycle of 48 to 72 hours)
• *Mycoplasma hominis*
• *Ureaplasma urealyticum*
• *Trichomonas vaginalis*
• Adenovirus
• HSV

Incubation period: 1–2 weeks.

Clinical Features

The patient comes with subtle complaints of burning micturition and genital discharge that is scanty, mucoid, odorless[Q] and more during mornings (Fig. 31.10). Other symptoms include:
• **Males:**
  – Asymptomatic in over 50% in community settings.
  – Dysuria (beware 'sterile pyuria'—it may be *Chlamydia*).
  – Urethral discharge, urethral discomfort, epididymo-orchitis, sexually acquired reactive arthritis.
  – Rectal infections usually asymptomatic, but may cause anorectal discomfort and discharge.

• **Females:**
  – Asymptomatic in 70%
  – Vaginal discharge
  – Postcoital or intermenstrual bleeding (always suspect *Chlamydia* especially if this is a new symptom in a young adult)
  – Dysuria (beware 'sterile pyuria' reported on an MSU—it may be *Chlamydia*)

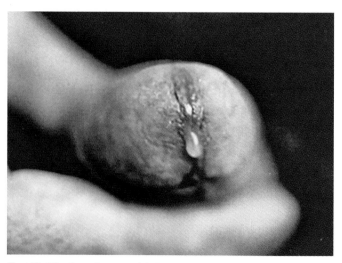

Fig. 31.10: Scanty mucoid discharge seen in non-gonococcal urethritis

- Lower abdominal pain
- Deep dyspareunia
- Cervicitis

Complications

- Pelvic inflammatory disease (PID): With no Rx, 10 to 40% will develop PID. PID can lead to tubal factor infertility, ectopic pregnancy and chronic pelvic pain
- Adult conjunctivitis: Unilateral or bilateral follicular conjunctivitis 1 to 2 weeks after exposure
- Neonatal conjunctivitis
- Sexually acquired reactive arthritis (SARA)
- Perihepatitis (Fitz-Hugh-Curtis syndrome)^Q: Inflammation of the hepatic capsule R^Q pain, sometimes referred to right shoulder. If chronic, adhesions (like *'violin strings'*)^Q may form between the liver capsule and abdominal wall. Usually seen with PID, suggesting intra-abdominal spread, but blood or lymph spread is a possibility.
- Pregnancy and the neonate:
  - *Increased risk* of premature rupture of membranes, preterm delivery and low birth weight, intra-partum pyrexia and late postpartum endometritis, postabortal PID.
  - Neonatal infections—exposed in birth canal during delivery 30 to 50% exposed infants develop infection. eyes, lungs, nasopharynx, genitals.

Investigation

1. Gram stain—reveals no diplococci but polymorpho-nuclear cells in abundance.
   Demonstration of more than 5 plus cells/oil immersion field is diagnostic.^{Q}
2. Urine routine microscopy—first void urine samples with 10–15 PMNs is also considered diagnostic.
3. Nucleic acid amplification techniques (NAATs)—a very sensitive way of detecting DNA^Q

Treatment

Therapy for NGU

Recommended regimens

- **Azithromycin** 1 g orally in a single dose or
- **Doxycycline** 100 mg orally twice a day for 7 days.

Alternative regimens

- **Erythromycin** base 500 mg orally four times a day for 7 days.
- **Levofloxacin** 500 mg orally once daily for 7 days.

Azithromycin and doxycycline are highly effective for chlamydial urethritis; however, infections with *M. genitalium* respond better to azithromycin.

Key Points in Urethral Discharge

- Non-gonococcal causes have a higher incidence
- Chlamydia is the commonest among them
- Profuse, purulent discharge is associated with gonorrhea, while scanty, mucoid discharge is associated with non-gonococcal urethritis
- Testis is not involved in gonococcal urethritis^Q
- Gram staining is the investigation of choice for gonococcal urethritis, culture is 'gold standard'
- NAAT done on urethral swab is the most sensitive and recommended test in non- gonococcal urethritis.

Treatment of Recurrent and Persistent Urethritis

Persistent urethritis after doxycycline treatment might be caused by doxycycline-resistant *U. urealyticum* or *M. genitalium*. *T. vaginalis* is also known to cause urethritis in men.

- **Metronidazole** 2 g orally in a single dose *or*
- **Tinidazole** 2 g orally in a single dose *plus*
- **Azithromycin** 1 g orally in a single dose (if not used for initial episode).

HUMAN PAPILLOMAVIRUS INFECTION

GENITAL/VENEREAL WARTS

Genital warts are one of the commonest STIs. Importantly, they constitute a leading, preventable cause of cervical cancer.

Causative agent: Human papillomavirus (DNA papova virus).

Non-oncogenic or low-risk HPV types (HPV types 6 and 11).

As well as oncogenic HPV types (HPV types 16 and 18).

Incubation period: 3 weeks to 8 months.

Most infections are subclinical, but generally speaking their incidence is on the rise. They are seen in the sexually active group of 15–25 years. These can also be transmitted through close skin to skin contact with an infected individual or even through fomites.

Pathogenesis

- HPV transmission is from direct skin to skin contact with apparent or subclinical lesions and/or contact with genital secretions microabrasions in the recipients skin.
- Poor initial immune response: HPV can persist as a latent infection, with no visible warts.
- Subsequently the immune system 'catches up': Local lymphocyte infiltration causes lesions to regress spontaneously (one-third of all visible warts disappear spontaneously).

Clinical Features

Asymptomatic single or multiple, finger like projections or greyish-brown papules or cauliflower-like growths seen over the mucocutaneous area of the genitalia. The commonly affected areas are penile shaft, foreskin, vulva, vagina, cervix, perineum and perianal region.

A pointed genital wart is also called condylomata acuminata[Q] (Fig. 31.11).

A large cauliflower-like mass on the genital mucosa, essentially a well-differentiated squamous cell carcinoma with only local invasion is called Buschke-Löwenstein tumor or giant condyloma.[Q]

Investigation

1. Acetowhitening[Q]—using 5% acetic acid on the lesion makes it clearly visible especially over areas like cervical mucosa.
2. HPV tests
3. Biopsy
4. Pap smear—this test is done over exfoliated cervical cells to look for premalignant changes.

Treatment

Rx options probably reduce, but may not eradicate HPV infectivity. Reassure patients that although wart clearance may take 1 to 6 months and recurrences may occur, complete clearance occurs in most, sooner or later. Generally, warts can recur in a quarter of cases after apparent clearance.

Principles of Treatment

1. While warts that are smaller than 1 cm² at the base can be treated by topical therapy, larger lesions require surgical intervention.
2. There is no evidence-based proof that any treatment is superior to any other.
3. No treatment is an option particularly for vaginal/anal warts.
4. Soft, non-keratinized warts respond well to podophyllin, while keratinized lesions are better treated with aggressive measures such as cryotherapy, trichloroacetic acid (TCA), excision or electrocautery.
5. Imiquimod may be suitable for both types.
6. Podophyllin should not be used in the anal and cervical area and TCA in the urethral meatus.[Q]
7. Women with external anogenital warts should have a speculum examination to check for vaginal/cervical lesions.

Agents

1. 5% imiquimod cream is a topical immune response modifier:[Q] It is applied alternate nightly for 3 nights a week (usually Mon/Wed/Fri) and then washed off each morning (total duration—16 weeks).
   Not approved for use in pregnancy.
2. Podophyllin resin (25%): It should be washed off after 6 hours and repeated weekly.
   It is contraindicated in pregnancy.
3. TCA (80–90%) destroys affected tissue by protein coagulation. While applying TCA, a barrier of petroleum jelly can be used to protect areas adjacent to the wart undergoing treatment.
4. Excision under local anesthetic: Useful if pedunculated warts, or small warts at anatomically accessible sites.
5. *Pregnancy*: As treatment does not reduce perinatal transmission, it is best to wait and intervene after pregnancy is over. Role of LSCS—bleeding or outlet obstruction.[Q]

   The safest modalities include cryotherapy, TCA, electrocautery and laser vaporisation.[Q] The use of imiquimod has not been approved in pregnancy.[Q]

   An overview of the therapeutic options is listed in Table 31.3.

Prophylaxis

Three types of vaccine against HPV are available:
- Bivalent (protective against HPV 16 and 18)
- Quadrivalent (protective against HPV 6, 11, 16 and 18)

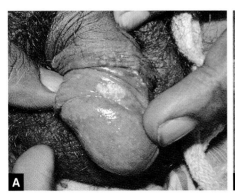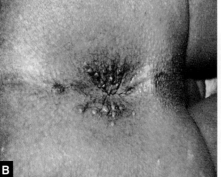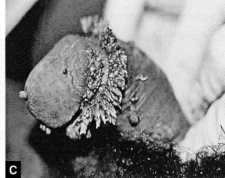

Fig. 31.11A to C: Various morphologies of genital warts ranging from verrucous (A), flat topped (B) and filiform (C) types

Table 31.3	Treatment of genital warts
Patient-applied	• Podofilox 0.5% solution or gel or • Imiquimod 5% cream or • Sinecatechins 15% ointment
Provider-administered	• Cryotherapy • Podophyllin resin 10–25% • Trichloroacetic acid (TCA) or • Bichloroacetic acid (BCA) 80–90% • Surgical removal
Cervical warts	• Biopsy evaluation to exclude high-grade SIL • Excision
Vaginal warts	• TCA 80–90% applied to warts • Cryotherapy
Urethral meatus warts	• Podophyllin 10–25% • Cryotherapy
Anal warts	• TCA 90% • Cryotherapy • Excision

• Nonavalent (protective against 6, 11, 16, 18, 31, 33, 45, 52 and 58)
  3 doses at 0, 2 and 6 months.

VAGINITIS

Vaginitis is characterized by vaginal discharge and odor, vulvar itching/irritation, dyspareunia, and dysuria. The three most common causes are:

1. **Bacterial vaginosis (BV):** Replacement of the vaginal flora (lactobacilli) by overgrowth of anaerobic bacteria including *Gardnerella vaginalis*,[Q] *Prevotella* sp., *Mobiluncus* sp., *Ureaplasma*, *Mycoplasma*; leads to foul smelling watery discharge; >20% clue cells[Q] on Gram-stain of vaginal smear (Fig. 31.12A and B). It is most common cause of altered vaginal discharge in women

Table 31.4	Amsel criteria[Q] for diagnosis of BV (three out of four criteria required)

1. Increased homogeneous thin vaginal discharge
2. Amine (fishy) odor when 10% KOH solution is added to a drop of vaginal secretions (Whiff test)
3. Presence of clue cells in vaginal smear (>20%)
4. Vaginal pH >4.5

of reproductive age group.[Q] The diagnostic criteria are listed in Table 31.4.

Treatment: Tab. metronidazole 500 mg po BD for 7 days; clindamycin and tinidazole.

2. **Vulvovaginal candidiasis (VVC):** Overgrowth of *Candida albicans* presents as thick curdy white adherent discharge associated with itching[Q] (Fig. 31.12C and D); pseudohyphae[Q] are seen on KOH smear. Common in women on long-term antibiotics, diabetics,[Q] immunocompromised or organ transplant recipients.

Treatment: Tab. fluconazole 150 mg stat; topical fluconazole.

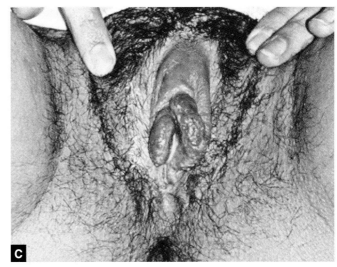

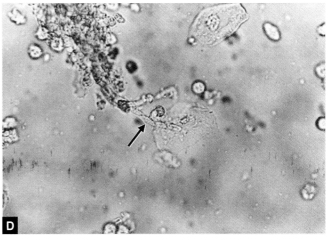

Fig. 31.12C and D: Candidiasis: (C) Lumpy white discharge with the consistency of a paste, wet talc or curdled milk, (D)10% KOH smear showing pseudohyphae

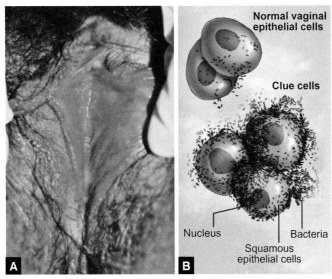

Fig. 31.12A and B: (A) White discharge that is *homogenous without* hyperemia of the mucosa seen in bacterial vaginosis; (B) A depiction of clue cells

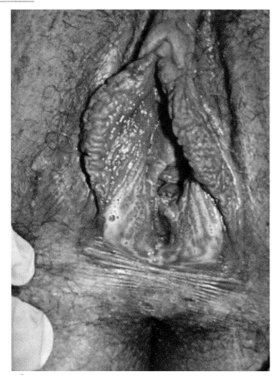

Fig. 31.12E: Frothy discharge suggestive of trichomoniasis

3. **Trichomoniasis:** Infection with *Trichomonas vaginalis*; greenish frothy discharge (Fig. 31.12E), and a strawberry cervix.ᵠ Mobile flagellate protozoaᵠ on wet saline smear.

Treatment: Tab. metronidazole 500 mg po BD for 7 days; tinidazole and secnidazole.

BV and VVC are not transmitted sexually, no partner treatment required.ᵠ

 Key Points in Genital Warts

- Imiquimod is generally considered to be drug of choice (works by stimulating toll like receptors 7 and 8).
- Podophyllotoxin acts as an antimitotic but is contraindicated in pregnancy.
- Interferon is a third line treatment in warts.
- Gental warts in pregnancy—cryotherapy is preferable to TCA.
- Routine cesarean section is not recommended for genital warts at labor although there appears to be a small risk of development of laryngeal papillomatosis of the newborn.
- Condylomata acuminata is a finger-like genital wart (e.g. Condylomata lata is a feature of secondary syphilis)
- Buschke-Löwenstein tumor is a giant condyloma and a well-differentiated squamous cell carcinoma with low metastatic rate.

Kit no.	Syndrome	Color	Contents
1.	Urethral discharge, cervicitis	**Grey**	Tab azithromycin 1 g (1) and Tab cefixime 400 mg (1)
2.	Vaginitis	**Green**	Tab secnidazole 2 g (1) and Tab fluconazole 150 mg (1)
3.	GUD	**White**	Inj. benzathine penicillin 2.4 mu (1) and tab azithromycin 1 g (1)
4.	GUD	**Blue**	Tab doxycycline 100 mg (30 doses) and tab azithromycin 1 g (1)
5.	GUD	**Red**	Tab acyclovir 400 mg (21 doses)
6.	LAP	**Yellow**	Tab cefixime 400 mg (1) and Tab metronidazole 400 mg (28 doses) and tab doxycycline 100 mg (28 doses)
7.	Inguinal bubo	**Black**	Tab doxycycline 100 mg (42 doses) and tab azithromycin 1 g(1)

Table 31.5 Color-coded STI/RTI drug kits available at suraksha clinics

SYNDROMIC MANAGEMENT OF STD

Due to paucity of resources in field settings and peculiar reluctance of STI patients to seek good quality care, as well as their reluctance in follow-up, government through National Aids Control Organization (NACO) promotes syndromic approach.

The syndromic management approach is based on the identification of groups of consistent symptoms and easily recognised signs (syndromes) and the provision of treatment that will deal with the majority of or the most serious organisms responsible for producing a syndrome. The various common syndromes and their treatment is given in Table 31.5. The aim of this approach is primarily to deal with the common STD seen and deal with them in the first visit.

The following are the syndromes:
- Urethral discharge
- Vaginal discharges
- Genital ulcer
- Inguinal buboes
- Lower abdominal pain
- Acute scrotal pain/scrotal swelling
- Genital skin conditions

The various color-coded kits that are part of this approach are given in Table 31.5.ᵠ

Therapeutics

CHAPTER 32

Medical Therapy

Chapter Outline

TOPICAL TREATMENTS

Introduction

The word 'Topical' derived from the Ancient Greek topos meaning 'place' or 'location'. Basic principle of topical therapy in dermatology is—'if lesion is wet, dry it or if lesion is dry, wet it'. Or more scientifically, 'if it's dry, use an ointment, if it's wet, use a cream.'

What Influences Absorption?

- *Body site*: The palm has very thick stratum corneum so absorbs little. The scrotum and periocular skin has a thin stratum corneum so absorbs more.
- *Stratum corneum function*: If the stratum corneum is moist (e.g. in body folds) much more will be absorbed than in dry exposed areas.
- *Influence of the disease*: If the stratum corneum is decreased absorption is easier. Thus, in treating psoriasis the drug gets in more easily at the diseased sites than the surrounding normal skin.
- *Size of what is being absorbed*: If the molecule is too large, very little will get in. Penetration enhancers such as propylene glycol may be added to topical drugs to increase drug absorption.

VEHICLES

Topical drugs are incorporated into 'vehicles'. They include all the constituents of formulation apart from active ingredients. An ideal vehicle should be non toxic, non-allergic, non-irritant, stable, chemically inert, cosmetically acceptable and should not inactivate the drug.

Vehicles may have non-specific beneficial effects like occlusion, hydration, cooling, soothing and astringent action. They form the reservoir of active agent.

Classification of Vehicles (Fig. 32.1A)

Galenics is the art to bring effective substances together with the desired vehicles into the correct mixture so that they reach their respective tissue. It is the most important aspect of topical dermatotherapy. In principle, there are different physicochemical characteristics of topical preparations which can be classified according to their nature with the so-called phase triangle according to Polano (Fig. 32.1A). These can then form various topical preparations.

- Monophasic vehicles: Powder, greases, liquids (gels, solution, lotion, tincture)
- Biphasic vehicles: Ointment (water in oil), cream (oil in water, shake lotion, paste).
- Triphasic vehicles: Foam/aerosols

Dosage forms

- *Solid*: Powder
- *Liquid*: Lotion, suspension, foam
- *Semisolid*: Paste, cream, ointment

Constituents of Vehicle

Lipids, emulsifiers, humectants, penetration enhancers, preservatives, solvents.

Important vehicles are listed in Table 32.1 and depicted in Fig. 32.1A.

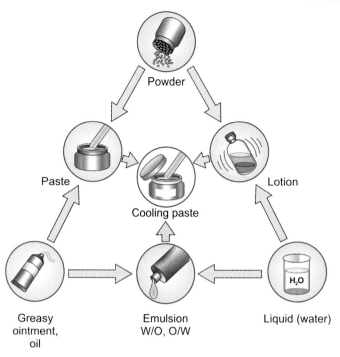

Fig. 32.1A: Phase triangle according to Polano for selection of vehicle in topical dermatotherapy (Ring, 2005);

Creams: A cream is a semi-solid mixture of water and lipids. Creams usually look opaque white (like fresh cream). Water and lipids do not blend, but can form an 'emulsion' in which small droplets of one are suspended in the other. If the cream is 'lipids in water' (e.g. aqueous cream), it will evaporate and so is cooling, and the cream will mix with water so it can be washed off. If the cream is 'water in lipids' (e.g. oily cream), it is more difficult to wash off.

Ointments are semi-solid mixtures of lipids (no water). They feel greasy and look transparent and grey. Drugs such as corticosteroids may be added to both cream and ointment bases. Ointments stick well to dry diseased skin.

An emollient ('moisturizer') is something that moisturizes and softens the skin surface. Both creams and ointments can be emollients.

PRESCRIPTION OF TOPICAL DRUGS

To be prescribed in right concentration of drug, required frequency of application, accurate quantity to be used, proper sites of application and precise timing of application.

Table 32.1 Overview of the various topical preparations

Type	Characteristic	Examples
Powder	They are solid vehicles that absorb moisture and decrease friction, maceration	Organic (starch, zinc/magnesium stearate) Inorganic powders (ZnO, titanium oxide, talc)
Lotion	It is finely divided insoluble drug dispersed in a liquid (water, alcohol or other)	Liquid soaps, shampoos (for scalp psoriasis, lice infestation, etc.), sunscreens
Shake lotions/ suspensions	They are lotion to which powder/solid particles is added to increase surface area of evaporation. Require shaking before use	Calamine lotion
Paste	It is a semisolid preparation, containing high concentration of powder up to 50% incorporated in ointment bases	Lassar's paste—used in psoriasis (anthralin, ZnO, corn starch, white soft paraffin and salicyclic acid)
Ointment	A semisolid dosage form, usually containing <20% water and volatiles and >50% hydrocarbons, waxes, or polyols as the vehicle. They are highly potent	Nitroglycerin ointment, mupirocin 2% ointment Tacrolimus 0.03% and 0.1% ointment In general useful for chronic scaling conditions like psoriasis, chronic eczema
Solution	It is a dissolution of two or more substances in homogenous clarity	Tincture, colloidions, liniments. Gauze dressings kept moist with dilute potassium permanganate solution (1:8000) or aluminium subacetate solution (8%) solutions providing antiseptic and astringent action.
Cream	It is a semisolid dosage form which, usually contains >20% water and volatiles and/or <50% hydrocarbons, waxes, or polyols as the vehicle It is a transition between lotions and ointments	Permethrin 5% cream Bezoyl peroxide cream 4% Clotrimazole 1% cream
Gel	A semisolid dosage form that contains a gelling agent to provide stiffness to a solution or a colloidal dispersion	Usually used in scalp solutions
Foam/aerosols	A product that is packaged under pressure and contains therapeutically active ingredients that are released upon activation of an appropriate valve system	Minoxidil foam, steroid foam, betamethasone foam 0.1%
Paint	It is a liquid preparation which is applied with brush to skin or mucous membrane	Castellani paint Wart paints contain salicylic acid and lactic acid

32

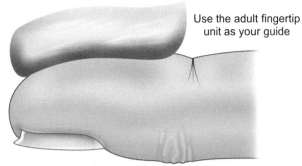

Use the adult fingertip unit as your guide

One adult fingertip unit

Fig. 32.1B: One fingertip unit (FTU) is the amount of cream/ointment squeezed from a tube from the distal interphalangeal joint to the end of the finger

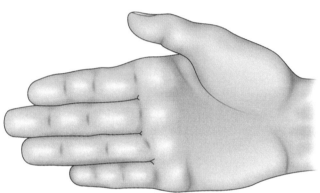

One hand print area is about 150 cm² in men and 120 cm² in women. This represents about 0.75% of total body surface area, but think of it as approximately 1%
Remember: One FTU covers 2 hand print areas

Fig. 32.1C: Rule of hand

Quantity can be determined by:

1. *FTU (fingertip unit)*: A fingertip unit (FTU) is the amount of ointment expressed from a tube with a 5 mm internal diameter nozzle applied from the distal skin-crease to the tip of the index finger. It is approximately 0.49 g in males and 0.43 g in females (Fig. 32.1B).

2. *Rule of hand*: States that 4 hand areas (adult) = 2 FTU = 1 g (Fig. 32.1C).

A general figurative guide to using this rule for the body is given in Fig. 32.1D and E.

If the patient does not improve with the topical treatment, it may be because of:

- Wrong diagnosis and inappropriate treatment
- Incorrect usage of the medication
- The condition is resistant to the drug
- An adverse effect from its use (e.g. contact allergy)

Adverse effects from topical drugs (Table 32.2): Adverse effects can be local or systemic.

Table 32.2	Adverse effects of topical agents
Adverse effects	*Characteristics*
Local	
Allergic contact dermatitis	Allergic eczematous rash at site of application, e.g. from neomycin, gentamicin
Irritant contact dermatitis	Irritant eczematous rash at site of application, e.g. from benzoyl peroxide
Photosensitivity	Erythematous or eczematous rash at sun-exposed site of application, e.g. antimicrobials, retinoids
Acneiform folliculitis	Acneiform rash at site of application, particularly in seborrheic areas
Others	Atrophy, comedogenicity, formation of telangiectases, pruritus, stinging and pain
Systemic	

Though generally safer than other routes of administration rare side effects can be observed like end-organ toxicity (CNS, cardiac, renal), teratogenicity, carcinogenicity, drug interactions

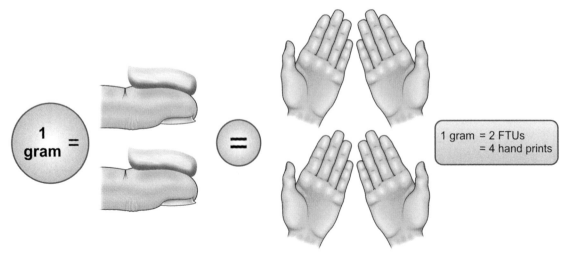

1 gram = = 1 gram = 2 FTUs = 4 hand prints

Fig. 32.1D: Figurative guide to FTU and rule of hand

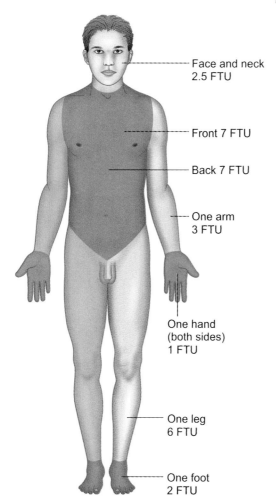

Fig. 32.1E: A depiction of FTU rule for various parts of the body

Labels on figure:
- Face and neck 2.5 FTU
- Front 7 FTU
- Back 7 FTU
- One arm 3 FTU
- One hand (both sides) 1 FTU
- One leg 6 FTU
- One foot 2 FTU

IMPORTANT TOPICAL AGENTS

Moisturizers

They are complex formulations designed to maintain hydration and integrity of skin. They contain varying combinations of emollients, occlusives and humectants to achieve beneficial effects by enhancing water holding capacity. An ideal moisturiser should mimic sebum.

Types of Moisturizer

- *Emollients*: Derived from 'mollire' meaning to soften. Emolliency is ability of a product to fill in the crevices between desquamating corneocytes.
- *Occlusives*: Oily substances which form a physical barrier and prevent evaporative water loss from skin, e.g. petrolatum.
- *Humectants*: These substances have high affinity for water, function to attract water from lower viable skin layers to stratum corneum, e.g. glycerin, honey.

Topical Corticosteroids

They are the most frequently used drugs for the treatment of patients with inflammatory skin diseases like psoriasis, eczematous skin conditions. Hydrocortisone acetate, the first topical corticosteroid developed for the treatment of inflammatory skin diseases, was introduced in 1952, by Sulzberger and Witten. In 1955, Fitzpatrick et al. first reported side effects from topical steroids.

They have specific and nonspecific effects like anti-inflammatory, immunosuppressive, antiproliferative and vasoconstrictive effects which are mostly mediated via the glucocorticoid receptor (GR). A major part of their action is inhibition of phospholipase A2-which is important in the generation of eicosanoid compounds involved in the inflammatory process.

Classification of Topical Steroids

British National Formulatory	American classification
1. Mild	Class 1: Superpotent
2. Moderate	Class 2: Potent
3. Potent	Class 3: Potent
4. Very potent	Class 4: Midstrength
	Class 5: Midstrength
	Class 6: Mild
	Class 7: Least potent

A few representative preparations are given below:
- *Mild potency*: Minimal risk of side-effects. Least effective, e.g. hydrocortisone 0.5%, 1.0%, 2.5%.
- *Moderate potency*: Minimal risk of side-effects. Mildly effective, e.g. clobetasone butyrate.
- *Strong potency*: Side-effects only if used daily for >2–3 weeks. Safe to use for few days in acute situations. Very effective, e.g. betamethasone valerate.
- *Very strong potency*: High risk of side-effects. Extremely effective, e.g. clobetasol propionate. Needed for resistant conditions (e.g. discoid lupus erythematosus), poor absorption sites (e.g. palms).

Adverse Effects

Local

1. Skin atrophy-thinning and striae, telengiactasias, purpura, ulceration, easy bruising.
2. Masked infection, particularly ringworm (tinea incognito), flaring up/increased incidence of infections, reactivation of Kaposi's sarcoma.
3. Acneiform eruptions: Rosacea—especially in fair skinned
4. Perioral dermatitis.
5. Hypertrichosis, hypopigmentation.
6. Delayed wound healing, genital ulceration burning, itching, irritation, dryness.

Topical Antimicrobial Agents

A list of the various antimicrobial agents that are used are listed in Tables 32.3 to 32.5.

Table 32.3 Topical antibacterial

Drug	Bacterial coverage	Mechanism of action
Bacitracin	Gram-positive and *Neisseria* species	Interferes with bacterial wall synthesis
Neomycin	Gram-positive and gram-negative bacteria; good *S. aureus* coverage	Inhibits protein synthesis
Mupirocin	Methicillin-resistant *S. aureus*; *S. pyrogenes*	Inhibits bacterial RNA and protein synthesis
Retapamulin	*S. pyogenes*, mupirocin-resistant and methicillin-resistant *S. aureus*, anaerobes	Inhibits bacterial RNA and protein synthesis; occurs by reversibly binding to bacterial isoleucyl transfer RNA synthetase
Gentamicin	Gram-positive and Gram-negative organisms; coverage includes *P. aeruginosa*	Inhibits bacterial protein synthesis; occurs by binding to protein L3 on 50s ribosomal subunit
Silver sulfadiazine	Gram-positive and Gram-negative organisms	Binds to bacteria DNA and inhibits its replication
Iodoquinol	Gram-positive and Gram-negative organisms	Unknown

Table 32.4 Topical antibacterial agents for acne and rosacea

Drug	Coverage	Mechanism of action
Benzoyl peroxide	Broad spectrum	Non-specific oxidizing activity
Clindamycin	Broad spectrum (*S. aureus*, streptococci, pneumococci, *B. fragilis*, *P. acnes*)	Reversibly binds to 50s subunit of ribosomal RNA subunit; net result is inhibition of protein synthesis
Erythromycin	Most Gram-positive bacteria and *P. acnes*	Reversibly binds to 50s subunit of ribosomal RNA subunit; net effect is inhibition of protein synthesis
Metronidazole	Gram-positive and Gram-negative bacterial coverage as well as anaerobic coverage	Disruption of mitochondrial respiration and DNA synthesis
Azelaic acid	Bacteriostatic and bactericidal against *P. acnes*	Disruption of mitochondrial respiration and DNA synthesis
Dapsone	Bacteriostatic against *Mycobacterium* species	Inhibition of dihydropteroate synthase and nucleic acid synthesis
Sodium sulfacetamide	Inhibition of dihydropteroate synthase and nucleic acid synthesis	Inhibits dihydropteroate synthase

Table 32.5 Topical antifungal agents

Drug	Coverage	Mechanism of action
Polyenes	Candida	Increase cell membrane permeability
Nystatin		
Azoles (mainly triazoles)	Inhibits ergosterol synthesis blocking 14α-demethylation of lanosterol	Dermatophytes, *M. furfur*, Candida
Miconazole, clotrimaxole, econazole, oxiconazole		
Allylamines and benzylamines	Inhibits sterol synthesis by blocking action of squalene epoxidase	Dermatophytes (both drugs) *Candida* (only terbinafine)
Terbinafine, naftifine		

SYSTEMIC TREATMENT

Even though topical treatments are extensively used and very effective for most of the dermatological conditions, systemic therapy is still required for many conditions and also in conditions unresponsive to topical treatment.

A few of the following considerations have to be kept in mind while choosing a systemic therapy:

- Higher chances of adverse side effects and so adverse profile of each drug and monitoring for the same is required.
- Appropriate dose to be administered to exert maximum effect with minimum adverse effects.
- Combination therapies of both topical and systemic drugs can also be administered.
- Usually for recalcitrant disorders systemic therapy is preferred (Table 32.6).

Table 32.6 Overview of common systemic agents used in dermatology

Drug	MOA	Main indications	Main adverse effects (A/E)	Dose	Remarks
Antifungal 1. Terbinafine	Inhibits sterol synthesis by blocking action of squalene epoxidase	• Dermatophytic infections • Systemic drug of choice in tinea infections • Dermatophyte onychomycosis (OM) of toenails/fingernails in adults (FDA approved)	• Gastrointestinal (GI) side effects (nausea vomiting, diarrhea, abdominal pain) • Headache • Rashes • Liver enzymes abnormality • Taste disturbance • Visual disturbances	250 mg, OD • Tinea pedis: 1–2 weeks • Tinea corporis: 2 weeks • Tinea unguium (OM): Fingernail: 6 weeks; toe-nails: 12 weeks	• Contraindicated (C/I) in allergic patients • Precautions required in liver and renal failure • Can be given in pregnant women
2. Azoles	Inhibits ergosterol synthesis blocking 14α-demethylation of lanosterol	**Fluconazole** • Candidiasis; vaginal candidiasis (FDA approved) • Other: P. versicolor, dermatophytic infection	• Very favorable side effect profile • GI Side effects (S/E)	• Acute vaginal candidiasis: 150 mg stat single dose • Recurrent vaginal: 150 mg/week for 6 weeks	• C/I in allergic patients and with drugs causing QTc prolongation • Avoid in pregnant and lactating women • Precaution in patients with renal, liver damage, pro-arrhythmic conditions
		Itraconazole • Candidiasis dermatophytic infections • OM (FDA approved)	• Headache • GI SEs	Vulvovaginal candidiasis: 200 mg, BD for 1 week • Oropharyngeal candidiasis: 100 mg OD for 1 to 2 weeks • Pityriasis versi-color: 200 mg OD for 1 week • OM: 200 mg, BD/week every month, for 2–3 cycles	• To be taken after food • Contraindicated in patients with ventricular arrhythmia and QTc interval prolongation • Caution in patients with hepatic impairment • Not recommended for children and in pregnant and lactating mothers
Corticosteroids	Mainly immuno-suppressive and anti-inflammatory	• Bullous disorders: pemphigus (FDA approved) pemphigoid • Autoimmune connective tissue disorders (AICTD): SLE, dermatomyositis, systemic sclerosis • Severe urticaria (FDA approved) • Extensive contact dermatitis (CD) • Stevens-Johnson syndrome (SJS), toxic epidermal necrolysis (TEN)	*Systemic side effects*: • HPA axis suppression • Infections—reactivation of TB and other opportunistic infections • Diabetes • Hypertension • Fluid electrolyte imbalance • Fat redistribution • Muscle wasting • Osteoporosis and vertebral collapse, avascular necrosis of head of femur • Growth retardation in children • Peptic ulcer disease, bowel perforation	Dosing (depends on the condition) • Daily/alternate day • Pulse therapy: Given as monthly 1–3 doses • Oral mini pulse: Given as weekly, single dose or on two consecutive days	C/I: Systemic fungal infections • Herpes simplex keratitis • Hypersensitivity • Long-term treatment to be tapered slowly to avoid adrenal insufficiency Supplementation to counteract A/E required: 1. Vit D, calcium, and bisphosphonates to prevent osteoporosis 2. Proton pump inhibitors

(Contd.)

Table 32.6   Overview of common systemic agents used in dermatology *(Contd.)*

Drug	MOA	Main indications	Main adverse effects (A/E)	Dose	Remarks
		• Vasculitis	• Psychiatric S/E • Cataracts, glaucoma *cutaneous side effects* *Common:* • Acneiform eruption • Fungal and bacterial infections • Impaired wound healing, skin atrophy, telangiectasia, purpura striae • Telogen effluvium		3. Potassium supplements 4. Salt restricted diet
Methotrexate	Inhibition of DNA synthesis, T cell inhibition, Immuno-suppressive and anti-inflamma-tory	• Psoriasis (FDA approved) • Bullous diseases: pemphigus vulgaris, pemphigoid; • AICTD: Dermato-myositis, systemic sclerosis, reactive arthritis • Vasculitis	• Hepatotoxicity • Pulmonary toxicity • Renal effects • Bone marrow suppression • Malignancy induction • Ulcerative stomatitis	5–25 mg/week or 0.3–0.5 mg/kg/week	• C/I in pregnancy and lactation • Caution in renal or hepatic • Impairment, alco-holics, active TB • Folic acid supplementation to reduce bone marrow suppression
Azathioprine	Purine antimetabolite, converted to 6-Mercaptopu-rine	• Bullous disorders: Pemphigus and pemphigoid • AICTD: Dermato-myositis, discoid LE • Photodermatoses • Dermatitis: Atopic dermatitis	• GI upset • Bone Marrow suppression • Malignancy induction • Hepatotoxicity • Hypersensitivity reactions	2–2.5 mg/kg/day or 50–150 mg/day	• C/I in pregnancy, hypersensitivity to azathioprine • Dose reduction in severe renal impair-ment, allopurinol use
Cyclosporine	Calcineurin inhibitor suppresses cellular and humoral immunity	• Psoriasis (FDA approved) • Atopic dermatitis • AICTD: Systemic LE • Bullous diseases: Bullous pemphigoid, pemphigus gp • Vasculitis • Photodermatoses	• Hepatic impairment • Renal impairment • Hypertension • GI side effects • Hypertrichosis • Gum hyperplasia • Tremors • Fluid electrolyte imbalance • Seizures, tremors	2–5 mg/kg/day	• Caution in severe renal impairment and uncontrolled hypertension • C/I hypersensitivity
Mycophenolate mofetil	Inhibition of T cell and B cell proliferation Inhibitor of IMP dehydro-genase	• Psoriasis • Atopic dermatitis • Bullous disorders • Pemphigus and pemphigoid • AICTD • Vasculitis	• Skin rashes: SJS, TEN • Headache • Malignant induction • Hepatitis • Neuropathy and neurological S/E • Myelotoxic • GI s/e	Dose: 50–150 mg daily	• C/I pregnancy, hypersensitivity • Caution in peptic ulcer disease, hepatic and renal dysfunction
Dapsone	Interferes with function of neutrophils and eosinophils Inhibition of folic acid syn-thesis by bacteria (bacteriostatic)	• Leprosy (FDA approved) • Bullous disorders: Dermatitis • Herpetiformis (FDA), chronic bullous dermatosis of childhood, pemphi-gus, linear IgA group • Vasculitis: Pyoderma gangrenosum • Lichen planus	• Haemolysis • Agranulocytosis • Methemoglobinemia sulfhemoglobinemia • Fixed drug, drug rash eruption • Hepatotoxic • Neurological S/E	50–100 mg/day	• C/I: Hypersensiti-vity reaction • Caution in G6PD

(Contd.)

Table 32.6	Overview of common systemic agents used in dermatology (Contd.)				
Drug	MOA	Main indications	Main adverse effects (A/E)	Dose	Remarks
Systemic* retinoids					
1. Acitretin	Analogue of retinoic acid	• Severe psoriasis • Disorders of keratinization like ichthyosis • Multiple nonmelanoma skin cancers	• Minor: Cheilitis, xerosis of oral/nasal/ocular mucosae, diffuse hair loss, paronychiae, itching • Serious: Teratogenicity, hepatotoxicity, bone marrow depression • Lipid derangement, hepatotoxic, bone toxicity	0.5–1.0 mg/kg, daily after food	
2. Isotretinoin	Inhibition of sebaceous gland function	• Moderate-severe acne vulgaris	• Same as above	Dose: 0.5–1 mg/kg, daily after food × 12–16 w	• Women in reproductive age must use effective contraception by two methods for 1 month before, during and for at least 1 m (for isotretinoin) and 3 years (for acitretin) after treatment and not donate blood during and for 1 m (for isotretinoin), 3 years (for acitretin) after treatment • Caution in renal, hepatic impairment or impaired lipid profile
Chloroquine/ hydroxychloroquine	Antimalarial which has immunosuppressive, anti-inflammatory, antiproliferative, antiviral, inhibition of thrombocyte aggregation effects	• Systemic and discoid lupus erythematosus (LE) • Polymorphous light eruption and photodermatoses • Granulomatous disorders • Porphyria cutanea tarda (PCT)	• Retinopathy, which may cause permanent blindness • Corneal deposits, loss of accommodation • Headaches • GI S/E • Hematotoxic • Pruritus and rashes • Worsening of psoriasis	Dose: 6.5 mg/kg day (200–400 mg) daily in LE • Lower dose in PCT	• C/I hypersensitive • Caution in severe blood dyscrasia, hepatic dysfunction, retinopathy, neurological S/E
Cyclophosphamide	Alkylating agent, non-cell cycle specific damage to DNA	• Bullous disorders: Pemphigus vulgaris • AICTD: SLE with renal involvement, dermatomyositis, system sclerosis • SJS, EM major	• Myelosuppression • Genitourinary: Amenorrheal, bladder toxicity, hemorrhagic cystitis, sterility • GI upsets • Carcinogenic: Bladder carcinoma, leukemia, lymphoma • Cutaneous: Alopecia, pigmentation of skin, photosensitivity	1–3 mg/kg/day	• Avoid in females of reproductive age

*Retinoids are small-molecule hormones that elicit their biologic effects by activating nuclear receptors and regulating gene transcription.

PROCEDURES IN DERMATOLOGY

Some common procedures are depicted here. The aim is not to discuss them in detail but to give a overview. Contrary to the placement of this chapter at the end of the book, dermatology and its practice follows the converse logic and most are interested in these aspects of the field.

It must be remembered that cosmetology is a 'grey zone' as multiple specialities like surgery, plastic surgery and gynaecology also can perform some of these procedures. Though it may seem attractive it has a flip side of medicolegal hazards.

We are descending into a field where many practitioners and beauty palour offer the same services. Thus it is up to the learner where he wants to place his skills and there is possibly no need to 'waste' 3 years in a MD degree, if cosmetology is the ultimate aim, as there is no prescribed degree in cosmetology.

SKIN BIOPSY

Skin biopsy serves as an integral component of the diagnostic armamentarium of a dermatologist and has the following uses:

- Diagnosis
- Study the evolution of a lesion
- Investigate a poor response to therapy
- Documentary evidence for the diagnosis and treatment (very important in today's scenario!!)

Selecting the Biopsy Site

- A primary lesion is generally preferred for the biopsy, as secondary changes such as lichenification, crusting, etc. may obscure the primary pathological process.
- A well-developed but 'fresh' lesion is usually chosen, as it will exhibit the most characteristic histopathology and immature or an old lesion may demonstrate non-specific changes. Exception to this is vasculitis, where lesions < 24 hrs old are preferred.
- The central aspect of a primary lesion is generally preferred for biopsy, except for:
  - Patterned alopecia: Active margin is preferred.
  - Ulcer: Wedge biopsy, including the edge and surrounding skin.
  - Direct immunofluorescence: Biopsy is obtained from the uninvolved perilesional skin (within 1 cm).

Biopsy Techniques (Fig. 32.2A to D)

Punch Biopsy (Fig. 32.3A to C)

Use: This is the most widely used technique and may be utilized both as a diagnostic and therapeutic tool. It is employed for any lesion that can be contained within the punch (Fig. 32.2C).

Method:

1. The area to be biopsied is punched out using a punch (disposable or metal). It is available in various sizes, and the 4 mm punch is most commonly used.
2. After infiltration of local anesthesia, the skin is stretched in a direction perpendicular to the resting skin lines.
3. The punch is pushed into the skin in a rotatory fashion until a 'give away' feeling is perceived (entry of the punch into the subcutaneous tissue plane).
4. The resultant wound can either be sutured or left as it is to heal by secondary intention.

Shave Biopsy (Fig. 32.2A)

Use: Superficial lesions such as seborrheic keratosis can be biopsied in this manner. However, it is better avoided as it does not include deeper tissues.

Method: Here, the portion of the lesion that is above the level of the surrounding skin is shaved off using a blade.

Saucerization (Fig. 32.2B)

Use: Suitable for the biopsy of vesiculobullous disorders and epidermal neoplasms.

Here, the plane of cleavage passes through the reticular dermis and occasionally through the subcutaneous tissue.

Method: Using a shaving blade, that is bent between the thumb and the index finger to form an arc and is introduced through the skin such that it goes through the dermis.

However, it may also be performed using a scalpel. The lesion is shaved completely in this manner and the wound is dressed to heal by secondary intention.

Incisional Biopsy (Fig. 32.2D)

It involves the removal of a portion of the lesion via a scalpel, using standard surgical techniques.

Excisional Biopsy

The entire lesion is completely removed till subcutaneous tissue plane and is preferred when a neoplasm is suspected.

ELECTROSURGERY

Definition and Types

Electrosurgery refers to a group of procedures, where tissue is removed or destroyed through the application of electrical current. In modern electrosurgery, high-frequency alternating current is converted to heat

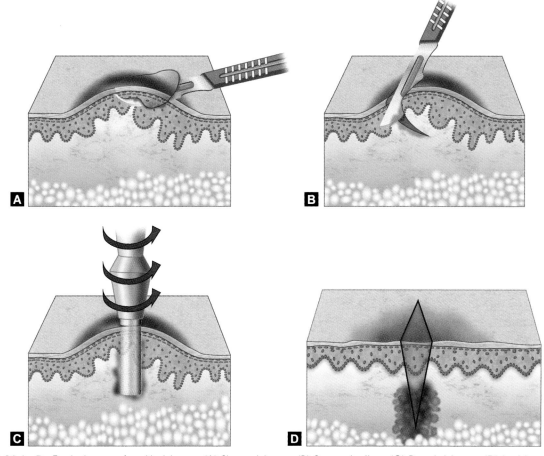

Fig. 32.2A to D: Techniques of a skin biopsy: (A) Shave biopsy; (B) Saucerization; (C) Punch biopsy; (D) Incisional biopsy

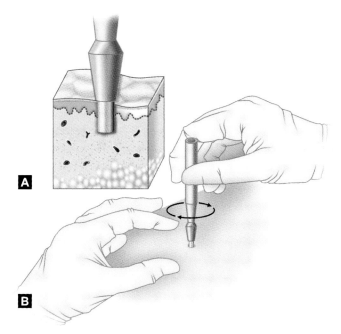

Fig. 32.3A and B: Punch biopsy: (A) This is the most widely employed skin biopsy technique where after infiltration of local anesthesia, the skin is stretched in a direction perpendicular to the resting skin lines; (B) The punch is pushed into the skin in a rotatory fashion until a 'give away' feeling is perceived. (entry of the punch into the subcutaneous tissue plane)

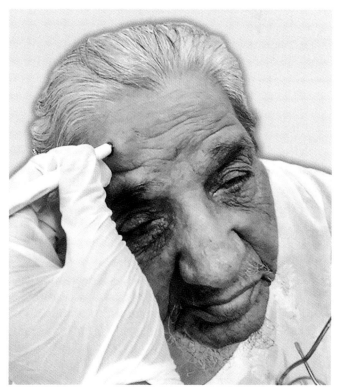

Fig. 32.3C: Punch bipsy being performed on the face (Dr Diksha Agrawal, RML Hospital)

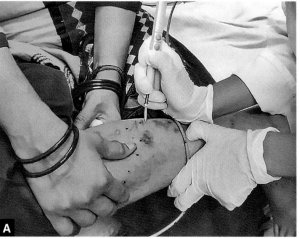 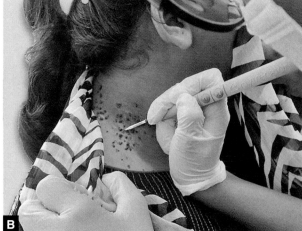

Fig. 32.4A and B: Electrosurgery for seborrheic keratosis (A) and epidermal nevi (B) (Dr Diksha Agrawal, RML Hospital)

within the treated tissues as a result of resistance to its passage and encompasses the following different techniques:

1. Electrodesiccation refers to superficial ablation via touching the tissue with a monoterminal device (Fig. 32.4).
2. Electrofulguration is superficial ablation by use of a monoterminal device whose electrode is held at a slight distance from the tissue, allowing a spark to jump to the tissue?
3. Electrocoagulation uses a biterminal device for deeper coagulation?
4. Electrosection uses a biterminal device to cut while achieving hemostasis by mild lateral heat spread.

Electrodessication and electrofulguration are superficial ablative procedures and result in minimal post-procedure scarring, while electrocoagulation causes deep ablation at the cost of the possibility of scarring, while electrosection allows tissue cutting for the surgical removal of lesions.

Electrosurgery has the inherent advantage of causing minimal bleeding, since the vessels can be simultaneously coagulated as the procedure is being carried out.

INTRALESIONAL STEROIDS

Definition

Intralesional steroid therapy refers to the injection of a steroid directly into skin lesions without significant systemic absorption and us based on the rationale of the establishment of a subepidermal depot, bypassing the superficial barrier zone. Steroids with a low solubility are preferred for their slow absorption from the injection site, promoting maximum local action with minimal systemic effect. Immunosuppression is the main mechanism of action.

Steroids Used

Triamcinolone acetonide is the most common agent used.

Triamcinolone acetonide is the preferred intralesional product because it is less atrophogenic.

Method

Generally, for most lesions, dose per session is generally 0.1–0.2 mL/cm of involved skin (<1–2 mL/dose) with an interval of 3–6 weeks between two consecutive injections. The maximum dosage of triamcinolone acetonide should not exceed 40 mg/mL/session. Corticosteroids can be injected in full strength or diluted with normal saline or local anesthetic (Fig. 32.5).

CHEMICAL PEELS

Definition

Chemical peeling refers to the application of a chemical agent to the skin, which leads to a controlled destruction of a part or the entire epidermis, with or without the dermis, leading to exfoliation and removal of superficial lesions, followed by regeneration of new epidermal and dermal tissues.

Indications

Pigmentary Disorders

- Melasma
- Postinflammatory hyperpigmentation
- Freckles
- Lentigines
- Facial melanoses

Acne

- Superficial acne scars
- Postacne pigmentation
- Comedonal acne

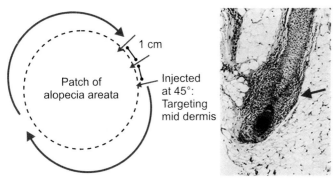

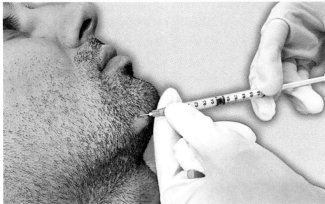

Fig. 32.5: Method of intralesional triamcinolone injection for alopecia areata: 4–6 weekly, injections of concentration 5–10 mg/mL, using a 30-gauge needle, as multiple 0.1 mL injections at 1 cm intervals, at mid-dermal level with a maximum of 3 mL dose per session

- Acne excoriee
- Acne vulgaris—mild to moderately severe acne

Esthetic
- Photoaging
- Fine superficial wrinkling
- Dilated pores
- Superficial scars

Epidermal Growths
- Seborrheic keratoses
- Actinic keratoses

Table 32.7 Types of peels based on depth

Type	Depth of penetration into skin
Superficial peels	
• Glycolic acid (20–70%)	Stratum corneum to papillary dermis
• Jessner's solution	
• Salicylic acid	
• Lipohydroxy acid	
• Solid CO_2 slush	
• Retinoic acid	
• TCA (10–25%)	
Medium-depth peels	
• TCA (35–50%)	Papillary dermis to upper reticular dermis
• 35% TCA + Jessner's solution	
• 35% TCA + 70% glycolic acid	
• 35% TCA + solid CO_2	
Deep peels	
• Baker-Gordon	Mid-reticular dermis
• 88% phenol	
• >50% TCA	

- Warts
- Milia
- Sebaceous hyperplasia
- Dermatoses papulosa nigra

Types of Peels

Chemical peels can be classified (Table 32.7) based on the depth of peel they generate as:
- Superficial peels (stratum granulosum)—it includes alpha hydroxy acids such as glycolic acid, lactic acid, citric acid, etc. and beta hydroxy acids such as salicyclic acid (Fig. 32.6).
- Medium depth peels (papillary dermis)—trichloroacetic (TCA) acid based.
- Deep peels (upper reticular dermis)—phenol or TCA based.

Additionally, a combination of peels can also be used for various indications.

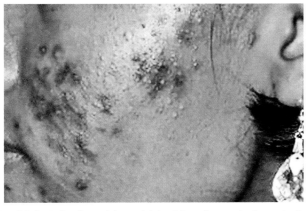
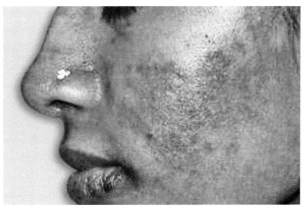

Fig. 32.6: Salicylic acid peel–ideal for pigmented and oily skin, here being used to decrease acne and pigmentation

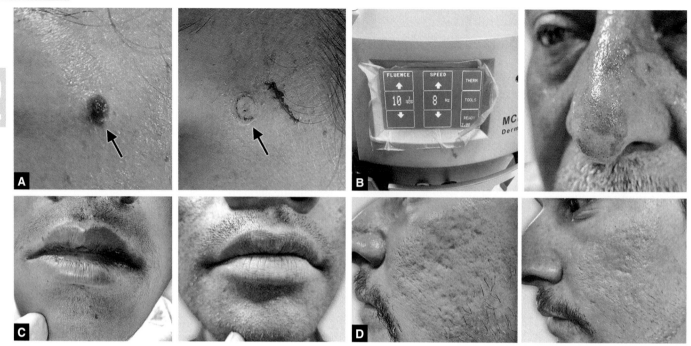

Fig. 32.7A to D: (A) Removal of a mole using the Er:YAG laser with minimal thermal damage or necrosis. Chromophore is water. Best for achieving scar free results; (B) Er:YAG for treating seborrheic keratosis; (C) Q-switched 532 nm laser used for lentigines on the lip; (D) Fractional ablative laser (Er:Glass) for treating case of acne scars

LASERS

LASER is an acronym for light amplification by stimulated emission of radiation. Laser light is generated by sending radiation through a crystal, gas, or liquid, thus bundling the rays. Laser emissions are always monochromatic and coherent with a small diameter.

Principles of Laser Therapy

The principle is to target a specific target called the chromophore which could be hemoglobin, melanin, tattoo pigment or vessels), which determines the appropriate wavelength, duration of pulse, and beam size.

The basic measure is the thermal relaxation time (TRT) which is the length of time, it takes for uptake of energy and transfer to adjacent tissues. If the exposure time is less than the TRT, the target tissue will be damaged without affecting the surrounding tissue. A continuous-wave (cw) laser releases a constant beam of light, where the duration of exposure determines the energy transmitted to tissue. Pulsed lasers can be long-pulsed, such as the pulsed dye laser working in the

millisecond range, or very short-pulsed such as the 'quality switch' (Qs) laser working in the nanosecond range both forms release very large amounts of energy over very short intervals.

The various indications are listed in Table 32.8 and depicted in Fig. 32.7A to D.

Table 32.8	Indications of various lasers in dermatology	
Ablative lasers	CW CO2 (10, 600 nm) Er:YAG (2940 nm)	Removal of benign lesions
Vascular lasers	Argon (418. 514 nm) Copper vapor (578 nm) PDL (585 nm)	Vascular lesions, rosacea, port-wine stain
Pigmented lasers	Q switched Nd:YAG (532 nm, 1064 nm) Q switched Ruby (694 nm) and Alex (755 nm)	Lentigines Freckles Tattoo Nevus of Ota
Hair removal lasers	Diode long pulse Nd:YAG IPL (intense pulse light)	In Indian skin long pulse Nd:YAG is ideal In a fair skin type Diode is a good option

Index